ULTRASONICS AND MATERIALS SCIENCE FOR ADVANCED TECHNOLOGY

ULTRASONICS AND MATERIALS SCIENCE FOR ADVANCED TECHNOLOGY

Editors

Giridhar Mishra

Punit K. Dhawan

Manish Kumar Gupta

Devraj Singh

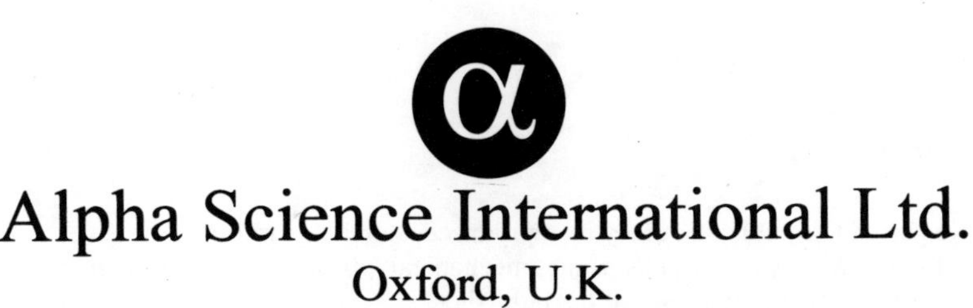

Alpha Science International Ltd.
Oxford, U.K.

Ultrasonics and Materials Science for Advanced Technology

424 pages

Editors
Giridhar Mishra
Punit K. Dhawan
Manish Kumar Gupta
Department of Physics
Veer Bahadur Singh Purvanchal University
Jaunpur

Devraj Singh
Department of Physics
AIAS, Amity University
Noida

Copyright © 2020

ALPHA SCIENCE INTERNATIONAL LTD.

7200 The Quorum, Oxford Business Park North
Garsington Road, Oxford OX4 2JZ, U.K.

www.alphasci.com

ISBN 978-1-78332-546-7

Foreword

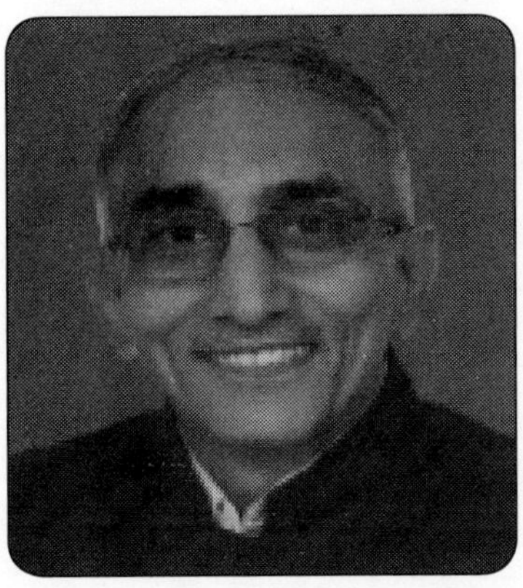

It is great pleasure to write the foreword for the book entitled *"Ultrasonics and Materials Science for Advanced Technology"* edited by Dr. Giridhar Mishra, Dr. Punit Kumar Dhawan, Dr. Manish Kumar Gupta and Dr. Devraj Singh.

The book covers various areas such as Ultrasonics, Acoustics, Instrumentation, Materials Science, Nanomaterials, Luminescent Materials, Biomaterials and Energy Materials. As evidence of that, a total seventy-nine chapters have been published. The authors of submitted papers are from India and abroad. The matter introduced in this book will be beneficial for the budding researchers with varied exposure of Ultrasonics and Materials Science and its usages through easy words and clear diagrammatic illustration. The high quality of the papers and the discussion represent the thinking and experience of experts in their particular fields.

The editors have done an admirable job and I am happy to recommend the book for all the researchers, postgraduate and graduate students of the above said topics.

Prof. (Dr.) Raja Ram Yadav
Vice Chancellor
V.B.S. Purvanchal University
Jaunpur-222003, India
Patron, ICUMSAT-2019

Preface

The materials science and characterization is a field concerned with inventing new materials and improving previously known materials by developing a deeper understanding of properties under different physical conditions. The properties of materials depend upon their composition, structure, synthesis and processing. Many properties of materials depend strongly on the structure, even if the composition of the material remains same. This is why the structure or microstructure property relationships in materials are extremely important.

Ultrasonic offers the possibility to detect and characterize micro structural properties as well as deformation processes in materials controlling materials behaviour based on the physical mechanism to predict future performance of the materials. Nanoscience and technology deals with the understanding and exploitation of new phenomena and properties that emerge at the molecular scale, so it requires atomic precision in the manipulation and control of the materials. Next to biotechnology, nanotechnology is going to make a significant impact on the life of human beings. The field of bionanotechnology requires expertise from both life sciences and physical sciences. Many of its applications are likely to be realize in medicines.

Keeping all these developments in mind, International Conference on Ultrasonics and Materials Science for Advanced Technology (ICUMSAT-2019) has been organized by Department of Physics, Prof. Rajendra Singh (Rajju Bhaiya) Institute of Physical Sciences for Study and Research, Veer Bahadur Singh Purvanchal University Jaunpur, U.P., India in collaboration with Ultrasonics Society of India (USI), New Delhi, during November 16-18, 2019 at VBSPU Jaunpur.

The conference provided a platform to the researchers in the field of Ultrasonics, Materials Scientists, Entrepreneurs, Young Budding Scientists for mutual exchange of views, knowledge and planning for the future development in the various area of Science and Technology. Ultrasonic Non-destructive Testing (NDT) is a useful technique that is being applied to a range of materials for the characterization of their microstructures, the appraisal of defects and determination of physical properties such as density, thermal conductivity and electrical resistivity. Ultrasonic measurements taken during the fabrication and heat treatment of materials are being used to ensure that the preferred microstructure is obtained and also to prevent the formation of defects in welds between two different materials. Insight into the interaction of ultrasound with microstructures is also important for resolving many materials problems. Now-a-days materials scientists are trying to find new generation of materials with quantifiably exact/desired properties such as nanomaterials or intelligent materials. Some relevant examples are: electronic materials for communication technology, bio-materials for better health care, energy materials for renewable energy and environment, different light alloys for better transportations, aeronautical applications etc. Keeping these aspects in mind a theme on Ultrasonics in Materials Science has been included in ICUMSAT- 2019. Mutual Stimulation by the interaction of different cultures and backgrounds is very effective for the promotion of scientific studies. The topics which have been covered in the conference were:

1.	Ultrasonic Instrumentation	2.	Nondestructive Evaluations/ Testing
3.	Industrial Ultrasound	4.	Sensors and Transducers
5.	Biomedical Ultrasound	6.	Physical Acoustics
7.	Signal Processing	8.	Under Water Ultrasonics
9.	Ultrasonics and Pharmaceutical Sciences	10.	Ultrasonic Standards and Calibrations
11.	Laser Ultrasonics	12.	Ultrasonics in Environmental Science & Technology
13.	Ultrasonic Spectroscopy	14.	Ultrasonics and Materials Science in Ancient India
15.	Nanoparticles- Liquid Suspensions	16.	Nanocomposite Materials
17.	Engineering Materials	18.	Materials for Defence Applications

19. Ultrasonics in Nanoscience and Technology
20. Materials Synthesis and their Applications
21. Advanced Functional Materials
22. Nano Materials and their Characterizations
23. Nanoscience and Technology in Ayurveda
24. Energy Materials and Bio-Materials
25. Luminescent Materials
26. Transport Phenomenon
27. Thermophysical Properties of Materials
28. Modelling and Simulations
29. Miscellaneous

The talks delivered in the conference created awareness and greatly benefited to youngsters and motivated them to excel in their scientific pursuits.

It is my pleasure to place on record our grateful thanks to my Gurudev, Prof. Dr. Raja Ram Yadav, Honourable Vice-Chancellor of Veer Bahadur Singh Purvanchal University, Jaunpur, U.P., India who has been my source of inspiration for showing keen interest, continued support, advice and encouragement.

I would like to express our hearty appreciation to our colleagues for their great contribution to the success of the event. In addition, I would like to offer our sincere thanks for the valuable help of supporting groups. My colleagues of Rajju Bhaiya Institute have done a marvellous job of putting together an exciting scientific program.

I thank the members of the advisory and organizing committee and sponsors for their support.

Finally, I am grateful to all the speakers and all others who have enthusiastically responded to our call, participated, and contributed greatly to the success of the conference.

Dr. Giridhar Mishra
Convener- ICUMSAT-2019

Contents

Ultrasonic Non-destructive Evaluation of Biological and Industrial Tissues

Nico F. Declercq[1], Esam T. Ahmed Mohamed[1], Pascal Pomarede[1], Nada Miqoi[1,2], Fodil Meraghni[2] and Jean-Marc Perone[3]

[1]Laboratory for Ultrasonic Nondestructive Evaluation LUNE, UMI Georgia Tech–CNRS 2958, 2 rue Marconi, 57070 Metz, France
[2]LEM3, UMR CNRS 7239, Art et Métiers Paris Tech, Metz, France
[3]Ophthalmology Department of the Regional Hospital Center of Metz-Thionville, 1 Allée du Château 57530 Ars-Laquenexy, cedex 03, 57085 Metz, France
declercq@gatech.edu

ABSTRACT

An overview is given of past and ongoing research at Declercq's laboratory at Georgia Tech Lorraine in Metz, France.

Current biomedical research in our lab is mainly involving gigahertz scanning acoustic microscopy (GHz-SAM), where subsurface imaging, utilizing the so-called V(z) is applied. Generally, V(z) has long been restricted to very stiff materials, in terms of acousto-mechanical impedance, such as metals. Our approach is based on quantifying the variations in the surface acoustic waves in the underlying substrates induced by the perturbations i nduced by the inspected sample. Our recent GHz-SAM data aims to contribute to gaining a further understanding of the alterations in the biomechanical properties in Descemet's membrane and endothelial cells of cornea tissue with Fuchs endothelial dystrophy (FECD, cornea Guttata).

As biological tissue can be processed to become composites, much of our lab's research is devoted to NDT of fiber reinforced composites. As the materials are more and more complex and the requirements in the quality of non-destructive evaluation (NDE) more and more stringent, it is necessary to consider several methods of NDE for a complete investigation of a given piece. For the composite materials, the evolution of the stiffness constants with different kinds of applied loading was measured and compared with the appearance of damage mechanisms observed with X-ray micro-tomography. The sensitivity of the Coda part (late arrival) and the non-linear frequency response with damage was investigated and was found to be valuable to obtain information about the early damage appearance on composite materials. Finally, it is worth mentioning that the special case of low-velocity impacted plates was studied with, for example, the analysis of the link between the size of the permanent indent resulting from the impact and the severity of the internal damage. These contemporary research topics will be explained in the framework of earlier research and in the context of future pathways yet to follow.

Keywords: *Ultrasound, non-destructive evaluation, composites, biology, industry, GHz-SAM.*

1. Ultrasonic Microscopy Non-destructive Evaluation of Biological Tissues

Biological tissues exhibit a varying degree of complexity to adapt the different physiological functions. The complexity emerges from theirheterogeneous structure involving different types of cells, and extracellular matrixconstituents[1].

High frequency (megahertz regime) ultrasonic imaging is nowadays a daily routine diagnostic and inspection modality, which depends on contrasts based mainly on the biomechanical variations detected during ultrasonic reflection off ortransmission through the tested object[2]. Ultrasound echoes recorded at Gigahertz frequency, can, however, provide a resolution comparable to that of optical imaging and can,therefore, contribute to the diagnosis at a cellular level besidesits efficiency in providing a quantitative biomechanical evaluation of a targeted tissue sample[3][4][5].

The V(z) technique [3] is well-established in Gigahertz-scanning acoustic microscopy (GHz-SAM) and known to be highly acclaimed for two main reasons: 1) It allows inspecting the subsurface of the material owing to the collection and analysis of the interfering surface acoustic waves (SAWs) with the specularly reflected waves, giving SAM its unique capability.2) It providesthe qualitative and quantitative signature of a material. Nonetheless, V(z) utility has long been restricted to very stiff materials, and since biological samples do not support SAWs, V(z) has seldom been usedto characterize biological samples[6][7].We have recently reported on the analysis of the changes that take place in the V(z) curves of the solid substrate underlying a biological sampledue to the perturbation caused by the presence of the biological sample.The variations on the micro-elastic properties could, thus, be extracted[8]. As an example,the analysis based on V(z) is shown below, where GHz-SAM could distinguish between cornea tissues with Fuchs' endothelial dystrophy (FECD, cornea Guttata) and normal tissues (figures 1 and 2). A discrepancyof 53±7 m/s in the velocities of Rayleigh surface acoustic waves (RSAW) was quantified and attributed to the variation in the micro-elastic properties.

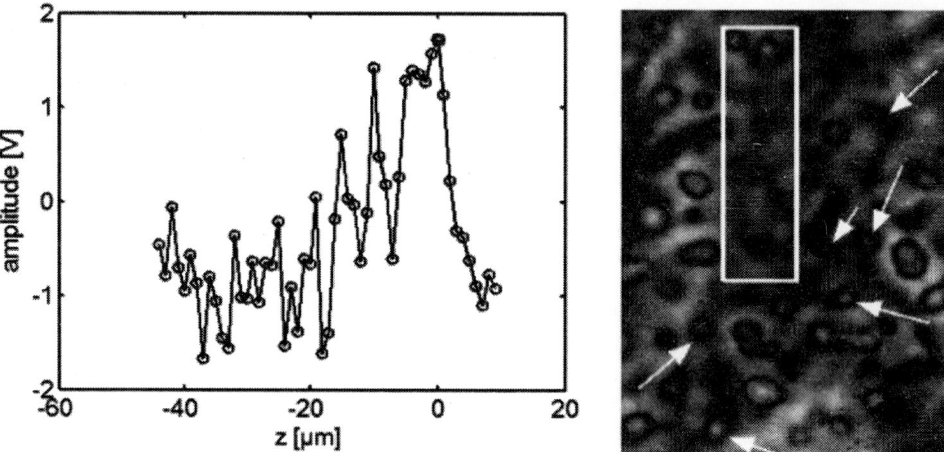

Figure 1. Acoustic micrograph (75μm ×103μm) of a sample of cornea tissue diagnosed with Fuchs' endothelialdystrophy (FECD, cornea Guttata)recorded at 1 GHz with the acoustic lens focused on the top surface of the glass substrate (left). The graph to the right is the corresponding V(z) curve extracted from the stack of images taken by translating the lens at different defocusing distances passing through the focus length (corresponding to zero μm).

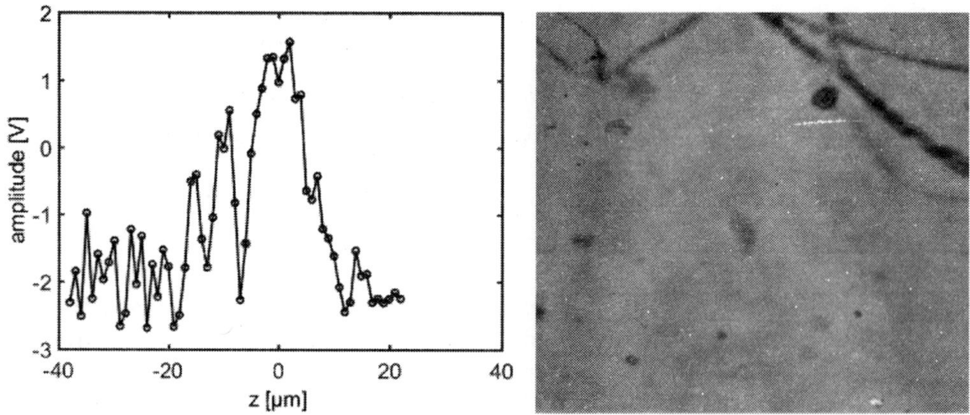

Figure 2. Acoustic micrograph (140μm ×135μm) of normal cornea tissueat 1 GHz with the acoustic lens focused on the top surface of the glass substrate and the corresponding V(z) curve.

2.   Stiffness Measurement and Damage Indicator for the Non-Destructive Evaluation of Plastic Reinforced Composites

In addition to our studies on biological samples, our team has made various researches on plastic reinforced composite materials known to be versatile for the industry. These studies took place in the framework of aerospace or automotive applications, among others. In these fields, there is a continuous need of light-but-stiff compositesthat are increasingly present, nowadays, in the production of planes and cars. Likewise, environmental standards become more stringent,therefore manufacturers introduce biological fibers in composite materials to improve the recyclability [9].

However, ultrasonic Non Destructive Evaluation (NDE) of fiber reinforced composite materials is still a great challenge. The presence of different components makesimaging and analysis complicated. Moreover, insome techniques, using low frequencies,the need to consider a homogenized version of the composite which should be carefully fabricated, emerges. Hence the need for new ultrasonic based NDE methods.

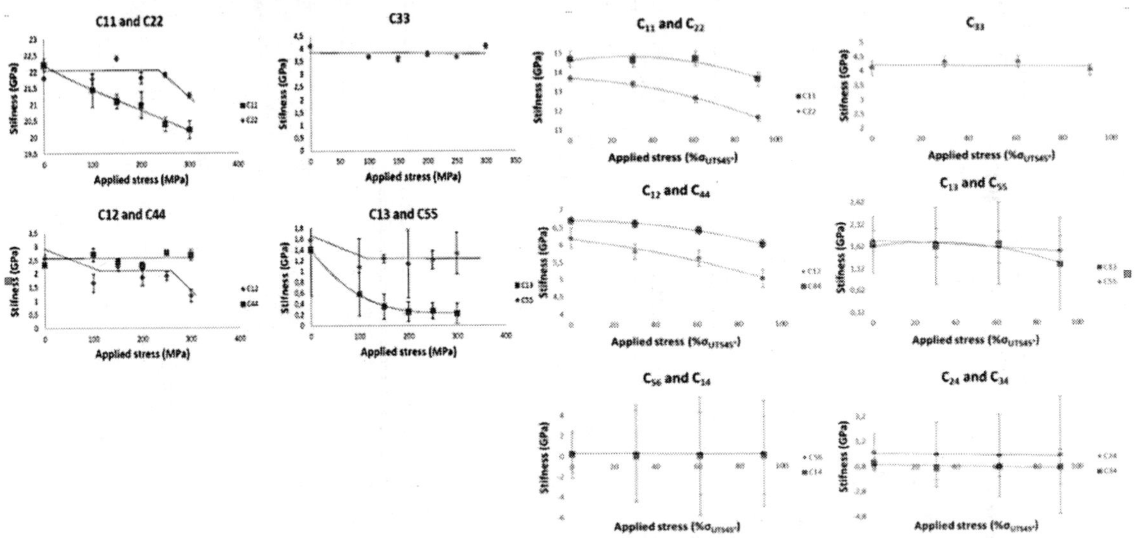

Figure 3. Evolution of the stiffness constants with the increase of the loading for (a) 0° oriented samples and (b) 45° oriented samples

The idea of the method is to perform ultrasonic acquisition in three principal planes of the composite and then, using an optimization algorithm (e.g. Levenberg-Marquardt), to determine the anisotropic stiffness tensor of the composite. We present results obtained on woven glass fiber reinforced polyamide 66/6. Traction loadingsand two loading orientations are considered (0° off the fiber axis and 45° off the fiber axis). Different levels of loading are considered to see the stiffness evolution, which evolves clearlyas a function ofthe fiber orientation. For 0°, the main decrease is in the loading direction '1', whereas for 45°, the decrease occurs in the'1' and '2'. In addition, the shearing components decrease with the traction loading.More details about the damage indicator and the method can be found in [10]. Emerging results on plates related to low velocity impact loading have also been analyzed. The data showa decrease ofalmost all of the computed stiffness components for impactvelocitiessufficiently high to cause internal damage.

3.   Nonlinear Ultrasonic Wave Spectroscopy for the Non-Destructive Evaluation of Plastic Reinforced Composites

The non-linear ultrasonic NDE method is utilized to investigate samples made of woven glass fiber reinforced vinyl-ester, damaged by traction. It is proven that the nonlinear response of an ultrasonic signal is sensitive to the appearance of small damages [11]. This approach consists of analyzing the nonlinear response, the evolution of the harmonics and sideband amplitude with increasing applied loading traction. We observed that the latter increases with increasing load [12]. A damage indicator was identified which isa function of these amplitudes, and is based on the definition of the Total Difference Frequency Distortion:

$$(TDFD) : TDFD = \frac{\sqrt{\Sigma_i A_i^2}\ \text{int}\,er\,\text{mod}\,ulation}{A_{excitation_1} + A_{excitation\,2}}$$

This parameter increases significantly with an increase in the applied loading.

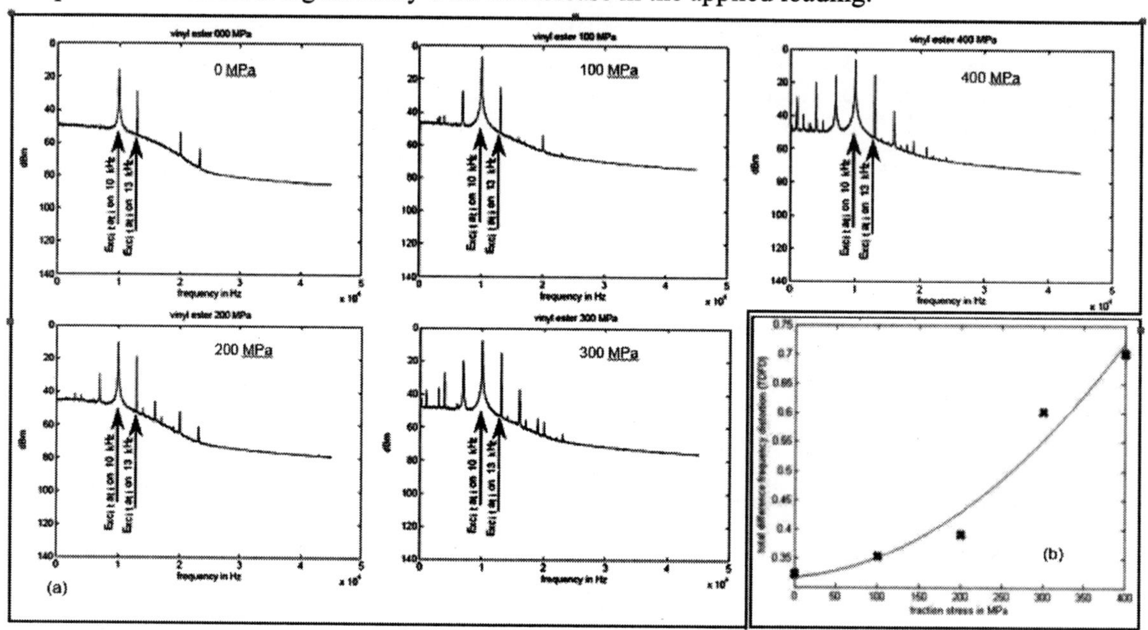

Figure 4. (a) Frequency spectra on tested composite samples and (b) Evolution of the TDFD after different levels of applied loadings

4.   Coda Wave Interferometry for the Non-destructive Evaluation of Plastic Reinforced Composite Materials

The approach is based on the analysis of the late part of ultrasonic signals, known as the Coda [13]. Here, the technique is applied to investigate samples of woven carbon fiber reinforced composite. Different levels of three-point-bending were applied before each ultrasonic acquisition. The focus is put on the difference of the relative velocity estimated using a cross-correlation between the signals before and after bending. Similar ultrasonic acquisitions were performed on an unloaded reference sample for comparison. The relative velocity decreases after a specific level of applied loading, whereas no major change is visible on the reference sample.The evolution of the relative velocity is then compared with the decrease of the bending modulus and a strong correlation is visible between the two indicators.

5.   Acknowledgement

Gratitude goes to the organizing committee of "ICUMSAT2019" for the invitation to Declercq to present this plenary lecture and also to Mr. M. Ficocelli for his technical advice and upgrade of the Ritec RAM 5000 snap in our laboratory.

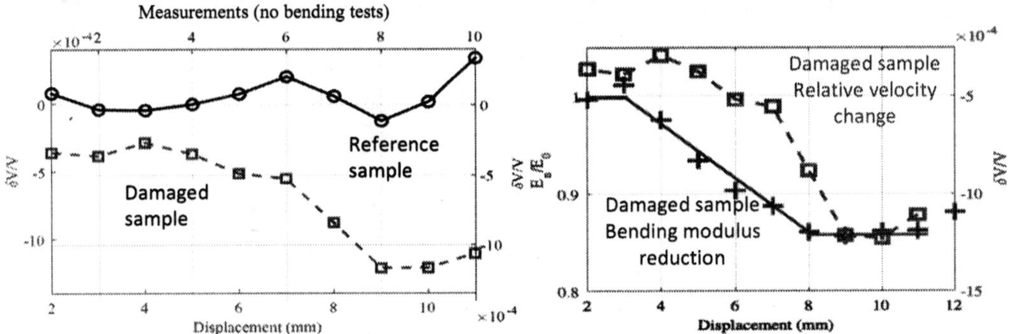

Figure 5. (a) Evolution of the relative velocity during the experiment for a reference sample and a sample with applied damage (b) Comparison of the relative velocity change with the decrease of the bending modulus

6. References

1. J. G. Betts, P. Desaix, E. Johnson, J. E. Johnson, O. Korol, D. Kruse, B. Poe, J. A. Wise, M. Womble, and K. A. Young, Anatomy & physiology. Houston: Rice University, 2013.

2. R. W. Cootney, "Ultrasound Imaging: Principles and Applications in Rodent Research," ILAR, vol. 42, no. 3, pp. 233–247, 2001.

3. A. Briggs, "Acoustic microscopy-a summary," Rep.prog.Phys;, vol. 55, pp. 851–909, 1992.

4. Y. Saijo, K. Kobayashi, T. Iwamoto, N. Okada, A. Tanaka, and N. Hozumi, "Recent progress of acoustic microscopy for medicine and biology," J. Acoust. Soc. Am., vol. 123, no. 5, pp. 2998–2998, 2008.

5. K. Miura, "Application of Scanning Acoustic Microscopy to Pathological Diagnosis Katsutoshi," in Microscopy and analysis, 2016, pp. 384–403.

6. T. Kundu, J. Bereiter-Hahn, and K. Hillmann, "Measuring elastic properties of cells by evaluation of scanning acoustic microscopy V(Z) values using simplex algorithm," Biophys. J., vol. 59, no. 6, pp. 1194–1207, 1991.

7. B. R. Tittmann, "Biomedical Acoustic Microscopy: Recent Results on Living Cells and Tissue," pp. 311–315, 2003.

8. E. T. Ahmed Mohamed, J. Perone, S. Brand, M. Koegel, and F. Nico, "Scanning acoustic microscopy comparison of descemet ' s membrane normal tissue and tissue with Fuchs ' endothelial dystrophy," Invest Ophthalmol Vis Sci., vol. 59, no. 13, pp. 5627–5632, 2018.

9. N. Perry, S. Pompidou, O. Mantaux, A. Gillet, N. Perry, S. Pompidou, O. Mantaux, A. Gillet, and C. Fiber, "Composite Fiber Recovery : Integration into a Design for Recycling Approach," in Technology and Manufacturing Process Selection, Springer, 2014, pp. 281–296.

10. P. Pomarède, F. Meraghni, L. Peltier, S. Delalande, and N. F. Declercq, "Damage Evaluation in Woven Glass Reinforced Polyamide 6 . 6 / 6 Composites Using Ultrasound Phase-Shift Analysis and X-ray Tomography," J. Nondestruct. Eval., vol. 37, no. 12, 2018.

11. M. Meo, U. Polimeno, and G. Zumpano, "Detecting damage in composite material using nonlinear elastic wave spectroscopy methods," Appl. Compos. Mater., vol. 15, pp. 115–126, 2008.

12. S. Eckel, F. Meraghni, P. Pomarède, and N. F. Declercq, "Investigation of Damage in Composites Using Nondestructive Nonlinear Acoustic Spectroscopy," Exp. Mech., 2016.

13. P. Pomarède, L. Chehami, N. F. Declercq, F. Meraghni, J. Dong, A. Locquet, and D. S. Citrin, "Application of Ultrasonic Coda Wave Interferometry for Micro-cracks Monitoring in Woven Fabric Composites," J. Nondestruct. Eval., vol. 38, no. 26, 2019.

Intrinsic Conducting Polymer Nanocomposites

V Brahmaji Rao

C.N.S.T Department of Physics, Gayatri Vidya Parishad College of Engineering (Autonomous) Madhurawada,
Visakhapatnam 530048, India
Email: prof.vrbr.160845@gmail.com

ABSTRACT

All carbon-based polymers were earlier regarded as insulators. But now a new class of polymers known as intrinsically conductive polymers or electroactive polymers have come on to the arena and find multiple applications. Their unique electronic, electrical, magnetic and optical properties [1] get them the name "Synthetic Metals". A Nanocomposite material contains more than one solid phase, metal, ceramic, or polymer, and one of these is compositionally or structurally has particulate-dimension of the nanometres range. The morphological modifications or electronic and magnetic interactions introduced between the components causes a host of versatile properties that make the Polymer Nanocomposites display an array of utilities technologically [2]. The electronically conducting polymers (ECPs), such as polypyrrole (PPy), polythiophene (PT) and polyaniline (PANI) possess unusually high electrical conductivity in the doped state with Nanomaterials [3] caused due to quasi particles like Polarons, Bipolarons &Solitons which are created in the polymeric structures. Graphene Oxide,[4] MWCNT, SWCNT, Diamond, graphite, fullerenes Metal/metal oxides doped Ferrites, Dendrimers and a host of similar materials find extensive application. Nanocomposites made up of polymer matrices and carbon nanotubes, Quantum dots, III-N semiconductors, are a class of advanced materials with great application potential in electronics packaging. Nano composites with carbon nanotubes as fillers have been designed with the aim of exploiting the high thermal, electrical and mechanical properties characteristic of carbon nanotubes. Graphene is extensively worked upon in the areas of Conducting polymer nanocomposites, finding use in super-capacitor devices, drug delivery systems, solar cells, memory devices, transistor devices, biosensors and electromagnetic/ microwave absorption shields and even in Theragnostic of Cancer as a nanomedical implement

1.   Introduction

Until about 30 years ago all carbon-based polymers were rigidly regarded as insulators. The notion that plastics could be made to conduct electricity would have been considered to be absurd. Indeed, plastics have been extensively utilized by the electronics industry for this very property. They are used as inactive packaging and insulating material. This very narrow perspective is rapidly changing as a new class of polymers known as intrinsically conductive polymers or electroactive polymers are being discovered. often referred as "Synthetic Metals". This class of polymer possess the unique electronic, electrical, magnetic and optical properties of a metal along with known advantages of conventional polymers like light weight, easy processability, resistance to corrosion and low cost etc. its infancy, much like the plastic industry was between the 1930's and 50's, the potential uses of these polymers are quite significant (Richard B. Kaner, Alan G. MacDiarmid, Scientific America , February 1988, p60 – 65).

A nanocomposite is defined as a material with more than one solid phase, metal ceramic, or polymer, compositionally or structurally where at least one-dimension falls in the nanometres range. Most of the composite materials are composed of just two phases; one is termed the matrix, which is continuous and surrounds the other phase, often called the dispersed phase and their properties are a function of properties of the constituent phases, their relative amounts, and the geometry of the dispersed phase. The combination of the nanomaterial with polymer is very attractive not only to reinforce polymer but also to introduce new electronic properties based on the morphological modification or electronic interaction between the two components. Depending on the nature of the components used and the method of preparation, significant differences in composite properties may be obtained. Nanocomposites of conducting polymers have been prepared by various methods such as colloidal dispersions, electrochemical encapsulation, coating of inorganic polymers, and in situ polymerization with nanoparticles and have opened new avenues for material synthesis [Shimizu, F. et.al., (1995). Synthetic Metals, 69(1-3), 43-44; Higashika, S. et.al.,(1999).Carbon, 37(2), 354-356.; Wang, H. et.al., Electrochemistry Communications, 11(6), 1158-1161].

The electronically conducting polymers (ECPs), such as polypyrrole (PPy), polythiophene (PT) and polyaniline (PANI) are known to possess unusually high electrical conductivity in the doped state. (Ding, K. et.al, (2011). Ind. Eng. Chem. Res., Vol.50, No.11, pp. 7077-7082). Among the conductive polymers, polyaniline and polypyrrole have drawn considerable interest because of their economic importance, good environmental stability and satisfactory electrical conductivity when doped. Therefore, find applications in electromagnetic interference (EMI) shielding, transparent packaging of electronic components, solar batteries, nonlinear optical display devices, 'smart' fabrics and recording, and so on.

Recently, electroluminescence from conjugated polymers opened up potential markets for organic light-emitting diodes(OLED) . This light-emitting polymer (LEP) technology is expected to provide an opportunity for the fabrication of flexible, full-colour displays with high luminescence, small power consumption and low-cost technology. The ECP films behave like a redox polymer and have potential applications in electrocatalysis, solar energy conversion, corrosion, electronics, etc. The redox polymer reaction is accompanied by a change in the electrical properties of the film from an insulator to an electrical conductor involving both electron and ion transport within the film (Kaplin, D.A. et.al., (1995). Polymer, Vol.36, No.6, pp.1275-1285, ISSN 0032-3861).

Conducting polymers can be synthesized either chemically or electrochemically. Electrochemical synthesis is the most common method as it is simpler, quick and perfectly controllable. PPy is one of the most interesting conducting polymers since it is easily deposited from aqueous and non-aqueous media, very adherent to many types of substrates, and is well-conducting and stable.

Electronically Conducting Polymers can be modified in several ways (Juttner et al., 2004) to obtain tailored materials with special functions: (i) derivatization of the monomer by introducing aliphatic chains with functional groups; (ii) variation of the counterion, incorporated for charge compensation during the polymerization process; (iii) inclusion of neutral molecules with special chemical functions and (iv) formation of compounds with noble metal nanoparticles as catalyst for electrochemical oxidation and reduction processes.

Depending on the nature of the components used and the method of preparation, significant differences in composite properties may be obtained. Nanocomposites of conducting polymers have been prepared by various methods such as colloidal dispersions, electrochemical encapsulation coating of inorganic polymers, and in situ polymerization with nanoparticles and have opened new avenues for material synthesis

Conducting polymer composites with graphite, CNT, Metal/metal oxides are studied a lot because of their usual electrical and mechanical properties. For example, In case of electromagnetic interference shielding application, the combination of magnetic nanoparticles with conducting polymer leads to form a ferromagnetic conducting polymer composite possessing unique combination of both electrical and magnetic properties. This type of materials can effectively shield electromagnetic waves generated from an electric source. When conducting polymers are combined with carbons material like CNT graphite and graphene, they show good thermal and electrical properties as electronic conduction occurs at long range.

Conducting polymers are polymers containing an extended π-conjugated system made up of overlap of singly occupied p-orbitals in the backbone of the polymer chain. Although conducting polymers possess a relatively large number of delocalized π-electrons, a fairly large energy gap exists between the valence band and the conduction band (greater than 1 eV), thus these polymers are considered to be semi-conducting at best. These polymers must be doped (to alter the number of π-electrons) in order to render the polymers truly conducting. The mechanism of conductivity in these polymers is based on the motion of charged defects within the conjugated framework. The charge carriers, either positive p-type or negative n-type are the products on oxidizing or reducing the polymer, respectively.

Three frequently used physical terms for describing conduction in solid are Soliton, Polaron and Bipolaron

'SOLITON', is recognised as a conjugational defect, and is an unpaired electron created in the polymer backbone during the synthesis of conductive polymer, in very low concentration. Conjugational defect is a misfit in the bond alternation so that two single bonds will touch. Soliton can be generated in pairs, as soliton and antisoliton. Chemical doping, Photogeneration and Charge injection are methods being used to generate additional solitons.

An electron will be accepted by the dopant anion to form a carbocation (positive charge) and a free radical during the chemical doping (oxidation) of the polymer chain. This carbocation is called **POLARON** by physicists. Both the soliton and polaron can be neutral or charged (positively or negatively) Thus, the charge coupled to the surrounding (induced) lattice distortion to lower the total electronic energy is known as polaron (i. e., an ordinary radical ion) with a unit charge and spin = ½. A **'BIPOLARON'** consists of two coupled polarons with charge = 2e- and spin = 0.

A novel type of supramolecular native cellulose nanofiber/nanocluster adduct was obtained by using poly (methacrylic acid) (PMMA) as the mediator between Ag nanocluster and cellulose. The PMMA not only stabilized the Ag nanoclusters but also allowed hydrogen bonding between the particles and cellulose. Another example reports Au and Ag NPs as colourfast colorants in cellulose materials for textiles with antimicrobial and catalytic properties Polymer-Graphene Nanocomposites is another type of Nanocomposites that are developed using Diamond, graphite, fullerenes, carbon nanotubes and newly discovered graphene are the most studied allotropes of the carbon family. The significance of these material can be understood by the fact that their discovery of fullerene and graphene has been awarded noble prizes in the years 1996 and 2010 to Curl, Kroto & Smalley and Geim & Novalec, respectively.

Graphene is a flat monolayer of carbon atoms tightly packed into a two-dimensional (2D) honeycomb lattice, completely conjugated sp2 hybridized planar structure and is a basic building block for graphitic materials of all other dimensionalities. It can be wrapped up into 0D fullerenes, rolled into 1D nanotube or stacked into 3D graphite.

Novoselov, Geim et al. reported on the unusual electronic properties of single layers of the graphite lattice. One of the most remarkable properties of graphene is that its charge carriers behave as massless relativistic particles or Dirac fermions, and under ambient conditions they can move with little scattering. This unique behaviour has led to a number of exceptional phenomena in graphene

(1)   Graphene is a zero-band gap 2D semiconductor with a tiny overlap between valence and conduction bands.

(2)   It exhibits a strong ambipolar electric field effect so that the charge carrier concentrations of up to 1013 cm-2 and room-temperature mobility of ~10000 cm-2s-1 are measured.

(3)   An unusual half-integer quantum Hall effect (QHE) for both electron and hole carriers in graphene has been observed by adjusting the chemical potential using the electric field effect.

(4)   It has high thermal conductivity with a value of ~ 5000 WmK−1 for a single-layer sheet at room temperature. In addition, graphene is highly transparent, with absorption of ~ 2.3% towards visible light; [Iijima, S. (1991). Nature, 354(6348), 56-58; Novoselov, K.S., et.al, (2004). Science, 306(5696), 666-669.; Ibid (2005). Two-dimensional gas of massless Dirac fermions in graphene, Nature,438(7065), 197-200.]

2.   Complex Permittivity and Permeability of ICNCP s

To investigate the possible mechanism and effects giving rise to improve microwave absorption, experimentally: the complex permittivity ($\varepsilon r = \varepsilon' - j\varepsilon''$) and permeability ($\mu r = \mu' - j\mu''$) of the samples have been calculated using scattering parameters based on the theoretical calculations given in Nicholson, Ross and Weir method , [Nicolson, A. M.et.al.,(1970). IEEE Trans Instrum Meas, 19-377; Weir. j (1974). Proceedings of the IEEE, 62-33; Ishino, K. et.al., (1987) Ceram Bull, 66-1469; Dimitrov, D. A. et.al., (1995). Phys Rev B, 51(11947); Shilov, V. P. et.al., (1999). J Appl Phys., 85(6642); Basavaraja, C. et.al., (2011). Materials Letters, 65(19-20), 3120-3123]. The dielectric performance of the material depends on ionic, electronic, orientational and space charge polarization. The contribution to the space charge polarization appears due to the heterogeneity of the material. The real (ε') and imaginary (ε'') part of complex permittivity vs. frequency has been shown in Fig. below. The real part (ε') is mainly associated with the amount of polarization occurring in the material while the imaginary part (ε'') is related with the dissipation of energy. In polyaniline, strong polarization occurs due to the presence of polaron/ bipolaron and other bound charges, which leads to high value of ε' & ε''. With the increase in frequency, the dipoles present in the system cannot reorient themselves along with the applied electric field as a result of this dielectric constant decreases.

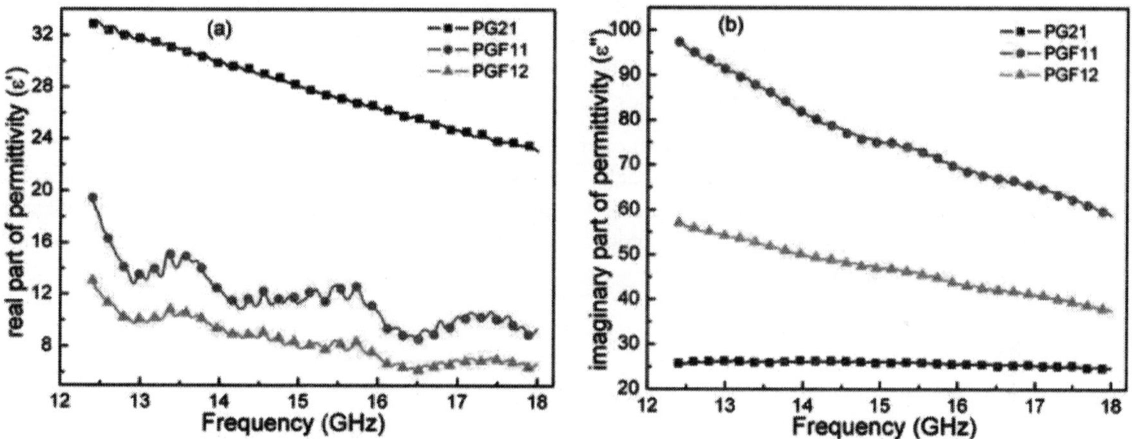

3.   COMPLEX Magnetic Permeability Studies

The main characteristic feature of GRAPHENE OXIDE is that it has high dielectric constant ($\varepsilon' \sim 32$) with dominant dipolar polarization and the associated relaxation phenomenon constitutes the loss mechanism. With the addition of GO and γ-Fe2O3 in polyaniline matrix, significant increase of the dielectric loss is attributed to the more interfacial polarization due to the presence of GO and γ-Fe2O3 particles which consequently leads to more shielding effectiveness due to absorption. Fig. below shows the variation of real part and imaginary part of magnetic permeability with frequency. The magnetic permeability of all the samples decreases with the increase in frequency whereas, higher magnetic loss has been observed for higher percentage of γ-Fe2O3 in the polymer matrix. The magnetic loss caused by the time lag of magnetization vector (M) behind the magnetic field vector. The change in magnetization vector generally brought about by the rotation of magnetization and the domain wall displacement. These motions lag behind the change of the magnetic field and contribute to the magnetic loss (μ''). The rotation of domain of magnetic nanoparticles might become difficult due to the effective anisotropy (magneto-crystalline anisotropy and shape anisotropy). The surface area, number of atoms with dangling bonds and unsaturated coordination on the surface of polymer matrix are all enhanced [Weir, (1974). Proceedings of the IEEE, 62-33.]

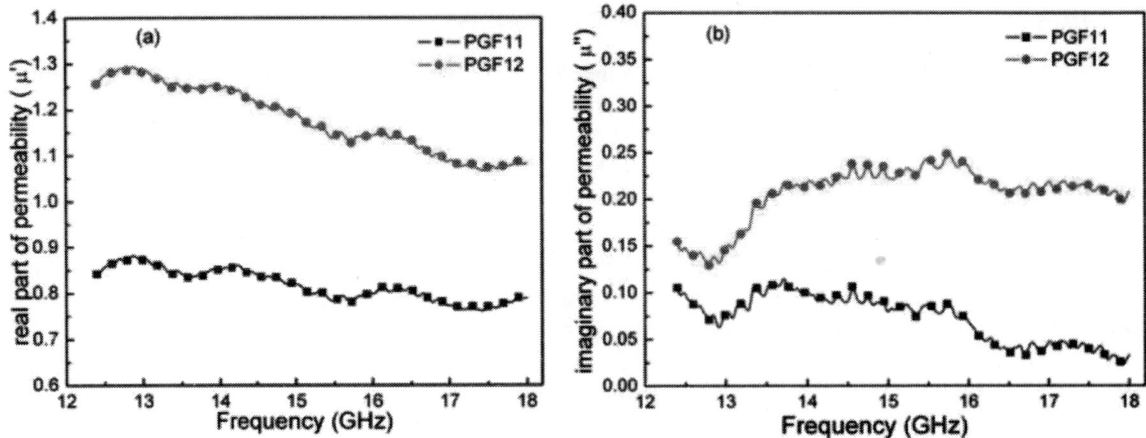

The attachment of functional groups to graphene also aids in dispersion in a hydrophilic or hydrophobic media, as well as in the organic polymer. Therefore, an efficient approach to the production of surface-functionalized graphene sheets in large quantities has been a major focus of many researchers. The goal is to exploit the most frequently proposed applications of graphene in the areas of polymer nanocomposites, super-capacitor devices, drug delivery systems, solar cells, memory devices, transistor devices, biosensors and electromagnetic/ microwave absorption shields

Nanocomposites made up of polymer matrices and carbon nanotubes, Quantum dots, III-N semiconductors, are a class of advanced materials with great application potential in electronics packaging. Nano composites with carbon nanotubes as fillers have been designed with the aim of exploiting the high thermal, electrical and mechanical properties characteristic of carbon nanotubes. [Stankevich S, et.al., Graphene-based composite materials. Nature 2006; 442:282–6.]

Ultrasonic Studies of the Nonlinear Behaviour of Solid Materials: A Brief Review

Devraj Singh

Department of Physics, AIAS, Amity University Uttar Pradesh, Noida-201313, India
dsingh13@amity.edu

ABSTRACT

In present work, the ultrasonic studies have been discussed for the numerous of materials such as metallic, intermetallics, semimetallics, semiconductors, metallic alloys, dielectrics in various crystalline structures materials e.g., face centered cubic (fcc), body centered cubic (bcc), hexagonal closed pack (hcp) under different physical conditions like temperature, pressure and size. These all the materials have been described in 4 phases of computation and discussion of: (1) higher order elastic constants; (2) mechanical Properties; (3) ultrasonic velocities and thermal properties (4) ultrasonic attenuation. The higher order elastic constants have been evaluated with different type of potential models (Coulomb & Born-Mayer potential; Morse potential; Lennard-Jones potential) according to their crystalline structure. The methods to compute the elastic constants have been examined and implemented for different types of materials. The mechanical constants of the materials were evaluated using the second order elastic constants. These constants provide the information about the intrinsic properties of the materials for example information about bonding, stability etc. Further the higher order elastic constants were applied for the computation of ultrasonic velocities for longitudinal and shear modes of propagation, Debye average velocity, Debye temperature, thermal relaxation time, acoustic coupling constants, thermal conductivity etc. Finally these all computed parameters have been utilized to compute ultrasonic attenuation due to electron-phonon interaction, phonon-phonon interaction and thermoelastic relaxation mechanisms. On the basis of the studies, the divisions of the materials have been provided and discussed.

Keywords: *Elastic properties, mechanical properties, thermal properties, ultrasonic properties.*

1.   Introduction

The elastic properties of the metallics, intermetallics, semimetallics, semiconductors, metallic alloys, dielectrics materials are suited for the study of phonon-phonon interaction which account for direct conversion of acoustic energy into thermal energy. These materials are suitable for the study of phonon-phonon interaction which has been discussed briefly here [1]. The knowledge of higher order elastic constants like the second and third order elastic constants is essential for the study of the anharmonic properties of solids. The elastic constants provide insight into the nature of the binding forces between atoms since they are represented by the derivatives of the internal energy (adiabatic constants) or of the free energy (isothermal constants) [2]. The second order elastic constants (SOECs) are used to determine the mechanical constants such as Young's modulus, bulk modulus, shear modulus, Poisson's ratio, Zener anisotropic ratio, Pugh's indicator, Breazeale's non-linearity parameters, Cauchy's pressure. The SOECs are also used to compute the ultrasonic velocity, thermal conductivity. The prediction about the future performance of the materials such as mechanical stability and bonding etc. is made on the basis these mechanical, thermal and ultrasonic properties. The ultrasonic velocity is a vital factor in characterization and can deliver evidence about crystallographic texture [3]. The thermal relaxation time of the material also give us information about the type of the material i.e, 10^{-11} s, 10^{-12}s and 10^{-12-13} s for metallic, intermetallic and semiconducting materials [4]. The ultrasonic attenuation study of the materials has gained novel height with the growth in materials science [5]. In the present paper, a general and brief review of the investigated structural materials has been present briefly.

2. Theoretical Background

The elastic energy density for a cubic crystal (face centered, body centered and hexagonal close packed) is defined in terms of expansion of strain, which defines the higher order elastic constants (second-, third- and fourth- order elastic constants) using the components of the strain tensor by the Brügger's definition. The elastic energy is well related to interaction potential. The inter-ionic potential used for a nondeformed crystal (face centred and body centered) is sum of electrostatic/Coulomb and repulsive/Born-Mayer potential [6, 7]. The theory to compute the second- and third- order elastic constants (SOECs and TOECs) of the b.c.c metals establishing the applicability of Morse potential function as described by Garifalco and Weizer [8]. The interaction potential for hexagonal close packed (hcp) is the many body interaction potential i.e., the Lennard-Jone potential [9].

The second order elastic constants (SOECs) are used to compute the mechanical properties such as Young's modulus (Y), bulk modulus (B), shear modulus (G), tetragonal modulus (Cs), Poisson's ratio (v), Pugh's indicator (B/G), Cauchy's pressure (Cp), Breazeale's non-linearity parameters, Vicker's hardness (Hv) for getting the information about brittleness or ductileness of the material. The SOECs is further apply to find out the values ultrasonic velocity and the Debye velocity for longitudinal modes of wave propagation along <100>, <110> and <111> orientations [10]. Further the Debye velocity is used to evaluate the Debye temperature of different types of materials on the basis of their atomic weight and number of atoms in unit cell. The second-, third- and fourth- order elastic constants (SOECs, TOECs and FOECs) have been used to compute the ultrasonic Grüneisen parameters (UGPs) [11].

All above achieved results of numerous parameters are finally used to estimate the acoustic coupling constants (D), thermal relaxation time (τ) and the ultrasonic attenuation (α). Many of the investigators have made physical properties of the face centered and body centered metals like theoretical dealing with electron-phonon interaction and its effects on the these metals have been reviewed by Maksimov et al. [12]. The temperature dependent part of ultrasonic attenuation has been explained in terms of the model, where the acoustic phonon interacts with number of thermal phonons in the lattice [5]. Many of the investigators [1, 13-15] have assumed three phonons interaction in which the low energy acoustic phonon interacts with one thermal phonon to produce another; both thermal phonons have the higher energy. All these studies indicate that major portion of attenuation is caused by direct conversion of acoustic energy into thermal energy via phonon-phonon interaction mechanism. The ultrasonic attenuation due to the thermoelastic phenomenon is caused by the thermal conduction between compressed and rarefied parts of the propagating wave.

3. Existing Results and Comments

3.1 Face centered cubic crystals (Rock salt type or B1 structured materials)

The rock-salt structured materials have been investigated extensively for the elastic, ultrasonic and the mechanical properties since 1993 by our Group Leader Professor Raja Ram Yadav at the Department of Physics, University of Allahabad. Initially he investigated lead monochalcogenides at room temperature using Coulomb and Born-Mayer potential on the basis of Mori and Hiki approach [16]. This paper was the mile stone to develop and apply the theory for B1 structured materials. In the continuation of this work, Prof. Yadav and me worked on gadolinium monopnictides in year 2000. Prof. Yadav presented this work in the 15th WCNDT at Roma during 15-21 October, 2000. After that we sent an Academic Paper on such materials in low temperature regime (electron-phonon interaction) in *Intermetallics (Elsevier)*. This paper was with much appreciation by Editor-in-Chief, a British Metallurgist Professor Robert Wolfgang Cahn, FRS. This was initial momentum for us especially for me [17, 18]. In this work, the SOECs have been computed in the temperature range 2-80K. These SOECs have been applied to evaluate the ultrasonic velocity, which in turn used to find the ultrasonic attenuation due to electron-phonon interaction. We found that coupling between electron and phonon ceases at 80K. The Coulomb and Born-Mayer potential has been applied to find out the temperature SOECs and TOECs for lanthanum monopnictides [19]. In this work, the main comment was for the fixed value of hardness parameter for the evaluation of the elastic constants. We successfully answered this by giving the equilibrium condition. In this work, the ultrasonic attenuation due to phonon-phonon interaction and thermoelastic relaxation mechanisms has been discussed in high temperature regime. The ultrasonic attenuation values have been increased with temperature. In year 2009, we apply Morse potential for face centred cubic (fcc) metals V, Nb and Ta to find the SOECs. Further, ultrasonic attenuation due to e-p interaction have been determined for these superconducting metals in temperature range 5-50K. The resistivity was the main dominating factor in this work [20]. In the same year, we did one of interesting problem on thulium monochalcogenides [4]. We found the classification of the materials on the basis of thermal relaxation time and ultrasonic attenuation. The order of the thermal relaxation time for TmTe, TmS, and TmSe were 10^{-11}s, 10^{-12} s, and 10^{-12}-10^{-13} s, respectively. This resolved with the finding that TmS, TmSe, and TmTe have metallic, intermettallic, and semiconducting behavior respectively. The acoustic attenuation has determined for the rare-earth monochalcogenides CeS, CeSe, CeTe, NdS, NdS, NdSe and NdTe at room temperature along different orientations [5]. The effect of platinum addition to coinage metals on their ultrasonic properties has been discussed for bimetallic alloys of coinage metals (copper, silver and gold) [3]. The thermal relaxation time was decreased with increasing platinum content in the alloys studied. The ultrasonic attenuation was also shown to decrease with increasing platinum content in these bimetallic alloys. The same theory was attempted to discuss the elastic, thermal and ultrasonic properties for dielectrics and semiconductors during 2001-2012. In year 2013, we (me and my Ph.D. students Dr. Vyoma Bhalla, Dr. Raj Kumar and Dr. Chinmayee Tripathi) changed the way to present the things and we published a research paper of 28 pages in *International Journal of Modern Physics B* [6]. We applied first time the elastic constants for finding the mechanical constants such as Y, B, G, B/G, Breazeale's non-linearity parameter, pressure derivatives and the lattice thermal conductivity with Slack and Berman approach for the praseodymium monopnictides. All these associated parameters have been used to get the relaxation time, acoustic coupling constants and ultrasonic attenuation for praseodymium monopnictides. On the basis of obtained results, we found that these materials are brittle, stable and semimetallic in nature. In year 2016, Dr. Vyoma Bhalla with me did an investigation on ultrasonic velocity and thermal conductivity of erbium nitride and erbium arsenide using the open source software MTEX 4.0.22 [21]. Dr. Vyoma Bhalla with us (me and Dr. S. K. Jain) first time presented the renormalized Pugh and Pettifor criteria for holmium nitride and Vicker's hardness [22]. We found that HoN a good candidate for cryocooler application. Mr. Sudhanshu Tripathi with us (me and Prof. R. Agarwal) first time presented frequency dependence of the ultrasonic attenuation in lead telluride as per suggestion by Dr. Sanjay Yadav, Senior Principal Scientist at CSIR-National Physical Laboratory, New Delhi. It has been found that the ultrasonic attenuation increases exponentially with an increase in frequency [23].

3.2   Body centered cubic crystals (CsCl-type type or B2 structured materials)

The SOECs and TOECs of the B2 structured intermetallics AgMg, CuZr, AuMg, AuTi, AuMn and AuCd have been computed by me and Dr. D. K. Pandey using simplified formulations, which is based on Coulomb and Born-Mayer potentials model and Brugger's definition of the elastic constant [24]. These materials have good mechanical strength compared to the Cs/Rb-halides. The nature of thermal relaxation time followed the reciprocal trend of the deviation number. The total attenuation provided direct information about the deviation number. Here the deviation number denotes the difference of column number of noble metal and secondary element. The thermal conductivity is high for lower deviation number. After 10 years, we (Mr. Chandreshvar P Yadav, Dr. D. K. Pandey and me) again attempted the elastic and ultrasonic properties on B2 structured TbZn, DyZn, HoZn, ErZn, TmZn, TbCu, DyCu, HoCu, ErCu, TmCu intermetallics and found that (i) these materials were mechanical stable; (ii) The thermal conductivity was predominantly affected by ultrasonic Gruneisen parameters (UGPs); (iii) The thermal relaxation time is mainly affected by the thermal conductivity [25]. Two of our papers on CsCl-type structured materials have been submitted in the Proceedings of ICUMSAT-2019 by my Ph.D. student Mrs. Jyoti Bala. The materials under studies are hafnium and boron monopnictides. Recently we (Mrs. Jyoti Bala, me, Mr. Chandreshvar P Yadav and Dr. D.K. Pandey) submitted a research article on scandium based intermetallic compounds ScM (M=Ru, Rh, Pd, Ag) in Canadian Journal of Physics [26]. Main findings of this investigation were given as: (i) The elastic properties of ScRu were predominant over that of ScRh, ScPd and ScAg; (ii) The hardness of the materials decreased on increasing the molecular weight of the materials; (iii) The chosen ScM intermetallics have covalent bond character and less ductile in nature (iv) The nature of ultrasonic velocity directly measured the elastic and mechanical characteristic of ScM intermetallics; (v) Thermal conductivity, thermal expansion coefficient and thermal relaxation time are found enhancement while melting temperature is found to decay with the lattice parameter of chosen ScM compounds; (vi) The order of relaxation time is of 10^{-11}s which confirms intermetallic nature of the materials; (vii) The lowest entropy producing intermetallic in selected ScM compounds was ScPd as it has minimum ultrasonic attenuation; (viii) Thermal properties of ScAg and mechanical properties of ScRu were quite good among ScM intermetallics (ix) The net attenuation value of ScPd showed its superior applicability for industrial purposes in comparison to other ScRu, ScRh and ScAg intermetallics.

3.3   Hexagonal closed packed (Wurtzite symmetry B4 structured materials; AB2: Laves phase)

First attempt has been made by us (Dr. D.K. Pandey, me and Prof. R. R. Yadav) in 2007 on hexagonal structured (wurtzite-w) third group nitrides (GaN, AlN and InN) to find their higher order elastic constant using Lennard-Jones potential and ultrasonic properties on the basis of Mason's approach. This work was published in *Applied Acoustics*. Here It is great pleasure to mention that this paper has been cited by 67 times [27]. Out of these materials AlN was more ductile. After 12 years, we (Mr. Sudhanshu Tripathi, me and Prof. R. Agarwal) described the elastic, mechanical and thermal behavior of w-BeO nanowires (NWs) [28]. The Pugh's indicator confirms the brittle nature of the chosen NWs. The comparative analysis of w-BeO NWs with other materials of wurtzite hcp structured indicated that w-BeO NWs has better acoustical behavior. The size dependent characterization is important for nanoelectromechanical systems (NEMS), nanogenerator, biosensor and other related areas at higher temperature regime. We recently published an academic piece of work on elastic, thermal and ultrasonic properties of w-zinc oxide NWs in *Johnson Matthey Technol. Rev.* [9]. The hcp structured stability criterion for mechanical stability is satisfied for ZnO-NWs. The thermal relaxation time for the equilibrium distribution of thermal phonons was found lowest for wave propagation along 45°. The order of relaxation is of picoseconds, which confirms the semiconducting nature of ZnO-NWs.

4.   Conclusion

On the basis of above discussion following points can be drawn:

- The computation of higher oder elastic constants has been utilized for fcc, bcc and hcp materials. It will be helpful to study any material in different phases with different types of interaction potential models.

- On the basis of materials' properties, we can classify the materials in different groups such as metals, dielectrics, semiconductor, semimetallic, intermetallic, metallic alloys.

- We can find different characteristics of any material along different crystallographic directions.

- The thermal conductivity and thermal relaxation time play an important role for total attenuation in the materials.

The elastic, mechanical, thermal and ultrasonic properties of the materials may be used for further investigation on their transport properties and in the manufacturing industries.

5.   Acknowledgements

I would like to express my special thanks of gratitude to Prof. S.K. Kor, Prof. R. R. Yadav, Dr. Ashok K. Chauhan, Dr. Atul Chauhan, Prof. B. Shukla, Dr. S. Ahmed, Dr. Ashok Kumar, Dr. S. K. Jain, Prof. R. Paikaray, Dr. Sanjay Yadav, Prof. V. Rajendran, Prof. R. K. Singh, Prof. R. Agarwal, Prof. S. Rattan, Dr. Y. K. Yadav, Dr. A. K. Tiwari, Dr. Priyanka Awasthi, Dr. D. K. Pandey, Dr. A. K. Gupta, Dr. D. K. Singh, Dr. P. K. Yadawa, Dr. A. K. Yadav, Dr. Giridhar Mishra, Dr. S. K. Verma, Dr. Meher Wan, Dr. P. K. Dhawan, Mr. Mohit Gupta, Dr A. K. Jaiswal, Dr. A. K. Verma, Mr. S. P. Singh, Mr. Navneet Yadav, Mr. Gaurav Singh, Dr. Raj Kumar, Dr. Shivani Kaushik, Dr. Vyoma Bhalla, Dr. Amit Kumar, Dr. Chinmayee Tripathy, Mr. C. P. Yadav, Mr. Sudhanshu Tripathi, Mrs. Bhawan Jyoti and Mrs. Jyoti Bala, who always encouraged and helped in doing a lot of research and I came to know about so many new things I am really thankful to them. I would also like to thank my family members, particularly my wife Mrs. Mamta and sons Shobhit and Parth, who helped me a lot for doing research work.

6.   References

1.   Mason W.P., Effect of impurities and phonon processes on the ultrasonic attenuation of germanium, crystal quartz and silicon, In Physical Acoustics, Vol. IIIB, Academic Press, New York, pp. 237- 286, 1965.

2.   Murnaghan F. D., Finite deformations of an elastic solid, Am. J. Math. 59 (1937) 235-260.

3.   Singh D. and Yadawa P.K., Effect of platinum addition to coinage metals on their ultrasonic properties, Platinum Metals Rev. 54 (2010) 172-179.

4.   Singh D., Pandey D. K. and Yadawa P.K., Ultrasonic wave propagation in rare-earth monochalcogenides, Cent. Eur. J. Phys. 7 (2009) 198-205.

5.   Singh D., Behaviour of acoustic attenuation in rare-earth chalcogenides, Mat. Chem. Phys. 115 (2009) 65-68.

6.   Bhalla V., Kumar R., Tripathy C. and Singh D., Mechanical and thermal properties of praseodymium monopnictides: an ultrasonic study, Int. J. Mod. Phys. B 27 (2013) 1350116 (28 pp.)

7.   Verma A. K., Kaushik S., Singh D. and Yadav R. R., Elastic and thermal properties of carbides of U, Pu and Am, J. Phys. Chem. Solids 133 (2019) 21-27.

8.   Garifalco L.A. and Weiser V.G., Application of the Morse potential function to cubic metals, Phys. Rev. 114 (1969) 687-690.

9.   Tripathi S, Agarwal R. and Singh D., Size dependent elastic and thermophysical properties of zinc oxide nanowires, Johnson Matthey Technol. Rev. 63 (2019) 166-176.

10.   Yadav C. P., Pandey D. K. and Singh D., Ultrasonic study of Laves phase compounds ScOs2 and YOs2, Indian J. Phys. 93 (2019) 1147-1153.

11.   Singh D., Mishra G., Kumar R. and Yadav R. R., Temperature dependence of elastic and ultrasonic properties of sodium borohydride, Commun. Phys. 27 (2017) 151-164.

12.   Maksinov E.G., Savrasov D.Y. and Savrasov S.Y., The electron-phonon interaction and the physical properties of metals, Phys. Usp. 40 (1997) 337-358.

13.   Kor S.K., Tandon U.S. and Rai G., Ultrasonic attenuation in copper, silver and gold, Phys. Rev. B 6 (1972) 2195-2197.

14.   Kor S.K., Mishra P.K. and Tandon U.S., Ultrasonic attenuation in aluminium, Solid Stat. Commun. 15 (1974) 499-501.

15.   Nava R., Vecchi M.P., Romero J. and Fernândez B., Akhiezer damping and the thermal conductivity of pure and impure dielectrics, Phys. Rev. B 14 (1976) 800-807.

16.   Yadav R. R.and Shanker K., Ultrasonic attenuation in normal valence semicondcutors, Ultrasonics International 93 Conference Proceedings, pp. 459-462.

17.   Yadav R. R. and Singh D., Ultrasonic characterization of intermetallics, 15th World Conference on Nondestructive Testing, Roma 15-21 October, 2000.

18.   Yadav R. R. and Singh D., Behaviour of ultrasonic attenuation in intermetallics, Intermetallics 9 (2001) 189-194.

19.   Yadav R. R. and Singh D., Ultrasonic attenuation in lanthanum monopnictides, J. Phys. Soc. Jpn. 70 (2001) 1825-1832.

20.   Singh D., Pandey D. K., Yadawa P.K. and Yadav A.K., Attenaution of ultrasonic waves in V, Nb and Ta at low temperature, Cryogenics, 49 (2009) 12-16.

21.   Bhalla V. and Singh D., Anisotropic assessment of ultrasonic velocity and thermal conductivity in ErX (X:N,As), Indian J. Pure Appl. Phys. 54 (2016) 40-45.

22.   Bhalla V., Singh D. and Jain S.K., Mechanical and thermophysical properties of rare-earth monopnictides, Int. J. Comput. Mat. Sci. Eng. 5 (2016) 1650012.

23.   Tripathi S, Agarwal R. and Singh D., Nonlinear elastic, ultrasonic and thermophysical properties of lead telluride, Int. J. Thermophys. 40 (2019) 78.

24.   Singh D. and Pandey D. K., Ultrasonic investigations in intermetallics, Pramana-J. Phys. 72 (2009) 389-398.

25.   Yadav C. P., Pandey D. K. and Singh D., Elastic and ultrasonic studies on RM (R= Tb, Dy, Ho, Er; M=Zn, Cu) compounds, Z. Naturforsch. 2019 (Article in press)

26.   Bala J., D.Singh, Pandey D. K. and Yadav C. P., Elastic and ultrasonic properties of ScM (M: Ru, Rh, Pd, Ag) intermetallics, Can. J. Phys. (Communicated).

27.   Pandey D. K., Singh D. and Yadav R. R., Ultrasonic wave propagation in IIIrd group nitrides, Appl. Acoust. 68 (2007) 766-777.

28.   Tripathi S, Agarwal R. and Singh D., Elastic, mechanical and thermal properties of wurtzite BeO nanowires, J. Pure Appl. Ultrason. 41(2019) 44-50.

Behaviour of Ultrasonic Attenuation in Semiconductors at Higher Temperatures

Arvind Kumar Tiwari

Department of Physics, B.S.N.V.P.G.College Lucknow-226001, India
E-mail: tiwariarvind1@rediffmail.com

ABSTRACT

Semiconductors provides an excellent opportunity for testing the basic concepts of the various processes which contribute to heat conduction and the different mechanism related to the scattering of phonons and electrons. Semiconductors are enabling the convergence of computing, communication and consumer electronics. The contribution of thermoelastic attenuation to total attenuation increases by about 20 times for metals as compared to alkali halides lattices. A thorough study of smooth variation of thermoelastic attenuation, the best approach is the study of semiconductors. In the paper the semiconducting materials FeO, TiO and VO are chosen for the study of the acoustical properties at the temperature range 100-500K along <111> direction. The higher order elastic constants are evaluated using Coulomb and Born-Mayer potential upto second nearest neighbour. The ultrasonic velocity, Debye average velocity, thermal relaxation time and specific heat are calculated using the higher order elastic constants and other related parameters. The obtained results are discussed in correlation with available results on these properties for the chosen materials.

Keywords: Elastic properties, ultrasonic velocity, specific heat, Akhieser loss

1. Introduction

The characterization of materials using non-destructive evaluation has been growing steadily with the advent of newer materials. Semiconductors provide an excellent opportunity for testing the basic concepts of the various processes which contribute to heat conduction and the different mechanism related to the scattering of phonons and electrons. The semiconductors are all around us. The compound semiconductors, for instance, provide the photons that are the vehicles that carry the information along optical fibre highways. The compound semiconductors also make possible the very high frequency device-Cell phones and pagers-used in today's wireless communications. The semiconductors are enabling the convergence of computing, communication and consumer electronics. The result is shaping the way we live and work. It is having a huge effect not only in our country but also around the world. Acoustic attenuation studies [1-4] has been made experimentally and theoretically both in solids and liquids in different ways. However, the results on ultrasonic propagation in semiconducting materials at different temperatures are rarely found in literature. In this paper we plan to study the variation in acoustic wave propagation in transition-metal oxides. Transition-metal oxides initially attracted interest because of the fact that it was generally acknowledged, the same electrons, those originally associated with the d-orbitals of the transition-metal ions, are responsible not only for the magnetic properties, but for the electrical and low energy optical properties as well [5]. This contrasts for example, with the transition-metals in which the d-electrons are primarily responsible for the magnetic properties, but the s-band overlaps the d band above and below, and the s band is primarily responsible for the metallic conductivity. Consequently, electrical studies of the transition-metals probe mainly the s band, and give us little information about the d band. The temperature dependent ultrasonic attenuation has been computed using Mason's theory to study the internal structure and inherent properties of the materials.

2.   Theory

Starting with hardness parameter and nearest neighbour distance and assuming Born-Mayer potential, the second and third order elastic constants are obtained at 0K following Brügger's definition [6]. The approach developed by Leibfried and Haln [7] and Mori and Hiki [8] is used here. Formulations for various elastic constants are found as:

$$C_{IJ} = C_{IJ}^0 + C_{IJ}^{Vib}$$
$$C_{IJK} = C_{IJK}^0 + C_{IJK}^{Vib}$$

Where superscript 0 has been used to denote SOEC and TOEC at 0K and superscript Vib. for temperature dependence SOEC and TOEC.

Theory of ultrasonic attenuation: Akhieser [9] first proposed the ultrasonic attenuation due to phonon-phonon interaction; which was modified by Woodruff and Ehrenreich [10], Bömmel and Dransfeld [11] and finally by Mason [12].

Formulations for the evaluations of ultrasonic absorption coefficient (α) and related parameters like non-linearity parameters (acoustic coupling constants) (D), velocity ($\overline{V}$), thermal relaxation time (τ_{th}) are given as

$$\tau_{th} = \tau_{shear} = \frac{1}{2}\tau_{long} = \frac{3K}{C_V \overline{V}^2}$$

K is the thermal conductivity, CV is specific heat per unit volume and $\overline{V}$ is the Debye average velocity of ultrasonic wave as

$$3/\overline{V}^3 = 1/V_l^3 + 2/V_s^3$$

Where V_l, V_s = longitudinal and shear wave velocity respectively

The thermal relaxation time for longitudinal wave is twice that of shear wave.

Thermo-elastic loss is obtained from

$$(\alpha/f^2)_{th} = \frac{4\pi^2 <\gamma_i^j>^2 KT}{2\rho V_{long}^5}$$

ρ is the density and T the temperature in Kelvin scale.

For the Akhieser loss (phonon-viscosity loss) one has to evaluate the anharmonic-parameter (acoustic coupling constant); which is the measure of the conversion of acoustic energy into thermal energy and is obtained from

$$D = 9 < (\gamma_i^j)^2 > - \frac{3<\gamma_i^j>^2 KT}{E_0}$$

E_0 is the thermal energy and is evaluated from the knowledge of specific heat (C_v).

The Akhieser loss is given by [9]

$$(\alpha/f^2)_{Akh.} = \frac{4\pi^2 \tau E_0 (D/3)}{2\rho V^3}$$

by determining D_{long} and D_{shear} for longitudinal and shear wave; $(\alpha/f^2)_{Akh.long}$ and $(\alpha/f^2)_{Akh.shear}$ can be obtained. Here V is the velocity of ultrasonic wave (longitudinal and shear wave).

3.   Results and Discussion

Second and third order elastic constants at the temperatures 100-500K are evaluated using nearest neighbour distance r_0=2.155A^0, 2.083A^0, 2.031A^0 for FeO, TiO and VO respectively and hardness parameter b= 0.313A^0 same for all the materials and are presented in Tables1, 2,and3.The comparison is made with other NaCl-type semiconducting materials PuS and PuSe [13,14]. The order of the values of the SOEC and TOEC are same [10^{11} Dyne/cm^2]. The attenuation due to both type of mechanisms viz. phonon viscosity effect and thermoelastic effect has been calculated in FeO, TiO and VO along <111> direction and presented in Table 4. As expected, the ultrasonic attenuation due to thermoelastic loss $(\alpha/f^2)_{th}$ in semiconductors is very small as compared to that in metals. Contribution of $(\alpha/f^2)_{th}$ to the total value of attenuation (α/f^2) at any temperature is intermediate to that of conducting (metals) and non-conducting materials (insulators). This is due to the fact that the thermal conduction and thermal expansion coefficient of semiconductors is intermediate between the two. In the present investigation it is pointed out that the values of attenuation varies with temperature T in the following manner: $a = a_0 T^n$ Where α_0 and n are constants. The values of $(\alpha/f^2)_l$ is greater than that of $(\alpha/f^2)_s$ along all the direction. This is what observed in other semiconductors experimentally [15]. The order of ultrasonic attenuation (α/f^2) in FeO is of the order of 10^{-20} Nps^2/cm. While in case of TiO and VO it is of the order of 10^{-16} Nps^2/cm and 10^{-18} Nps^2/cm respectively at all the temperature range. This is because of the different nature of variation in thermal conductivity values of these materials in the temperature range. Although generally much more complicated than the transition metals, the transition metal oxides are simpler in one respect- the 'S-band' spreads from antibonding orbitals between anions and cations, and pushed up in energy, so that it is empty and begins a few eV above the Fermi energy. The only band of interest associated with the oxygen ions is the '2p band', which arises from the bonding orbitals, is filled, and ends a few eV below at Fermi energy. The only state near the Fermi energy thus are d-electron states, and all low energy experimentals probe only the d-band. FeO with 6d-electrons undergo small distortions below their Neel temperatures, and it is possible, in principle, that splitting resulting from these could lead to FeO being a Mott insulator. In TiO nature of thermal conductivity is metallic, which increases with increase in temperature. In VO at low temperature it has low conductivity which increases exponentially with increasing temperature, just as in an ordinary semiconductors. In conclusion it can be said that the thermal conductivity of the semiconducting materials at different temperatures which is well connected to electronic structural change at particular temperature is the governing parameter to the temperature dependence of ultrasonic attenuation arising from interaction between acoustical phonons and lattice phonons. The results may be directly applicable for the processing industries.

Table1 SOEC & TOEC in 10^{11} Dyne/cm^2 of FeO at temperature range 100-500K

SOEC &TOEC	100K	200K	300K	400K	500K
C_{11}	7.108	7.239	7.424	7.626	7.836
C_{12}	4.811	4.725	4.636	4.548	4.459
C_{44}	4.926	4.939	4.957	4.975	4.994
C_{111}	-96.809	-97.034	-97.609	-98.316	-99.081
C_{112}	-19.651	-19.428	-19.186	-18.944	-18.703
C_{123}	6.907	6.551	6.197	5.844	5.490
C_{144}	7.304	7.345	7.389	7.433	7.478
C_{166}	-20.010	-20.049	-20.104	-20.166	-20.230
C_{456}	7.256	7.256	7.256	7.256	7.256

Table 2: SOEC & TOEC in 10^{11} Dyne/cm^2 of TiO at temperature range 100-500K.

SOEC &TOEC	100K	200K	300K	400K	500K
C_{11}	7.303	7.432	7.619	7.826	8.041
C_{12}	5.586	5.498	5.407	5.317	5.227
C_{44}	5.707	5.722	5.741	5.762	5.783
C_{111}	-97.804	-97.988	-98.537	-99.225	-99.977
C_{112}	-22.722	-22.506	-22.267	-22.029	-21.793
C_{123}	7.972	7.624	7.277	6.932	6.586
C_{144}	8.365	8.410	8.458	8.506	8.555
C_{166}	-23.092	-23.132	-23.192	-23.259	-23.329
C_{456}	8.313	8.313	8.313	8.313	8.312

Table3: SOEC & TOEC in 10^{11} Dyne/cm^2 of VO at temperature range 100-500K

SOEC &TOEC	100K	200K	300K	400K	500K
C_{11}	7.329	7.459	7.648	7.857	8.076
C_{12}	6.246	6.157	6.065	5.974	5.883
C_{44}	6.371	6.387	6.408	6.430	6.453
C_{111}	-96.849	-97.019	-97.552	-98.227	-98.965
C_{112}	-25.309	-25.099	-24.865	-24.632	-24.402
C_{123}	8.867	8.528	8.191	7.855	7.519
C_{144}	9.253	9.301	9.352	9.403	9.455
C_{166}	-25.681	-25.723	-25.787	-25.859	-25.934
C_{456}	9.197	9.197	9.197	9.197	9.197

Table 4: $(\alpha/f^2)_{Akh.long}$ and $(\alpha/f^2)_{Akh.shear}$ and $(\alpha/f^2)_{th.}$ of the semiconductors the temperature range 100-500K along <111> direction in 10^{-18} Nps^2/cm.

Material	Temp.(K)	$(\alpha/f^2)_{th}$	$(\alpha/f^2)_{Akh.long}$	$(\alpha/f^2)^*_{Akh.shear}$
FeO	100	0.00017	0.00038	0.00016
	200	0.00094	0.00402	0.00182
	300	0.0033	0.0201	0.0099
	400	0.0061	0.0474	0.0259
	500	0.0092	0.0859	0.0517
TiO	100	0.165	0.246	0.061
	200	0.498	1.402	0.377
	300	0.773	3.252	0.985
	400	1.024	5.734	2.015
	500	1.948	13.615	5.402

VO	100	0.199	0.151	0.019
	200	0.475	0.752	0.113
	300	0.615	1.649	0.302
	400	0.689	2.658	0.586
	500	0.759	3.866	1.006

*Shear wave polarized along $<\bar{1}10>$ direction

4.   References

1.   Yu. V. Shaldin, I. Warchulska and Yu. M. Ivanov, Semiconductors-Vol. 38(2), 169-174 (2004).

2.   F. Gamiz, Semicond. Sci. Technol. 19, 393-398 (2004).

3.   R. K. Das, S. Sahoo, and G. S. Tripathi, Semicond. Sci. Technol. 19, 433-441 (2004).

4.   V. P. Matsokin and G. A. Petchenko, Low. Temp. Phys. 26, 517 (2000).

5.   D. Adler, Solid State Physics 21(1), (1968a); Rev. Mod. Phys. 40, 714 (1968b).

6.   K. Brugger, Phys. Rev. A133,1611(1964).

7.   G. Leibfried and H.Haln, Z.Phys. 150, 497(1958).

8.   S.Mori and Y.Hiki, J.Phys.Soc.Jpn. 45,1449 (1978).

9.   A.Akhieser, J.Phys.(USSR) 1,277 (1939).

10.   T.O. Woodruff and H.Ehrenreich, Phys.Rev. 123,1553 (1961).

11.   H. E. Bömmel and K.Dransfeld, Phys.Rev. 117,245 (1960).

12.   W.P. Mason, Physical Acoustics (Academic Press,New York 1965), Vol.IIIB p.237.

13.   D. S. Puri and M. P. Verma, Solid State Commn. 18, 1295 (1976).

14.   J. Shanker and G. D. Jain, Phys. Rev. B27, 2515 (1983).

15.   S. S. Shukla and Y. S. Yun, J. Acoust. Soc. Am. 70, 1723 (1983).

MTHFR Gene A1298C Polymorphism and Alzheimer's Disease Susceptibility

Vandana Rai

Department of Biotechnology V B S Purvanchal University Jaunpur-222003,UP
raivandana@rediffmail.com

ABSTRACT

Methylenetetrahydrofolate reductase (MTHFR) is a crucial enzyme involved in homocysteine/methionone metabolism. It catalyzes the conversion of 5,10methlenetetrahydrofolate in to 5methyltetrahydrofolate. A number of studies have examined the association of MTHFR A1298C polymorphism as risk factor for Alzheimer's disease (AD), but the results were contradictory. To clarify the influence of MTHFR A1298C polymorphism on Alzheimer's disease (AD), a meta-analysis of ten case-control studies was carried out. Four electronic databases were searched up to August, 2019 for suitable articles. The pooled odds ratios (ORs) with 95% confidence intervals (95% CIs) were used to evaluate the association. All statistical analyses were performed by MetaAnalyst program.

The results of meta-analysis suggested that except allele contrast model, A1298C polymorphism is not risk for Alzheimer's disease using overall comparisons in three genetic models (C vs. A: OR= 1.26, 95%CI= 0.912-1.76, p= 0.04; CC+AC vs. AA: OR= 1.43; 95%CI= 0.85-2.44; p=0.05; CC vs. AA: OR= 1.16, 95%CI = .88-1.55, p= 0.51; AC vs. AA: 1.55; 95%CI= 0.81-2.93,p=0.07). Publication bias was absent in all five genetic models. In conclusion, results of present meta-analysis showed no significant association between MTHFR A1298C polymorphism and AD risk.

Keywords:Alzheimer's disease, MTHFR, A1298C, Polymorphism

1. Introduction

Alzheimer's disease (AD) is one of the major neurodegenerative diseases in elderly population. It is the most common form of dementia, affecting 1 in 8 individuals older than 60 years of age. Most AD cases are late in onset and are probably influenced by both genetic and environmental factors. Epidemiological studies have demonstrated that elevated levels of plasma homocysteine (Hcy) may play an important role in the pathogenesis of AD [1-3].

Folic acid/folate is essential for cellular methylation, DNA synthesis, and homocysteine metabolism. MTHFR and methionine synthase reductase (MTRR) are two important enzymes of folate pathway and dysfunction of these genes increases plasma homocysteine concentration [4,55). Both genes show polymorphism as MTHFR C677T, A1298C [6-9] and MTRR A66G [10-12] and frequency of these polymorphisms varies greatly word wide. MTHFR enzyme required for the conversion of 5,10-methylene-tetrahydrofolate to 5-methyltetrahydrofolate (5THF), 5THF is the methyl donor for synthesis of methionine from homocysteinine [13]. The MTHFR gene is present on short arm of chromosome 1 at position p36.3. MTHFR A1298C polymorphism is associated with reduced MTHFR enzyme activity and hyperhomocysteinemia [5].

In A1298C polymorphism, A is substituted with C nucleotide at position 1298 [5], leading to substitution of glutamate by alanine s (Glu429Ala) in the MTHFR enzyme. Glu429Ala in MTHFR enzyme, reduces 40% enzyme activity. Frequency of 1298C allele differs greatly in various ethnic groups of the world. The prevalence of the mutant CC homozygote variant genotype ranges from 7 to 12% in Europe, 4 to 5% in Hispanics and 1 to 4% in Asian populations (1 to 4%) [14]. Several studies have reported A1298Cpolymorphism as risk factor for several diseases like- cleft lip and palate, Down syndrome, neural tube defects, and psychiatric disorders etc [14]. MTHFR polymorphisms were studied as risk for AD by several researcher but their results were controversial. Hence, the aim of present meta-analysis was to conclude the role of MTHFR A1298C polymorphism in AD risk.

2.   Methods

Article search was carried out in electronic databases up to August, 2019 using key terms - MTHFR', 'A1298C' , and 'Alzheimer's disease'. Criteria for inclusion of studies were as follows; (i) studies should be case-control association study; and (ii) the articles must report the sample size, distribution of alleles or genotypes for estimating the odds ratio (ORs) with 95% confidence interval (CIs). Studies were excluded if one of the following existed: (i) case-only studies, and (ii) editorial, case reports or reviews. Meta- analysis was carried out according to the method of Rai et al [15] (.2014). Publication bias was calculated according to the method of Egger et al. [16] . All statistical analysis was done by MetaAnayst.

3.   Results

Total ten studies [17-26] were found suitable for the inclusion in the meta-analysis. In incuded ten studies number of cases was 1067and number of contro was 1527. The lowest sample size was 43 [23] and highest sample size was 162 [20, 21] in included studies (Table 1). Total cases genotype percentage of AA, AC and CC was 55.34%, 44.65% and 11.84% respectively. The controls genotypes percentage of AA, AC and CC were 55.34%, 44.65% and 11.84% respectively.

Table 1. The distributions of MTHFR A1298C genotypes and allele number in Alzheimer's disease cases and controls

Study	Country	No. of Case/ Controls	Case Genotypes			Control Allele Genotypes			Allele Case		Allele Control		P value HWE
			AA	AC	CC	AA	AC	CC	A	C	A	C	
Wakutani et al.,2002	Japan	241/352	174	51	16	210	127	15	399	83	547	157	0.44
Bosco,2004	Italy	140/136	69	67	16	59	61	16	205	99	179	93	0.96
Ravaglia et al.,2004	Italy	63/122	26	18	4	52	63	7	70	26	167	77	0.03
Linnebank et al.,2004	Germany	162/169	75	68	19	71	71	27	218	106	213	125	0.19
Anello et al., 2004	Italy	162/190	83	78	19	82	89	19	244	116	253	127	0.46
Silva et al.,2006	Brazil	49/50	21	21	1	27	22	1	63	23	76	24	0.14
Dorszewska et al., 2007	Poland	43/50	13	18	7	21	23	6	44	32	65	35	0.93
Gledraltis et al.,2009	Sweden	92/238	32	41	12	176	18	44	105	65	370	106	0
Mansoori et al.,2012	India	61/120	20	41	19	44	59	17	81	79	147	93	0.69
Mansouri et al.,2013	Tunisia	38/100	15	23	0	93	7	0	53	23	193	7	0.71

In allele contrast (A vs C) meta-analysis, mutant C allele showed significant association with AD in random effect (OR= 1.26, 95%CI= 0.912-1.76, p= 0.04) models (Figure 1). Unlike to allele contrast meta-analysis, pooled odds ratio for homozygote genotype (CC vs. AA) did not show any association with AD adopting random (OR= 1.16, 95%CI= .88-1.55, p= 0.51) effect models. Association of mutant heterozygous genotype (AC vs. AA; co-dominant model) aso did not show any association with AD using random effect models (OR= 1.55; 95%CI= 0.81-2.93). Dominant mutant genotypes (CC+AC vs. AA) showed no association with AD using random (OR= 1.43; 95%CI= 0.85-2.44; p=0.05) effect models. Allele contrast cumulative meta-analysis showed that after inclusion of Gledraltis et al. [24] study, odds ratio increased to 1.029 and after then it increased to 1.26 (Figure 2). As evident by funnel plot the publication bias was not observed in any genetic model.

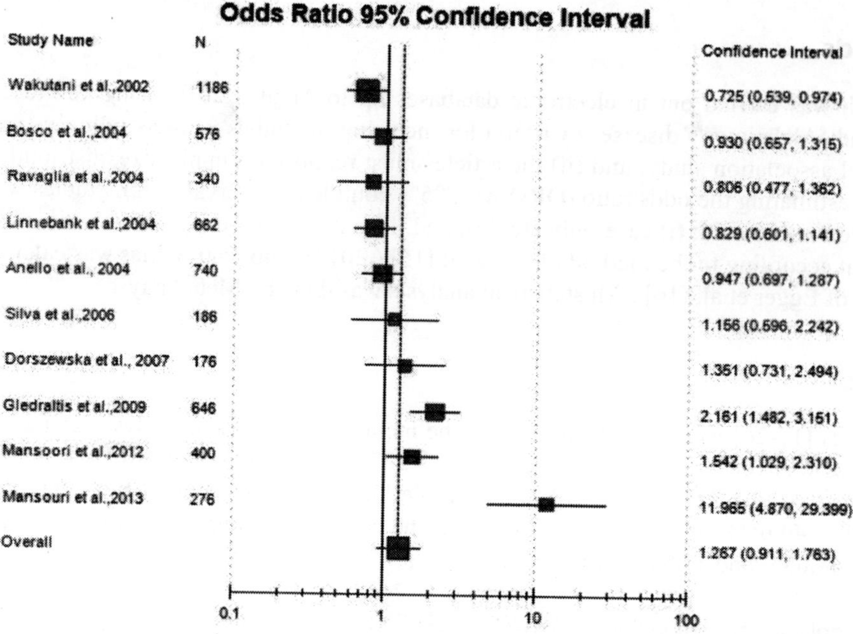

Figure 1. Allele Contrast (A vs C) Random Effect Forest Pot of Ten Studies

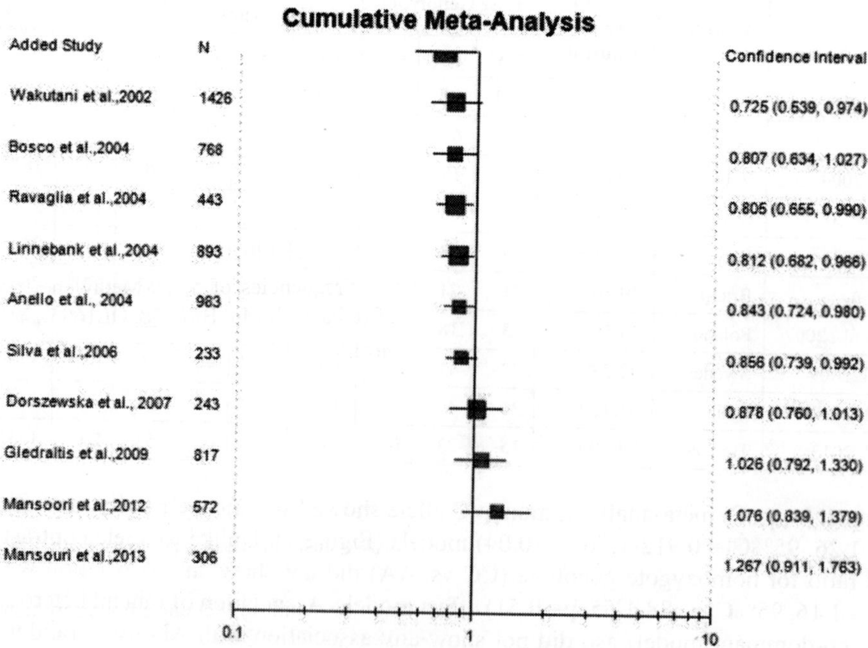

Figure 2. Allele Contrast Cumulative Meta-analysis

4. Discussion

Results of present meta-analysis showed no association between MTHFR A1298C polymorphism and Alzheimer's disease. Elevated Hcy has been reported to be a risk factor for several psychiatric and neurodevelopmental disorders like neural tube defects, schizophrenia, bipolar disorder and depression. Hcy is implicated in increased oxidative stress, DNA damage, the triggering of apoptosis and excitotoxicity, all important mechanisms in neurodegeneration [27,28].

Meta-analysis is a statistical tool, which is successfully used for the compilation of contradictory results of small effect/power case-control studies. Several meta-analysis were published which evaluated risk of small effect gene polymorphism for different disease and disorders like- epilepsy [29], Alzheimer's disease [30], G6PD [31], Down syndrome [32-34], Uterine Leiomyoma [35], orofacial cleft [36,37], depression [38], schizophrenia [39,40], autism [41, , male infertility [42] digestive tract cancer [43], lung cancer [44], endometrial cancer [45], breast cancer [46,47], prostate cancer [48], colorectal cancer [49], and esophageal cancer [50] etc.

Limitations of the study should be acknowledged like—(i) unadjusted crude OR is used, (ii) study number (only ten studies) and sample size are small, (iii) gene–gene or gene-environment interactions may modify the AD risk and; however, such stratified analysis could not be performed owing to lack of data.

5. References

1.   Fernandez, L.L., Scheibe, R.M. Is MTHFR polymorphism a risk factor for Alzheimer disease like APOE? Arq Neuropsiquiatr 63,1–6 (2005).

2.   Wingo, T.S., Lah, J.J., Levey, A.I., et al. Autosomal recessive causes likely in early-onset Alzheimer disease. Arch Neurol. 69,59–64 (2012).

3.   Quadri, P., Fragiacomo, C., Pezzati, R., et al. Homocysteine, folate, and vitamin B-12 in mild cognitive impairment, Alzheimer disease, and vascular dementia. Am J Clin Nutr. 80,114–22 (2004).

4.   Frosst, P., Blom, H.J., Milos, R., et al. A candidate genetic risk factor for vascular disease: A common mutation in methylenetetrahydrofolate reductase. Nat Genet 10, 111–113 (1995).

5.   Weisberg, I., Tran, P., Christensen, B., et al. A second genetic polymorphism in methylenetetrahydrofolate reductase (MTHFR) associated with decreased enzyme activity. Mol Genet Metab. 64, 169–72 (1998).

6.   Rai V, Yadav U, Kumar P, Yadav SK. Methyleletetrahydrofolate reductase polymorphism (C677T) in Muslim population of Eastern Uttar Pradesh, India. Ind J Med Sci. 64(5),219–23 (2010).

7.   Rai, V., Yada, U. Kumar, P. Genotype Prevalence and Allele Frequencies of 5, 10-Methylenetetrahydrofolate Reductase (MTHFR) C677T Mutation in two Caste Groups of India. Cell Mol Biol. 58, OL1695- 701 (2012).

8.   Rai, V., Yadav U, Kumar P. Prevalence of methylene tetrahydrofolate reductase C677T polymorphism in Eastern Uttar Pradesh. Indian J Hum Genet. 18(1), 43-46 (2012).

9.   Yadav, U., Kumar, P., Gupta, S., Rai, V. Distribution of MTHFR C677T Gene Polymorphism in Healthy North Indian Population and an Updated Meta-analysis. Ind J Clin Biochem. 32(4),399-410 (2017).

10. Rai, V., Yadav, U., Kumar, P., Gupta, S. Methionine Synthase Reductase (MTRR) A66G Polymorphism in Rural Population of Uttar Pradesh (India).   Biotechnology 10(2), 220-223 (2011).

11. Rai, V., Yadav, U., Kumar, P. MTRR A66G polymorphism in two caste groups of Uttar Pradesh (India). Indian J Med Sci. 66(5-6), 136-40 (2012).

12. Rai, V., Yadav, U., Kumar, P., Yadav, S.K. Analysis of methionine synthase reductase polymorphism (A66G) in Indian Muslim Population. Indian J Hum Genet. 19(2), 183-187 (2013).

13. Goyette, P., Pai, A., Milos, R., et al. Gene structure of human and mouse methylenetetrahydrofolate reductase (MTHFR). Mamm Genome. 9, 652–6 (1998).

14. Botto, L.D., Yang, Q. 5,10-Methylenetetrahydrofolate reductase gene variants and congenital anomalies: A HuGE review. Am J Epidemiol. 151,862–77 (2000).

15. Rai, V., Yadav, U., Kumar, P., et al. Maternal methylenetetrahydrofolate reductase C677T polymorphism and Down syndrome risk: A meta-analysis from 34 studies. Plos One 9 (9), e108552 (2014).

16. Egger, M., Dave Smith, G., Schneider, M., Minde, C. Bias in meta-analysis detected by a simple, graphical test. BMJ 315, 629–634 (1997).

17. Wakutani, Y., Kowa, H., Kusumi, M., et al. Genetic analysis of vascular factors in Alzheimer's disease. Ann N Y Acad Sci 977, 232–238 (2002).

18. Bosco, P. Association of IL-1 RN*2 allele and methionine synthase 2756 AA genotype with dementia severity of sporadic Alzheimer's disease. J Neurol Neurosurg Psychiatry. 75, 1036–1038 (2004).

19. Ravaglia, G., Forti, P., Maioli, F., et al. Common polymorphisms in methylenetetrahydrofolate reductase (MTHFR): relationships with plasma homocysteine concentrations and cognitive status in elderly northern italian subjects. Arch Gerontol Geriatr Suppl 9, 339–348 (2004).

20. Linnebank, M., Linnebank, A., Jeub, M., et al. Lack of genetic dispositions to hyperhomocysteinemia in Alzheimer disease. Am J Med Genet A 131,101–102 (2004).

21. Anello, G., Gueant-Rodriguez, R.M., Bosco, P., et al. Homocysteine and methylenetetrahydrofolate reductase polymorphism in Alzheimer's disease. Neuroreport 15, 859–861.

22. da Silva, V.C., Ramos, F.J., Freitas, E.M., et al. Alzheimer's disease in Brazilian elderly has a relation with homocysteine but not with MTHFR polymorphisms. Arq Neuropsiquiatr 64, 941–945 (2006).

23. Dorszewska, J., Florczak, J., Rozycka, A., et al. Oxidative DNA damage and level of thiols as related to polymorphisms of MTHFR, MTR, MTHFD1 in Alzheimer's and Parkinson's diseases. Acta Neurobiol Exp (Wars) 67,113–129 (2007).

24. Giedraitis, V., Kilander, L., Degerman-Gunnarsson, M., et al. Genetic analysis of Alzheimer's disease in the Uppsala longitudinal study of adult men. Dement. Geriatr Cogn Disord 27, :59–68 (2009).

25. Mansoo, N., Tripathi, M., Luthra, K, et al. MTHFR (677 and 1298) and IL-6-174 G/C genes in pathogenesis of Alzheimer's and vascular dementia and their epistatic interaction. Neurobiol Aging 33,1003 e1001-1008 (2012).

26. Mansouri L, Fekih-Mrissa N, Klai S, et al. Association of methylenetetrahydrofolate reductase polymorphisms with susceptibility to Alzheimer's disease, Clin Neurol Neurosurg 115, 1693-1696 (2013).

27. Mattson, M.P., Shea, T.B. Folate and homocysteien metabolism in neural plasticity and neurodegenerative disorders. Trends Neurosci. 26,137–46 (2003).

28. Sachdev, P.S. Homocysteine and brain atrophy. Prog Neuropsychopharmacol Biol Psychiatry 29,1152–61(2005).

29. Rai, V., Kumar, P. Methylenetetrahydrofolate reductase C677T polymorphism and susceptibility to epilepsy. Neurol Sci. 10.1007/s10072-018-3583-z (2018).

30. Rai, V. Folate pathway gene methylenetetrahydrofolate reductase C677T polymorphism and Alzheimer disease risk in Asian population. Indian J Clin Biochem 31,245-52 (2016).

31. Kumar, P., Yadav, U., Rai, V. Prevalence of glucose-6-phosphate dehydrogenase deficiency in India: an updated meta-analysis. Egypt J Med Hum Genet, 17, 295–302 (2016).

32. Rai, V. Polymorphism in folate metabolic pathway gene as maternal risk factor for Down syndrome. Int J Biol Med Res 2(4), 1055-1060 (2011).

33. Rai, V., Yadva, U., Kumar, P. Null association of maternal MTHFR A1298C polymorphism with Down syndrome pregnancy: An updated meta-analysis. Egypt J Med Hum Genet. 18, 9-18 (2017).

34. Rai, V., Kumar, P. Fetal MTHFR C677T polymorphism confers no susceptibility to Down Syndrome: evidence from meta-analysis. Egyptian J Med Hum Genet. 19, 53-58 (2018).

35. Kumar, P., Rai, V. Catechol-O-Methyltransferase Val158Met polymorphism and susceptibility to Uterine Leiomyoma. Jacobs Journal of Gynecology and Obstetrics 5(1), 043 (2018).

36. Rai, V. Maternal methylenetetrahydrofolate reductase (MTHFR) gene A1298C polymorphism and risk of nonsyndromic Cleft lip and/or Palate (NSCL/P) in offspring: A meta-analysis. Asian J Med Sci. 6 (1), 16- 21 (2014).

37.   Rai, V. Strong association of C677T polymorphism of methylenetetrahydrofolate reductase gene with nosyndromic cleft lip/palate (nsCL/P). Ind J Clin Biochem 33(1), 5-15 (2018).

38.   Rai, V. Genetic polymorphisms of methylenetetrahydrofolate reductase (MTHFR) gene and susceptibility to depression in Asian population: a systematic meta-analysis. Cell Mol. Biol. 60 (3), 29-36 (2014).

39.   Yadav, U., Kumar, P., Gupta, S., Rai, V. Role of MTHFR C677T gene polymorphism in the susceptibility of schizophrenia: An updated meta-analysis. Asian J Psychiatry 20, 41–51 (2016).

40.   Rai, V., Yadav, U., Kumar, P., et al. Methylenetetrahydrofolate Reductase A1298C Genetic Variant and Risk of Schizophrenia: an updated meta-analysis. Indian J Med Res. 145(4), 437-447 (2017).

41.   Rai, V., Kumar, P. Methylenetetrahydrofolate reductase A1298C Polymorphism and Autism susceptibility. Austin J Autism and Related Disabilities 4, 1048-1053 (2018).

42.   Rai, V., Kumar, P. Methylenetetrahydrofolate reductase C677T polymorphism and risk of male infertility in Asian population. Indian J Clin Biochem 32(3), 253–60 (2017).

43.   Yadav, U., Kumar, P., Rai, V. NQO1 Gene C609T Polymorphism (dbSNP: rs1800566) and Digestive Tract Cancer Risk: A Meta-Analysis. Nutr Cancer. 70(4), 557-568 (2018).

44.   Rai, V. Folate Pathway Gene MTHFR C677T Polymorphism and Risk of Lung Cancer in Asian Populations. Asian Pac J Cancer Prev. 15 (21), 9259-9264 (2014).

45.   Kumar, P., Singh, G., Rai, V. Evaluation of COMT Gene rs4680 Polymorphism as a Risk Factor for Endometrial Cancer. IJCB 10.1007/s12291-018-0799-x (2018).

46.   Rai, V. Methylenetetrahydrofolate reductase A1298C polymorphism and breast cancer risk: a meta-analysis of 33 studies. Annals of Medical and Health Sciences Research 4 (6), 841-851 (2014).

47.   Rai, V., Yadav, U., Kumar, P. Impact of catechol-O-methyltransferase Val 158Met (rs4680) polymorphism on breast cancer susceptibility in Asian population. Asian Pac J Cancer Prev. 18(5), 1243–50 (2017).

48.   Yadav, U., Kumar, P., Rai, V. Role of MTHFR A1298C gene polymorphism in the etiology of prostate cancer: A systematic review and updated meta-analysis. Egyptian J Med Hum Genet 17, 141-148 (2016).

49.   Rai, V. Evaluation of the MTHFR C677T Polymorphism as a Risk Factor for Colorectal Cancer in Asian Populations. Asian Pac J Cancer Prev 16 (18), 8093-8100 (2016).

50.   Kumar, P., Rai, V. Methylenetetrahydrofolate reductase C677T polymorphism and risk of esophageal cancer: An updated meta-analysis. Egypt J Med Hum Genet 19(4),: 273-284 (2018).

Development of Ultrasonic Instrumentation for Inspection of Concrete Structures using a Pulse-Echo Technique

Harshit Jain[1,2*] and V.H. Patankar[1,2]

[1]Homi Bhabha National Institute (HBNI), Mumbai-400094, India
[2]Electronics Division, Bhabha Atomic Research Centre (BARC), Mumbai-400085, India
*Email: harshitj@barc.gov.in

ABSTRACT

In this paper, NDT of non-homogeneous structures like concrete/ RCC has been carried out using ultrasonic pulse-echo (P-E) mode. P-E mode is a very difficult mode for inspection of concrete, as far as penetration and flaw detection sensitivity are concerned. Ultrasonic Imaging of concrete blocks, using various pairs of low frequency transducers in P-E mode has been carried out to acquire B-scan images. A concrete block with simulated defects have also been inspected by acquiring A-scan data and B-Scan images of the test specimens using commercially available HV Pulser and ultrasonic imaging system in-house developed at Electronics Division, BARC. Earlier, authors of this paper have carried out B-scan imaging of concrete blocks using conventional T-R mode, on defective regions of the test block. Now in this paper, non-homogeneous materials such as concrete\RCC have been inspected having access from one side and by using, a very difficult mode to implement namely Pulse-Echo mode, using contact technique.

Keywords: Ultrasonic testing, concrete, pulse-echo, NDT, contact method, A-scan, B-scan image.

1.   Introduction

Concrete/RCC structures are non-homogeneous and porous materials which comprise aggregates bound with cement paste. Aggregates include gravel, crushed stone, sand etc. which make up 60-80% of concrete mix. They provide compressive strength to concrete. Despite having a high durability and high compressive strength, concrete structures get affected by many processes such as mechanical loading and harmful chemical reactions because of environmental effects, which result in the deterioration of concrete structures. Concrete structures deteriorate slowly at first and then progress fast to failure [1]. Therefore, to avoid any failure of the concrete structure, the defects inside the structure are examined using two types of techniques namely Destructive and Non-Destructive Testing (NDT). As the destructive testing provides direct, precise and reliable information about the structural integrity and quality of the concrete structure but still this technique is avoided because to inspect the structure it requires few small samples from the structure which degrades the structure. Conversely, NDT is a harmless method which provides the indirect information about the health of the structure and such information needs further post-processing. Now-a-days different NDT methods are used for the inspection of concrete structures out of which Ultrasonic Pulse Velocity (UPV) test is most preferred [2]. In UPV test, Time of Flight (TOF) of Ultrasonic pulse travelling through concrete is measured. The TOF and acoustic velocity in the concrete provides information about defects and strength of the concrete structure [3]. When an ultrasonic pulse is transmitted in the concrete, then three types of scans can be obtained at the receiver side. These scans are called A-scan, B-scan and C-scan. When the amplitude of the ultrasonic wave is plotted with respect to time, then the scan obtained is called as A-scan waveform [4]. The A-scan waveform depicts the information about the size of discontinuity which can be estimated by comparing the amplitude of ultrasonic signal received from a reference defect in the sample of concrete to that received from defect portion. When the TOF of the ultrasonic wave is plotted with respect to the linear position of the transducer then the scan obtained is called B-scan image. B-scan is a 2-D presentation which displays the cross-sectional front view of the test specimen. The C-scan presentation is a top view 2D presentation that is possible for automated two-dimensional scanning systems that provides a plan view of the location and size of defect. Ultrasonic inspection of concrete is carried out by using two modes namely Through-transmission UPV mode and Pulse–Echo (PE) mode. In Through-transmission UPV mode, access from both the sides of the structure is required whereas for PE mode only one side access is sufficient. The through-transmission UPV method is mostly employed in the construction industry. Traditionally, inspection of concrete structure was carried out using UPV test but now-a-days A-scan waveforms and B-scan images are acquired for the inspection [5]. In this paper, the PE technique is used to develop the Ultrasonic instrumentation system for inspection of concrete structures. The A-scan waveforms are acquired and displayed on the computer screen using three different frequencies of ultrasonic transducers and also B-scan imaging is carried out to indicate the presence of defects in the sample concrete blocks.

2. System Design

The measurement is carried out on a concrete block of size 150mm × 150mm × 150mm with the two artificially generated holes in it. The two holes with 1″ diameter each have been artificially generated in the concrete test-block at two different depths, one at 4″ deep from the top and other at 2″ deep as shown in Fig.1(a). The concrete sample is the standard concrete block having high strength. All the measurements were made using high power ultrasonic imaging system developed by Electronics Division, BARC [6]. Authors developed imaging software specifically for concrete structures. The ultrasonic imaging system as shown in Fig.1(b) consists of the commercially available high power pulser-receiver, in-house developed 100 MSPS @ 8 bits high speed digitizer, commercially available USB controller module and the host PC. The Ultrasonic A-scan and B-scan imaging software has been developed using Visual C#. The USB Controller has USB 3.0/2.0 Interface with host PC through windows Dynamically Linked Libraries (DLL) based interface program.

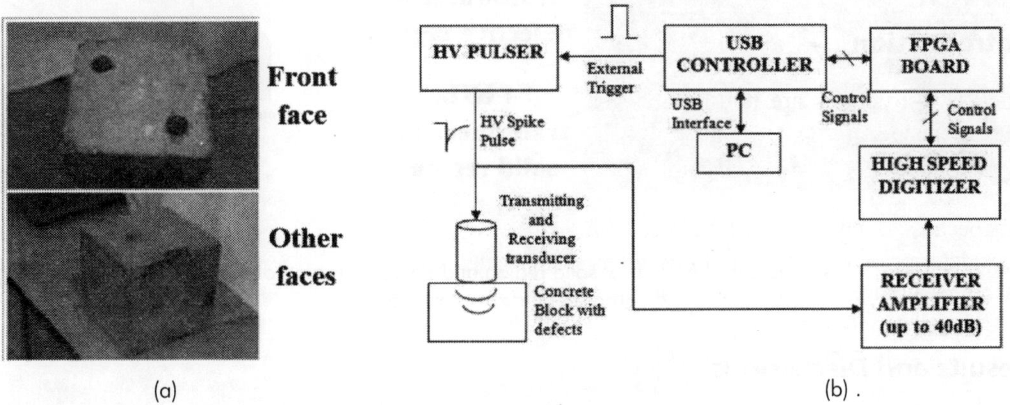

Figure 1. (a) Concrete test block with two artificially generated holes, (b) Schematic Block Diagram of Ultrasonic Imaging system for inspection of concrete block in P-E mode.

USB Controller generates trigger pulses through FPGA board with desired pulse width and pulse repetition frequency (PRF) when acquisition is initiated through the GUI on the PC. The high voltage pulser is a spike pulser which generates high voltage pulses of maximum 1100 V in response to the trigger pulses to energize the ultrasonic transducer which generates the longitudinal waves inside the concrete block. For ultrasonic inspection of concrete structures, low frequency ultrasonic transducers are utilized because high frequency ultrasonic waves get attenuated in the concrete due to scattering in the aggregate [7]. The ultrasonic signal received by receiving transducer needs to be amplified and processed for better SNR with the intent to suppress spurious artifacts. The ultrasonic signals received from the transducer in P-E mode are amplified, filtered using a band pass filter and then digitized and displayed on the computer screen for measurement of TOF. The B-scan imaging, on the concrete structure is performed using three types of transducers with a frequency of 54 kHz, 108 kHz and 250 kHz respectively. The HV pulser provides a fixed PRF of 10 Hz. For data acquisition, Spartan 6 FPGA and a USB Controller are used. The data is acquired at 1 MSPS with 8-bit resolution using in-house developed flash ADC.

3.   Experimental Setup

Ultrasonic data is acquired in the form of A-scan waveforms and B-scan images using three different types of low frequency transducers. The inspection is carried out across the depth of the artificially generated hole in the concrete test block as shown in Fig.3. The A-scan waveforms and B-scan images at the solid region of concrete are compared with the defect region having holes in the concrete block. The quality of the received signal also depends on the coupling between the transducer and the concrete surface. Various coupling agents such as gel, vaseline, water, glycerin, grease or oils of different viscosity, etc. are used to eliminate the presence of air pockets between the transducer front face and the concrete surface. We used grease as a coupling agent. For acquiring the B-scan images, the excitation voltage of the pulser was fixed at 50V for all the three frequencies and the amplifier gain was also 20dB for all the three frequencies. The pulse repeating frequency (PRF) for triggering the pulser was fixed at 10Hz.

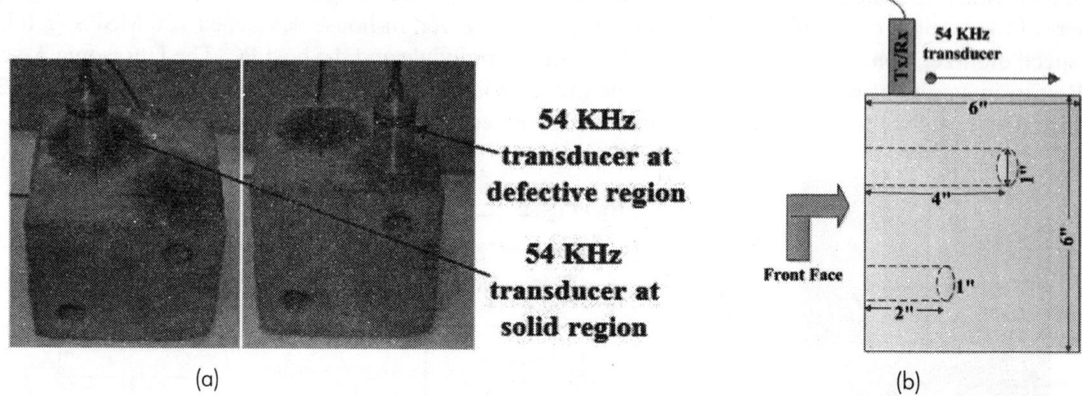

Figure 2. (a) Ultrasonic transducer of 54 KHz at solid region and defective region of concrete block, (b) Schematic diagram of ultrasonic test setup

4.   Results and Discussions

Ultrasonic Pulse-Echo method is a useful tool to detect voids and porosities inside the concrete structure [8]. The laboratory experiments were carried out to detect the void inside the sample concrete block. Both A-scan waveforms and B-scan images were obtained as shown in Fig.4 and Fig.5 respectively.

In Fig.4, bottom side of the image depicts the A-scan waveforms at defect region and upper side of the image depicts the A-scan waveforms at solid region. It can be seen that there is a drastic change in the waveform at the defect region when compared with the solid region which indicates the presence of void or porosity inside the concrete sample. Large attenuation in the waveform is observed at the defect region. As the ultrasonic pulse travels slowly in the air as compared to that in the concrete, there is an increase in the TOF and decrease in the energy of ultrasonic pulse which causes attenuation in the resulted A-scan waveform.

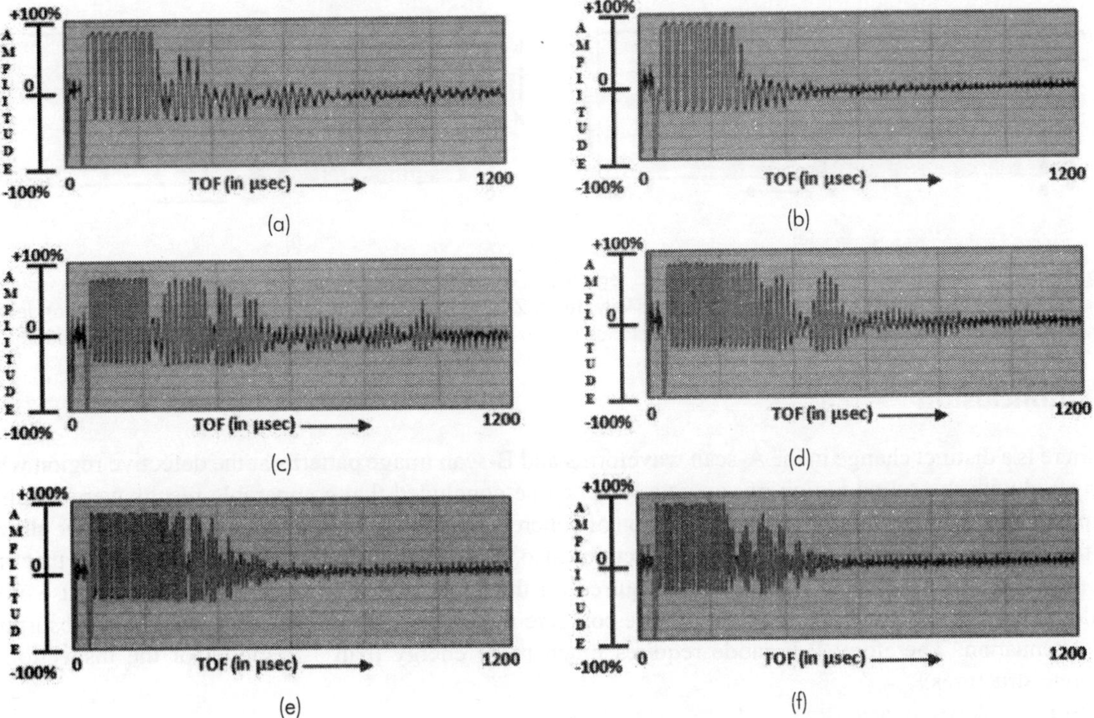

Figure 4 (a),(b) A-scan acquired using 54 KHz transducer at solid region and at defect region respectively;
(c), (d) A-scan acquired using 108 KHz transducer at solid region and at defect region respectively;
(e), (f) A-scan acquired using 250 KHz transducer at solid region and at defect region respectively

In Fig.5, B-scan images have been plotted at the solid as well as defect region. The bottom side images depict the B-scan images at defect region and upper side images depict the B-scan images at solid region. Similar to A-scan waveforms, here also there is a significant change in the pattern of the image at the defect region when compared with the solid region due to the increase in the attenuation and scattering at the defect region which indicates the presence of void or porosity inside the concrete sample. When compared with the conventional UPV test, these B-scan images are more revealing about the defects and are sensitive to the defects.

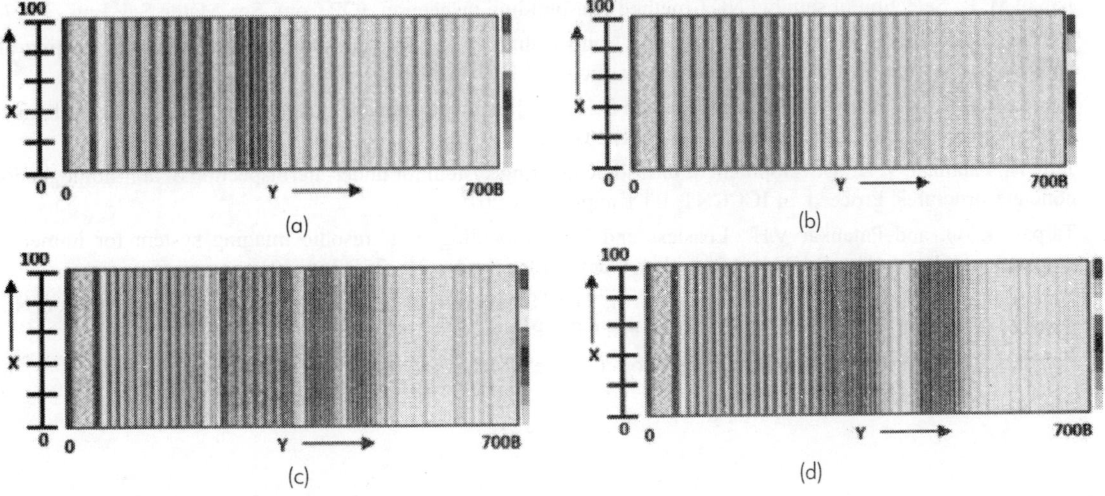

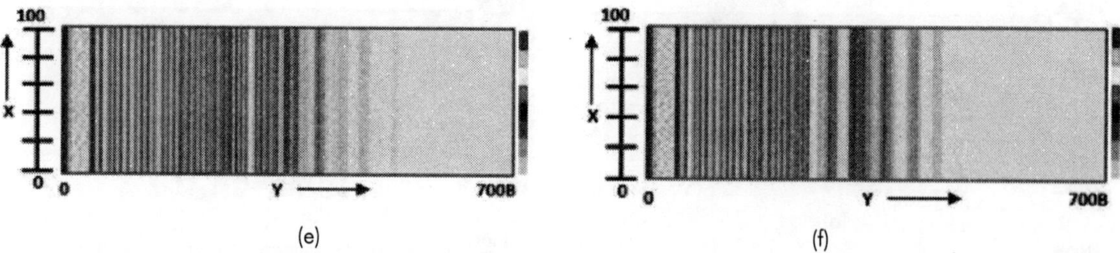

(e)   (f)

Figure 5 (a),(b) 54 KHz transducer: B-scan at solid region and at defect region respectively; (c),(d) 108 KHz transducer: B-scan at solid region and at defect region respectively; (e),(f) 250 KHz transducer: B-scan at solid region and at defect region respectively. [X-axis: Transducer travel distance in mm and Y-axis: Number of samples in Bytes along depth]

5. Conclusion

As there is a distinct change in the A-scan waveforms and B-scan image patterns at the defective region when compared with the sound region of concrete so it can be concluded that comparable results were obtained from the Pulse Echo technique for the inspection of concrete structures. This technique can be further utilized for the under-water inspection of concrete structures also. The advantage of using this technique is that only one side access of the concrete structure is required for the inspection. There is a difficulty in the use of PE mode because of the large heterogeneity of the concrete material which causes wave scattering, absorption and attenuation. Therefore, P-E mode requires much more energy than T-R mode for the inspection of concrete structures.

6. Acknowledgement

Authors are thankful to Mrs. Anita Behere, Head, Electronics Division, BARC, for providing support and guidance for this work.

7. References

1. Karaiskos, G.; Deraemaeker, A.; Aggelis, D.; Van Hemelrijck, D. Monitoring of concrete structures using the ultrasonic pulse velocity method. Smart Mater. Struct. 2015, 24, 113001.

2. Ismail M. P., Selection of suitable NDT methods for building inspection, IOP Conf. Ser. Mater. Sci. Eng., 2017.

3. Martínez A., Estrella J. H. L., Medrano A. S., and Galiana F. J., Relationship between ultrasonic testing and compressive strength in different age concrete structures, 7, 89–93, 2018.

4. Iyer S., Sinha S.K., Pedrick M.K. and Tittmann B.R., Evaluation of ultrasonic inspection and imaging systems for concrete pipes, Autom. Construct., 22, 149-164, 2012.

5. Jain, H., Patankar, V. H., Development of ultrasonic imaging system for under-aterinspection of non-homogeneous concrete structures, Proceed. of ICCCNT, IIT Kanpur, July 2019.

6. Tarpara E. G. and Patankar V.H., Lossless and lossy modeling of ultrasonic imaging system for immersion applications: Simulation and experimentation, Comp. Elec. Engi, 71, 251-264, 2018.

7. Naik T. R., Malhorta V. M. and Popovics J. S., The Ultrasonic Pulse Velocity Method in Handbook on Non-destructive Testing of Concrete, Boca Raton, FL: CRC Press, 2004, 384.

8. Schickert M., Progress in ultrasonic imaging of concrete". Mat Struc 38, 807–815, 2005.

Ultrasonic Properties of Rare Earth DyX (X: S, Se and Te) Chalcogenide Compounds

Bhawan Jyoti[1,*] and Devraj Singh[2,3]

[1]University School of Information and Communication Technology, Guru Gobind Singh Indraprastha University, Sector 16 C, Dwarka, New Delhi, Delhi 110078, India
[2]Amity School of Engineering & Technology Delhi, AUUP Premises, Noida-201313, India
[3]Department of Physics, AIAS, Amity University Uttar Pradesh, Noida-201313, India
*E-mail: aabru_sharma@yahoo.co.in

ABSTRACT

We have investigated the temperature dependent elastic, mechanical, thermal and ultrasonic properties of dysprosium chalcogenides, DyX (X = S, Se and Te) along crystallographic directions <100>, <110> and <111>. First of all, we computed the second and third order elastic constants using the Mori and Hiki approach. These elastic constants are applied to compute the mechanical properties, ultrasonic velocities and thermal conductivity. Finally all the computed parameters are used to find out ultrasonic attenuation in these materials. Obtained results have presented and discussed with available theoretical results of different approximations.

Keywords: Dyprosium chalcogenides, elastic constants, thermal conductivity, ultrasonic properties

1. Introduction

The monochalcogenide compounds like YX, BeX, NpX (X = S, Se and Te) have attracted the much interest for researchers because of their fascinating structural, electronic, magnetic, mechanical and thermal properties [1–7]. The major advantages of monochalcogenide compounds is its scope in the fabrication of supercomputing machines and spintronic devices [2]. Many studies on high magnetic ordering and valence behaviour reveal that these materials are suitable for modulators and magneto-optic memory devices [5].

The ultrasonic properties of crystals are important for studying their solid-state characteristics, such as the energy density, specific heat, thermal relaxation time, and thermal conductivity [8]. Various elastic and mechanical parameters such as Young's modulus, Zener anisotropy ratio, shear modulus, bulk modulus, Poisson's ratio, ductility/brittleness ratio (Pugh's indicator), and Vicker's hardness are crucial for determining the nature and quality of crystals in response to external stress [9,10]. Linear elastic constants such as the second order elastic constants (SOECs) are related to the response of stress to strain [11]. Nonlinear elastic constants such as the third order elastic constants (TOECs) are connected with the mechanical and an harmonic properties of solids. These elastic constants provide valuable information regarding the mechanical strength, nature of atomic bonding, nonlinearity, and empirical interatomic potentials [12]. Temperature-dependent anisotropic studies of these elastic constants can help to understand the dynamic thermo-mechanical characteristics of crystals and they play crucial roles in the design of industrial equipment with desirable physical properties under ambient operating conditions.

This motivated us to conduct a study of the ultrasonic and thermal properties of DyS, DySe, and DyTe . In the present work, we computed the temperature dependence of the second and third order elastic constants (SOECs and TOECs), bulk modulus (B), shear modulus (G), Young's modulus (Y), Poisson ratio (v), Pugh's indicator (G/B), Zener anisotropy ratio (A), ultrasonic velocities of these materials.

2.   Theory

The elastic constants at higher temperature are calculated using the method developed by Mori and Hiki [13]. The detailed expressions to find out SOECs and TOECs have been given in literature [14]. The shear modulus (G), bulk modulus (B), Zener's anisotropy (A), Poisson's ratio (v) and tetragonal moduli (C_s) for YCh are also evaluated using SOECs. The expressions for these mechanical constants are given in literature [14]. V_D is the Debye average velocity and is dependent on the longitudinal (V_L) and the shear (V_S) wave velocities [14]. The expressions of the ultrasonic velocities have been given in literature [14].

3.   Results and Discussion

3.1   Second and Third order elastic constants

The SOECs and TOECs are computed in the temperature range 100-300K using two parametes the Nearest-neighbour distance and the hardness parameter. The nearest- neighbour distance for DySe, DyS and DyTe 2.695 Å, 2.875 Å, 3.06 Å respectively and hardness parameter 0.292 Å for all the chosen materials.

Table 1. Elastic constant of DyX (in the unit of 10^{11} dynes/cm ^{2})

Material	Temp. [K]	C_{11}	C_{12}	C_{44}	C_{111}	C_{112}	C_{123}	C_{144}	C_{166}	C_{456}
DyS	100	6.22	1.69	1.79	-99.63	-6.59	2.76	2.99	-7.30	2.97
	200	6.39	1.60	1.80	-99.64	-5.52	2.96	3.01	-7.33	2.97
	300	6.59	1.51	1.80	-99.93	-4.53	3.07	3.03	-7.36	2.97
DySe	100	5.48	1.26	1.35	-91.01	-4.72	2.10	2.31	-5.46	2.29
	200	5.65	1.17	1.35	-91.03	-3.65	2.27	2.32	-5.48	2.29
	300	5.84	1.08	1.36	-91.36	-2.67	2.36	2.34	-5.50	2.29
DyTe	100	4.18	0.98	1.05	-69.17	-3.53	1.77	1.80	-4.26	1.78
	200	4.35	0.91	1.05	-69.45	-2.73	1.84	1.81	-4.28	1.78
	300	4.51	0.84	1.06	-69.81	-1.96	1.89	1.83	-4.30	1.78

The computed values of temperature dependent SOECs and TOECs have been presented in Table 1. It is seen that the values of C_{11}, C_{44}, C_{111}, C_{166}, C_{144} and C_{123} increase with temperature while the values of C_{12}, C_{112} decrease with rise in temperature. The value of C_{456} is not vary with temperature. If the interatomic distance increases or decreases with temperature then the interaction potential decreases or increases, which causes decreases or increases in elastic constants. This type of behavior of SOECs and TOECs is already found in other rare earth material such as lanthanum monochalcogenides [15]. The SOECs and TOECs also supply significant evidence regarding the character of the forces working in crystalline materials. In particular, SOECs and TOECs offer information on the stiffness and stability of rare earth DyX (X: S, Se and Te) chalcogenide with the application of Coulomb and Born–Mayer potential.

3.2   Mechanical properties

The mechanical constants like Zener anisotropic ratio(A), Young's modulus(Y), shear modulus(G), Poisson's ratio(v) and Pugh's ratio (B/G) ratio at room temperature are obtained by using SOECs values at room temperature and these values are given in Table 2. The Pugh's ratio have been found less than 1.75, which confirms that the materials are brittle in nature. Since, the values $B > 0$, $C_{44} > 0$, $C_S > 0$ and $C_{12} < B < C_{11}$, so these compounds are mechanical stable as per Born criteria. The bond character and ductile/brittle nature is further determined by Cauchy's pressure ($C_{12} - C_{44}$), which is negative confirms the brittle nature. Poisson's ratio $v < 0.26$, indicate brittle nature of materials.

Table 2. Mechanical properties of DyX, Bulk modulus B, Young's modulus E, Shear modulus G, Poisson ratio v, Anisotropy factor A.

Material	G(GPa)	A	B(GPa)	v	Y (GPa)	B/G	$C_{12} - C_{44}$
DyS	207	0.7090	321	0.23	511.19	1.55	-0.29
DySe	170	0.5706	267	0.24	421.42	1.57	-0.28
DySe	132	0.5785	206	0.24	327.21	1.56	-0.22

The propagation velocities for the longitudinal wave and shear waves of DyX (X: S,Se,Te) along three crystallographic direction <100>,<110> and <111> are calculated using the expressions for computation of wave velocities [14]. The computed values of ultrasonic velocities along different crystallographic directions are given in Table 3. From Table 3, it is observed that highest velocity is for longitudinal mode of wave propagation along <100> direction for DyS, DySe and DyTe.

Table 3 Ultrasonic velocities V_L, V_s, V_m (cm/s) for DyS, DySe, DyTe at room temperature

Material		<100>	<110>	<111>
DyS	V_L	2.68×10^5	2.64×10^5	2.63×10^5
	V_{S1}	1.54×10^5	1.53×10^5	1.58×10^5
	V_{S2}	1.54×10^5	1.61×10^5	1.58×10^5
	V_m	1.71×10^5	1.53×10^5	1.75×10^5
DySe	V_L	2.45×10^5	2.31×10^5	2.26×10^5
	V_{S1}	1.29×10^5	1.29×10^5	1.45×10^5
	V_{S2}	1.29×10^5	1.52×10^5	1.45×10^5
	V_m	1.43×10^5	1.32×10^5	1.59×10^5
DyTe	V_L	2.32×10^5	2.11×10^5	2.03×10^5
	V_{S1}	1.12×10^5	1.12×10^5	1.37×10^5
	V_{S2}	1.12×10^5	1.48×10^5	1.37×10^5
	V_m	1.26×10^5	1.18×10^5	1.49×10^5

4.   Conclusion

On the basis of obtained results for DyX materials and their discussion, we conclude the following points:

- SOECs and TOECs of have been computed successfully using Coulomb and Born-Mayer potential model.

- The fracture/toughness ratio have been found less than 1.75, which confirms that the materials are brittle in nature.

- Since, the values $B > 0$, $C_{44} > 0$, $C_S > 0$ and $C_{12} < B < C_{11}$ are greater than unity. So these compounds are mechanical stable as per Born criterion.

- The Cauchy's pressure (C_{12} - C_{44}), is found to be negative, this confirms the brittle nature of the DyX.
- Poisson's ratio $\nu < 0.26$, indicates brittle nature of material.

5. References

1. L Petit, Z Szotek, M Luders and A Svane, J. Cond. Mater. 28 22 (2016)

2. M A Kuroda, Z Jiang, M Povolotskyi, G Klimeek, D M Newns and G J Martyna, Phys. Rev. B90 245124 (2014)

3. L Yang, D Liu, D Chen and L Zou, Chin. Phys. B25 027401 (2016)

4. S Qaisi, M S Abu-Jafar, G K Gopir and R Khenata, Phase Trans. 89 1155 (2016)

5. V Srivastava, S Bhajanker and S P Sanyal, Physica B406 2158 (2011)

6. L Hasni, M Ameri, D Bensaid, I Ameri, S Mesbah, Y Al-Douri and J Coutinho, J. Supercond. Nov. Magn. 17 4130 (2017)

7. S N Tripathi, V Srivastava and S P Sanyal, J. Supercond. Nov. Magn. 31 3925 (2018)

8. X.H. Li, C.H. Xing, H.L. Cui, R.Z. Zhang, J. Phys. Chem. Solids 126 65–71(2019).

9. M. Shafiq, S. Arif, I. Ahmad, S.J. Asadabadi, M. Maqbool, H.A.R. Aliabad, J. Alloy. Comp. 618, 292–298(2015).

10. O. Gomis, F.J. Manjón, P. Rodríguez-Hernández, A. Muñoz, J. Phys. Chem. Solids 124 111–120 (2019).

11. J.M. Winey, A. Hmiel, Y.M. Gupta, J. Phys. Chem. Solids 93 118–120(2016).

12.   L. Liu, G. Xu, A. Wang, X. Wu, R. Wang, J. Phys. Chem. Solids 104 243–251(2017).

13. S.Mori .,Y. Hiki, J. Phys. Soc. Jpn. 45, 1449-1456 (1978).

14. V. Bhalla, D.Singh, S.K. Jain, Int. J. Thermophys. 37, p.33, (2016).

15. R.R. Yadav and D.Singh, J. Phys. Soc. Jpn. 70 1825-1832 (2001).

Investigation of Phase, Microstructural and Dielectric Behavior of Manganese Doped CaCu$_3$Ti$_4$O$_{12}$ Synthesized by a Semi-wet Route

Santosh Pandey[*] and K.D. Mandal

¹Department of Chemistry, Indian Institute of Technology (BHU), Varanasi - 221005, India
*Email: santoshpandey.rs.chy17@itbhu.ac.in

ABSTRACT

The manganese doped CaCu$_3$Ti$_3$MnO$_{12}$ (CCTO) ceramics have been successfully synthesized through a semi-wet route and sintered at 1323 K for 8 h. The phase, as well as microstructure, was confirmed by XRD and SEM analysis, respectively. The average crystallite size was calculated from XRD is 30 ± 10 nm. The grain size was found to be 1.36 µm. The dielectric constant of silver-coated cylindrical pellets was measured by LCR meter (PSM1735, NumetriQN$_4$L, and U.K.) After Mn doping, the dielectric constant of CCTO decreases from 10^4 to 10^2. The dielectric constant increases with increasing temperature. The investigated dielectric constant, as well as tangent loss, was found to be 100 and 0.1, respectively. The dielectric constant and tangent loss decreases due to decreasing of grain size and increasing the density on grain boundaries. The CCTO ceramic shows the semiconducting grain and insulating boundaries which is responsible for the dielectric behavior.

Keywords: Semi-wet route, ceramic, dielectric behavior.

1. Introduction

The ACu$_3$Ti$_4$O$_{12}$ ceramics (Where A= Y$_{2/3}$, Bi$_{2/3}$, Gd$_{2/3}$) was discovered in 1967 [1]. Which have the ability to produce high dielectric constant used in many applications? From the last decade, scientists across the globe used BaTiO$_3$ as a relaxer ferroelectric such as Pb(Mg$_{0.33}$Nb$_{0.66}$)O$_3$(PMN), Pb(Zn$_{0.33}$Nb$_{0.66}$)O$_3$(PZN) [2] which possess high permittivity constant ($\varepsilon r \approx 10^2 - 2 \times 10^4$). The main problems with BaTiO$_3$ (a ferroelectric type of perovskite) are instability due to the reason of phase transition and dielectric constant variation at high temperatures which made it a bad candidate for study at high temperature. Due to these drawbacks, Subramanian et al discovered firstly ACu$_3$Ti$_4$O$_{12}$ perovskite oxide with a high dielectric constant which is greatly utilized from the last two decades for such study [3, 4]. Scientists' have reported that the microstructure and impedance properties of CCTO ceramics influenced by the synthesis route [5, 6]. Seriously, The major problems in the application of CCTO. So, high dielectric loss and urgently need to developing stable processing method. Till now, some theoretical method has been suggested to explain the origin of giant dielectric constant and high dielectric loss and finally assist to develop applications of CCTO perovskite material. These methods are internal domain [7], electrode polarization effect [8], bimodal grain size model [9], internal barrier layer capacitance (IBLC) [10], and nanoscale barrier layer capacitance model (NBLC) [11]. The property of abnormal behavior of CCTO ceramics most successfully explained by internal barrier layer capacitance (IBLC) model [12], which recommended that n-type semiconducting grains are separated by insulating barrier corresponding to Ti-rich secondary phase observed in grains boundaries [13].

In the present work, we have synthesized CCTMO via a semi-wet route and studies of phase, microstructure and dielectric behavior of Manganese doped CCTO sintered at 1323 K for 8h.

2.   Experimental

2.1   Materials synthesis

CCTMO was synthesized through a semi-wet route. In this method, chemicals calcium nitrate, $Ca(NO_3)_2.4H_2O$ (98% Merck, India), Copper nitrate, $Cu(NO_3)_2.3H_2O$ (99% Merck, India), Manganese acetate, $Mn(CH_3COO)_2.4H_2O$ (99% Merck, India), and titanium oxide, TiO_2 (99% Merck, India), was taken in stoichiometric amount in molar ratio. The solution of $Ca(NO_3)_2. 4H_2O$, $Cu(NO_3)_2.3H_2O$, and $Mn(CH_3COO)_2.4H_2O$ were prepared in distilled water. All the solutions were mixed together in a beaker and stoichiometric amount of solid TiO_2 was added in solution. The calculated amount of citric acid (99.5%, Merck India) equivalent to metal ions was dissolved in distilled water and mixed with the solution. The resulting solution was heated on a hot plate magnetic stirrer at 343 K to evaporate water and allows for self-ignition. A fluffy mass of CCTMO powders was obtained after removal of a lot of gases. Citric acid used as a complexing agent that acts as fuel in the ignition step. The resulting CCTMO powder was ground with the help of agate and mortar to make a fine powder. The Powder was calcined at 1323 K for 6 h. Calcined powder was used to make for cylindrical pellets with the using of 2% PVA as a binder on applying 5 tons of pressure using hydraulic pressure for 75 seconds. Finally, the CCTMO pellets were sintered at 1323 K for 8 h.

2.2   Characterizations

The crystalline phase of CCTMO ceramic sintered sample was identified by X-ray diffractometer (Rigaku mini flex 600, Japan) applying Cu-kα radiation with wavelength 1.5418 A⁰. The microstructure and elemental composition were examined by scanning electron microscope (SEM) (ZEISS; model EVO18 research, Germany) attached with energy-dispersive X-ray (EDX) analyzer (Oxford instrument, USA). The dielectric data of silver-coated cylindrical pellets were examined by LCR meter (PSM1735, NumetriQN$_4$L, and U.K.).

3.   Results and Discussion

Figure 1(a) presents the X-ray Diffraction pattern of CCTMO ceramics sintered at 1323K for 8 h. The whole diffraction pattern is properly matched with the JCPDS (card no.21-0140), confirmed the phase formation of manganese doped CCTO ceramic having body cantered cubic structure along with the minor secondary phase JCPDS (card no.46-1238) of TiO2. The crystalline size (D) of manganese doped CCTO was calculated by using Debye Scherrer formula.

$$D = \frac{k\lambda}{\beta\cos\theta} \qquad (1)$$

where D is crystallite size, k is constant equal to 0.89, λ is the wavelength of X-ray, θ is the Bragg diffraction angle and β is the full width at half maximum (FWHM) in radians. For the calculation of correct value of crystallite size, the line broadening due to instrument effect eliminated by using standard sample for XRD data. The average crystallite size of CCTMO calculated from XRD data is 30 ± 10 nm.

The SEM micrograph of sintered pellets of CCTMO depicts in Fig. 1(b). The average grain size measured by SEM was found to be 1.40 μm. It is confirmed from SEM micrograph smaller grains observed in nanometre and bigger grain in micrometer range. The grains and grains boundaries are separated which confirmed by SEM micrograph. Fig. 1(c & d) depicts the permittivity (ε_r) result of CCTMO sample 100Hz to 1 MHz data indicate that Mn doping CCTO shows low value of dielectric constant (10^2 at 1 MHz).The decreasing behavior of dielectric constant explained by Maxwell-Wagner phenomenon. The dielectric constant was found less than 100 at all measured temperatures. The low value of dielectric function of manganese doped CCTO ceramic is due to low conductivity nature of Mn-doped CCTO ceramic.

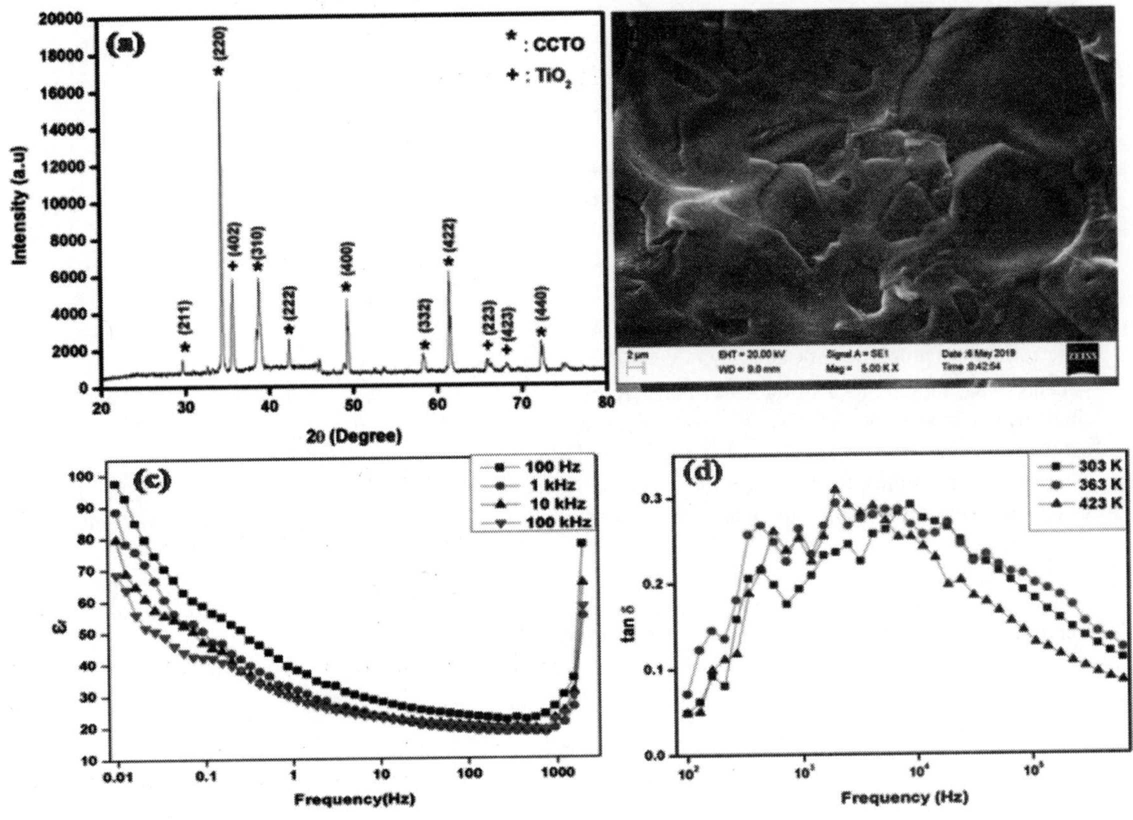

Figure 1(a) XRD pattern (b) SEM micrograph (c) frequency dependent dielectric function (d) frequency dependent tangent loss of Mn doped CCTO.

4. Conclusion

In this work, Mn-doped $CaCu_3Ti_3MnO_{12}$ (CCTMO) was successfully prepared by using a semi-wet route. The Phase formation of CCTMO ceramic was confirmed by XRD and the average crystallite size obtained from the XRD results was found to be 30 ± 10 nm. The average grain size of sintered materials observed by SEM analysis was 1.40 μm. The value of dielectric function (ε_r) and tangent loss (tan δ) were found to be 100 and 0.1, respectively at 303 K and 100 Hz.

5. References

1. Bochu, B., Deschizeaux, M.N., Joubert, J.C., Collomb, A., Chenavas, J. and Marezio, M.: Synthèse et caractérisation d'une série de titanates perovskites isotypes de CaCu3.(Mn4) O12. J. Solid State Chem. **29**(2), 291-298 (1979)

2. Windlass, H., Raj, P.M., Balaraman, D., Bhattacharya, S.K., Tummala, R.R.: Colloidal processing of polymer ceramic nanocomposite integral capacitors. IEEE Trans. Adv. Packag. **26**, 100-105 (2003)

3. Li, J., Subramanian, M.A., Rosenfeld, H.D., Jones, C.Y., Toby, B.H., Sleight, A.W.: Clues to the giant dielectric constant of $CaCu_3Ti_4O_{12}$ in the defect structure of $SrCu_3Ti_4O_{12}$. Chem. Mater. **16**(25), 5223-5225 (2004)

4. Ramirez, A.P., Subramanian, M.A., Gardel, M., Blumberg, G., Li, D; Vogt, T., Shapiro, S.M.: Giant dielectric constant response in a copper-titanate. Solid State Commun.**115**(5), 217-220 (2000)

5. Huang, Y., Shi, D., Li, Y., Li, G., Wang, Q., Liu, L., Fang, L.: Effect of holding time on the dielectric properties and non-ohmic behaviour of $CaCu_3Ti_4O_{12}$ capacitor-varistors. J Mater Sci-Mater EL. **24**(6), 1994-1999 (2013)

6. Ouyang, X., Habib, M., Cao, P., Wei, S., Huang, Z., Zhang, W., Gao, W.: Enhanced extrinsic dielectric response of TiO2 modified CaCu3Ti4O12 ceramics. Ceram. Int. **41**(10), 13447-13454 (2015)

7. Fang, T. T., Liu, C. P.: Evidence of the internal domains for inducing the anomalously high dieectric constant of $CaCu_3Ti_4O_{12}$. Chem. Mat., 17(20), 5167-5171 (2005).

8. Lunkenheimer, P., Fichtl, R., Ebbinghaus, S. G., & Loidl, A.: Nonintrinsic origin of the colossal dielectric constants in $CaCu_3Ti_4O_{12}$. Phys. Rev. B, 70(17), 172102 (2004).

9. Pan, M. J., Bender, B. A.: A bimodal grain size model for predicting the dielectric constant of calcium copper titanate ceramics. J. Am. Ceram. Soc., 88(9), 2611-2614 (2005).

10. Senda, S., Rhouma, S., Torkani, E., Megriche, A., Autret, C.: Effect of nickel substitution on electrical and microstructural properties of $CaCu_3Ti_4O_{12}$ ceramic. J. Alloys Comp., 698, 152-158 (2017).

11. Bueno, P. R., Tararan, R., Parra, R., Joanni, E., Ramírez, M. A., Ribeiro, W. C., Varela, J. A.: A polaronic stacking fault defect model for $CaCu_3Ti_4O_{12}$ material: an approach for the origin of the huge dielectric constant and semiconducting coexistent features. J. Phys. D: Appl. Phys., 42(5), 055404 (2009).

12. Fiorenza, P., Lo Nigro, R., Bongiorno, C., Raineri, V., Ferarrelli, M. C., Sinclair, D. C., West, A. R.: Localized electrical characterization of the giant permittivity effect in $Ca\,Cu_3\,Ti_4\,O_{12}$ ceramics. App.Phys. Lett., 92(18), 182907 (2008).

13. Fernandez, J. F., Leret, P., Romero, J. J., De Frutos, J., De La Rubia, M. Á., Martín González, M. S., García, M. Á.: Proofs of the coexistence of two magnetic contributions in pure and doped $CaCu_3Ti_4O_{12}$ giant dielectric constant ceramics. J. Am. Ceram. Soc., 92(10), 2311-2318 (2009).

Two-Dimensional Materials via Ultasonication Assisted Liquid-phase Exfoliation

T. P. Yadav

Department of Physics, Institute of Science, Banaras Hindu University, Varanasi-221005, India
Email: yadavtp@gmail.com

ABSTRACT

Two-dimensional (2-D) materials are containing unique structure and excellent properties and it rapidly became a research hotspot in the fields of materials, chemistry, physics, and engineering. Currently, there are many methods for preparing 2-D materials, such as ball milling method, chemical oxidation-reduction, chemical vapor deposition, and liquid-phase exfoliation. Among these methods, liquid-phase exfoliation is the most important preparation method. Large-size 2-D materials are successfully prepared by ultrosonic assisted liquid phase exfoliation process.

Keywords: 2-D materials, 2-D quasicrystal, icosahedral phase, decagonal phase quasicrystalline monolayer ordering.

1. Introduction

Over the past two decades nanomaterials have attracted major attention due to their fascinating properties and wide range of potential applications. Nanomaterials are typically defined as materials that have at least one dimension in the range of 1-100 nm. There are two categories of nanomaterials: organic (mostly carbon allotropes) and inorganic nanomaterials (iron, silver, gold, boron nitride nanosheets, molybdenum disulfide, and tungsten disulfide). The nanomaterials have completely different properties than the bulk parent materials; these properties include high surface area, conductivity, mechanical strength, and transparency. Nanotechnology is expanding in academic research and also moving into industry in recent years. When the size or dimension of a material is continuously reduced from a large or macroscopic size, such as a meter or a centimeter, to a very small size, the properties remain the same at first, then small changes begin to occur, until finally when the size drops below 100 nm, dramatic changes in properties can occur. If one dimension is reduced to the nanorange while the other two dimensions remain large, then we obtain a structure known as a quantum well. If two dimensions are so reduced and one remains large, the resulting structure is referred to as a quantum wire. The extreme case of this process of size reduction in which all three dimensions reach the low nanometer range is called a quantum dot.The word quantum is associated with these three types of nanostructures because the changes in properties arise from the quantum-mechanical nature of physics in the domain of the ultra small [1].

2. Preparation of Nanostructures

One approach to the preparation of a nanostructure, called the bottom-up approach, is to collect, consolidate, and fashion individual atoms and molecules into the structure. This came out by a sequence of chemical reactions controlled by catalysts for example, in biology, catalysts called enzymes assemble amino acids to construct living tissue that forms and supports the organs of the body. The opposite approach in the preparation of nanostructures is called the top-down method, which starts with a large-scale object or pattern and gradually reduces its dimension or dimensions.e.g.-litho-graphy technique which shines radiation through a template on to a surface coated with a radiation-sensitive resist; the resist is then removed and the surface is chemically treated to produce the nanostructure. A typical resist material is the polymer polymethyl methacrylate [2]

2.1   Two dimensional materials

When one dimension is of nonorange, while others two are large, then this is 2-D nanostructure. Since 400 C.E., people have been harnessing properties of layered materials; Layered materials are those crystals which form strong in-plane chemical bonds but weak out-of-plane van der Waals interaction. These kinds of materials can allow people to exfoliate into so-called nanosheets which less than one nanometer is thick.

2.2   Exfoliation

Exfoliation is defined as the process that changes the pristine bulky materials to Nano-scale thin sheets. After exfoliation, the nanosheets will not retain all the original properties from the pristine bulky crystal. However, some new properties will occur that are very different from the bulky one which makes the nanosheets so unique for applications. There are many kinds of layered materials. One of the simplest and most common are the graphene and hexagonal boron nitride.Transition metal halides (such as $TiCl2$), transition metal oxides (such as $MoO3$, $TiO2$) and metal double hydroxides[such as $Mg6Al2(OH)16$] also represent diverse layered structures, clays, layered silicates and other layered minerals are the members of the layered materials family. And nowadays one of the most popular layered materials are the transition metal dichalcogenides (such as $MoS2$, $WS2$) [3]. After graphene, Transition metal dichalcogenides have attracted many research interests due to their unique electrochemical and mechanical properties [4]. After exfoliation, the accessible surface area of the material will dramatically increase, so it can be used as surface-active or catalytic chemicals. Recently, another effect of exfoliation has been reported that the band gap of the transition metal dichalcogenide will change after the exfoliation, this allows electronic response to be chosen at will [5].

As for the exfoliation of layered materials, graphene exfoliated by mechanical force such as scotch tape was reported at first. These mechanical forces can obtain highquality graphene which has outstanding properties; however, low yield and production rate limited their applications. After some great research works, people developed some exfoliation methods that were done in the solution which can give us large quantities, high-quality and sizable few layer or monolayer materials. The earliest liquid-phase method of exfoliation is the chemical oxidation of graphite. Natural graphite was treated with oxidizers such as sulfuric acid and potassium permanganate. These oxidation will add hydroxyl and epoxide groups to the basal plane of graphite which makes the graphite become hydrophilic. Then water intercalation or ultrasonication can be used to yield large scale monolayer graphene oxide which is stable in solution. Afterwards the thin graphene oxide can be easily reduced chemically in the liquid-phase but will be no longer stable and aggregate unless polymer or surfactant stabilizers are present. However, although graphene oxide can be reduced to graphene easily, the structural defects will remain and cause low quality which will narrow its application [6]. Recently, a new method has been developed as to exfoliate layered materials that is to use ultrasonic waves in solvent. These kind of powerful ultrasonic beam can generate cavitation bubbles that can collapse into high-energy jetswhich can break the van der Waals interaction between the layers of the materials so as to produce single layer materials. Graphite, hexagonal boron nitride, transition metal dichalcogenides and some of transition metal oxides can be exfoliated by this method. On the other hand, due to the power of the ultrasonic waves, the size of single layer flakes is relatively small and cannot be controlled [7].

Another liquid-phase method of exfoliation of layered materials is called intercalation. Because of the weak van-der-waals interaction between the layers, layered materials can strongly absorb the small molecules into the space between layers. This introduced another method of exfoliation of layered materials called intercalation, which has been widely applied in the exfoliation of graphite and transition metal dichalcogenides.

The intercalation of molecules will enlarge the space between sheets and weaken the interlayer adhesion so as to reduce the energy of exfoliation. Some intercalation species such as IBr can transfer the charge to the layers resulting the reducing of interlayer binding. Further treatment such as low-power ultrasonication or thermal shock will be applied to exfoliate the intercalated layered materials. Intercalation can give high quality materials but have some drawbacks such as sensitivity to the ambient conditions. For the transition metal oxides and clays, ion exchange has become a developed method of exfoliation [5]. Since these kinds of layered materials contain some exchangeable interlayer of cationic ions. Those ions can be exchanged for protons by soaking in acidic solutions. The protons can be exchanged for bulk organic ions leading to substantial swelling. Then low-power ultrasonication is applied to exfoliate the materials into nanosheets. Among the methods that have been developed to exfoliate layered material, mechanical exfoliation are most common.

2.3   Liquid-phase exfoliation via ultrasonication

The liquid-phase exfoliation methodology to prepare graphene sheets generally involves three steps: i) dispersion of the starting material in a liquid medium, ii) exfoliation via ultrasonication and iii) purification. To achieve an effective exfoliation of layered materials the strategy needs to be scalable and efficient. Ultrasonication processes have been widely exploited to produce 2D layered materials in liquid media. Shear forces and cavitations produced due to the propagation of high amplitude sonication waves act on the surface of bulk materials inducing its exfoliation. In order to stabilize the as-produced 2D sheets, the interfacial tension between the materials and the liquid medium needs to be minimized, thus reflecting the existence of good interactions. Hence, the choice of liquid systems for the dispersion of the materials is crucial on the effectiveness of the methodology.

2.4   Ultrasonication process

Ultrasonication has emerged as one of the most powerful strategies to overcome the van der Waals interactions and produce 2D layered structures from 3D crystals. Ultrasound is defined as a sound wave that is transmitted through any substance (solid, liquid or gas) with elastic properties. During ultrasonication of materials, physical phenomena, mainly acoustic cavitation, are manifested influencing the related sonochemical events. According to these phenomena, the sonication process has been divided in different steps: i) generation of nuclei on cavitation bubbles; ii) bubble growth due to gas diffusion; iii) damage of bulk materials due to intense shock-waves or high-speed jets; iv) formation of high-velocity interparticle collisions and; v) increase of surface area of solid materials because of their fragmentation. Evidently, for an efficient and scalable sonication scheme several parameters should be considered, from sonication time to cavitation intensity.

2.5   Purification

The preparation of 2D layered materials with well-defined size is of crucial importance for the control of their physico-chemical properties and applications. After sonication, the majority of the material in the dispersions is composed of nanosheets with different size and thickness, which can be separated by different approaches based on differential centrifugation strategies. Among these strategies the most widely used is sedimentation-based separation (SBS), with or without a density gradient medium (DGM), where nanosheets are separated by sedimentation after selecting the appropriate range of centrifugal forces. By transmission electron microscopy (TEM) it has been found that centrifugation at higher rates results in a dispersion of small flakes . Nevertheless, separation by centrifugation is strongly dependent on the concentration of the material in the dispersions.

3. Transition Metal Dichalcogenides

Over the past decade an ever-increasing interest in the remarkable properties of graphene at the scientific and technological levels has triggered a new wave of attention towards other 2D layered materials, such as the transition metal dichalcogenides (TMDs). The potential of 2D nanostructures arises from their dimensionality as well as the composition and arrangement of the atoms in single layers. TMDs adopt the general formula MX_2, where M represents a transition metal element (usually Mo, W, Nb, Ti, Ni or V) while X is a chalcogen (S, Se or Te), consist of hexagonal layered structures of the form X-M-X. The bulk 3D crystals are formed in different polytypes, varying on the stacked planes, covalently bonded, and the van der Waals interactions between adjacent layers. Hence, the lamellar structure of TMDs, analogous to that of graphite, can be exfoliated into single- and few-layer nanosheets. It is worth noting that exfoliated TMDs are chemically reactive and possess unique electronic, electrochemical and photonic properties, due to their high surface area and quantum confinement effects, not observed in their bulk counterparts. Nevertheless, the exceptional properties of exfoliated TMDs show a strong layer dependency. For instance, when MoS_2 is exfoliated, its electronic properties change from an indirect band gap of 1.2 eV in its bulk state, to a direct gap semiconductor of 1.8 eV for a monolayer. As a result of this upshift, a strong photoluminescence in single-layer MoS_2 is observed which was otherwise absent in thicker crystals. One of the main advantages of these layered materials, that have to be remarked, pertains to their functional diversity. Depending on the combination of the transition metal and chalcogen, these materials behave as insulators (HfS_2), semiconductors (MoS_2, WS_2), semimetals (WTe_2, $TiSe_2$), metals (NbS_2, VSe_2) and superconductors ($NbSe_2$, TaS_2). As a consequence, the exciting electronic and physicochemical properties of atomically thin 2D TMDs have aroused tremendous research interest for applications in photovoltaic devices, transistors, supercapacitors, lithium ion batteries, heterogeneous catalysis, sensors, and storage devices.

3.1 Liquid-phase exfoliation of TMDs

The isolation of high-quality single-layer TMDs has increased the interest of the scientific community since the discovery of the extraordinary properties of single-layer graphene. In TMDs, as the number of layers is reduced, dramatic changes in the electronic structure and properties are observed. As in the case of graphene, two main strategies have been developed for the production of atomically thin 2D TMDs; bottom-up and top-down. Liquid-phase exfoliation of 2D TMDs has emerged as a leading method to obtain mono- and few layer nanosheets in a wide range of solvents. The direct band gap of MoS_2 nanosheets can be potentially used in transistors, light-emitting diodes, solar cells, and field-effect transistors (FET), ultra-high strength nanocomposites. WS_2 is a potential semiconducting material for solar energy conversion and also extensively used as electrode in lithium batteries, shock absorbers, and hydrogen storage. hBN is electrical insulator and widely used as gate dielectrics in capacitors. For some time there has been a wide interest in two-dimensional systems from both a theoretical and experimental point of view. Exfoliation of layered materials such as graphite and transition metal dichalcogenides into mono- or few-layers is of significant interest for both fundamental studies and potential applications. Two-dimensional layered materials are characterized by their strong in-plane bonding and weak van der Waals coupling between the layers. Exfoliation can be achieved mechanically to yield 2D nanosheets of high quality but is generally limited by its lack of scalability. Sonication assisted liquid-phase exfoliation of layered compounds in appropriate solvents or an aqueous surfactant solution is one of the most promising and simplest routes for the production of 2D materials on a large scale. Sonication results in the exfoliation of the layered crystal into single- and multilayer nanosheets that are then stabilized by interaction with the solvent or the surfactant present in the dispersion. The method has the advantage of extreme simplicity and scalability and is the method of choice for the production of nanosheets for fabrication as films or composites. Liquid-phase exfoliation has the advantage over lithium intercalation– exfoliation methods in that it is not an air-sensitive process nor does it involve chemical reactions and consequently provides 2D nanosheets with high crystallinity [8]. In this regard there has been considerable interest in the transition metal dichalcogenide layered compounds, a group of materials which are often considered to be two-dimensional because of the high anisotropy resulting from strong bonding within the layers and weak interlayer interactions. Additional interest in layered compounds arises from the fact that they can be intercalated with a variety of metals and compounds. We report here on the exfoliation of the semiconducting layered compound MoS2 using liquid exfoliation technique.

3.2   Exfoliation of MoS2 in Dimethyl Formamide solution by liquid exfoliation through ultrasonication

10 mg freshly prepared MoS2 powder was measured through electronic weighing machine which is of company Shimadzu Corporation Japan and least count of electronic machine is 0.0001 g and maximum capacity is 200g and measured MoS2 was put into 100 ml DMF (Dimethyl Formamide) solution for exfoliation. The ultrasonic vibration for exfoliation of layered MoS2 was carried out for 10 hrs. Water was regularly changed in the regular interval of 15 min so that it did not get heat up. After complete dispersion of layered MoS2, the resulting liquid was characterized by X-ray diffraction (XRD), SEM, EDX and TEM.

4.   Results and Discussions

4.1   X –Ray Diffraction of MoS2 before and after exfoliation

XRD spectra were taken through PANalytical XRD system. The XRD pattern of bulk MoS2 (Figure 1(a)) shows the diffraction peaks with an especially sharp and strong peak at $\Theta=13.8843°$ which is due to (002) plane indexed in accordance with the rhombohedral lattice parameters. Standard data was taken from JCPDS space group-R3mH with lattice parameters, a=b= 3.17 Å, c=18.34 Å. For taking the XRD of exfoliated MoS2 which is in liquid form, we first deposited our sample over glass sample holder by drop casting method and sample was dried over glass holder (diameter 1.5cm and thickness 1 mm) by RT- elite heater. For the exfoliated MoS2 only broad peaks could be observed (Figure 1(b)). MoS2 Peaks of (004) was absent. These results indicate that the exfoliated MoS2 crystal is very fine.

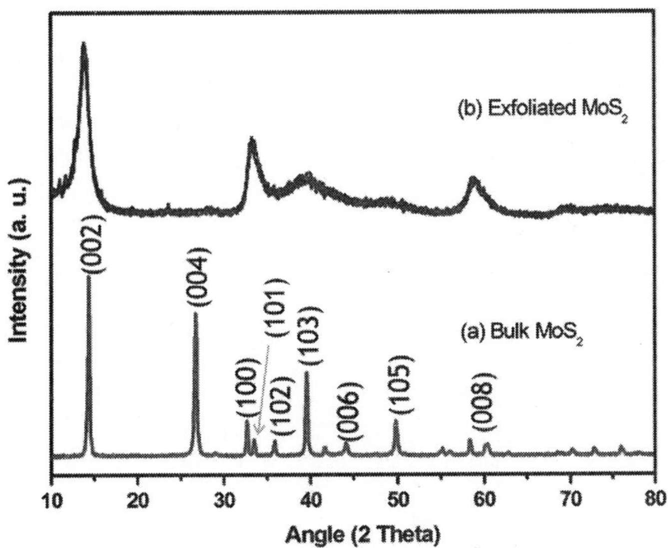

Figure 1. XRD of bulk and exfoliated MoS2.

4.2   SEM image of exfoliated MoS2

SEM image was obtained using QUANTA-200 with tungsten filament as an electron source. Electron accelerated voltage was 20kV and base vacuum was 10^{-6} mbar during the SEM observation. The exfoliated sample (MoS2) was deposited over Si/SiO2 by drop casting method and it was dried with the help of table lamp. When sample was completely dried over SiO2, SiO2 was gently transferred over carbon tape with the help of forcep and all together were put on SEM holder. From SEM image (Figure 2), it is clear that few layer of MoS2 have been exfoliated.

Figure 2. SEM of exfoliated MoS2

5.   References

1.   Jonathan N. Colemn et al., Two –dimensional nanosheets produced by liquid exfoliation of layered materials, Science, 331, 568-571 (2011).

2.   Valeria Nicolosi et al., Liquid exfoliation of layered materials Science 340, 1226419 (2013).

3.   M.P. Lavin-Lopez et al., Solvent-Based Exfoliation via Sonication of Graphitic Materials for Graphene Manufacture, Ind. Eng. Chem. Res. 55, 845–855 (2016).

4.   Claudia Backes et al. Guidelines for exfoliation, characterization and processing of layered materials produced by liquid exfoliation, Chem. Mater. 29, 243–255 (2017).

5.   J.R. Brent et al., Synthetic approaches to two dimensional transition metal dichalcogenides nanosheets,Prog. Mater. Sci. 89, 411–478 (2017).

6.   Per Joensen et al., Single layer MoS2, Mat. Res. Bull. 21, 457-461(1986).

7.   Ali Jawid et al., Mechanism for liquid phase exfoliation of MoS2, Chem. Mater. 28, 337–348 (2016).

8.   A. Gupta et al. Liquid-phase exfoliation of MoS2 nanosheets: The Critical Role of Trace Water, J. Phys. Chem. Lett. 7, 4884–4890 (2016).

Elastic, Mechanical, Thermal and Ultrasonic Properties of InP Nanowires

Sudhanshu Tripathi[1, 2, *], Rekha Agarwal[3], Devraj Singh[4]

[1]University School of Information Communication and Technology, Guru Gobind Singh Indraprastha University, Dwarka, Delhi-110078, India [2]Department of Instrumentation and Control Engineering, Amity School of Engineering and Technology, Sector-125, Noida-201313, India [3]Department of Electronics and Communication Engineering, Amity School of Engineering and Technology, Sector-125, Noida-201313, India
[4]Department of Physics, AIAS, Amity University, Uttar Pradesh, Noida-201313, India
*E-mail:-tripathisudhanshu@gmail.com

ABSTRACT

We have computed elastic, mechanical, thermal and ultrasonic properties of wurtzite InP nanowires in high temperature regime using Lennard Jones potential model. The ultrasonic parameters such as ultrasonic wave velocities, ultrasonic Grüneisen parameter, ultrasonic attenuation have obtained with the help of elastic constants, density, etc. The obtained results are discussed in correlation with available experimental and theoretical results.

Keywords: Indium phosphide, mechanical properties, thermal properties, ultrasonic properties

1. Introduction

Indium Phosphide (InP) is one of the most popular material among the III-V group semiconductor materials because of its unique electrical and thermophysical properties [1-3]. Furthermore, the new design parameters and parameters modification may open new dimensions e.g. modification in nanowire diameter, variation of physical phenomenon, crystalline structure change under varying physical conditions. Recently solar cell performance has been characterized by utilizing InP nanowire array[4]. Z. Liu et al. [5] discussed the mechanical and fracture mechanism of InP nanowires. They investigated the impact of changes in diameter of nanowire on the elastic moduli. The ab-intio study on electrical properties, structural properties and electronic properties were discussed using local density approximation (LDA) and generalized gradient approximation (GGA) of the InP. The density function theory (DFT) based study reveals that the change in pressure affects the chemical bonding leading to phase transition in the material and change in the physical properties of the InP[6]. Luca et al. [7] discussed in detail the growth process, optical and structural characteristics of w-InP nanowires. Recently the thermoelectric properties of InAs/InP nanowires have been studied in high temperature regime [8]. Göransson et al. [9] has demonstrated the measurement of strain and band gap in InAs-InP core shell nanowires for w-crystal phase. In the present work we had estimated the elastic and mechanical behavior of w-InP nanowires (w-InP-NWs) at room temperature and analyzed the ultrasonic and thermophysical characteristics with temperature and size variations of nanowires.

2. Theory

The w-InP-NWs considered under study is of wurtzite crystalline structured hexagonal closed packed (hcp) material. The elastic constants of hcp structured material can be estimated using the interaction potential model, with the help of developed formulations [10]. The formulated six second order elastic constants (SOECs) and ten third order elastic constants (TOECs) strongly depend on the interaction potential, which in turn depends on harmonic and anhormonic parameters of the material. The value of these harmonic and anhormonic parameters may be evaluated using the values of integers, unit cell parameters and the Lennard-Jones parameter (b_0) for the materials under observation [11]. The ultrasonic velocity has been computed using the expressions available in literature. The Debye average velocity is obtained ,from the summation of the original slopes along the three acoustical branches by the integration over all directions [12]. The values of the mechanical parameters have been computed using the formulated values of SOECs[13].The phonon-phonon interaction (PPI), electron-phonon interaction (EPI) and thermoelastic relaxation mechanism plays a vital role in ultrasonic attenuation. At higher temperature the PPI is also termed as Akhieser loss (α) Akhieser loss and thermoelastic attenuation (α)th in subscript please i.e. (α)th are prominent factor for appreciable ultrasonic attenuation[14,15].

The thermal relaxation loss depends on the thermal conductivity, Grüneisen parameter and temperature respectively [16,17]. The Grüneisen number $\left\langle \gamma_i^j \right\rangle$ for hcp structured materials is directly consequences of SOECs and TOECs [18]. The deviation in the elastic modulus $\Delta C (= 3E_0 \left\langle (\gamma_i^j)^2 \right\rangle - \left\langle \gamma_i^j \right\rangle^2 C_V T)$ because of applied strain, depends on the E_0, C_V, $\left\langle \gamma_i^j \right\rangle$. Here C_V is the specific heat per unit volume. The acoustical energy transformed to thermal energy being measured by acoustic coupling constant $D(=3\Delta C/(E_0))$. The thermal relaxation time with the assumption ωτ less than unity is directly dependent on thermal conductivity and varies inversely with Debye average velocity square. Slack and Berman [19-21] had proposed the model for the computation of lattice thermal conductivity.

3.   Results and Discussion

The elastic constants of w-InP-NWs calculated at room temperature (300K). The resistance variation toward linear compression along the unique axes can be measured using second order elastic constants(SOECs). Figure 1 shows the deviation plot of SOECs for w-InP-NWs computed using simple interaction potential model. The value of the Lennard Jones parameter for w-InP-NWs is found to be 1.3284×10^{-63} erg-cm⁷, measured under the equilibrium conditions. The low value of C_{11} in comparison to C_{33} indicates that a-axis is more compressible in comparison to the c-axis. The third order elastic constants (TOECs) of w-InP-NWs has been reported first time. As depicted in Fig.1 the similarities of SOECs values, validates our approach for elastic properties estimation of w-InP-NWs.

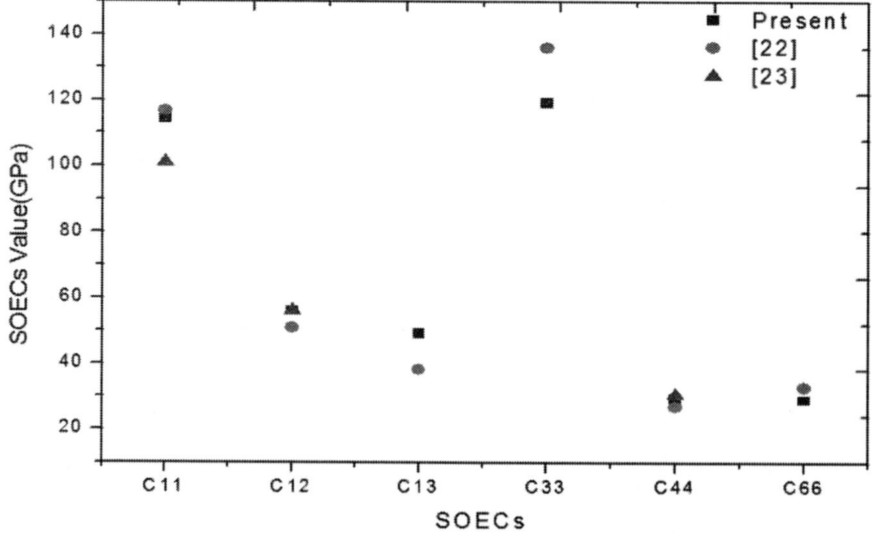

Figure 1. Deviation plot of SOECs of present work with previous works

Table 1 represents the obtained values of TOECs and mechanical parameters e.g. bulk modulus (B), Young's modulus (Y), shear modulus (G) and Poisson's ratio. The obtained values of bulk modulus is similar to that reported experimentally and theoretically [5]. The theoretical estimated values of Young modulus lying in the range 120±10 GPa match with our findings 124.1 GPa. The other thermophysical properties of the InP like $C_V, E_0, \theta_D, D_L, D_S, V_1, V_2, V_D$, has been depicted in Table 2.

Table 1. TOECs, B,Y,G (GPa) and ν of w-InP-NWs at room temperature

C_{333}	C_{222}	C_{155}	C_{144}	C_{344}	C_{133}	C_{123}	C_{113}
-1527.8	-1476.1	-62.3	-93.5	-378	-403.2	-80.2	-63.1
C_{112}	C_{111}	B	Y	G	ν		
-295.7	-1865.6	73	124.1	30.4	0.31		

Table 2. C_V, E_0, D_L, D_S, V_L, V_S, and V_D of w-InP-NWs at room temperature

$C_V (10^6 Jm^{-3}K^{-1})$	$E_0 (10^6\ Jm^{-3})$	θ_D (K)	D_L	D_S	$V_L (10^3 ms^{-1})$	$V_S (10^3 ms^{-1})$	$V_D (10^3 ms^{-1})$
0.74	143.03	407.8	419.19	7.92	4.99	2.48	2.78

The obtained value of longitudinal ultrasonic velocity for w-InP-NWs is similar to the values reported in literatures [24] validating our approach for computation of ultrasonic properties. The $D_L > D_S$ indicates that energy transformation in w-InP-NWs is more prominent when ultrasonic wave propagates along the length of nanowire rather than surface. The picoseconds order of thermal relaxation time confirms the semiconducting nature of w-InP-NWs. The ultrasonic attenuation for longitudinal mode of ultrasonic wave is dominant in comparison to the ultrasonic attenuation due to shear wave. It has been observed that the thermal conductivity of the nanowire increases with increase in diameter of the nanowire. Since the ultrasonic attenuation depends on the thermal conductivity of the material, thus the total ultrasonic attenuation founds to be increasing with increase in size on the nanowire.

4.   Conclusion

Based on the discussion made above following points are concluded:

- The theoretical model used for nonlinear elastic and ultrasonic properties estimations of w-InP-NWs is validated.
- The order of thermal relaxation time indicates the semiconducting nature of w-InP-NWs.
- The Born mechanical stability criterion approves the mechanical stability of w-InP-NWs.
- The diameter dependent study of InP nanowire indicates the ultrasonic attenuation in w-InP-NWs increases with increase in nanowire diameter.

The observed results for w-InP-NWs may be further utilized for research and industrial applications.

5.   References

1.   Kempa, T.J., Cahoon, J.F., Kim, S.K., Day, R.W., Bell, D.C., Park, H.G. and Lieber, C.M.: Coaxial multishell nanowires with high-quality electronic interfaces and tunable optical cavities for ultrathin photovoltaics. Proceedings of the National Academy of Sciences, 109(5), 1407-1412 (2012).

2.   Yan, X., Li, B., Lin, Q., Liu, P., Luo, Y., Lu, Q., Zhang, X. and Ren, X.: High performance transistors and photodetectors based on self-catalyzed zinc-blende InP nanowires. Appl. Phys. Lett. 114(24), 243106 (2019).

3.   Lee, R., Jo, M.H., Kim, T., Kim, H.J., Kim, D.G. and Shin, J.C.: Photoresponse and Field Effect Transport Studies in InAsP–InP Core–Shell Nanowires. Electron. Mater. Lett., 14(3), 357-362 (2018).

4.   Otnes, G., Barrigón, E., Sundvall, C., Svensson, K.E., Heurlin, M., Siefer, G., Samuelson, L., Åberg, I. and Borgström, M.T.: Understanding InP nanowire array solar cell performance by nanoprobe-enabled single nanowire measurements. Nano Lett., 18(5), 3038-3046 (2018).

5.   Liu, Z., Papadimitriou, I., Castillo-Rodríguez, M., Wang, C., Esteban-Manzanares, G., Yuan, X., Tan, H.H., Molina-Aldareguia, J.M. and LLorca, J.:Mechanical behavior of InP twinning superlattice nanowires. Nano Lett. 19,4490-4497(2019).

6.   Baida, A., Ghezali, M.: Structural, electronic and optical properties of InP under pressure: An ab-initio study. Comput. Conden. Matter, 17, 00333 (2018).

7.   Luca, M. De, Polimeni, A.: Electronic properties of wurtzite-phase InP nanowires determined by optical and magneto-optical spectroscopy. Appl. Phys. Rev. 4, 041102 (2017).

8.   D. Prete, P.A. Erdman, V. Demontis, V. Zannier, D. Ercolani, L. Sorba, F. Beltram, F. Rossella, F. Taddei, S. Roddaro, Thermoelectric Conversion at 30 K in InAs/InP Nanowire quantum dots. Nano Lett. 19(5), 3033-3039 (2019).

9.   D.J.O. Göransson, M.T. Borgström, Y.Q. Huang, M.E. Messing, D. Hessman, I.A. Buyanova, W.M. Chen, H.Q. Xu: Measurements of strain and bandgap of coherently epitaxially grown wurtzite InAsP–InP core–shell nanowires. Nano Lett. 19(4) 2674-2681(2019).

10.   Mori. S., Hiki, Y.: Calculation of the third-and fourth-order elastic constants of alkali halide crystals. Phys. Soc. Jpn. 45(5), 1449-1456 (1978).

11.   Pandey, D.K., Singh, D. and Yadav, R.R.: Ultrasonic wave propagation in IIIrd group nitrides. Appl. Acoust. 68(7),766-777 (2007).

12.   Rosen, M., Klimker, H.: Low-temperature elasticity and magneto-elasticity of dysprosium single crystals. Phys. Rev. B 1(9), 3748(1970).

13.   Rahman, M.A., Rahaman, M.Z., Ali, M.L. and Ali, M.S.: The physical properties of ThCr2Si2-type nickel-based superconductors BaNi2T2 (T= P, As): An ab-initio study. Chin. J. Phys. 59, 58-69(2019).

14.   Mason, W.P., Rosenberg, A.: Thermal and electronic attenuations and dislocation drag in the hexagonal crystal Cadmium. J. Acoust. Soc. Am. 45(2), 470-480 (1969).

15.   Yadav, R.R., Singh,D.: Effect of thermal conductivity on ultrasonic attenuation in praseodymium monochalcogenides. Acoust. Phys. 49(5), 595-604(2003).

16.   W.P. Meson, Phys. Acoust. Vol. III B ,Academic Press, New York, (1955).

17.   Kor, S.K., Mishra, P.K., Tandon,U.S.: Ultrasonic attenuation in aluminum. Solid State Commun. 15(3), 499-501(1974).

18.   Rajagopalan, S., Nandanpawer, M.: Gruneisen number in hexagonal crystal. J. Acoust. Soc. Am. 71(6), 1469-1472(1982).

19.   Oligschleger, C., Jones, R.O., Reimann, S.M., Schober, H.R.: Model interatomic potential for simulations in selenium. Phys. Rev. B. 53(10), 6165 (1996).

20.   Slack, G.A.: The thermal conductivity of nonmetallic crystals. In Solid State Physics, Academic Press 34,1-71 (1979).

21.   Berman, R., Klemens, P.G.: Thermal conduction in solids. Physics Today, 31, 56 (1978).

22.   Hajlaoui, C., Pedesseau, L., Raouafi, F., Larbi, F.B.C. , Even, J., Jancu, J.M. : Ab initio calculations of polarization, piezoelectric constants, and elastic constants of InAs and InP in the wurtzite phase. J.Exp. Theo. Phys. 121(2) 246-249 (2015).

23.   Ehsanfar, S., Kanjouri, F., Tashakori, H., Esmailian, A.: First-principles study of structural, electronic, mechanical, thermal, and phonon properties of III-phosphides (BP, AlP, GaP, and InP). J. Elect. Materi.46(10) (2017) 6214-6223.

24.   Cui, H., Zhang, Y., Kang, Q., Chang, H.M., Zhang, X.B., Zhai, R.H., Wang, G.Q.: Bandgaps properties of III-phosphides (BP, AlP, GaP, InP) materials excited by ultrasonic. Optik: Int. Light Electron Opt. 177, 58-63 (2019).

Ionic Interaction in Aqueous L-Alanine Through Gibb's Free Energy

A.T. Shende[1,*], N.T. Tayade[2], M. P. Tirpude[3], V.A. Tabhane[4]

[1] Department of Physics, Dr. S.D. Devsey, Arts College and Commerce and Science College, Wada, Palghar, Maharashtra
[2] Department of Physics, Institute of Science, Nagpur, Maharashtra, [3] Vartak college of Arts, K. M. College of Commerce and E .S. Andrades College of Science, Vasai Road (W), Palghar, Maharashtra (India),
[4] Department of Physics, University of Pune, Pune, Maharashtra (India)
*E-mail: amardeepshende@gmail.com

ABSTRACT

L-Alanine in water forms stable Zwitrteions and the Gibb's free energy is a crucial factor for determining the molecular/ionic interaction in aqueous system. This paper deals with the analysis of non-covalent ionic interaction between water molecule and L-Alanine through this Gibb's free energy. The Gibb's free energy obtained by the ultrasonic experimental method was compared with the reported value and with the DFT method utilized in this study. The variations in it have been analyzed and discussed with respective to expected suitable possibilities of interactions between two types of molecules. The structure of L-Alanine in water has been optimized for it using the different functionals, and analyzed its density of states and interactions. The obtained thermo-chemistry at temperature 298.15K has also revealed the other thermodynamic parameters

***Keywords:** Gibb's free energy, L-alanine, ionic interaction, ultrasonic method, DFT.*

1. Introduction

L-Alanine (ALA) (CH_3CHNH_2COOH) is color less, odorless, sweet taste amino acids occurred in orthorhombic crystal structure solid [1]. It has applications in pharmaceuticals, biochemistry, biotechnology, medicine, etc. [2,3,4] also it is a NLO material [5,6]. ALA possesses relaxed structure in solid states but its water solubility [7] transform it into its transition phase 'zwitterions' due to the transfer of proton (hydrogen atom) from carboxylic group (COOH) to amine group (NH_2) causes COOH becomes COO^- and NH_2 becomes NH_3^+. It makes polar molecule in aqueous so that the resultant charges become zero having hydrophobic $-CH_3$ group. Their thermo-acoustical parameters have been reported using the ultrasonic method [8, 9, 10] and also using computer simulation [11](seen separately) for such binary solution. These different forms of ALA have not been examined by experiment (ultrasonic method) and computational combine in a point of view of the change in Gibb's free Energy (ΔG) on an ionic interaction issue and using the hybrid and double-hybrid functional with the CPCM solvation models to Hatree contribution in DFT results. Therefore the present work focuses on the molecular/ionic interaction using change in Gibb's free Energy (ΔG) for aqueous ALA using DFT and an ultrasonic method which added novelty to this work and making base for further extensions from the findings.

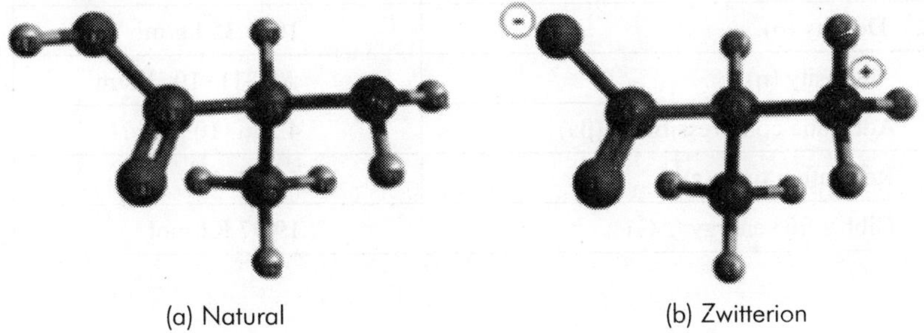

Figure 1. Two Forms of ALA

2. Material and Methods

ALA (E- Merck AR grade) with 0.009 Molar concentration of solution prepared in triple distilled water (Grade I) for the Ultrasonic characterization Method. The density is determined by using density bottle with plunger method and the viscosity by Oswald Viscometer. The Pulse Echo Overlap method is used to measure ultrasonic velocities and attenuation by AUAR-102 with 4 MHz. All measurements were done at 298.15K. The change in Gibb's free energy (ΔG) calculated by using Eyring-Polanyi equation as -

$$\Delta G = -2.303 \, RT \log_{10}\left(\frac{h}{k_B T_t}\right)\left(\frac{J}{mol}\right) \tag{1}$$

-where, R-real gas constant, T - temperature 298.15K, k_B - Boltzmann's constant, h-Plank's constant and τ-relaxation time. The relaxation time can be calculated by -

$$\tau = \frac{4}{3}\eta\beta_a \, (\text{sec}) \tag{2}$$

-where, η- viscosity, β_a- adiabatic compressibility. The adiabatic compressibility was calculated experimentally by finding ultrasonic velocity (u), density (ρ) and viscosity (η) for the molar concentration of ALA in an aqueous solution.

DFT method has been implemented in ORCA program [12] using GUI Avogadro [13] and plotted in Multiwfn [14]. Two functional, B3LYP and PBEh-3c (hybrid) with basis sets def2-SVP [15,16], def2/J [17] implemented in CPCM solvation models [18] (constructed using the GEPOL algorithm [19, 20, 21] and calculated as per in [22] and [23] involving the atom-pair wise dispersion correction D3BJ [24,25]). Vibrational entropy computed according to the QRRHO method of S. Grimme [26].

3. Results and Discussion

3.1 Experimental Study

The ten samples were randomly selected from the each from the five-five's four groups of samples from the prepared 20 sample with molar concentration 0.009M in the water solution. After measurement of velocity for these selected samples, the mean was calculated has been used shown in Table1. The Gibbs energy, truncated on 4th decimal, calculated as 19.97 KJ/mol from it along with all other parameters shown in Table1. This energy is the difference between two transition phases of ALA i.e., between normal ALA and zwitterions shown in Fig.1

Table 1. Experimental results of ALA in aqueous solution at T = 298.15K for 0.009 M

	Expt. Parameters	Values
1.	Ultrasonic velocity(u)	1517 m/s
2.	Density (ρ)	1021.35 kg/m^3
3.	Viscosity (η)	89.311×10^{-2} Ns/m^2
4.	Adiabatic compressibility (βa)	4.256×10^{-10} m^2/N
5.	Relaxation time (τ)	5.068×10^{-10} s
6.	Gibb's free energy (ΔG)	19.97 KJ/mol

3.2   Computational study

The result obtained from DFT method using two different functional for the zwitterions and Natural forms of ALA at temperature 298.15 K and at pressure 1.00 atm are given in Table 2 with its formulae. The change in Gibb's free energy of the reaction (given in sixth row) is calculated from the fifth row of Table 2 for functional. The reaction is mention as -

$$C_2H_3NH_2\ COOH + H_2O \rightarrow C_2H_4NH_3^+\ COO^- + H_2O$$

$$C_2H_3NH_2\ COOH\ (aq) \overset{\Delta G_r}{\longleftrightarrow} C_2H_4NH_3^+\ COO^-\ (aq)$$

Table 2. Thermo-chemistry of ALA in Normal and Zwitterion form at T = 298.15 K by DFT

Entities from DFT (Formula)	Natural/Normal ALA		Zwitterions ALA	
	B3LYP	PBEh-3c	B3LYP	PBEh-3c
1. Single Point Energy ($E_{el} = E_{kin\text{-}el} + E_{n\text{-}el} + E_{e\text{-}e} + E_{n\text{-}n}$)	-840737.31	-839995.01	-840753.63	-840015.20
2. Internal Energy ($U = E_{el} + E_{ZPE} + E_{vib} + E_{rot} + E_{trans}$)	-840440.36	-839688.28	-840454.76	-839704.09
3. Enthalpy ($H = U + k_B T$)	-840437.90	-839685.82	-840452.30	-839701.64
4. Final Entropy ($TS = T(S_{el} + S_{vib} + S_{rot} + S_{trans})$)	98.80	97.84	97.47	98.57
5. Final Gibbs free enthalpy ($G_N = H - TS$)	-840536.70	-839783.67	-840549.78	-839800.21
6. $\Delta G_r = G_N$ (Zwit) - G_N (Nat)	-13.08		-16.54	
7. For completeness ($G_{fZ} = G_N - E_{el}$)	200.61	211.34	203.86	214.99

Note: All Energies unit are in KJ/mole. TS is in energy unit. (Suffixes meaning: el-electronic, kin-kinetic, n-nuclear, ZPE-zero point energy, vib-vibrational, rot-rotational, trans-translational. k_B–Boltzmann's constant, T-Temperature in K)

B3LYP is seems to be accurate method in literature but it is fail to reach (due to basic sets or other variations in present work or CPCM model) to the good approximation here, where as PBEh-3c's value has shown better i.e., -16.54(6) kJ/mol with favorable positive entropy. Change in entropy (0.0231 KJ/mol) and change in enthalpy (26.8 KJ/mol) by experiment found larger compared to observe in DFT calculation.

The computed frequencies (IR) are illustrated in Fig .2(a) show drastic changes in fingerprint region for both structures. The 'h-3c' contribution introduces some changes. The peaks near and below 2000cm^{-1} reports the red shift for Zwitterions (polar) in both functional cases than ALA(aq). The dipole moment has been observed 13.449990 Debye in zwitterions which is more than four times of ALA(aq) i.e 3.398190 Debye. At the functional part of spectrum shows not-much-philic nature. However the enhancement of a peak between 2800 cm-1 and 3200 cm-1 observed in PBEh-3c. Hatree term seems significance over the merely hybrid functional for obtaining approximate values in term of the modes of vibrations and rotation due to the non-ionic and ionic interaction. From electronic density of state, (DOS), the band gap is found more in case of zwitterions compare to the natural state of ALA(aq) for both functional as illustrated in Fig.2(b) (agree with [6,7,8,27,28]). However PBEh-3c has highest one compare to B3LYP.

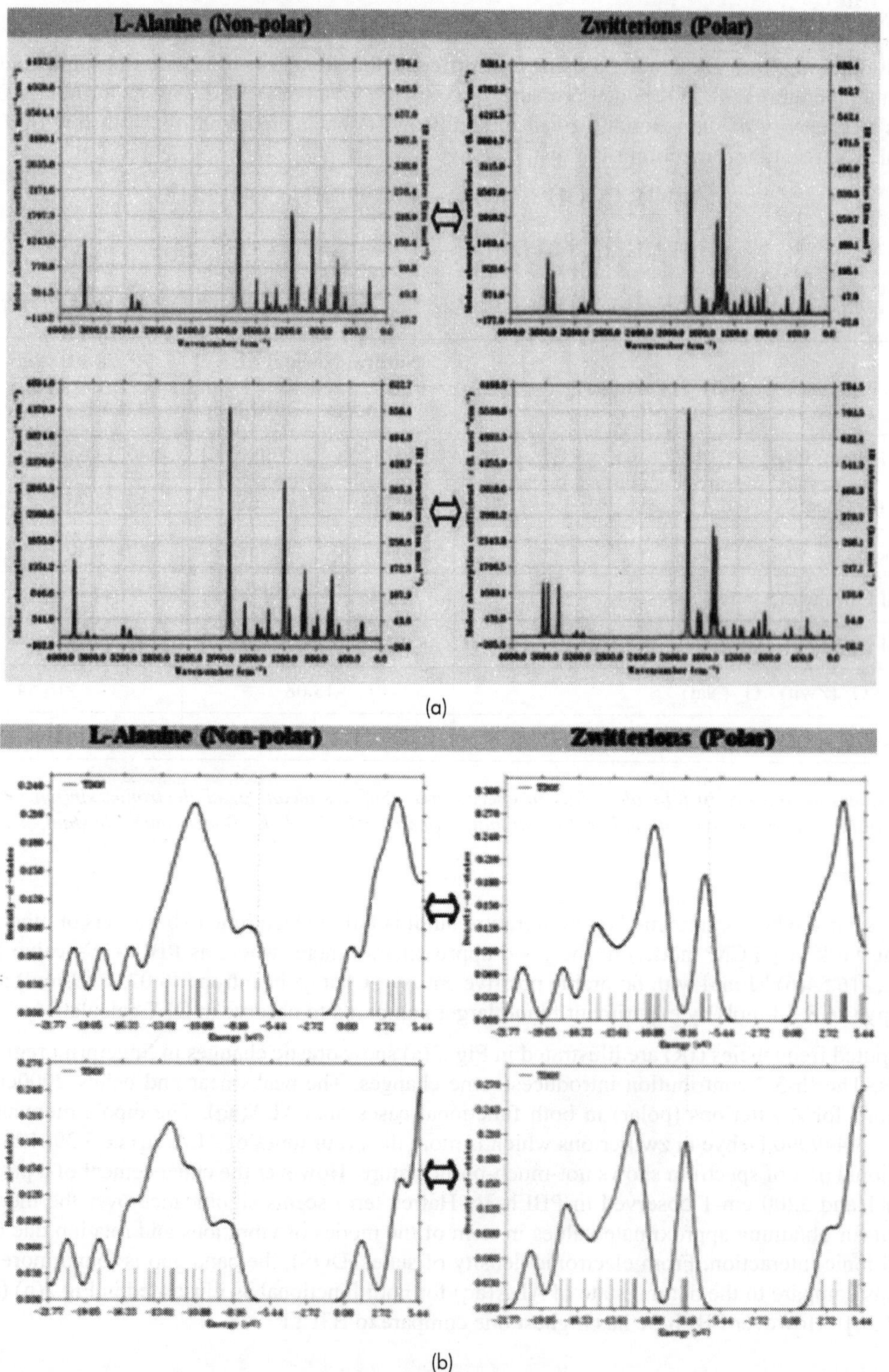

(a)

(b)

Figure 2: (a) Comparison of IR frequencies of Two Forms (/states) of ALA in water for different Functional and (b) electronic DOS of two forms (/states) of ALA for the band-gap comparison.

3.3   Interaction Perspective

Zwitterion in water is in a ground state and it is supposed to be maintaining the bonding (covalent or non-covalent). It is reported that the change in Gibb's free energy (ΔG) for various chemical bonds varies with molecular interactions [29] in the range as, for covalent bond -210 to -420 kJ/mol, for weak interactions -4 to -30 kJ/mol, for ionic interactions - 20 to -30 kJ/mol and for Van der Waal's interactions - 3 to -4 kJ/mol [31]. The interactions are slightly ionic and mostly weak type from the magnitude of ΔG in both experimental (19.97 kJ/mol) and computed cases but experimental value is positive and computed is negative. The negative and positive signed is the indication of transformation for normal to zwitterions and zwitterions to normal forms respectively. Overall perspectives can be explained as a following predictable mechanism. 'The ΔG approaching to -20KJ/mol indicates the spontaneously irreversible ionic interaction [30]. Atleast four to nine water molecules needed to begin stabilization of the ALA-zwitterions (shown in the establishment of orientations of functional sites in earlier ab initio studies) in water [3,4,31,32]. The application of ultrasonic wave to this zwitterions solution trying to break an interaction between ALA and water or detaching Hydrogen from the carboxylic group to transfers it to amine group (or both). Eventually this brings the ALA to its normal form from the zwitterionic form and the reaction becomes reversible (eg. 19.97 KJ/mol in experiment). Along with ionic, weak interactions also might be dominating. The formation of Zwitterions is spontaneous and irreversible, and justifiable with the negative value of Gibb's free energy (for eg. -16.54 KJ/mol in DFT). The ultrasound energy provides in this (i.e., $+\Delta G$) to revert the state (to a un-relaxed).' Conversely, the non-polar form (ALA(aq)) can be converted to polar Zwitterions form by utilizing its own Gibb's free energy revert by bringing back the non-polar form from polar by merely giving the 20KJ/mol energy. These differences mainly attribute the hydrogen bonding interaction in addition to small amount of ionic type interaction which renders the study to non-covalent or weak interaction.

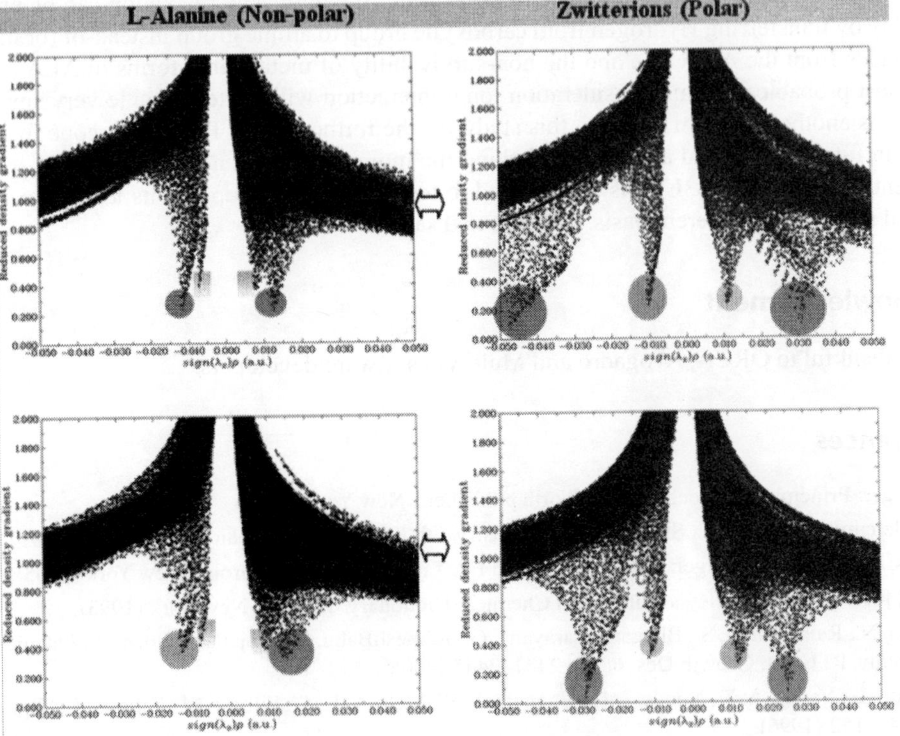

Figure 3. RDG as a function of sign(λ_2)ρ for the non-covalent & the weak interactions. (Bluish color oval shows hydrogen bonding interaction, Reddish oval shows satiric interaction and Greenish rectangular shows Van der Wall interaction. Bigger size shows dominating interaction and darker in color shows higher strength.)

3.4   Weak Interaction

For the more clear perspective using DFT data, we are analyzing the *Reduced Density Gradient* (*RDG*) verses $sign(\lambda_2)\rho$ plot as shown in Fig.4. The downward peaks at both sides far from the centre of $sign(\lambda_2)\rho$ in Fig.4 indicates the hydrogen bonding (left) and satiric effect (right) are dominated. But it is not as stronger, as strengthened and interactive as obtained for the zwitterions. In case of normal ALA (polar), the downward peaks of RDG observed between 0.2 to 0.4 isosurface for repulsion and attraction around 0.005 to 0.01 a.u. $sign(\lambda_2)\rho$. In case of zwitterions (polar) the downward peaks of RDG observed between 0.02 to 0.3 isosurface for repulsion around the 0.012 and 0.025 a.u $sign(\lambda_2)\rho$ and attraction around the 0.012 and 0.028 a.u. $sign(\lambda_2)\rho$ in PBEh-3c and the peaks of RDG observed between 0.04 to 0.2 isosurface for repulsion around 0.011 and 0.031 a.u. $sign(\lambda_2)\rho$ and for attraction around 0.011 and 0.047 a.u. $sign(\lambda_2)\rho$ in B3LYP. This study suggests domination of dipole-dipole, ion-dipole interaction than ion-ion interaction between ALA and water from DFT and confirmed the agreement with experiment.

4.   Conclusions

The present work concluded that the values of magnitude of ΔG from ultrasonic method and DFT methods show its dependencies on the functional in computation and on a molar concentration experimentally. It can't be denied that the repulsive and attractive bonding interactions of zwitterions with water get disturbed (due to the absorption of an ultrasonic wave) and destabilized into the ALA's natural form by utilizing the ΔG_r and got activated on the basis of experimental and DFT results. Mechanism has predicted and given on the basis of different sign of ΔG_r from it. The charges on zwitterions' groups are merely self-induced to stabilize it in a non-acidic and non-basic equilibrium state of polar water medium. The relaxation can be predicted to be done probably by transferring Hydrogen from carboxylic group to amine group instead-of (or in-added-with) water molecules from the ΔG_r value and the non-survivability of meta-stable forms of ALA (cation, anion) are found most probable. On this consideration ionic interaction with water became very small. Testing of its evidences is another problem found in this study for the further work. There is a scope for experimental verification in future works and as well as checking the more different functional for close approximations to experimental results. The B3LYP is also needed to test for entropy-drop and its less consistency with an experimental result using different basis, methods and salvation models.

5.   Acknowledgement

Authors are thankful to ORCA, Avogadro and Multiwfn software developers.

6.   References

1.   Lehninger: Principles of Biochemistry, Worth publishers, New York (1984).

2.   Berg, Jeremy, Tymoczko, J., Stryer L.: Biochemistry. 7th Edn. W.H. Freeman and Company, (2012).

3.   Hames, Daivd, Hooper, Nigel: Biochemistry. 3rd Ed. Taylor and Francis Group, New York (2005).

4.   Lewis, R.J.: Sr (Ed), Hawley's Condensed Chemical Dictionary. 12th Ed. New York (1993).

5.   Vijayan, N., Rajasekaran, S., Bhagavannarayana, G., RameshBabu, R., Gopalakrishnan, R., Palanichamy, M., and Ramasamy, P.: Cryst. Growth Des. 6(11), 2441–2445 (2006).

6.   Misoguti, L., Varela, A. T., Nunes, F. D., Bagnato, V. S., Melo, F. E. A., Filho J. M., Zilio, S. C., Opt. Mater (Amst) 6(3), 147–152 (1996).

7.   Clark, J.: An introduction to amino acids. (2004). www.chemguide.co.uk/organicprops/aminoacids/ (accessed: July 2019)

8.   Shende, A.T., Chinchkhede, N.D., Tabhane , V.A.: Int. Jr. of Scientific Res. in Sci. and Tech 4(3), 65-69 (2018).

9.   Shende, A.T.: Intern. J. of Res. in Bios., Agri. & Tech. 2(3), 270-273 (2015).

10.   Shende, A.T., Tabhane, P.V., Chimankar, O.P., Tabhane V.A.: Biotechnology-An Indian J. 6(10), 332-336 (2012).

11.   Degtyarenko, I.M., Jalkanen, K. J., Gurtovenko, A.A., Nieminen, R.M.: J. Phys. Chem. B 111, 4227-4234 (2007).

12.   Neese, F.: Wiley Interdiscip. Rev. Compu. Mol. Sci. 2(1), 73–78 (2012).

13.   Hanwell, M. D., Curtis, D. E., Lonie, D.C., Vandermeersch, T., Zurek, E., Hutchison, G. R.: J. Cheminformatics 4, 17 (2012).

14.   Tian Lu, Feiwu Chen: J. Comput. Chem. 33, 580-592 (2012).

15.   R. Ahlrichs and F. Weigend, Phys. Chem. Chem. Phys. 7, 3297 2005.

16.   Weigend F. and Ahlrichs, R., Phys. Chem. Chem. Phys. 7, 3297 (2005).

17.   F. Weigend, Phys. Chem. Chem. Phys. 8, 1057 (2006).

18.   Barone, V., Cossi, M. ; (1998) J. Phys. Chem. A 102, (1995).

19.   Pascual-Ahuir, J. L. Silla, E. J.: Comput. Chem. 11, 1047 (1990).

20.   Pascual-Ahuir, J. L., Silla, E., Tunon, I.; J. Comput. Chem. 12, 1077 (1991).

21.   Pascual-Ahuir, J. L., Silla, E., Tunon, I. J.: Comput. Chem. 15, 1127 (1994).

22.   Truong, T. N., Stefanovich, E. V.: Chem. Phys. Lett. 240, 253 (1995).

23.   Truong, T. N., Stefanovich, E. V.: Chem. Phys. Lett, 240, 253 (1995).

24.   Grimme, S., Ehrlich, S., Goerigk, L.: Comput. Chem., J. 32, 1456-1465 (2011).

25.   Grimme, S., Antony, J., Ehrlich S., Krieg, H.: J.Chem.Phys. 132, 154-104 (2010).

26.   Grimme, S.: Chem. Eur. J. 18, 9955 (2012).

27.   Tayade, N.T., Shende, A.T., Tirpude, M.P.: Int. J. Scientific Res. Phys. and App. Sci. 6(4), 23-27 (2018).

28.   Tayade, N.T., Shende, A.T., Tirpude, M.P.: Int. J. Scientific Res. Phys. and App. Sci. 4(3), 57-61 (2018).

29.   https://s10.lite.msu.edu/res/msu/botonl/b_online/e18/18c.htm, (accessed: June 2019).

30.   Chemical_equilibrium, OCN623, 2013 (accessed: June 2019). http://www.soest.hawaii.edu/oceanography/courses/OCN623/Spring2013/

31.   Tajkhorshid, E., Jalkanen K. J, Suhai, S.: J. Phys. Chem. B 102, 5899 (1998).

32.   Frimand, K., Bohr, H., Jalkanen Suhai, K. J., S.: Chem. Phys. 255, 165 (2000).

Cyclic Time Reduction in Precision Component Manufacturing

Deep Prakash Singh*, Sandip Kumar Singh, Hemant Kumar Singh

Department of Mechanical Engineering, U.N.S.I.E.T., V.B.S. Purvanchal University, Jaunpur
*E-mail:deepkantsingh@gmail.com

ABSTRACT

These days the need for short setups is bigger than before. The SMED method, developed by Shingo, for reducing setup times is already known in industry for about 20 years. This project report will present a study of setup time reduction in a leading Aircraft component manufacturer involved in the machining of Precision components in small batches with large variety. Single Minute Exchange of Dies mainly concerned with the recognition of internal and external activities. It is mainly concerned with transferring internal activities into external ones particularly in as many numbers as possible, by also minimizing the internal ones. The validity of the method and procedures are verified by an application of components manufacturing on DMU 100T and DMU 60T, five axis CNC milling machine where setup times are critical for time reduction. Significant time savings have been achieved with minimum take.

It is observed that setup time significantly changes when parallel operations are implied. The change over process becomes more controlled when fixtures are enabled the setup time improves significantly. The investment on fixtures causes high production capacity even without increasing the number of machines, and without compromising the quality. The payback periods also very small. On the basics of these results some recommendations are suggested for continuous improvement.

1. Introduction

Market competitiveness, customer's responsiveness and market demand are the key factors responsible for the implementation and adoption of lean manufacturing techniques in industry. Survival of any industry depends on response time, production costs and flexibility in manufacturing. Due to customer's complexity and demand behaviour, better changeover or setup time reduction enables better response and small batch manufacturing. Reducing setup time leads to increased manufacturing flexibility and capability, shorter lead time, reduced inventory levels and production costs. Short setup time reduces wastes and defects, and thereby improved product quality. Reducing setup time will boost, company's capacity, increases manufacturing flexibility, and help increase overall output. Setup time can be reduced by using Single Minute Exchange of Die (SMED) concepts, which can be achieved through better planning, process redesign and product. The ultimate goal of SMED is to perform machine setup and changeover operations in less than ten minutes.

2. Methodology

A complete study of recorded setup changeover data process and implementation of SMED principles and Quick Die Change (QDC)technology to reduce setup time. A design of plan has been developed to reduce setup time.

2.1 Data Collection, Designing of Fixture's and Supporting Component

Statistical data is collected and analyzed to measure the machine setup time. First, data check sheet is prepared or developed prior to data collection and measured by using a stop watch. The production flow and standard operation procedure is briefly reviewed before developing the data collection check sheet. Based on actual production, data is collected on the daily basis to monitor different type of time loss in setup and tool changeover process.

Initially complete setup data is recorded and SMED principles are implemented in recorded data. Single minute exchange of die is a philosophy to reduce setup time in less than 10 minute or single digit of minutes. The clamping and dialling of unfinished component or raw material/fixture on the machine bed was the critical issue as it takes maximum time in one complete changeover. Then few sub plate/riser blocks and clamp is to be designed to overcome this problem. We have forced to design two sub plates because of difference in bed size of DMU100T and DMU60T.Every sub plate has a series of threaded holes and reamed holes on its top surface. On the bottom side, every sub plate is having two locating slot and a location bung. With the help of location bung and location slot sub plate is fixed on to machine bed with required accuracy. Once the sub plate is fixed and dialled on the machine bed, no more dialling is required when we change the fixture to machine different component. Threaded hole on the sub plate is used to clamp the fixture and reamed hole is used to locate the fixture with respect to sub plate dialling face as these holes are made parallel to dialling face of sub plate with required accuracy.

2.2   Clamping of Fixture and Raw material

Threaded T-bolts are used to clamp the fixture manually and several other bolts are required for the clamping of fixture of different size and shape. Manual clamping of fixture is to be replaced with the clamping of sub plate block to reduce the clamping time. Sometimes first operation to be carried out on raw material is on Computer Numeric Control (CNC) milling centre. This raw material obviously does not have any clamping on locating feature. Therefore this raw material has to clamp on the machine bed directly with the help of T-bolt and nuts. The slots on machine bed are limited in nos. and there relative position is fixed. Due to the fixed position of slot some time very big clamps are required to clamp the small parts which need lot of readjustment and manipulation. To overcome this problem we have designed some system or process improvement so that raw material/small parts can be clamped on machine bed in an efficient manner.

After examinations of tool setup changeover process it is found that movement of worker from machine to tool crib is more than 20 times for bringing the tools regarding to changeover. To eliminate this time a tool holder trolley is designed and all tools and required components like clamps, nut, and bolt for new Part/Fixture in SMED are placed in tools trolley.

3.   Data Collection

Statistical data is collected and analyzed to measure the machine setup time at high speed CNC machining centres. Firstly, the production flow and standard operation procedure is reviewed and a data collection check sheet is developed. To measure different type of time loss in tool/fixture changeover/setup process at high speed CNC machining centres; daily actual production data is collected by using a stop watch and video recording. Data for varying shape and size machine component is collected and averaged to determine the acceptable value. Also, each setup operation is examined and record the time in data check sheet. Recording procedure is repeated should be done after implementing the method to establish the efficiency in both applying the method and achieving the result (SMED).

3.1   Changeover Data of DMU100T

All setup changeover data is video recorded and complete work activity sequence is written down manually and the time of manual recorded activity is noted down with stop watch, while setup changeover performed. The recorded average changeover data of all activities at DMU100T is shown in Table 1.

Table 1. Activity duration table of DMU100T

S. No.	Activity/Operation	Actual Time(min)
1	Unloading of Job from Fixture	05.0
2	Unloading of Fixture from Machine Bed	10.0
3	Unloading of tool holder from machine's Tool Magazine	05.0
4	Transportation of tool holder to tool crib	20.0
5	Removal of cutting tool from tool holder and setup of new tool in tool holder as per the requirement new component to be machined	30.0
6	Transportation of tool holder from tool crib to machine centre and its loading on machine magazine	20.0
7	Loading of tool holder in machine's Tool Magazine	05.0
8	Clamping and dialling of new fixture on Machine Bed	30.0
9	Clamping of job on Fixture	05.0
10	Loading of CNC Program on machine and Start of machine	05.0
	Total Time	135.00

3.2   Changeover Data of DMU60T

All changeover data is video recorded and complete work activity sequence is written down manually and the time of manual recorded activity is noted down with stop watch while setup changeover performed. The recorded average changeover data of all activities at DMU100T is shown in Table 2.

The used fixture which is to be removed and new fixture mounted at machine is milling fixture. In the recoded data clamping and dialling of new fixture on machine bed take maximum time 25% of total setup time. These setup operations have more scope to reduce time. Second most time consuming activity is the movement of worker from machine to tool crib due to transportation of tool holder to tool crib and back to the machine after fitting of new cutting tool as per the requirement of new part to be manufactured and it take 34% of total setup time. Third most time consuming activity is removal of cutting tool from tool holder and setup of new tool in tool holder as per the requirement new component to be machined which consumes 17% of the total setup time.

Table 2. Activity duration table of DMU60T

S. No.	Activity/Operation	Actual Time(min)
1	Unloading of Job from Fixture	05.0
2	Unloading of Fixture from Machine Bed	05.0
3	Unloading of tool holder from machine Tool Magazine	05.0
4	Transportation of tool holder to tool crib	20.0
5	Removal of cutting tool from tool holder and setup of new tool in tool holder as per the requirement new component to be machined	20.0
6	Transportation of tool holder from tool crib to machine centre and its loading on machine magazine	20.0
7	Loading of tool holder in machine's Tool Magazine	05.0
8	Clamping and dialling of new fixture on Machine Bed	30.0

9	Clamping of job on Fixture	05.0
10	Loading of CNC Program on machine and Start of machine	05.0
	Total Time	120.0

4.   Comparison of Setup Changeover Time at CNC Milling Centre

It is observed from the recorded data that DMU100T used to takes more setup time compared to DMU60T. DMU100T takes maximum time in removal of cutting tool from tool holder and setup of new tool in tool holder as per the requirement new component to be machined compare to DMU60T because it has 32 tool magazine as compared to DMU 60T which is having 24 tool magazine, so by virtue in the increase in of no. of tool to be fitted in magazine, time required to perform the operation increases. Clamping and dialling of new fixture on machine bed takes same time on both the machine as lot of trial and error operation has to perform before getting the desired accuracy due to generic nature of machine bed. It is one of the most time consuming activity also. Transportation of tool holder to tool crib, tool setup in tool crib and transportation of tool holder back to the machine consume a major part of setup time on both the machine. After all this comparison the conclusion is that setup operation on both the machine are more or less is same, therefore the problem to reduce the setup time on both the machine can be solve by applying the same method. Fixture designed to reduce the setup time on DMU100T can also be used on DMU 60T after scaling down to suit the DMU60T bed and tooling. The current setup time in all processes at CNC milling centre was noted down and analyzed thoroughly to investigate the bottleneck process. There are many causes of more changeover time are type of setup operations, setting of tools in tool holder, transportation of tool, clamping of work piece, dialling of work piece, worker skill and tools availability.

4.1   Machine Specification (DMU100T and DMU60T)

DECKEL MAHO made DMU100T and DMU60 CNC milling machine are used for setup time reduction study. DMU100T has the bed size of 1080 X 710 mm whereas DMU60TZ has the bed size of 630 X 560 mm. The magazine pocket of DMU100T can accommodate 32 tools whereas the capacity of DMU60T is 24 tools. DMU100T is a five axis machine and DMU60T is a four axis machine.

Table 3. Detail specification of DMU100T and DMU60T

Sr. No.	Feature	DMU100T	DMU60T
1.	General	Simultaneous 5-axis movement 2D & 3D graphic simulation 15.1" TFT colour flat screen; Memory: 6GB	Simultaneous 4-axis movement 2D & 3D graphic simulation 15.1" TFT colour flat screen Memory: 6GB
2.	Feed Drive	Digital AC Servo motor For axis X, Y, Z. Feed rate: X, Y, Z axis variable input-20-15000 mm/min Rapid feed: X Y and Z axis-30 m/min Setup mode: X Y and Z axis-20-2000 mm/min	Digital AC Servo motor For Axis X, Y, Z. Feed rate: X,Y, Z axis variable input-20-10,000 mm/min Rapid feed: X & Y axis-26 m/min, Z axis – 20 m/min Setup mode: X Y and Z axis- 20-2000 mm/min
3.	Path measuring system	Resolution: X, Y, Z axis-0.001 mm Least input increment: X, Y, Z axis-0.001 mm Positioning Tolerance: X, Y, Z axis-0.010 mm	Resolution: X, Y, Z axis-0.001 mm Least input increment: X, Y, Z axis-0.001 mm Positioning Tolerance: X, Y, Z axis-0.010 mm
4.	Work range	Travelling distance: X axis -1080 mm, Y axis - 710 mm, Z axis - 710 mm	Travelling distance: X axis - 630 mm, Y axis - 560 mm, Z axis - 560 mm
5.	Tool Capacity	Pick up system-vertical Magazine Pockets for - 32 tools	Pick up system-vertical Magazine Pockets for 24 tools

5.   Result

Due to implementation of new design of sub plate, clamps and procurement of transportation trolley for tool holder and spare tool holder and implementation of SMED methodology, the changeover time is reduced from 135 min to 17 min for DMU100T and from 120 min to 16 min for DMU60T. The results of this proposed method application has improved the machine flexibility and increased the machine utilization. The improvement in terms of time available for the actual machining operation before and after implementation of SMED. The existing time of complete changeover was 135 minute for DMU100T and 120 minute for DMU60T. After all improvement setup time is reduced up to 17 and 16 minutes and saving of time in one setup is 118 minutes and 104 minute for DMU100T & DMU60T respectively. The minimum change over required per month is 65 for DMU100T and 148 for DMU60T according to production record of CNC shop. Since the machine is available 24 hr/dayandthereare26workingday/month, the total available hour for machine is 624 hr. /month. The time available for machining/month is increased 16% for DMU100T and 34% for DMU60T after the improvement.

6.   References

1.   Deros B.M, Mohamad D, Idrish M.H.M., Rahman M.N.A. Ghani J.A, Ismail A.R.: Cost Saving In An Automotive Battery Assembly Line Using Setup Time Reduction, Department of mechanical & material Engineering & built environment University Kebangsaan Malaysia,49, 144-148 (2011)

2.   M. Perinic,M.ikonic, CS.Maricic.: Die Casting Process Assessment Using Single Minute Exchange of Dies (SMED) Method, Journal of Competitveness,48,199-202,(2009)

3.   Abhijit Shashikant Kulkarni: Implantation Of Jit System at High Speed Press, By Identifying & Eliminating All Forms Of Waste, M.S. thesis, Birla Institute of technology and Science, [April 2010].

4.   Tarcisio Abreu Saurin, Cleber Fabrico Ferreira.: International Journal of Industrial Ergonomics, 39, 403-412 (2009).

5.   M. cakmakci, MK Karasu.: International Journal of advanced manufacturing technology, 33, 334-344,(2007).

Estimation of Some Important and Useful Thermodynamic, Thermophysical and Thermoacoustical Properties of Different Types of Honey Sample

Rupali Sethi*, J. D. Pandey

Department of Chemistry, University of Allahabad, Prayagraj-211002 (INDIA)
*sethirupali.au@gmail.com

ABSTRACT

The aim of the present study is to investigate the influence of temperature (293.15, 298.15, 303.15, 308.15, 313.15, 318.15 and 323.15) K and change in physical properties (density, ultrasonic velocity and viscosity) measurement of seven types of honey samples taken from literature. The thermodynamic, thermophysical and thermoacoustical properties such as thermal expansion coefficient (α), isothermal compressibility (β_T), internal pressure (P_{int}), specific heat ratio (γ), pseudo-Grüneisen parameter (Γ) and solubility parameter (δ) were computed at different temperature and varying concentration. The results found were excellent. It predicts the quality of the types of honey with the exception of Baker's honey (Indian honey) which always show variation opposite to other six types owing to origin. The non-linearity parameter and internal pressure of seven types of honey samples the present study shows strong interactions among atoms and functional group due to prevalence of ion-ion, ion-dipole and dipole-dipole interactions.

The experimental data of surface tension (σ) confirm that temperature has minimal effect on the above properties and relevance of high viscosity of seven types of honey.

Keywords: honey, ultrasonic velocity, viscosity, density, non-linearity parameter, internal pressure, solubility parameter.

1.   Introduction

Honey produced by honey bees, Apis mellifera is produced globally in thousands of flavors and color depending on the blossoms visited by the honey bees. Single varietal honeys result when the honey bees gather nectar from the same type of flowers. Chemically honey contains fructose, glucose [1, 2, 3] and the amount and type of amino acids and organic acids vary by floral source which in turn determines the flavor of honey. The species of honey popular worldwide are Algerian honey [3], Australian honey [4], Millefiori honey [5], Israeli honey [6], Baker's honey (popularly known as Indian honey) [7], Romanian honey [8] and Spanish honey [9]. Raw honey is the best, as it is not adulterated.

Commercial honey has to be analyzed for its food and medicinal value (Figure 1) as more the medicinal value [11] more is its cost. Due to high anti-bacterial properties [12] New Zealand's Manuka [13], Malaysia's Tualang honey, Yemeni Sidr honey and European honeydew honey are 20 times costlier and kept as a treasure for treating burns, cuts, coughs, sore-throat, eye infection, insomnia, arthritis, diabetes [13, 14, 15], acid reflux, anticancer [13, 16, 17, 18] and other ailments.

Organic honey is also effective as it is certified by organic standard tests. Honey when mixed with a few spices act as medium for taking the medicine from the source to the place of infection and aids in its cure. It is a wonderful cosmetology base and is widely suggested by skin experts for cure of skin diseases. Pharmaceutical companies use it as a medium in some skin ointments.

Chemistry Involved in honey production

Bees harvest nectar, sucrose, a disaccharide which is stored in their honey stomachs and when mixed with enzymes break into smaller monosaccharide units namely glucose and fructose.

The nectar is deposited in the honeycomb and the bee fans it for fast evaporation of water till the water content falls to 17%. Since the water content is so low it draws water from surrounding i.e. dehydrates bacteria preventing it from spoilage. Apart from this gluconic acid, produced by bee secretion on glucose maintains a low pH of honey (pH = 3 − 4) and hydrogen peroxide prevents bacterial growth responsible for its long shell life.

Viscosity and surface tension are one of the most important properties of honey. The moisture content plays a key role in honey processing as it increases or decreases the viscosity of honey [20]. Apart from viscosity, water content is solely responsible of its storage conditions [21]. The rheological properties depend on temperature and composition. The presence of disaccharides alongwith monosaccharide increases the viscosity of honey.

In the present work, ultrasonic velocity, density data and viscosity measurements of seven types of honey done by M. Oroian [10] have been successfully used by us to predict the thermodynamic, thermophysical and thermoacoustical properties and also employed there property to study the nature of molecular interactions prevalent between them.

2. FORMULATION

Based on the dimensional analysis [22-25] following correlations between ρ-u thermodynamic properties are used:-

Isobaric thermal expansivity (Thermal expansion coefficient)

$$\alpha = \frac{1}{V}\left(\frac{\partial V}{\partial T}\right)_P = \frac{75.6\times10^{-3}}{T^{3/10}u^{1/2}\rho^{1/4}} \tag{1}$$

Isothermal Compressibility

$$\beta_T = \frac{1}{V}\left(\frac{\partial V}{\partial P}\right)_T = \frac{1.71\times10^{-3}}{T^{1/9}\rho.u^{3/2}} \tag{2}$$

Specific Heat Ratio

$$\gamma = C_P/C_V = \beta_T/\beta_S = \frac{17.1}{T^{4/9}\rho^{1/3}} \tag{3}$$

Internal Pressure

$$P_{int} = \alpha.T/\beta_T = 44.2\times u^{3/2}\rho.T^{4/3} \tag{4}$$

Pseudo-Grüneisen parameter

$$\Gamma = \frac{\gamma-1}{\alpha.T} \tag{5}$$

Solubility parameter

$$\delta = \sqrt{P_{int}} \tag{6}$$

Free length

$$L_f = k'(\beta_s)^{1/2} \tag{7}$$

where $k' = (93.875 + 0.375T) \times 10^{-8}$

Acoustic impedance

$$Z = \rho.u \tag{8}$$

The thermoacoustic non-linear parameter, (B/A) [26-28] has been obtained from the following different equations:

Hartmann-Balizer [26]

$$\frac{B}{A} = 2 + \left[\frac{0.98 \times 10^4}{u}\right] \tag{9}$$

Ballou [27]

$$\frac{B}{A} = -0.5 + \left[\frac{1.2 \times 10^4}{u}\right] \tag{10}$$

Johnson et al [28]

$$\left(\frac{B}{A}\right) = \gamma(C_1 - 1) - (\gamma - 1)(\delta - 1) \tag{11}$$

where, $\gamma = C_p/C_v$, C_1 = Moelwyn-Hughes parameter, δ = Anderson-Grüneisen parameter given respectively by

$$C_1 = \frac{13}{3} + (\alpha.T)^{-1} + \frac{4}{3}(\alpha.T) \tag{12}$$

$$\delta = \frac{10}{3} + 2(2\alpha.T)^{-1} + \frac{4}{3}\alpha.T + 1 \tag{13}$$

3. Results and Discussion

The density (ρ), ultrasonic velocity (u) and viscosity (η) data of seven types of honey namely Australian honey [4], Millefiori honey [5], Israeli honey [6], Baker's honey (popularly known as Indian honey) [7], Romanian honey [8], Spanish honey [9] and Algerian honey [3] have been taken from the paper of Oroian [10] at seven different temperatures (293.15, 298.15, 303.15, 308.15, 313.15, 318.15 and 323.15) K. The calculated values of thermal expansion coefficient (α), isothermal compressibility (β_T), heat capacities ratio (γ), internal pressure (Pint), pseudo-Grüneisen parameter (Γ), solubility parameter (δ), free length (Lf) and acoustic impedance (Z) of seven types of honey using empirical correlations (1-8) are reported in Table 1 at seven different temperatures mentioned earlier.

Table 1: Calculated values of Thermal expansivity (α), Isothermal Compressibility (β_T), Heat capacities ratio (λ) Internal pressure (P_{int}), pseudo-Grüneisen parameter (Γ), Solubility parameter (δ), Free Length (L_f) & Acoustic Impedance (Z) at different temperatures.

$\alpha \times 10^{-7}$	$\beta_T \times 10^4$	Γ	$P_{int} \times 10^4$	$\Gamma \times 10^3$	$\delta \times 10^7$	$L_f \times 10^{-2}$	$Z \times 10^6$
K^{-1}	TPa^{-1}		atm		$Pa^{1/2}$	Nm	$kgm^{-2}s^{-1}$
T=293.15K							
1.014	1.845	1.228	4.188	7.675	6.557	4.505	6.958
1.012	1.841	1.228	4.197	7.678	6.564	4.500	6.970
1.010	1.836	1.227	4.209	7.674	6.574	4.493	6.987
1.007	1.829	1.227	4.225	7.688	6.586	4.485	7.006
1.003	1.817	1.226	4.253	7.671	6.608	4.470	7.045

0.993	1.795	1.224	4.306	7.698	6.649	4.442	7.112
0.988	1.783	1.223	4.334	7.708	6.671	4.428	7.148
T=298.15K							
1.015	1.851	1.220	4.261	7.285	6.614	4.520	6.926
1.013	1.846	1.220	4.274	7.280	6.624	4.514	6.943
1.011	1.842	1.220	4.283	7.282	6.632	4.509	6.955
1.009	1.838	1.219	4.293	7.285	6.639	4.504	6.967
1.004	1.824	1.218	4.325	7.286	6.663	4.487	7.008
0.995	1.803	1.216	4.376	7.292	6.703	4.461	7.073
0.990	1.791	1.216	4.405	7.300	6.725	4.446	7.109
T=303.15K							
1.016	1.859	1.213	4.332	6.922	6.669	4.537	6.889
1.015	1.856	1.213	4.337	6.918	6.673	4.534	6.897
1.014	1.853	1.213	4.344	6.917	6.679	4.531	6.906
1.011	1.845	1.212	4.363	6.907	6.693	4.521	6.930
1.006	1.832	1.210	4.396	6.895	6.718	4.504	6.974
0.997	1.811	1.209	4.445	6.906	6.755	4.479	7.033
0.992	1.797	1.207	4.480	6.897	6.782	4.461	7.080
T=308.15K							
1.374	2.518	1.206	3.262	4.856	5.787	5.290	5.614
1.018	1.865	1.205	4.404	6.544	6.724	4.553	6.860
1.016	1.861	1.205	4.414	6.547	6.732	4.548	6.872
1.014	1.855	1.204	4.427	6.541	6.742	4.541	6.889
1.012	1.847	1.203	4.447	6.520	6.757	4.531	6.916
0.908	1.357	1.089	6.052	3.184	7.882	3.884	9.384
0.996	1.811	1.201	4.536	6.537	6.824	4.486	7.023
T=313.15K							
1.020	1.874	1.199	4.471	6.214	6.775	4.572	6.820
1.019	1.871	1.198	4.477	6.210	6.779	4.569	6.828
1.017	1.866	1.198	4.489	6.216	6.789	4.562	6.843
1.014	1.860	1.197	4.504	6.212	6.800	4.555	6.861
1.011	1.850	1.196	4.527	6.207	6.818	4.543	6.890
1.001	1.826	1.194	4.586	6.190	6.862	4.514	6.963
0.997	1.817	1.194	4.611	6.199	6.880	4.502	6.991
T=318.15K							
1.022	1.882	1.192	4.538	5.891	6.826	4.590	6.785
1.018	1.875	1.191	4.555	5.902	6.839	4.581	6.803
1.018	1.872	1.191	4.562	5.898	6.843	4.578	6.811
1.016	1.869	1.191	4.569	5.895	6.849	4.574	6.820
1.012	1.860	1.190	4.593	5.914	6.867	4.563	6.846

1.006	1.843	1.189	4.634	5.895	6.897	4.542	6.896
1.001	1.828	1.187	4.671	5.859	6.925	4.524	6.945
T=323.15K							
1.023	1.888	1.185	4.610	5.589	6.880	4.606	6.753
1.020	1.883	1.184	4.623	5.594	6.889	4.599	6.767
1.019	1.880	1.184	4.631	5.591	6.895	4.596	6.776
1.017	1.874	1.184	4.644	5.585	6.905	4.589	6.793
1.015	1.866	1.182	4.665	5.563	6.921	4.579	6.820
1.008	1.848	1.180	4.710	5.536	6.954	4.557	6.876
0.997	1.826	1.180	4.766	5.579	6.995	4.530	6.934

Table 1 indicates that with change in temperature from 293.15 to 328.15 K the value of thermal expansion coefficient (α) increases slightly showing that the fluidity of honey is minutely affected till 303.15 K but at 308.15 K there is a sharp increase in value if thermal expansion coefficient (α) indicating that Baker's honey fluidity increases manifolds, due to lesser interaction between the honey molecules & larger intermolecular space (voids). These two factors make the baker's honey less viscous at 313.15 K & 318.15 K. There is again a fall in value of thermal expansion coefficient (α), thereby decreasing the viscosity.

In the case of isothermal compressibility (β_T) similar trend is obtained which means that Baker's honey is most compressible with temperature rise making it stickier and most crystalline with adverse temperature range. The heat capacity ratio (γ) is constantly decreasing throwing light on the fact that specific heat at constant volume (C_v) is decreasing constantly at elevated temperatures. The internal pressure (P_{int}) values are high with regular rise with temperature till 303.15 K with the exception of Baker's honey at which it falls sharply and then rise constantly showing less repulsion between atoms of honey. Lesser repulsion is attributed to the fact of existence of a strong intermolecular hydrogen bonding.

In the case of pseudo-Grüneisen parameter (Γ) the value is falling constantly till 308.15 K then rising, reverse of thermal expansion coefficient (α) as they are inversely proportional to each other.

Solubility parameter (δ) is very high in all type of honey with increase in value till 303.15 K then falling at 308.15 K (Baker's honey) and again increasing makes it miscible in water easily and far more soluble.

Free length (L_f) values constantly increase and at its peak at 308.15 K indicating more mobility. The acoustic impedance is decreasing constantly i.e. the existence to flow of Honey is decreases constantly till 308.15 K then a sharp increase is shown marked by less resistance and more viscous flow.

Table 2 indicates the calculated values of non-linearity parameter (B/A), from equation (9-13), internal Pressure (P_{int}) and surface tension (σ) at seven different temperatures.

Table 2: Calculated values of non-linearity parameter (B/A), internal pressure (P_{int}) and surface tension (σ) at 293.15 K – 323.15 K temperature range

Hartmann		Ballou		Johnson		
B/A	P_{int}	B/A	P_{int}	B/A x10^4	P_{int} x10^{-3}	x10^{-3}
	atm		atm		atm	Nm^{-1}
T=293.15K						
3.952	6.961	1.850	12.093	3.364	1.025	3.275
3.950	6.982	1.848	12.136	3.370	1.026	3.282
3.948	7.009	1.846	12.188	3.377	1.027	3.292

3.944	7.048	1.841	12.266	3.387	1.029	3.304
3.941	7.107	1.836	12.379	3.402	1.032	3.326
3.929	7.234	1.822	12.634	3.436	1.038	3.367
3.924	7.301	1.815	12.768	3.454	1.041	3.390
T=298.15K						
3.954	6.919	1.853	12.016	3.305	1.037	3.277
3.952	6.946	1.850	12.067	3.312	1.039	3.286
3.950	6.967	1.848	12.110	3.317	1.040	3.294
3.948	6.989	1.846	12.153	3.323	1.041	3.301
3.943	7.059	1.839	12.292	3.341	1.044	3.325
3.933	7.174	1.827	12.519	3.371	1.050	3.364
3.927	7.241	1.820	12.652	3.388	1.053	3.387
T=303.15K						
3.956	6.873	1.855	11.930	3.247	1.049	3.276
3.955	6.884	1.854	11.952	3.250	1.050	3.280
3.954	6.899	1.853	11.981	3.253	1.051	3.285
3.951	6.937	1.850	12.055	3.263	1.053	3.299
3.946	7.006	1.843	12.187	3.279	1.057	3.324
3.937	7.115	1.832	12.404	3.308	1.062	3.361
3.931	7.191	1.825	12.554	3.326	1.066	3.388
T=308.15K						
4.393	4.207	2.390	6.692	2.363	0.960	2.427
3.960	6.825	1.860	11.836	3.188	1.062	3.276
3.958	6.846	1.858	11.879	3.194	1.063	3.284
3.956	6.873	1.855	11.930	3.200	1.064	3.293
3.954	6.909	1.853	11.998	3.208	1.067	3.308
3.943	9.453	1.839	16.460	3.576	1.306	4.502
3.937	7.105	1.832	12.387	3.258	1.076	3.374
T=313.15K						
3.963	6.772	1.863	11.738	3.132	1.073	3.273
3.962	6.784	1.862	11.760	3.134	1.074	3.277
3.959	6.812	1.859	11.815	3.142	1.075	3.286
3.957	6.841	1.856	11.873	3.149	1.077	3.297
3.953	6.889	1.851	11.966	3.161	1.080	3.314
3.944	7.009	1.840	12.200	3.189	1.086	3.358
3.939	7.062	1.834	12.307	3.203	1.089	3.375
T=318.15K						
3.966	6.722	1.867	11.642	3.077	1.085	3.270
3.962	6.759	1.862	11.717	3.087	1.087	3.282
3.961	6.770	1.861	11.739	3.089	1.087	3.287
3.960	6.785	1.860	11.767	3.093	1.088	3.292
3.954	6.839	1.853	11.876	3.108	1.090	3.309
3.948	6.918	1.846	12.030	3.126	1.095	3.339
3.944	6.987	1.841	12.160	3.141	1.100	3.366

T=323.15K						
3.968	6.681	1.870	11.566	3.026	1.097	3.270
3.965	6.708	1.866	11.621	3.033	1.098	3.280
3.964	6.723	1.865	11.649	3.037	1.099	3.285
3.962	6.749	1.862	11.699	3.043	1.101	3.295
3.960	6.785	1.860	11.767	3.050	1.103	3.309
3.954	6.869	1.853	11.929	3.069	1.109	3.341
3.941	6.995	1.836	12.184	3.103	1.114	3.381

Table 2 focuses on non-linearity parameter (B/A) and internal pressure (P_{int}) by Hartmann, Ballou and Johnson methods. By Hartmann and Ballou methods, B/A decreases constantly with viscosity & internal pressure is increasing showing more interaction between the atoms of honey making it stronger in interaction intensity. In Johnson method the B/A and P_{int} are constantly increasing indicating the role of specific heat capacity ratio (γ) in seven types of honey undertaken in our study.

The temperature change results in increase in B/A value & decrease in internal pressure as the intermolecular spaces increases and interaction decreases.

The surface tension (σ) increases with viscosity increase making the outer layer less susceptible to interaction. The cohesive force becomes far more than adhesive force creating tension into the outermost layer. This does not allow bacteria to incubate on honey. Killing the bacteria at the surface & in turn the shell life of honey is enhanced with increasing surface tension.

The temperature rise has no impact on the surface tension of honey or very minimal change is observed which can be omitted.

4.   Conclusion

The uniqueness is in the fact that Baker's honey has a characteristics feature which is an exception in all properties discussed in our study due to the types of honey bee present in Indian climate conditions.

Rests of the honey varieties are less susceptible to climate change. The quality of honey is affected by change in density, viscosity, ultrasonic velocity and surface tension effect. Our aim is to establish that thermodynamic and thermoacoustical properties support the experimental findings as honey is a thick fluid and shows all characteristics of liquid state. We have incorporated relevant structure for better understanding of the work.

5.   References

1.   Nagai, T., Inoue, R., Inoue, H., Suzuki, N., 2002. Scavenging capacities of pollen extracts from Cistus ladaniferus on autoxidation, superoxide radicals, hydroxyl radicals and DPPH radicals. Nutrition Research 22, 519–526.

2.   Terrab, A., Vega-Pe´rez, J.M., Diez, M.J., Heredia, F.J., 2001. Characterisation of northwest Moroccan honeys by gas chromatographic-mass spectrometric analysis of their sugar components. Journal of the Science of Food and Agriculture 82, 179–185.

3.   Ouchemoukh, S., Louaileche, H., Schweitzer, P., 2007. Physicochemical characteristics and pollen spectrum of some Algerian honeys. Food Control 18, 52–58.

4.   Bhandari, B., D'Arcy, B., Chow, S., 1999. Rheology of selected Australian honeys. Journal of Food Engineering 41 (1), 65–68.

5.   Blasa, M., Candiracci, M., Accorsi, A., Piacentini, M.P., Albertini, M.C., Piatti, E., 2006. Raw Millefiori honey is packed full of antioxidants. Food Chemistry 97, 217–222.

6.   Cohen, I., Weihs, D., 2010. Rheology and microrheology of natural and reduced calorie Israeli honeys as a model for high-viscosity Newtonian liquids. Journal of Food Engineering 100 (2), 366–371.

7.   Kumar, J.S., Mandal, M., 2009. Rheology and thermal properties of marketed Indian honey. Nutritional Food Science 39 (2), 111–117.

8.   Oroian, M., 2012. Physicochemical and rheological properties of Romanian honeys. Food Biophysics 7 (4), 296–307.

9.   Oroian, M., Amariei, S., Escriche, I., Gutt, G., 2013. Rheological aspects of Spanish Honeys. Food and Bioprocess Technology 6 (1), 228–241.

10.   Oroian, M., 2013. Measurement, prediction and correlation of density, viscosity, surface tension and ultrasonic velocity of different honey types at different temperatures. Journal of Food Engineering 119, 167–172.

11.   Alvarez-Suarez, J.M., Gasparrini, M., Forbes-Hernández, T.Y., Mazzoni L., Giampieri F., 2014. The Composition and Biological Activity of Honey: A Focus on Manuka Honey. Foods 3(3), 420–432.

12.   Ramalivhana, J.N., Obi, C.L., Samie, A., Iweriebor, B.C., Uaboi-Egbenni, P., Idiaghe, J.E., Momba, M.N.B., 2014. Antibacterial activity of honey and medicinal plant extracts against Gram negative microorganisms. African Journal of Biotechnology 13(4), 616-625.

13.   Roberts, A.E.L., Brown, H.L., Jenkins, R.E., 2015. On the antibacterial effects of Manuka honey: mechanistic insights. Research and Reports in Biology 6, 215-224.

14.   Sampath Kumar, K.P., Bhowmik, D., Chiranjib, Biswajit, Chandira, M.R., 2010. Medicinal uses and health benefits of Honey: An Overview. Journal of Chemical and Pharmaceutical Research 2(1), 385-395.

15.   Erejuwa, O.O., 2014. Effect of honey in diabetes mellitus: matters arising. Journal of Diabetes & Metabolic Disorders 13, 23.

16.   Bobiş, O., Dezmirean, D.S., Moise, A.R., 2018. Honey and Diabetes: The Importance of Natural Simple Sugars in Diet for Preventing and Treating Different Type of Diabetes. Oxidative Medicine and Cellular Longevity 2018, Article ID 4757893, 12 pages.

17.   Porcza, L.M., Simms, C., Chopra, M., 2016. Review- Honey and Cancer: Current Status and Future Directions. Diseases 4, 30.

18.   Ahmed, S., Othman, N.H., 2017. The anti-cancer effects of Tualang honey in modulating breast carcinogenesis: an experimental animal study. BMC Complementary and Alternative Medicine 17(1), 208.

19.   Timmins, K.A., Hulme, C., Cade, J.E., 2013. Dietary value for money? Investigating how the monetary value of diets in the National Diet and Nutrition Survey (NDNS) relate to dietary energy density. Proceedings of the Nutrition Society 72 (OCE4), E295.

20.   Yanniotis, S., Skaltsi, S., Karaburnioti, S., 2006. Effect of moisture content on the viscosity of honey at different temperatures. Journal of Food Engineering 72, 372–377.

21.   Trávníček, P., Vitez, T., Pridal, A., 2012. Rheological properties of honey. Scientia Agriculturae Bohemica 43(4), 160-165.

22.   Pandey, J.D., Gautam, P.K., Pandey, M.K., Sunil, 2013. Relationships of Some Useful Thermodynamic Properties of Liquid with Sound Velocity and Density Data. Journal of International Academy of Physical Science 17, 403-408.

23.   Pandey, J.D., Dubey, G.P., Tripathi, N., Singh, A. K., 1997. Evaluation of Internal pressure of Multicomponent Liquid Mixtures Using Velocity and Density Data. Journal of International Academy of Physical Science 1, 117-124.

24.   Pandey, J.D., Dey, R., Soni, N.K., Mishra, R.K., Dwivedi, D.K., 2006. Modified Flory theory and pseudo spinodal equation of state for the evaluation of isothermal compressibility, isentropic compressibility, internal pressure and pseudo Grüneisen parameter of binary liquid mixtures at elevated pressure. Indian Journal of Pure and Ultrasonics 28, 20-28.

25.   Pandey, J.D., Chhabra, J., Dey, R., Sanguri, V., Verma, R., 2000. Non-linearity parameter B/A of binary liquid mixtures at elevated pressures. Pramana – Journal of Physics 55(3), 433-439.

26.   Hartmann, B., Balizer, E., 1987. Calculated B/A parameters for n-alkane liquids. The Journal of the Acoustical Society of America 82, 614-620.

27.   Hartmann, B., 1979. Potential energy effects on the sound speed in liquids. The Journal of the Acoustical Society of America 65, 1392-1396.

28.   Johnson, I., Kalidoss, M., Srinivasamoorthy, R., 2003. Evaluation of thermo-acoustic parameters of some binary liquid mixtures from volume expansivity data. Journal of Pure and Applied Ultrasonics 25, 136-142.

Computation of Nonlinearity Acoustic Parameter for Pure Organic Liquids at Different Temperatures

Subhash Chandra Shrivastava[*] and Shekhar Srivastava

Department of Chemistry, University of Allahabad, Prayagraj-211002 (U.P.) India
[*]getsubhash77@gmail.com

ABSTRACT

In original Beyer's thermodynamic method for the determination of acoustic nonlinearity parameters B/A and C/A, the values of temperature and pressure derivatives of sound speed, the heat capacity at constant pressure (C_p) and thermal expansivity (α) are needed. After this some empirical and semi empirical approaches have been proposed. In these methods, the nonlinearity parameter can be obtained only from density and sound speed data. In the present we have used such methods for the computation of B/A for five pure organic liquids (n-hexane, n-heptane, n-dodecane, cyclohexane and toluene) at different temperatures (283.15 to 333.15) K. The experimental values of density and sound speed were taken from the literature [Phys. Chem. Chem. Phys., 3, 5230 (2001)]. Four different methods (Hartmann, Ballou rule, Johnson et al & Tong-Dong method) were used to compute to the values of B/A.

Keywords: Nonlinearity parameter; pressure; sound speed.

1. Introduction

The nonlinearity parameter B/A is a measure of the nonlinearity of the equation of state for a fluid. It plays a significant role in acoustics, from underwater acoustics to biology and medicine. The nonlinearity parameter is important because it determines dislocation of a finite amplitude wave propagating in the fluid. The parameter B/A determines the nonlinear correction to the velocity due to the influence of nonlinear effects caused by the propagation of finite amplitude wave. Moreover, it can be related to the molecular dynamic of the medium and it can provide information about structural properties of medium, internal pressure, clustering and inter-molecular sparing etc. Importance of the B/A parameter increases with the development of the high – pressure technologies of food processing and preservation.

The parameter B/A is very important in the medical applications of ultrasound, both in diagnosis and therapy. In diagnostic applications knowledge of B/A is necessary in design and optimization of the ultrasound imaging devices. In therapy it enables to predict the temperature in the tissue during ultrasonic hyperthermia treatment. During nonlinear wave propagation the harmonic frequencies are generated and they are absorbed more quickly than the fundamental one [1, 2]. The experimental technique for the B/A parameter measurement can be classified by two basic approaches; thermodynamic method and finite-amplitude method. In the first method, B/A is evaluated using sound speed as a function of pressure and temperature [3-8].The second method is more reliable for measuring the nonlinearity parameter B/A [10].

In the present work the B/A values of pure organic liquids namely n-hexane, n-heptane, n-dodecane, cyclohexane and toluene with carbon chain length $C_6 – C_{10}$ are taken in consideration. The density (ρ) and sound speed (u) have taken from literature [11].

The method used are Hartmann, Ballou, Johnson et al and Tong & Dong method at temperature ranging from 283.15K to 333.15K.

2.   Theory

Hartmann-Balizer [12]

$$\frac{B}{A} = 2 + \left[\frac{0.98 \times 10^4}{u}\right] \tag{1}$$

Ballou [13]

$$\frac{}{A} = -0.5 + \left[\frac{1.2 \times 10}{u}\right] \tag{2}$$

Johnson et al [14]

$$\left(\frac{B}{A}\right) = \gamma(C_1 - 1) - (\gamma - 1)(\delta - 1) \tag{3}$$

where, $\gamma = C_p / C_v$, C_1 = Moelwyn-Hughes parameter, δ = Anderson-Grüneisen parameter given respectively by

$$C_1 = \frac{13}{3} + (\alpha.T)^{-1} + \frac{4}{3}(\alpha.T) \tag{4}$$

$$\delta = \frac{10}{3} + 2(2\alpha.T)^{-1} + \frac{4}{3}\alpha.T + 1 \tag{5}$$

α being the thermal expansivity

Tong & Dong Method [15]

$$\frac{B}{A} = \left(1 - \frac{1}{\gamma}\right)\frac{u^2 \rho \beta_T}{\alpha T} + \frac{2(3 - 2x)^2}{3(x-1)(6-5x)} \tag{6}$$

where all the symbols have their usual notations, and $x = \dfrac{M}{\rho b}$, b the van der Waals constant

The above equations, for convenience, can be written as

$$\frac{B}{A} = J_{(0)} + J_{(x)} \tag{7}$$

where

$$J_{(0)} = \left(1 - \frac{1}{\gamma}\right)\left(\frac{u^2 \rho \beta_T}{\alpha T}\right) \tag{8}$$

$$J_{(x)} = \frac{2(3 - 2x)^2}{3(x-1)(6-5x)} \tag{9}$$

3.   Results and Discussion

The calculated value of B/A using equation (1), (2), (3) and (6) are tabulated in Table 1.

Table 1. Calculated values of nonlinearity parameter B/A by Hartmann, Ballou, Johnson et al and Tong & Dong Method for different organic liquids (n-hexane, n-heptane, dodecane, cyclohexane and toluene) at varying temperatures ranging from 283.15K to 333.15K.

T (K)	B/A Hartmann	B/A Ballou	B/A Johnson et al	B/A Tong & Dong method
		n-hexane		
283.15	11.79	11.49	6.40	10.40
288.15	11.90	11.63	6.38	10.25

293.15	12.01	11.75	6.37	9.87
298.15	12.22	12.02	6.31	10.00
303.15	12.44	12.29	6.27	9.44
308.15	12.67	12.56	6.19	9.49
313.15	12.90	12.85	6.14	9.54
318.15	13.11	13.10	6.05	9.17
333.15	13.30	13.34	5.94	9.08
n-heptane				
283.15	11.25	10.83	6.71	10.62
293.15	11.43	11.05	6.59	10.94
298.15	11.61	11.27	6.52	10.21
303.15	11.78	11.48	6.44	10.13
308.15	11.97	11.71	6.41	10.12
313.15	12.18	11.97	6.34	9.76
318.15	12.31	12.12	6.30	9.72
333.15	13.03	13.01	6.15	9.30
n-dodecane				
283.15	9.96	9.25	7.44	15.06
288.15	10.09	9.41	7.33	14.57
293.15	10.22	9.57	7.26	13.75
298.15	10.35	9.72	7.18	13.70
308.15	10.62	10.05	7.07	13.45
313.15	10.73	10.19	7.00	13.47
318.15	10.82	10.30	6.95	12.60
333.15	11.27	10.85	6.79	12.15
Cyclohexane				
283.15	10.24	9.58	6.83	11.14
288.15	10.49	9.90	6.76	10.29
293.15	10.69	10.14	6.68	10.88
298.15	11.04	10.57	6.57	10.17
308.15	11.36	10.96	6.44	9.63
313.15	11.55	11.19	6.37	10.28
318.15	11.73	11.41	6.33	9.47
333.15	12.32	12.14	6.23	9.62
Toluene				
283.15	10.04	9.34	7.10	11.97
288.15	10.22	9.57	7.02	11.09
293.15	10.58	10.00	6.94	10.47
298.15	10.66	10.10	6.87	11.06
313.15	10.77	10.24	6.72	10.26
333.15	10.79	10.26	6.56	9.96

From the date of Table 1 it is observed that the value of B/A in case of Hartmann & Ballou shows increase with temperature whereas the trend is reversed in case of Johnson et al and Tong & dong indicating that clustering of molecules is more in case of Hartmann and Ballou and hence less spacing at low temperature whereas in case of Johnson and Tong & Dong, less luster at low temperature hence high value of B/A & less interaction.

With increasing carbon chain length, the B/A value decreases as more intermingling and overlapping occurs leading to large voids hence less density in case of Hartmann & Ballou while the order is reverse in case of Johnson et al and Tong & Dong.

4.   Conclusion

B/A is a very important tool in characterization of molecular properties of liquids. Nonlinearity parameter is related to internal pressure, free energy of binding, effective van der Waals constant in case of pure liquids & also mixtures, emulsions & solution.

5.   References

1.   Duck, F.A.: Nonlinear acoustics in diagnostic ultrasound. Ultrasound in Medicine and Biology 28(1), 1–18 (2002).

2.   Liu, X., Gong, X., Yin, C., Li, J., Zhang, D.: Noninvasive estimation of temperature elevation in biological tissues using acoustic nonlinearity parameter imaging, Ultrasound in Medicine and Biology. 34(3), 414–424 (2008).

3.   Beyer, R.T.: Parameter of nonlinearity in fluids. J. Acoust. Soc. Am. 32, 719–721 (1960).

4.   Zorębski, E., Zorębski, M.: Acoustic nonlinearity parameter B/A determined by means of thermodynamic method under elevated pressure for alkanediols. Ultrasonics 54(1), 368– 374 (2014).

5.   Beyer, R.T.: The parameter B/A, in Nonlinear Acoustics. M.F. Hamilton and D.T. Black- stock [Eds.], Academic Press, New York, 1998.

6.   Khelladi, H., Plantier, F., Daridon, J.L., Djelouah, H.: Measurement under high pressure of the nonlinearity parameter B/A in glycerol at various temperatures. Ultrasonics 49, 668–675 (2009).

7.   Coppens, A.B., Beyer, R.T., Seiden, M.B., Donohue, J., Guepin, F., Hodson, R.H., Townsend, Ch.: Parameter of nonlinearity in fluids. J. Acoust. Soc. Am. 37, 797–804 (1965).

8.   Zhu, Z., Roos, M.S., Cobb, W.N., Jensen, K.: Determination of the acoustic nonlinearity parameter B/A from phase measurements. J. Acoust. Soc. Am. 87(5), 797–804 (1983).

9.   Adler, L., Hiedemann, E.A.: Determination of the nonlinearity parameter B/A for water and m-Xylene. J. Acoust. Soc. Am. 34, 410–412 (1962).

10.   Law, W.K., Frizzell L.A., Dunn, F.: Comparison of thermodynamic and finite amplitude methods of B/A measurement in biological materials. J. Acoust. Soc. Am. 74, 1295– 1297 (1983).

11.   Cerdeiriña, C. A., Tovar, C. A., González-Salgado, D., Carballo, E., Romaní, L.: Isobaric thermal expansivity and thermophysical characterization of liquids and liquid mixtures. Physical Chemistry Chemical Physics 3(23), 5230–5236 (2001).

12.   Hartmann, B.: Potential energy effects on the sound speed in liquids. J. Acoust. Soc. Am. 65, 1392-1396 (1979).

13.   Bayer, R.T.: Nonlinear Acoustics (U.S. Government Patenting Office, Washington, DC, 1974) 0-596-215, 89-102 (1974).

14.   Johnson, I., Kalidoss, M., Srinivasamoorth, R.: Evaluation of thermo-acoustic parameters of some binary liquid mixtures from volume expansivity data. J. Pure Appl. Ultrason. 25, 136-142 (2000).

15.   Pandey, J.D., Dey, R., Sanguri, V., Soni, N.K., Yadav, M.K., Pandey, N.: Non-linearity parameter (B/A) of cyclohexanes at varying temperatures and pressures. J. Indian Chem. Soc. 83, 649-651 (2006).

Comparative Studies of Aqueous Solution of Anta Acids by Ultrasonic Interferometry at 2 MHz

A.B. Dhote[1,*], G. R. Bedare[2,**]

[1] Department of Chemistry, N. S. Science and Arts College, Bhadrawati Dist– Chandrapur (M. S), (India) 442902
[2] Department of Physics, N. S. Science and Arts College, Bhadrawati Dist– Chandrapur (M. S), (India) 442902
E-mail: *dhoteaparna71@gmail.com; **gr.bedare@gmail.com

ABSTRACT

Rabeprazole sodium, Omeprazole sodiumare used to treat certain stomach and esophagus problems. The amount of acid that stomach make is decrease by these anta acids. Pantoprazole sodium reduces the amount of acid your stomach makes. In the present work we measured ultrasonic velocity, density and viscosity of aqueous solution of these drugs at different concentration and at different temperatures. The acoustical parameters as relative association, acoustic impedance, and free volume were calculated. Changes in concentration and temperature affect molecular interaction present in the solution. From the acoustic parameters, reactivity of the anta acids predicted.

Key words: acoustical parameters, acoustic impedance, Rabeprazole sodium, Omeprazole sodium, Pantoprazole sodium

1.   Introduction

Physico-chemical behavior of liquid mixture can be studied by using sound wave. Ultrasonic velocity measurements are helpful to interpret solute-solvent,ion-solvent and solvent-solvent interaction in aqueous and non aqueous medium.[1-5] Antacids are a group of medicines which help to neutralise the acid content of your stomach Rabeprazole sodium is used to treat certain stomach and esophagus problems (such as acid reflux, ulcers). It works by decreasing the amount of acid your stomach makes.Rabeprazole, like other proton pump inhibitors such as omeprazole, is used for the purposes of gastric acid suppression[6] This effect is beneficial for the treatment and prevention of conditions in which gastric acid directly worsens symptoms, such as duodenal and gastric ulcers[6] Pantoprazole is used to treat certain stomach and esophagus problems (such as acid reflux). It works by decreasing the amount of acid your stomach makes. This medication relieves symptoms such as heartburn, difficulty swallowing, and persistent cough. It helps heal acid damage to the stomach and esophagus; helps prevent ulcers, and may help prevent cancer of the esophagus. Pantoprazole belongs to a class of drugs known as proton pump inhibitors (PPIs)[7].

In the present study we are trying to study molecular interaction of three drugs from acoustic parameters such as acoustic impedance, relative association and free volume. From these parameters we predict reactivity of the drugs.

Rabeprazole Sodium

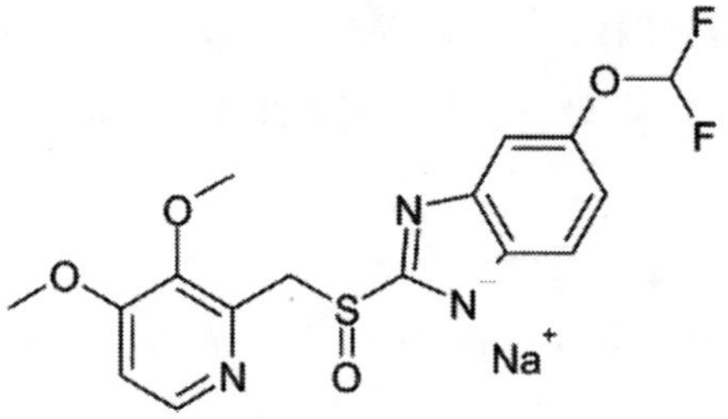

Pantoprazole Sodium

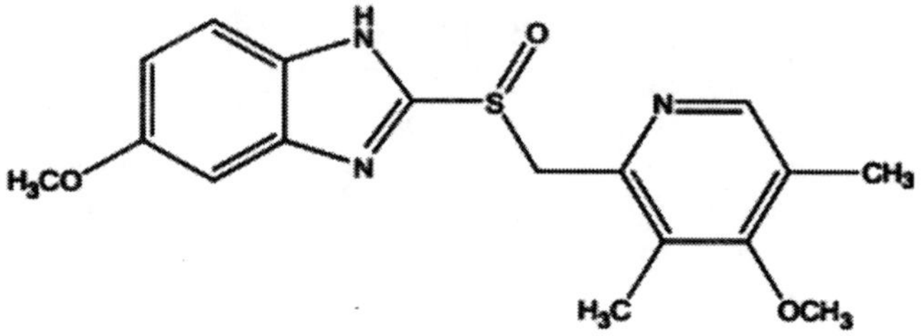

Omeprazole

2.   Materials and Methods

The ultrasonic velocity (U) in liquid mixtures which prepared by taking purified AR grade samples, have been measured using an ultrasonic interferometer (Mittal type, Model F-81) working at 2MHz frequency and at temperature 298K. The accuracy of sound velocity was ± 0.1 ms^{-1}. An electronically digital operated constant temperature water bath has been used to circulate water through the double walled measuring cell made up of steel containing the experimental solution at the desire temperature. The density of pure liquids and liquid mixtures was determined using pycknometer by relative measurement method with an accuracy of ± 0.1Kgm^{-3}. An Ostwald's viscometer was used for the viscosity measurement of pure liquids and liquid mixtures with an accuracy of ± 0.0001NSm^{-2}. The temperature around the viscometer and pycknometer was maintained within ± 0.1K in an electronically operated constant temperature water bath. All the precautions were taken to minimize the possible experimental error.

Using the experimental data of Density (ρ), Ultrasonic velocity (U), various acoustical parameters such as Relative Association (RA), free volume (V$_f$)and Specific acoustical impedance (Z)have been calculated from the measured data using the following standard expressions:

$$RA = (\rho / \rho_0)\,(U_0 / U)^{1/3} \tag{1}$$

$$V_f = (M_{eff}\,U/\eta K)^{3/2} \tag{2}$$

$$Z = U\,\rho \tag{3}$$

Where, K is constant, $M_{eff} = \Sigma x_i m_i$, where x_i is the mole fraction and m_i is the molecular weight of the component.

3.   Results and Discussion

The experimentally measured values of Density (ρ), Ultrasonic velocity (U) and the calculated values of Relative Association (RA), free volume (V$_f$), and Specific acoustical impedance (Z) for aqueous solution of

Rabeprazole sodium, Pantoprazole sodium and Omeprazol sodium at different concentrations at temperatures 298 K at 2MHz frequency are presented in Table-1.

Table-1 clearly shows that, density increases with increasing concentration of aqueous solution of Rabeprazole sodium, Pantoprazole sodium and Omeprazol sodium at temperatures 298K. The ultrasonic velocity values also have the same trend in the system. Velocity increases in this system, suggesting thereby more association between solute and solvent molecules[8].

The property which can be studied to understand the interaction is relative association (RA). It can be explained by two factors[9], the breaking up of solvent molecules on addition of solute to it and solvation of the solute molecule. The former leads to decrease and the latter to the increase of relative association. In the present study the values of RA decreases in aqueous solution of Rabeprazole sodium with increase in the solute concentration. It is due to solvation of the solute molecule.The molecules of a liquid are not quite closely packed and there are some free spaces between themolecules for movement and the volume V_f is called the free volume. The free volume as the effective volume in which particular molecule of the liquid can move and obey perfect gas laws is defined by Eyring and Kincaid. The free volume is increased with increasing concentration shows weak molecular interaction The aqueous Pantoprazol solution has high value of effective mass shows weak interaction. There is relation between acoustic impedance and elastic property of the solution. Non linear behavior in acoustic impedance shows molecular interaction present in the solution

Table 1: The experimentally measured values of Density (ρ), Ultrasonic velocity (U) and calculated values of Relative Association (RA), free volume (V_f), and Specific acoustic impedance (Z) for aqueous solution of Rabeprazole sodium, Pantoprazolesodium and Omeprazolat different concentrations at 298 K at 2MHz.

	At	**298.15K**	**Rabeprazol**	**Sodium**	
Concentration (M)	Velocity U (m/s)	Density ρ (kg/ m^3)	Relative Association	Free Volume $M_{effe}*10^{-8}$	Acoustic impedance Zx 10^4 (kg m-2sec-1)
0.001	1564.15	1310.01	1.334	2.16	204.90
0.01	1610.20	1314.15	1.334	2.28	211.55
0.1	1625.08	1317.25	1.333	2.37	214.06
	At	298.15K	Pantoprazole	Sodium	
Concentration (M)	Velocity U (m/s)	Density ρ (kg/ m^3)	Relative Association	Free Volume $M_{effe}*10^{-8}$	Acoustic impedance Zx 10^4 (kg m-2sec-1)
0.001	1455.23	1500.00	1.5753	2.38	218.28
0.01	1469.10	1502.00	1.5725	2.42	220.65
0.1	1488.23	1504.60	1.5681	2.53	223.91
	At	298.15K	Omeprazol	Sodium	
Concentration (M)	Velocity U (m/s)	Density (kg/ m^3)	Relative Association	Free Volume $M_{effe}*10^{-8}$	Acoustic impedance Zx 10^4 (kg m-2sec-1
0.001	1408.65	1396.00	1.482	2.038	196.64
0.01	1469.23	1398.05	1.463	2.180	205.39
0.1	1499.75	1400.01	1.455	2.303	209.96

4.   Conclusion

It is observed that ultrasonic velocityis highand free volume values are low in the solution of Rabeprazole sodium than pantaprole sodium and omeprazole which indicates strong molecular interaction present in aqueous solution of Rabeprazole sodium.

5.   References

1.   A. K. Dash and R. Paikaray, "Acoustical study in binary liquid mixture containing dimethyl acetamideusingultrasonic and viscosity probes", Der Chem. Sinica, 5 (1), pp. 81-88. 2014

2.   R. Paikaray and N. Mohanty, "Evaluation of Thermodynamical Acoustic Parameters of Binary mixture of DBP with Toluene at 308K and at Different Frequencies", Research Journal of Chemical Sciences, vol. 3(5), pp. 71-82,2013.

3.   R. Palani, S. Saravanan and R. Kumar, "Ultrasonic studies on some ternary organic liquid mixtures at 303,308 and 313K", RASAYAN J. Chem., 2(3), pp. 622-629, 2009.

4.   A. B. Dhote, G. R. Bedare, 'Research Journey' Special Issue 110 (B): February -2019 PP: 37-39.

5.   A. A. Mistry, V. D. Bhandakkar and O. P. Chimankar, "Acoustical studies on ternary mixture of toluene incyclohexane&nitrobenzene at 308k using ultrasonic technique", J. of Chem.andPharm.Res., vol. 4(1),pp. 170-174, 2012.

6.   Dadabhai, Alia; Friedenberg, Frank K (17 January 2009). "Rabeprazole: a pharmacologic and clinical review for acid-related disorders". Expert Opinion on Drug Safety. 8 (1): 119–126. doi:10.1517/14740330802622892

7.   A. B. Dhote, G. R. Bedare, acoustic parameters of pantoprazole solution at different concentration, INTERNATIONAL JOURNAL OF CURRENT ENGINEERING AND SCIENTIFIC RESEARCH (IJCESR), 6(1), 216-281,2019.

8.   A. B. Dhote, G. R. Bedare, Rabeprazol sodium, Pantoprazole Sodium and Omeprazole Sodium at DifferentTemperatures, IOSR Journal of Engineering (IOSRJEN) www.iosrjen.orgISSN (e): 2250-3021, ISSN (p): 2278-8719PP 01-02,2019.

9.   P. B. Agarwal, I. M. Siddiqui, and M. L. Narwade, "Acoustic properties of substituted thiadiazoles and methyl-5-carboxylates in dioxan-water, ethanol-water and acetonewater mixtures at 298.5±0.1 K," Indian Journal of Chemistry, vol. 42, no. 5, pp. 1050–1052, 2003.

Anharmonic Characteristics of Thorium Selenide Using Ultrasonic Method

P. D. Nagaich[1,*] and Kailash[2,**]

[1]Department of Physics, Bundelkhand University, Jhansi, 284128, India
[2]Department of Physics, BNV College, Rath; Hamirpur-210431, India
E-mail: *padmanagayach@gmail.com; **kailashrath@gmail.com

ABSTRACT

Many anharmonic properties of Thorium Selenide are used elastic constants to study and exact evaluation is essential. The elastic energy density for a crystal can be expressed as a power series of strains using Taylor's series expansion. The Thorium Selenide is a face centered cubic crystal. The expansion related to nearest neighbour distance and hardness parameter using long and short range potentials can be got for the face centered. We have extant this method to evaluate the temperature dependent elastic constants for Thorium Selenide crystal. Anharmonic properties as specific heat at higher temperature, thermal expansion, temperature variation of ultrasonic velocity and attenuation, first order pressure derivatives of second order elastic constants are directly related to second and third order elastic constants. To evaluate second order elastic constant (SOECs) third order elastic constants (TOECs) and fourth order elastic constants (FOECs) of Thorium Selenide crystal at higher temperature are computed. These results are used to calculate their pressure derivatives and results are discussed.

Keywords: elastic constants, Anharmonic characteristics nearest neighbour distance.

1. Introduction

Thorium is a radioactive and actinide series element so it has many properties and uses in different field. The elastic constants give a total representation of the elastic response for a deform crystal. The linear elastic stress strain response is described by the second order elastic constants for single crystals, including the propagation velocity along different crystallographic directions (1-5). The non linear characteristics of the Thorium Selenide are declared by higher order elastic constants, such as TOECs and FOECs, inclusive of changes in acoustic velocities due to elastic strain. The elastic constants values are very useful for multi purposes. In this research paper, we use the previous approach to give a valuable method for obtaining the SOECs, TOECs and FOECs starting from nearest neighbour distance using long and short range potentials. The theory of finite deformation of definite functions can be determined and represented in terms of second third and fourth order elastic constants.

The purpose of this research paper is the study of non linear characteristics of Thorium Selenide crystal. The first and second order pressure derivatives (FOPDs and SOPDs) of second order elastic constants (SOECs) of Thorium Selenide structure materials have been computed from room temperature to up to its melting point temperature. The higher order elastic constants such as SOECs, TOECs and FOECs and their pressure derivatives gives very valuable information about inter atomic forces and anharmonic properties of solids (6-10).

2. Methodology

The elastic energy density for a deform crystal expanded as a power series of strain the coefficients of quadratic, cubic and quartic terms known as the second, third and fourth order elastic constants. An important role by SOECs TOECs and FOECs for ultrasonic parameter investigation is played. We computed SOECs, TOECs and FOECs Brugger's notation of elastic constants at absolute zero (C_{IJ}^0 & C_{IJK}^0).

$\Phi(r)$ is the interaction potential equal to sum of electrostatic and Born Mayer potential (11).

$$\Phi(r) = \pm\left(\frac{e^2}{r}\right) + A\exp\left(\frac{-r}{b}\right)$$

In this equation e is the charge, r is nearest neighbour distance A and b is strength and hardness parameters. The elastic strain energy for a crystal can be expanded as:

$$
\begin{aligned}
U_0 \;=\;& U_2 + U_3 + U_4 \\
=\;& [1/2!]\,C_{ijkl}\,X_{ij}X_{kl} + [1/3!]\,C_{ijklmn}\,X_{ij}X_{kl}X_{mn} + [1/4!]C_{ijklmnpq}\,X_{ij}X_{kl}X_{mn}X_{pq} \\
=\;& 1/2C_{11}(X_{11}^2 + X_{22}^2 + X_{33}^2) + C_{12}(X_{11}X_{22} + X_{22}X_{33} + X_{33}X_{11}) + 2C_{44}(X_{12}^2 + X_{23}^2 + X_{31}^2) \\
& + 1/6C_{111}(X_{11}^3 + X_{22}^3) + 1/2\,C_{112}[X_{11}^2(X_{22} + X_{33}) + X_{22}^2(X_{33} + X_{11}) + X_{33}^2(X_{11} + X_{22})] + C_{123}X_{11}X_{22}X_{33} \\
& + 2C_{144}(X_{11}X_{23}^2 + X_{22}X_{31}^2 + X_{33}X_{12}^2) + 2C_{166}[X_{12}^2(X_{11} + X_{22}) + X_{23}^2(X_{22} + X_{33}) + X_{31}^2(X_{33} + X_{11})] \\
& + 8C_{456}X_{12}X_{23}X_{31} + 1/24\,C_{1111}(X_{11}^4 + X_{22}^4 + X_{33}^4) + 1/6C_{1112}[X_{11}^3(X_{22} + X_{33}) + X_{22}^3(X_{33} + X_{11}) \\
& + X_{33}^3(X_{11} + X_{22})] + 1/4\,C_{1122}(X_{11}^2X_{22}^2 + X_{22}^2X_{33}^2 + X_{33}^2X_{11}^2) + 1/2C_{1123}X_{11}X_{22}X_{33}(X_{11} + X_{22} + X_{33}) \\
& + C_{1144}(X_{11}^2X_{23}^2 + X_{22}^2X_{31}^2 + X_{33}^2X_{12}^2) + C_{1155}[X_{11}^2(X_{31}^2 + X_{12}^2) + X_{22}^2(X_{12}^2 + X_{23}^2) + X_{33}^2(X_{23}^2 + X_{31}^2)] \\
& + 2C_{1255}[X_{11}X_{22}(X_{23}^2 + X_{31}^2) + X_{22}X_{33}(X_{12}^2 + X_{23}^2)] + 2C_{1266}(X_{11}X_{22}X_{12}^2 + X_{22}X_{33}X_{23}^2 + X_{33}X_{11}X_{31}^2) \\
& + 8C_{1456}X_{12}X_{23}X_{31}(X_{11} + X_{22} + X_{33}) + 2/3C_{4444}(X_{12}^4 + X_{23}^4 + X_{31}^4) + 4C_{4455}(X_{12}^2X_{23}^2 + X_{23}^2X_{31}^2 \\
& + X_{31}^2X_{12}^2)
\end{aligned}
$$

Where C_{ijkl}, C_{ijklmn} and $C_{ijklmnpq}$ are SOEC, TOEC and FOEC in tensorial form, X_{ij} are the Lagrangian strain components (12-16).

The FOPDs of the SOECs and SOPDs of the SOECs of Thorium Selenide are presented by following expression;

$$dC_{11}/dP = (C_{11} + C_Q + C_{111} + C_{112})C_0 \; ; \; C_Q = C_{11} + 2C_{12}$$

$$dC_{12}/dP = -(-C_{11} + C_{12} + C_{123} + 2C_{112})\,C_0; \; C_0 = 1/C_Q$$

$$dC_{44}/dP = -(C_Q + C_{44} + C_{144} + 2C_{166})\,C_0;$$

$$d^2C_{11}/dP^2 = [(1 + 3C_P)C_{11} + (4 + 3C_P)(C_{111} + 2C_{112}) + C_{1111} + 4C_{1112} + 2C_{1122} + 2C_{1123}]C_0^2;$$

$$d^2C_{12}/dP^2 = [(1 + 3C_P)C_{12} + (4 + 3C_P)(2C_{112} + C_{123}) + 2C_{1122} + 5C_{1123}]C_0^2;$$

$$d^2C_{44}/dP^2 = [(1 + 3C_P)C_{44} + (4 + 3C_P)(C_{144} + 2C_{166}) + C_{1144} + 2C_{1166} + 4C_{1244} + 2C_{1266}]\,C_0^2;$$

$$C_P = (4C_{11} + C_{111} + 6C_{112} + 2C_{123})\,C_0$$

3.   Evaluation

We have calculated elastic constants and their pressure derivatives starting from nearest neighbour distance and basic potentials. The SOECs C11, C12 and C44, TOECs C111, C112, C123, C144, C456 and C166 and FOECs C1111, C1112, C1122, C1123, C1144, C1155, C1255, C1266, C1456, C4444 and C4455 have been computed. In this paper three second order, six third order and 11 fourth order elastic constants have been obtained. The values of partial contraction also computed.

Table 1: nearest neighbour distance and repulsive parameter in 10^{-8} cm SOECs in 10^{11} dyne/cm^2 at 0 k.

R	Q	C_{11}^{0}	C_{12}^{0}
2.8563	0.345	14.721	5.899

Table 2: Temperature coefficients Gn,N and natural frequency w in 10^{13} /sec.

G1	G11	G2	G21	G3	G4	G22	W
-16.39	4.743	141.3	-32.01	-1364	467.3	233.7	2.703

Table 3: SOECs and TOECs in 10^{11} dyne/cm^2 at 300 k.

C_{11}	C_{12}	C_{44}	C_{111}	C_{112}	C_{123}	C_{144}	C_{456}	C_{166}
15.384	5.728	5.927	-233.44	-235.22	8.491	9.463	9.406	-24.209

Table 4 (a): FOECs in 10^{11} dyne/cm^2 at 300 k.

C_{1111}	C_{1112}	C_{1122}	C_{1123}	C_{1144}	C_{1155}
2912.1	-63.673	-47.841	-197.47	-22.157	111.73

Table 4 (b): FOECs in 10^{11} dyne/cm^2 at 300 k.

C_{1255}	C_{1266}	C_{1456}	C_{4444}	C_{4455}
-22.066	134.27	-21.975	134.69	-21.992

Table 5: First order pressure derivatives of SOECs.

dC_{11}/dP	dC_{12}/dP	dC_{44}/dP
-8.88	1.79	0.23

Table 6: First order pressure derivatives of TOECs.

dC_{111}/dP	dC_{112}/dP	dC_{123}/dP	dC_{144}/dP	dC_{166}/dP	dC_{456}/dP
-74.66	13.14	22.12	-1.23	5.49	2.40

Table 7: second order pressure derivatives in 10^{-10} of SOECs.

d^2C_{11}/dP^2	d^2C_{12}/dP^2	d^2C_{44}/dP^2
1.52	-0.001	0.17

Table 8: Partial contraction in 10^{13}.

Y_{11}	Y_{12}	Y_{44}
0.217	-0.121	1.507

4.   Results and Discussion

The SOECs, TOECs and FOECs and their first order pressure derivatives (FOPDs) and second order pressure derivatives (SOPDs) for Thorium Selenide are given in these tables. Some theoretical results are also presented. Due to lack of experimental data of SOECs, TOECs and FOECs for Thorium Selenide crystal the comparison is not made. In this research paper SOECs, TOECs and FOECs have been obtained. The partial contractions for Thorium Selenide are also expressed in this paper. Computed results of SOECs, TOECs and FOECs for different temperatures are also mentioned. For Thorium Selenide we obtain that elastic constants and anharmonic properties are most sensitive to temperature.

5.   References

1.   Kailash, Acta Phys. Pol. A 89 ,75(1996).

2.   R Kotze, J Wiklund - Measurement Science and Technology, (2014)

3.   Kumar J, Shrivastava S K and Kailash, J. Pure Appl. Ultrasonics, 38 ,1(2016).

4.   K Lingtong, H U Hua, W Tianyou, D Huang - Journal Of Rare Earths, Elsevier (2011).

5.   J Li, X Xu, Y Wang, TRen - Tribology International, Elsevier (2010).

6.   M Salavati, G Hosseinzadeh, F Davar - Journal Of Alloys And Compounds, Elsevier (2011).

7.   Kumar J,Kumar V, Kailash and Srivastava S K, J. Pure Appl. Ultrasonics, 34 ,30 (2013).

8.   S Khanjani, AMorsali - Journal Of Molecular Liquids, Elsevier (2010).

9.   J. Huang, C. Li, L. Tao and H. Zhu, Journal of Molecular Structure, 1146, 853, (2017).

10.   Y. Zhou, W. Min Huang, Y. Zhao, Z. Ding and Y. Li, Journal of Alloys and Compounds,672,131, (2016).

11.   Kailash, Raju K M, Shrivastava S K and Kushwaha K S, Physica B 390,270 (2007).

12.   J. Yang, M. Shahid, M. Zhao, and X. Ren, Journal of Alloys and Compounds, 654, 435, (2016).

13.   E. Flage-Larsen, O. Martin Lovvik and J. Tafto, Computational Materials Science, 47, 752, (2010).

14.   P. Thamilmaran, M. Arunachalam, S. Sankarrajan and K. Sakthipandi, Physica B, 466, 19, (2015).

15.   X. Diez-Betriu, J. E. Garcia, C. Ostos, A. U. Boya and D. A. Ochoa, materials Chemistry and Physics, 125, 493,(2011).

16.   S. Khanjani and A.Morsali, Jouranl of Molecular Liquids, 153, 129,(2010).

Prediction of Vision Parameters of Surface Roughness and Wire Wear in Wire-EDM of Al-10 wt.% Si$_3$N$_4$ MMC Material using ANN

H. R. Gurupavan*, H. V. Ravindra, T.M. Devegowda

Department of Mechanical Engineering, P.E.S College of Engineering, Mandya, Karnataka, 571401, India
*E-mail: gpavan1989@gmail.com

ABSTRACT

Present study outlines the estimation of machine vision parameters of surface roughness and wire wear in wire EDM of Al-10wt. % Si$_3$N$_4$ metal matrix composite material using artificial neural network. Al-10wt. %Si$_3$N$_4$ material was selected as a work material. WEDM Parameters such as pulse-on time, pulse-off time, current and bed speed were considered. This work material was machined by varying pulse-on time and bed speed. The images of wire electrode and machined surface specimens were acquired using the machine vision system. The wire wear in WEDM and surface roughness (Ga) of a machined component is measured based on the analysis of the distribution of light intensity. The Artificial Neural Network is used to study and predict the machining responses. Input data are fed into the neural network and corresponding weights and bias are extracted. Then weights and bias are integrated in the program which is used to calculate and predict the machining responses. Estimation of machine vision parameters of surface roughness and electrode wear were obtained by using ANN for various cutting conditions. From the results it was observed that, measured and estimated machine vision parameters of surface roughness and electrode wear values were correlates well with ANN. From the predicted values, wire electrode status monitoring in WEDM can be successfully accomplished by analyzing the surface image data.

Keywords: WEDM, machine vision, MMC, ANN

1. Introduction

The need for composite material has increased in various sectors due to the technological developments and requirement of complex shapes in manufacturing sectors. Metal matrix composites are the most widely used composite materials. Wire cut EDM is quite efficient for machining such materials and it provides good solution for machining harder materials with complex shapes. Machine Vision system is a subfield of many engineering disciplines viz., computer science, industrial automation, optics and mechanical engineering. Machine vision system is the application of image processing to manufacturing industries. Manufacturer's favors vision system for visual inspections that require high-speed, high-magnification, 24-hour operation and repeatability of measurements. Under a given cutting conditions precise estimation of cutting tool life is one of the important issues in the metal cutting process. An integrated "Intelligent Sensor System" consisting of signal conditioning devices, signal processing algorithms, sensing elements, interpretation and decision makes procedure. In recent years, image analysis is easier and more flexible due to the advent of high-speed digital computers and vision systems. Stylus instruments measure surface roughness along a single line where as computer vision systems have the advantage of measuring surface roughness across the area [1]. It was found that vision parameters are affected by the roughness of the surface. For smooth surfaces coefficient of variance parameter is having more correlation than other parameters and the vision parameter, arithmetic gray level average (Ga) is having better correlation for rough surfaces [2]. The acquired images from modern cameras may be contaminated due to the various noise sources and very low intensity. Hence, to evaluate the roughness of the machined surfaces the evolvable hardware technique can be used. Further study is to be focused on artificial neural network (ANN) to estimate surface roughness parameters using image features as input [3].

2.   Experimental Work

The experiments were conducted on CONCORD DK7720C four axes CNC Wire-cut EDM. Wire electrode, a servo control system, a work table, dielectric supply system and a power supply are the basic parts of the Wire-cut EDM. Based on the material and height of the components the input parameters are selected in CONCORD DK7720C by the operator. The Wire-cut EDM has several special features. Unlike other Wire-cut EDM's, it uses the reusable wire technology. i.e., wire can't be thrown out once used; instead it is reused adopting the re-looping wire technology. The gap between wire and work piece is 0.02 mm and is constantly maintained by a computer-controlled positioning system. Molybdenum wire having diameter of 0.18 mm was used as an electrode. Experiments were conducted on machining of Al-10wt.%Si$_3$N$_4$ composite material. The input parameters were pulse-on time, pulse-off time, bed speed and current. Response variables were wire electrode status and Surface roughness. Surface roughness and wire electrode status were measured using machine vision system, then it is compared with the surfcom flex 50-A and digital micrometer; which are conventional measuring instruments for measuring Surface roughness and wire electrode status respectively.

3.   Results and Discussion

Vision parameters of workpiece surface roughnes (SR) and electrode wear (EW) models were defined utilizing feed forward neural networks based on back propagation algorithm. For the designed neural network, the cutting test data were provided in order to train, validate and test them. Several configurations of networks, characterized by different number of hidden layers and number of neurons in the hidden layers, were trained for carrying out the best arrangement for the status parameters prediction, in terms of resulting errors. The Neural Network Toolbox of Matlab software was used for developing artificial neural network and the Levenberg-Marquardt back propagation algorithm was chosen. The input pattern had to be divided in two sets for training and validating the network. The Matlab toolbox was programmed to divide the input pattern as: the 70% for training the network and the 30% for validating it. After these two first phases, the ANNs giving the lowest MSE were chosen as the right predictive instruments. In particular, vision parameters of workpiece surface finish and electrode status data of experiments were utilized. ANN architecture provided the best results for surface finish and electrode wear prediction. The results of experimental and theoretical analysis are presented in the following graphs so that a clear insight can be obtained about the various signals. Functional relationships between the parameters obtained have been shown to derive a basis for a more detailed analysis. Experiments were done for various cutting conditions. The experimental results are presented below. Figs. 1-2 and Figs. 3-4 shows the ANN estimates of vision parameters of electrode wear and surface finish respectively for different cutting condition.

Some established observation from the estimation by ANN study were found to produce a regression coefficient closer to 1 and mean squared error closer to 0. Hence this particular topology of ANN was found to be feasible. The training and estimation has generated closer outputs. Analyzing the graphs, it was seen that most of the estimates represent the observed trend of machine vision parameters. The trend observed was same with other cutting conditions. Better correlation was obtained at high bed speeds. Under these conditions, there will be a large-scale variation in electrode wear, resulting in more vision values. Due to higher values, correlation may have been better. Similar trend was observed for other cutting conditions.

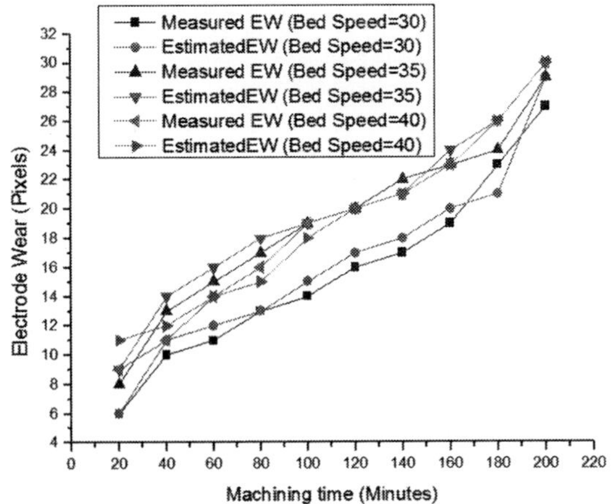

Figure 1. ANN estimates of EW at P-on $=20\mu$Sec, P-off$=5\mu$Sec & current$=4$mA

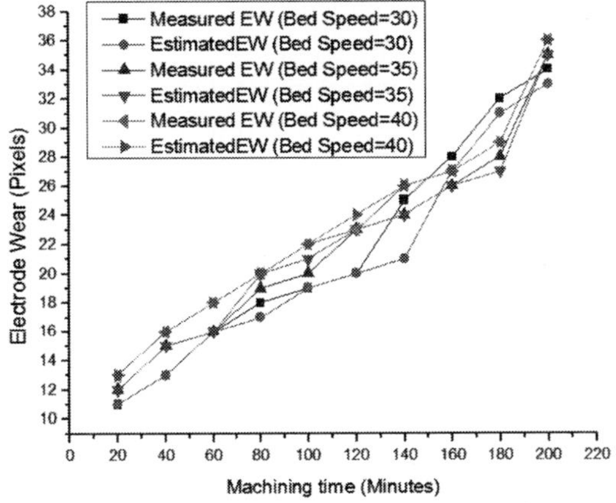

Figure 2. ANN estimates of EW at Pulse-on $=28\mu$Sec, P-off$=5\mu$Sec ¤t$=4$mA

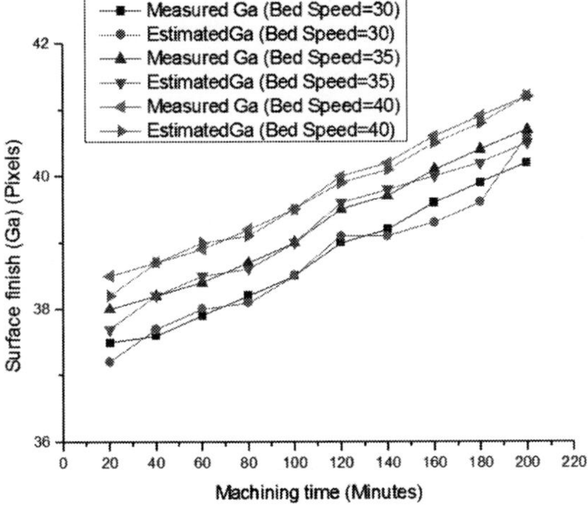

Figure 3. ANN estimates of SR (Ga) at P-on$=20\mu$Sec, P-off$=5\mu$Sec & current$=4$mA

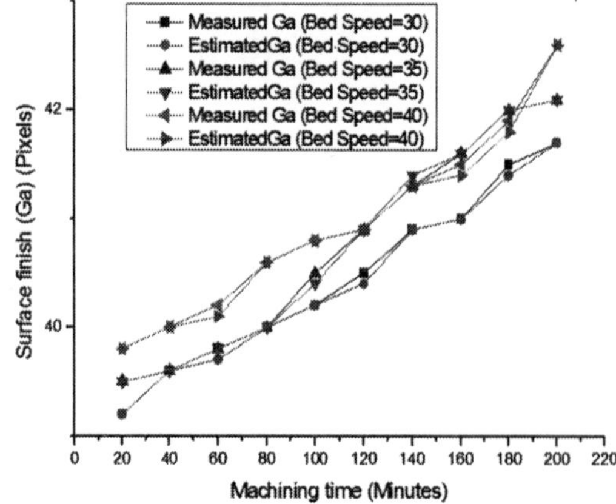

Figure 4. ANN estimates of SR (Ga) at P-on=28μSec, P-off=5μSec & current=4mA

4. Conclusion

In this paper, a machine vision system has been implemented on Wire EDM machine to measure wire electrode status and surface finish of the workpiece. With the aid of image-processing software, this developed vision system has been well constructed to precisely measure the wire electrode status and surface finish of the workpiece. For real time surface texture condition monitoring with non-contact techniques, the image processing algorithms can be used for enhancing the automation proficiency in unmanned tool

From analysis of results obtained in estimation of vision parameters in machining of Al-10 wt.%Si_3N_4 with molybdenum electrode at different cutting conditions investigated, the following conclusions can be drawn:

➢ Regression coefficient closer to 1 and mean squared error closer to 0, were found to produce with 4 input parameters, 2 hidden layers and 10 hidden neurons. Hence this particular topology of Artificial Neural Network was found to be feasible.

➢ The training and estimation have generates closer outputs with 4 input parameters, 2 hidden layers and 10 hidden neurons.

➢ ANN estimates have good correlation at higher bed speed.

➢ The use of vision signal of electrode status and workpiece surface finish has proved to be more efficient than conventional monitoring.

5. References

1. Shivanna.D.M, Kiran M.B. and Kavitha S.D, Evaluation of 3D surface roughness parameters of EDM components using vision system, Proced. Mat. Sci. 5, 2132 – 2141(2014) .

2. Babu G. D., Babu K. S. and Gowd B. U. M., Evaluation of surface roughness using machine vision, IEEE, International Conference on Emerging Trends in Robotics and Communication Technologies (INTERACT-2010)

3. Narayanan M.R., Gowri S. and Krishna M.M., On line surface roughness measurement usingimageprocessing and machine vision, Proceedings of the World Congress on Engineering, London, U.K, Vol 1 (2007).

4. Samtas G., Measurement and evaluation of surface roughness based on optic system using image processing and artificial neural network, Int. J. Adv. Manuf. Techn. 73,353–364 (2014).

Physical Properties of Mixed Spinel Ferrite Nano-particles: Effect of Calcination Temperature

Dilip S. Badwaik[1,*], P. S. Hedaoo[1], S. S. Suryawanshi[1], V. D. Badwaik[2], V. A. Tabhane[3]

[1]Department of Physics, Kamla Nehru Mahavidyalaya, Nagpur-440025, India
[2]Nutan Bharat College, Abhyankar Nagar, Nagpur-440010, India
[3]Department of Physics, Savitribai Phule Pune University, Pune-411007, India
*E-mail: badwaik_ds@rediffmail.com

ABSTRACT

Nano-crystalline NiCoZn mixed ferrite powder with chemical composition $Ni_{0.3}Co_{0.3}Zn_{0.4}Fe_{1.8}Cr_{0.2}O_4$ has been synthesized by sol-gel auto combustion method assisted by micro-wave with frequency 2.45 GHz and characterized to investigate the effect of heat treatment on the structural and optical behavior of the synthesized powder. The structural and optical properties were determined by X-ray diffraction (XRD) and FTIR. The powder was calcinated at 500°C, 700°C, 900°C and 1000°C. Analysis of results indicated that thermal heat influences the magnitude of structural parameters. The crystallite size is found to increase with calcinations temperature and in the range 68 – 123 nm. Slight increase in lattice parameter is also observed. The FTIR spectra shows the two strong absorption bands in the wave number range 400 - 600 cm^{-1} arising due to the inter-atomic vibrations in the tetrahedral and octahedral coordination compounds.

Keywords: Sol-gel auto combustion; nano-ferrite; XRD; FTIR.

1. Introduction

Spinel ferrites have been widely used in numerous technological applications due to their excellent electrical, magnetic and optical properties [1, 2]. Recent advances in the synthesis techniques for the production of ferrites have initiated interest in ferrites in order to improve their physical properties and expand their applications [1]. With the fast growing technology, the electronic components with small size, high efficiency, and low cost are urgently demanded [3]. Ferrites are technologically important and have been used in many applications like magnetic recording media for the storage and/or retrieval of information, magnetic resonance imaging (MRI) enhancement, magnetically guided drug delivery, sensors, catalysis, pigments, transformer cores, multilayer chip inductor, etc. [4,5]. Requirement of desirable microstructure: a high sintered density, a small particle size and a narrow particle size distribution is important in such applications [6]. The physical properties of nano materials are often different from those of the bulk materials due to large surface area to volume ratio [7]. Among ferrites, Cobalt ferrite based nano-materials are known to be the good candidates for magneto optical recording and high density storage [8, 9]. On the other hand, Ni- Zn ferrite offers high resistivity but relatively low permeability at high frequencies. For high-frequency magnetic application, ferrites with high permeability as well as high resistivity are indispensable. Phase formation, particle size and morphology of the ferrite powder depend on pH value of the initial solution, molar ratio of the ions and calcinations temperature. Various preparation methods have been developed to obtain nano-sized ferrite particles, including a chemical process, co-precipitation, mechanical alloying, sol–gel method, hydrothermal and ball milling methods [10]. In every synthesis route, process parameters are responsible for the difference in the microstructure and properties of the final product. In the present study, ferrite with chemical composition $Ni_{0.3}Co_{0.3}Zn_{0.4}Fe_{1.8}Cr_{0.2}O_4$ has been synthesized by sol-gel auto combustion method assisted by micro-wave. Advantage of the sol-gel method is not only to lower the calcinations temperature but also has better control over the micro structure and homogeneity. Objective of this work is to study the effect of calcinations temperature on the structural and optical properties of prepared sample.

2.   Experimental Methodology

Mixed spinel ferrite with composition $Ni_{0.3}Co_{0.3}Zn_{0.4}Fe_{2-x}Cr_xO_4$ was prepared by sol gel auto combustion method assisted by microwave. The starting chemicals used were analytical grade cobalt nitrate, nickel nitrate, zinc nitrate, ferric nitrate, chromium nitrate and urea as a fuel. Take Stoichiometric amount all chemicals and dissolve one after another in minimum amount of distilled water. The solution stirred continuously for 30 minutes to become homogeneous solution, then add urea into the beaker and slowly heated with continuous stirring at about 60^0C.to obtain gel. Beaker containing gel is kept in domestic microwave with operating frequency of 2.45GHz. After few minute of exposure to microwave dark brown fumes started coming out and finally gel gets fired in self propagating manner. Foamy dark brown powder obtained is grinded in pestle mortar for 1 hour to obtained uniform powder. It is then calcinated at four different temperatures $500°C$, $700°C$, $900°C$ and $1000°C$ under atmospheric conditions for 6 hours. The calcined powder is again grinded for 1 hour and now ready for characterizations.

X-ray diffraction (XRD) was used to investigate the structure, structural parameters and space group symmetry of synthesized nano-ferrites. The Fourier Transform Infrared (FTIR) spectra were recorded using FTIR spectrometer in the wave number range 4000 cm−1 to 400 cm−1 using KBr pellets to confirm formation of the spinel structure of the samples.

3.   Results and Discussion

3.1   Structural Analysis

The powder x-ray diffraction patterns of Ni0.3Co0.3Zn0.4Fe1.8Cr0.2O4 nano ferrite calcinated at $500°C$, $700°C$, $900°C$ and $1000°C$ is shown in Fig. 1. The peaks were indexed as (111), (220), (311), (222), (400), (422), (511), (440) belong to the cubic spinel phase structure with space group Fd3m, in agreement with JCPDS – ICDD Cards, for Co- ferrite (22- 1086) and for Zn- ferrite (89-1009). Thus XRD Patterns confirmed that all samples calcinated at different temperature have single phase cubic spinel structure and the absence of any additional peaks confirms their purity and monophasic nature. The peak broadening hints towards the nano-crystalline nature of prepared sample. The unit cell dimensions are determined from the d-spacing of a most intense peak (311) by making use of the cubic formula for inter-planer spacing.

$$a = d\ (h^2 + k^2 + l^2)^{1/2}$$

Where,

a = lattice constant; d = inter planer distance; (h k l) is the miller indices of the crystal planes.

The theoretical density (X-ray density) was calculated from XRD data during the following equations.

$$D_s = ZM/Na^3$$

Where,

Z = No. of atoms per unit cell (Z = 8)

M = Molecular weight of the sample; N = Avogadro's number; a = Lattice constant.

The crystallite size has been calculated from the most intense diffraction peak (311) by Scherrer formula,

$$D = k\lambda/\beta\ Cos\theta$$

Where

D = Crystallite Size.

λ = Wavelength of incident X-rays.

θ = Diffraction angle.

β = Full width at half-maximum, (FWHM), and

K = Shape factor, about 0.9 for spherical shaped particles.

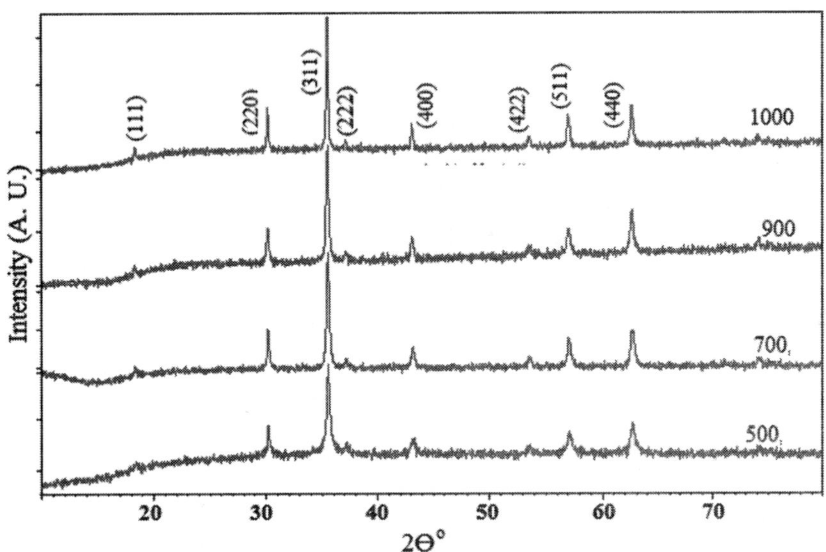

Figure 1. XRD micrograms of $Ni_{0.3}Co_{0.3}Zn_{0.4}Fe_{1.8}Cro_{0.2}O_4$ calcinated at different temperaturre

The calculated values of lattice parameter, crystallite size and x-ray density are shown in Table 1. The crystallite size and lattice parameter of the samples were found to be 68.33 nm, 78.58 nm, 81.98 nm, 123.72 nm and 8.3734 Å, 8.3784 Å, 8.3877 Å, 8.3887 Å corresponding to calcinations temperature of 500 °C, 700 °C, 900 °C and 1000 °C respectively. The lattice parameter and x-ray density are in close agreement with earlier reported values [11]. The reflection peaks were slightly shifted to lower angles and intensity was increased due to crystal growth. The broadness of diffraction peak decreases with increasing calcinations temperature, result into increasing crystallite size. Thus crystallite size is very sensitive to the calcination temperature. In addition, the calcination temperature also led to a slight change in the lattice parameter. This is attributed to the heat coupling in the sample at higher temperature allowing the diffusion of metals into their octahedral sites [12].

Furthermore, the results XRD peak intensity I220/I222 and I422/I222 show the distribution of cations in octahedral and tetrahedral sites, respectively. The XRD peak intensity ratios for both I220/I222 and I422/I222 obtained are 4.91 and 1.11, 4.46 and 1.13, 4.24 and 1.03 respectively, corresponding calcinations temperature of 700°C, 900°C and 1000°C. The experimental results for 1000°C offers very close to the numerical calculated results i.e. I220/I222 is equal 4.1 and I220/I422 is 1.3 where Co^{2+} and Fe^{3+} completely separate at tetrahedral and octahedral sites[13]. The modification of the peak XRD intensity ratio indicates that the calcination temperature affects cation distribution for both tetrahedral and octahedral sites.

The X-ray diffraction data is further used to calculate the octahedral and tetrahedral sites ionic radii (r_B, r_A), the bond length on octahedral (B-O) and tetrahedral (A-O) sites, hoping length in octahedral sites (L_B) and in tetrahedral sites (L_A) by using standard equations [14]. It is observed from Table II, that with increasing the calcination temperature, the ionic radii (r_B, r_A) and bond length (B-O, A-O) increases. This could be due to increase in lattice parameter with calcination temperature. The hopping lengths in the octahedral site (L_B) and tetrahedral site (L_A) which is nothing but the distance between the magnetic ions are also increases with temperature. This shows that more energy is required for jumping of electrons between A and B-sites. Jump lengths are directly related with lattice constants. So increase of the lattice constant values consequently increases the jump lengths.

Table 1. Structural parameters calculated from XRD of the $Ni_{0.3}Co_{0.3}Zn_{0.4}Fe_{1.8}Cr_{0.2}O_4$

Sr No	Calcination temperature	Lattice parameter (a) in Ao	Crystallite size in nm	Molecular wt.	X-ray density gm/cm3	Intensity ratio 220/222	Intensity ratio 422/222
1	500	8.3734	68.33	236.37	5.347	--	---
2	700	8.3784	78.58	236.37	5.337	4.91	1.11
3	900	8.3877	81.981	236.37	5.320	4.46	1.13
4	1000	8.3887	123.72	236.37	5.318	4.24	1.03

Table 2. Different parameters calculated from XRD data of $Ni_{0.3}Co_{0.3}Zn_{0.4}Fe_{1.8}Cr_{0.2}O_4$

Calcination temperature	r_A	r_B	A-O	B-O	L_A	L_B
500	0.460	0.743	1.8108	2.0934	3.626	2.960
700	0.461	0.744	1.8118	2.0946	3.628	2.962
900	0.463	0.746	1.8138	2.0969	3.632	2.965
1000	0.464	0.747	1.8141	2.0972	3.632	2.965

3.2   FTIR Analysis

Fig. 2 shows the FTIR absorption spectra of $Ni_{0.3}Co_{0.3}Zn_{0.4}Fe_{1.8}Cr_{0.2}O_4$ nano-ferrite calcinated different temperature in the wave number ranging from 400 to 4000 cm^{-1}. The FTIR spectroscopic technique is a very important tool to obtain the structural features and redistribution of cations between tetrahedral and octahedral sites of spinel ferrite nanoparticles [15]. In general the FT-IR spectra show two strong band assignments in the range below 1000 cm^{-1}, attributed to the band assignment between inorganic elements and oxygen ions [16]. Normally, the higher frequency band is observed in the range of 550–600 cm^{-1}, corresponds to vibrations of the A-site [M tetra O] and the lower frequency band observed in the range of 400–450 cm^{-1}, due to the vibrations of the B-site groups [M octa O]. These two bands are common features for all ferrites [17]. The vibration of band in the tetrahedral sites occurs at higher wave number than octahedral sites, which is due to the smaller bond length of tetrahedral positions compared to the octahedral sites [18]. Thus FTIR spectra confirmed the formation of spinel structure in the prepared samples

In prepared $Ni_{0.3}Co_{0.3}Zn_{0.4}Fe_{1.8}Cr_{0.2}O_4$ samples, the tetrahedral frequency band v_1 is observed at 590, 591, 587 and 591 cm^{-1} whereas the octahedral frequency band v_2 is observed at 430, 428, 426 and 428 cm^{-1} in the calcination temperatures of 500, 700, 900, and 1000 °C, respectively. As shown in Fig.2, slight variations of band positions are observed with increasing calcination temperatures. It mainly attributes the variation in ion distribution between tetrahedral and octahedral sites with calcination temperatures [19].

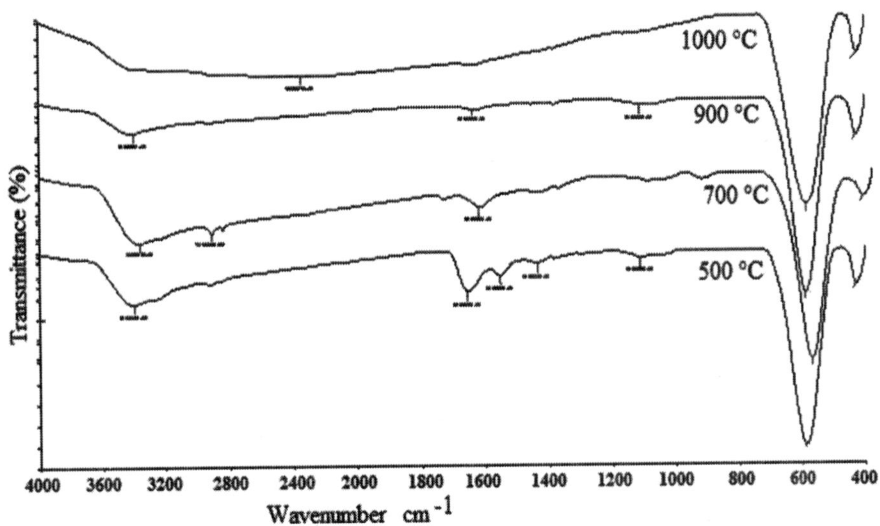

Figure. 2 FTIR spectra of $Ni_{0.3}$ $Co_{0.3}$ Zn0.4 Fe1.8 Cr0.2O4 nano ferrites at different calcinaton temperature

4.   Conclusion

Nano-crystalline ferrite powder $Ni_{0.3}Co_{0.3}Zn_{0.4}Fe_{1.8}Cr_{0.2}O_4$ has been successfully synthesized by micro-wave assisted sol-gel auto combustion method at much lower temperature of 500°C. The crystallite size and lattice parameter increases with calcination temperature. The changes in the reflection plane intensity ratio of I220/ I222 and I422/I222 indicates that the calcination temperature affects cation distribution for both tetrahedral and octahedral sites. Two strong absorption band one in the range of 400–450 cm^{-1} and other the range of 550–600 cm^{-1} confirmed the formation of spinel structure in the prepared samples.

5.   References

1.   Y. Ahn and E.J. Choi, Magnetization and Mossbauer study of nanosize $ZnFe_2O_4$ particles synthesized by using a microemulsion method, Journal of the Korean Physical Society, 41, 123-128(2002).

2.   P. Laokul, V. Amornkitbamrung, S. Seraphin and S. Maensiri, Characterization and magnetic properties of nanocrystalline $CuFe_2O_4$, $NiFe_2O_4$, $ZnFe_2O_4$ powders prepared by the Aloe vera extract solution, Current Applied Physics, 11, 101-108 (2011).

3.   X.W. Qi, J. Zhou, Z.X. Yue, L.T. Li and Z.L. Gui, Room temperature preparation of nanocrystalline MnCuZn ferrite powder by auto-combustion of nitrate-citrate gels, Key Engineering Materials, 593-596 (2002).

4.   S. Maensiri, C. Masingboon, B. Boonchom and S. Seraphin, A simple route to synthesize nickel ferrite ($NiFe_2O_4$) nanoparticles using egg white, Scripta Materialia, 56, 797–800, (2007)

5.   B. Li, Z.X. Yue, X.W. Qi, J. Zhou, Z.L. Gui and L.T. Li, High Mn content NiCuZn ferrite for multiplayer chip inductor application, Materials Science and Engineering B 99, pp. 252-254 (2003).

6.   E.J. Choi, Y. Ahn and E.J. Hahn, Size dependence of the magnetic properties in super-paramagnetic zinc-ferrite nanoparticles, Journal of the Korean Physical Society, 53, 2090-2094 (2008).

7.   Ahmad, M. Ali, I., Aen, F., Islam, M.U., Ashiq, M.N., Atiq, S., Ahmad, W. and Rana, "Effect of sintering temperature on magnetic and electrical properties of nano-sized Co2W hexaferrites", Ceramics International, 38, 1267-1273 (2012).

8.   R.N.Panda, J.C.Shih and T.S. Chin, Magnetic properties of nano-crystalline Gd- or Pr-substituted $CoFe_2O_4$ synthesized by the citrate precursor technique, J. Magn. Magn. Mater. 257, 79-86 (2003).

9.   A.M.Abo EI Ata, S .M. Attia and T.M. Meaz, The frequency dependence of dielectric loss tangent (tan δ) is found to display, Solid State Sci. 6, 61(2004).

10.   A. Kumar, D. Singh and V. Agarwala, Effect of particle size of Ba $Fe_{12}O_{19}$ on the microwave absorption characteristics in x band, Progress In Electromagnetics Research, 29, 223-236 (2013).

11.   P.S. Hedao, D.S. Badwaik, S.M. Suryawanshi, K.G. Rewatkar, Structural and magnetic studies of Zn doped nickel nanoferrites synthesize by sol-gel auto combustion method, Materials Today: Proceedings 15, 416–423 (2019)

12.   Abubakar Yakubu1, Zulkifly Abbas, Nor Azowa Ibrahim and Mansor Hashim, "Effect of temperature on structural, magnetic and dielectric properties of cobalt ferrite nanoparticles prepared via Co precipitation method", Physical Science International Journal 8(1): 1-8, (2015), Article no.PSIJ.18787.

13.   Ajroudi, L., Mliki, N., Bessais, L., Madigou, V., Villain, S., Leroux, C., Magnetic, electric and thermal properties of cobalt ferrite nanoparticles,. Mater. Res. Bull.59, 49–58 (2014).

14.   Nasrin S., Hoque S. M., Chowdhury F. U. Z., Hossen M. M. , Influence of Zn substitution on the structural and magnetic properties of Co1-XZnXFe2O4 nano-ferrites, IOSR Journal of Applied Physics, 6, III (2014).

15.   Ateia, E., Effect of gamma Irradiation on the structural and electrical properties of Co0.5Zn0.5CeyFe2-yO4, Egypt J. Solids 29, 317-328 (2006).

16.   Modi KB, Shah SJ, Pujara NB, Pathak TK, Vasoya NH, Jhala IG, Infrared spectral evolution, elastic, optical and thermo-dynamic properties study on mechanically milled Ni0.5Zn0.5Fe2-O4 spinel ferrite, J Mol Struct 1049, 250–262 (2013).

17.   Waldron RD, Infrared spectra of ferrites, Phys Rev 99, 1727–1735

18.   Pradeep A, Priyadarshini P, Chandrasekaran G, Structural, magnetic and electrical properties of nanocrystalline zinc ferrite. J Alloys Compound 509, 3917–3923 (2011).

19.   Effects on structural, optical, and magnetic properties of pure and Sr-substituted $MgFe_2O_4$ nanoparticles at different calcination temperatures, Appl Nanosci 6, Kumar, 629–639 (2016).

Optimization of P-GMAW Welding Output Parameters Using Taguchi Technique for SS 304 Material

Rudreshi Addamani* and H V Ravindra

Department of Mechanical Engineering, P.E.S College of Engineering, Mandya-571401, India
*E-mail: rudreshaddamani@gmail.com

ABSTRACT

The pulsed gas metal arc welding (P-GMAW) process is one of the most vital arc welding processes, used in high-technology industrial applications. P-GMAW is widely used in process, especially in thin sheet metal industries. It offers an improvement in quality and productivity over regular gas metal arc welding (GMAW). The process enables stable spray transfer with low mean current and low net heat input. Cost, quality and productivity of welding are the important factors which are affected by the P-GMAW in put parameters. In order to control and understand the P-GMAW process parameters, it is necessary to determine the input and output relationship of the welding processes. This paper describes the influence of welding input parameters like welding current (amp), gas flow rate (GFR, ltrs/min) and wire feed rate (WFR, mm/min), etc. on weld strength for SS 304 pipes. The parameters can be optimize and having the best parameters combination to get good quality weld bead joint by using DOE method. A plan of experiments based on Taguchi technique has been employed to acquire the data. An Orthogonal array of L27 and analysis of variance (ANOVA) are adopted to investigate the welding characteristics of SS 304 material and optimize the welding parameters. The response parameters considered are Ultimate Tensile Strength (UTS, N/mm2), Yield Strength (YS, N/mm2) and % of elongation. Finally the conformations tests have been carried out to compare the predicated values with the experimental values to confirm its effectiveness in the analysis of weld bead joint strength.

Keywords: P-GMAW, SS304, Taguchi technique, ANOVA.

1. Introduction

The pulsed gas metal arc welding (P-GMAW) is broadly used fabrication process, particularly in thin metal sheet industries. It offers an enhancement in quality and productivity over regular gas metal arc welding (GMAW). The process enables stable spray transfer with low mean current and low net heat input. It applies waveform control logic (Fig. 1) to produce a very precise control of the arc through a broad wire feed/speed range. With precise control of arc dynamics, P-GMAW welding can be used as a high deposition rate at high travel speeds, or it can be run as a fast-follow process with fast-fill process. A variation of the spray transfer mode, pulse-spray is based on the principles of spray transfer but uses a pulsing current to melt the filler wire and allow one small molten droplet to fall with each pulse. This feature of current pulsating reduces net heat input to the base metal, so decreases undesirable effects of comparatively high heat input in MIG welding. The main setting parameters which influence weld quality or wire melting are background current (Ib), peak current (Ip), background time (Tb) and peak time (Tp). Pulsed current metal inert gas welding is commonly used for root pass welding of tubes and pipe welding.

A research work carried out on the optimization of MIG welding parameters using Taguchi design method. The input parameters considered are viz., welding voltage, current, speed of welding and depth of penetration.

MS C20 was selected as work piece material. A plan of experiments based on Taguchi technique has been used to acquire the data. An orthogonal array, signal to noise(S/N) ratio and analysis of variance (ANOVA) were employed to investigate the welding characteristics of MS C20 material and optimize the welding parameters. Their experimentation results that the lower current [1]. Some of the researchers performed their analysis on optimization of resistance spot welding parameters using Taguchi method. The experiments were conducted under varying pressure, welding current and welding time. The output characteristic considered was tensile strength of the welded joint. The material used was low carbon steel sheets of 0.9mm. Their conclusion leads that the contribution of welding current holding time and pressure towards tensile strength is 61%, 28.7% and 4 % respectively as determined by the ANOVA method[2]. Sum researchers have obtained the use of Taguchi's parameter design methodology for parametric study of gas metal arc welding of stainless steel and low carbon steel. The input process variables considered here include welding current, welding voltage and gas flow rate. A total number of 9 experimental runs were conducted using an L9 orthogonal array, and calculate the signal-to-noise ratio. Subsequently, using analysis of variance ANOVA) the significant coefficients for each input parameter on tensile strength and Hardness (PM, WZ and HAZ) were determine[3]. A work has done on optimization of MIG welding parameters in order to improve yield strength of AISI 1040 mild steel. The process parameters welding current, voltage, gas flow rate and wire speed were studied. The experiments were conducted based on four factors, three level orthogonal arrays. The empirical relationship can be used to predict the yield strength of welded material [4].

2.   Experimental Setup

The experiments have been carried out using a pulsed current lorch welding machine with air type cooling and automated welding set up having 400 amperes maximum current. Trials are conducted based on Taguchi L27 orthogonal array. Trial specimens are having dimension of 25 mm outer diameter, 22 mm inner diameters and 3 mm wall thickness. Each specimen is cut in to 150 mm long and tack welded before welding. Single pass butt welding is done on SS 304 by varying the process parameters, having edge preparation with 45o angle. Welding process was carried out by using Argon (85%) and CO_2 (15%) gas mixture. The working ranges for the process parameters were selected based on expert's advice, literature review and with the american welding society (AWS) handbook.

3.   Taguchi Methodology

3.1.   S/N Ratio

The Signal to Noise ratios (S/N), which are log functions of desired output, serve as the objective functions for optimization, help in data analysis and the prediction of the optimum results. There are 2 Signal-to-Noise ratios of common interest for optimization of Static Problems.

1.   Smaller the better is given by $\eta = -10 \log [(\Sigma Yi2/n]$

2.   Larger the better is given by $\eta = -10 \log [(\Sigma 1/Yi2)/ n]$

Where, η = Signal to Noise ratio, Yi = ith observed value of response, n = no. of observations in a trial, y = average of observed response.

3.2   ANOVA

The purpose of the analysis of variance (ANOVA) is to examine which design parameters significantly affect the quality characteristic. This is accomplished by separating the total variability of the S/N ratios, which is measured by the sum of the squared deviations from the total mean S/N ratio, into contributions by each of the parameters and the error.

4.   Result and Discussion

4.1   Optimum parameter selection from S/N ratio for UTS (N/mm²)

Ultimate Tensile Strength is larger-the-better type quality characteristic. Therefore higher values of Ultimate Tensile Strength are considered to be optimal. It is clear from Fig.3, that Ultimate Tensile Strength is highest at third level of welding current, first level of GFR and first level of WFR (A3B3C3).

4.2   Optimum parameter selection from S/N ratio for YS (N/mm²)

Yield Strength is larger-the-better type quality characteristic. Therefore higher values of yield strength are considered to be optimal. It is clear from Fig. 4, that Ultimate Tensile Strength is highest at third level of welding current, first level of GFR and first level of WFR (A3B2C3).

4.3   Optimum parameter selection from S/N ratio for % of elongation

% of elongation is smaller-the-better type quality characteristic. Therefore smaller values of % of elongation are considered to be optimal. It is clear from below Fig. 5, that % of elongation is highest at second level of welding current, first level of GFR and third level of WFR (A1B1C3).

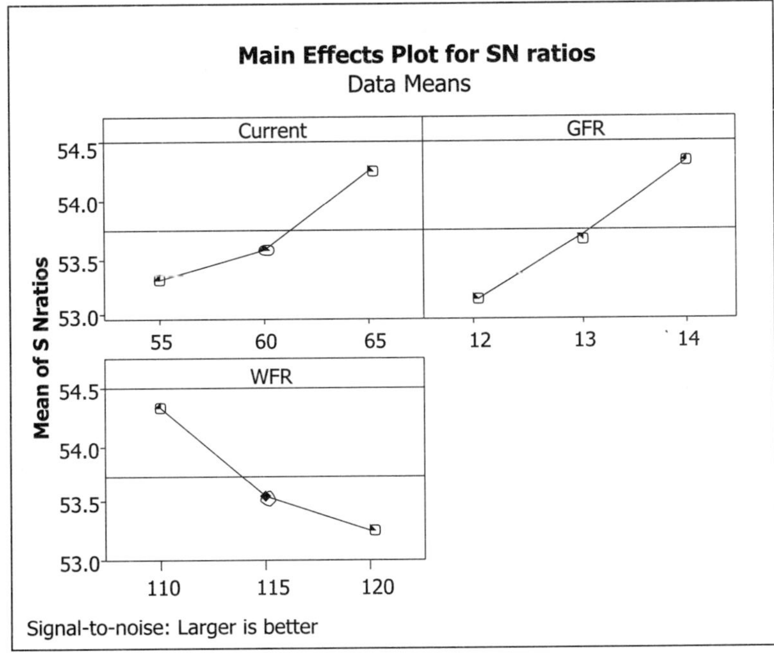

Response plot on UTS (N/mm²)

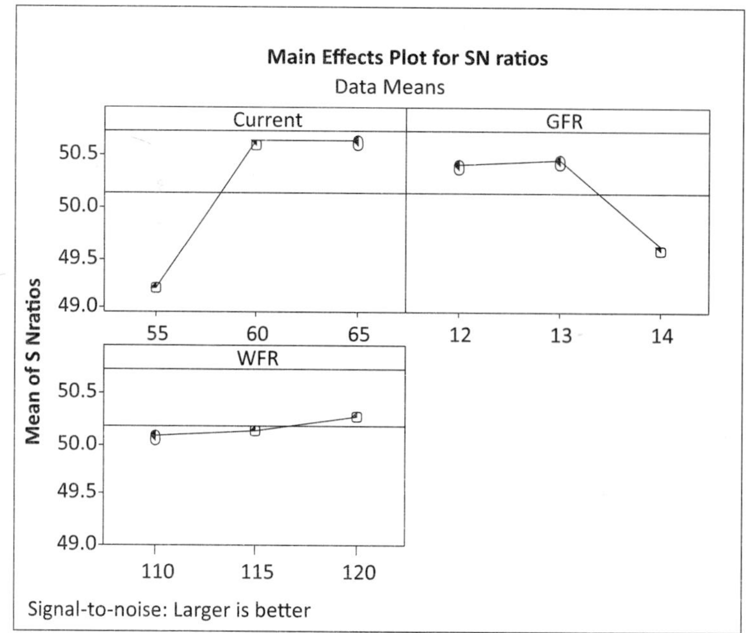

Response plot on YS (N/mm²)

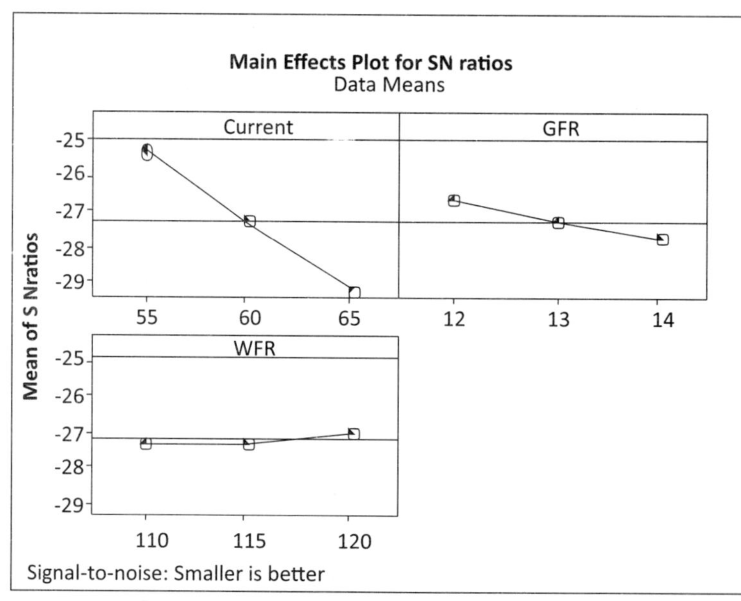

Response plot on % of Elongation

5.   CONCLUSION

In this present work the optimization of the process parameters of P-GMAW for SS 304 pipes with larger the better for UTS, YS and smaller the values with % of elongation have been reported. A Taguchi orthogonal array, the signal-to-noise (S/N) ratio and Analysis of Variance (ANOVA) were used for the optimization of welding parameters and it is found that i) optimum condition for maximum UTS is (A3B3C3) i.e. current = 65 amp, GFR = 14 LPM and WFR = 120 mm/min ii) optimum condition for maximum YS is (A3B2C3) i.e. current = 65 amp, GFR = 13 ltrs/min and WFR = 120 mm/min and iii) optimum condition for minimum % of elongation is (A1B1C3) i.e. current = 55 amp, GFR = 12 LPM and WFR = 120 mm/min . ANOVA for UTS shows that current is the most significant factor, followed by GFR. ANOVA for YS indicates that GFR influences most significantly, followed by current and ANOVA for % of elongation indicates that WFR influences most significantly. Conformation experiment was also conducted and verified the effectiveness of the Taguchi optimization method.

6.   Acknowledgement

The work reported in this paper is supported by P E S College of Engineering, Mandya-571401, through the Technical Education Quality Improvement Program [TEQIP-III] of the MHRD, Government of India.

7.   References

1.   S.V Sapakal, M.T. Telsang,(2012),Parametric optimization of MIG welding using Taguchi design method. Int. J. Adv. Eng. Res. Stud., pp. 28-30.

2.   A.K. Panday, M.I. Khan, K.M. Moeed, (2013), Optimization of resistance welding parameters using Taguchi method. Int. J. Eng. Sci. Tech., pp. 243-240.

3.   Kumar P, Roy DB, Parameters optimization for gas metal arc welding of austenitic stainless steel (AISI 304) and low carbon steel using Taguchi s technique, Int J Eng, 3:2250–0758.

4.   A. Hooda, A.i Dhingra and S. Sharma, (2012) , Optimization of welding process parameters to predict maximum yield strength in AISI 1040, Int. J. Mech. Eng. Robot. Res. India, pp. 204-212.

Acoustic and Refractive Behaviour of the Binary Mixture of 1-Butyl-3-methylimidazolium Tetrafluoroborate with 1-Alkanol at 298.15 to 313.15 K

Ankit Gupta, Vikas Singh Gangwar, Ashish Kumar Singh and Sandeep Kumar Singh*

Department of chemistry, VSSD College, Kanpur-208002 India.
*E-mail:dr.sksingh76@rediffmail.com

ABSTRACT

Densities, refractive indices and speeds of sound and their excess properties for 1-butyl-3-methylimidazolium tetrafluoroborate [Bmim][BF4] with 1-pentanoll over the entire range of mole fraction are reported at temperatures ranging from 298.15 K to 313.15 K and atmospheric pressure. Isentropic and excess isentropic compressibilities for ionic liquids with 1–alcohols were calculated from the experimental results. Deviation properties were further correlated using the Redlich-Kister polynomial. The measured speeds of sound were compared to the values obtained from Schaaffs' collision factor theory, Jacobson's intermolecular free length theory of solutions and Nomoto's relation. In addition, the experimentally obtained refractive indices were compared to the calculated values using Lorentz-Lorenz, Dale-Gladstone and Eykman mixing rules.

Keywords:, Density, Refractive index, speed of sound, ionic liquids, 1–alkanols, binary mixtures

1. Introduction

Ionic liquids (ILs) have recently emerged as environment friendly solvents for their use in the industrial manufacture of chemicals. In the past decade, ILs have been increasingly used for diverse applications such as organic synthesis, catalysis, electrochemical devices, and solvent extraction of a variety of compounds [1−4]. The interest in ILs was initiated because of their advantageous physico−chemical properties. ILs are composed of cations and anions having a low melting point. The physico−chemical properties of the ILs can be tuned by changing the cation or the anion. Thus, novel solvents can be formed and can be used for a specific application which cannot be done with the use of conventional organic solvents. The information regarding the thermo-physical properties of pure ILs as well as their mixtures with other compounds is essential for the design and development of equipment for commercial applications.[Bmim][BF4] is most efficient in the removal of dibenzothiophene (DBT) containing liquid fuels [5]. Pentanol is used as co-solvent in the petroleum industry to increase the selectivity and solvent power for extracting aromatic hydrocarbons.

The present work is aimed at studying the molecular interactions in the binary mixture of the IL 1-butyl-3-methylimidazolium tetrafluoroborate [Bmim][BF4] with 1-Alconol. Isentropic and excess isentropic compressibilities for ionic liquids with 1–alconols were calculated from the experimental results. Excess and deviation properties were further correlated using the Redlich-Kister polynomial [6]. The measured speeds of sound were compared to the values obtained from Schaaffs' collision factor theory(CFT) [7], Jacobson's intermolecular free length theory(FLT) [8] of solutions and Nomoto's relation (NR) [9]. In addition, the experimentally obtained refractive indices were compared to the calculated values using Lorentz-Lorenz [10], Dale-Gladstone [11] and Eykman mixing rules [12]. Experimental values and excess thermodynamic properties of IL systems allow researchers to draw information on the structure and interactions of liquid mixtures. The corresponding excess molar volume and excess isentropic compressibility and coefficients of thermal expansion were calculated. Furthermore, the Redlich and Kister (R–K) polynomial was used to obtain the coefficients and to estimate the standard deviations for the calculated excess and deviation properties. Moreover, the effect of the alkyl chain in ILs, chain length of 1–alkanol and the temperature on the excess and deviation properties are investigated.

2. Experimental

2.1 Materials

[Bmim][BF4] (mass fraction, 0.99) is procured from Merck, Germany, and is used without further purification. 1-Pentanol (mass fraction 0.97) is procured from Sigma-Aldrich, USA, and is purified by the fractional distillation method under reduced pressure. The water content is checked by conductometric titration with platinum electrode. The purity of the chemicals was ascertained by comparing the experimental values of density, refractive index and speed of sound, at temperatures T = (298.15 to 313.15) K with the literature.

2.2 Apparatus and Procedure

The binary mixture is prepared by weighing appropriate amounts of pure liquids on a digital electronic balance model Shimadzuax-200 with an uncertainty of $\pm$ $1 \cdot 10^{-4}$kg. Before each series of experiments, we calibrated the instrument at atmospheric pressure with doubly distilled water. The average uncertainty in the composition of the mixtures was estimated to be less than $\pm$0.0001.A crystal controlled variable path ultrasonic interferometer supplied by M/s Mittal enterprises (model-05F), New Delhi (India), operating at a frequency of 2 MHz was used in the ultrasonic measurements. The reported uncertainty is less than $\pm$ 3% which is the highest uncertainty found from all the data points. Refractive index was measured by Abbe refractometer (Agato 3T, Japan). Refractive index data were accurate to $\pm$0.0001units. The purity of chemicals used was confirmed by comparing the densities and ultrasonic speeds with those reported in the literature as shown in Table 1.The uncertainty in the density measurement was within $\pm$ 0.7 kg.m^{-3} (about 0.06%).The densities of the pure components and their mixtures were measured with the bi-capillary pyknometer. The liquid mixtures were prepared by mass in an air tight stopped bottle using an electronic balance model Shimadzuax-200 accurate to within $\pm$0.1 mg. Isentropic compressibility, k_s, were calculated from the relation,

$$k_s = u^{-2}\rho^{-1} \tag{1}$$

where ρ is the density and u is the ultrasonic velocity.

3. Results and Calculations

The experimental density, speed of sound, and refractive index values for binary systems of 1-butyl-3-methylimidazolium tetrafluoroborate with 1–pentanol are reported at T = (298.15 to 313.15) K and atmospheric pressure are listed in Table 2. The excess volume, V^E and excess isentropic compressibility values were calculated from the relation as;

$$V^E = \sum_{i=1}^{n} \frac{x_I M_I}{\rho} - \sum_{i=1}^{n} \frac{x_I M_I}{\rho} \text{ and } k_s^E = k_s - k_s^{idl} \tag{2}$$

where, $k_s^{idl} = k_s x_1 + k_s x_2$ $\tag{3}$

and volume fractions, Φ were calculated from the relation; $\Phi = \dfrac{x_i V_I}{\sum_{i=1}^{n} x_i V_I}$ $\tag{4}$

The dependency of V^E on composition is shown in figure 1 where all V^E values are negative for all systems under study and this is due to the interstitial accommodation of ILs into alkanols structure [13]. The negative V^E trend reflects the formation of hydrogen bonded hetero associations and the dissociation of alkanol structure as the chain length increases. This is conformed from the previously reported studies [2,3,5]. In addition as expected, V^E becomes less negative as the temperature increases for ILs with 1–propanol. The excess isentropic compressibility values k_s^E were calculated from relations by Benson et al. [14] where κ_s^{id} is the isentropic compressibility of the ideal solution, κ_s is the isentropic compressibility and it is calculated using the Laplace–Newton $V = 1/u^2\rho$ where the relation is judged to be valid and therefore the speed of sound may be regarded as a thermodynamic quantity. The excess isentropic compressibility are negative for the system under study and exhibited a similar trend as the excess volume (see figure 2) while κ^E becomes more negative as the temperature increases as shown in Table 2. which suggest the dominance of interstitial of accommodation of the components effect over the dissociation effect. The calculated excess properties were fitted to the Redlich-Kister (R–K) polynomial equation Schaaff's Collision Factor Theory (CFT), Jacobson's Free Length Theory (FLT) and Nomoto's relation (NR) [7-9] were used to predict the speed of sound (u_m) for 1-Butyl-3- methylimidazolium Tetrafluoroborate + 1-Pentanol binary systems. The critical temperatures for the pure ILs were predicted using available surface tension data [15] since they are needed for CFT,

$$u = u_\infty \sum_{i=1}^n \frac{(x_i s_i)\left(\sum_{i=1}^n x_i B_i\right)}{V} \tag{5}$$

where $u_\infty = 1600 \ \mathrm{m \cdot s^{-1}}$, S_i and B_i are the space filling factor and the actual volume of the molecule per mole of pure component i in the mixture. Jacobson's Free Length Theory(FLT) can be expressed as;

$$u = \frac{K}{L_f \rho^{1/2}} \tag{6}$$

where K is the Jacobson's constant and $L_{f,m}$ is the intermolecular free length of the binary mixture and Nomoto's relation as;

$$u = \left[\frac{\sum_{i=1}^n (x_i u_i)}{\sum_{i=1}^n (x_i V_i)}\right]3 \tag{7}$$

In addition, Lorentz-Lorenz (L–L), Dale-Gladstone (D–G) and Eykman (Eyk) mixing rules [10-12] were used to predict refractive indices for studied system. They are given as;

$$\frac{n^2-1}{n^2+2} = \sum_{i=1}^n \varnothing\left[\frac{n^2-1}{n^2+2}\right]; \ n-1 = \sum_{i=1}^n [\varnothing_i(n-1)]; \ \frac{n^2-1}{n^2+0.4} = \sum_{i=1}^n \varnothing_i\left[\frac{n^2-1}{n^2+0.4}\right] \tag{8}$$

The comparison shows that Nomoto's relation for predicting speed of sound is the best among the relations used in the case of 1-Butyl-3- methylimidazolium Tetrafluoroborate + 1-Pentanol while both Nomoto's and Schaaff's Collision Factor Theory are also comparable. As for the refractive index mixing rules, all rules used showed good agreement with the experimental data for the system under study.

4.   Conclusion

Density, speed of sound and refractive index and their excess or deviation properties of ILs with 1–pentanol binary mixtures have been reported at different temperatures and atmospheric pressure. Although ILs show stronger hydrogen bonding with 1–pentanol than conventional solvents. Prediction of the speed of sound can be obtained using Nomoto's relation and Schaaff's Collision Factor Theory while refractive index can be predicted using Lorentz-Lorenz, Dale-Gladstone and Eykman mixing rules for systems containing ionic liquids. In addition, The calculations showed a systematic dependence of excess and deviation properties on the chain length and on temperature for all investigated mixtures.

Table 1. Comparison of Experimental Density (ρ_{exp}), Refractive Index (n_{exp}) and Speed of Sound (u_{exp}) of Pure Components with Literature (lit) Values at Temperatures from T = (298.15 to 313.15) K

Components	T/K	ρ/kg·m^{-3}		n		u/m·sec^{-1}	
1-butyl-3-ethylimidazolium tetrafluoroborate	298.15	1198.78	1200.57[b]	1.42058	1.4197[e]	1565.09	1565.1
	303.15	1195.18	1196.98	1.41913	1.4181	1553.15	1552.6
	308.15	1191.60	1194.2	1.41764	1.4166	1541.35	1540.3
	313.15	1188.04	1189.86	1.41621	1.4155	1529.69	1528.3
1-pentanol	298.15	811.00	81099	1.408	1.40784	1276	1275.4
	303.15	807	80711	1.407	1.4065	1259	1262
	308.15	803	8036	1.406	1.4047	1242	1245
	313.15	800	7999	1.404	1.40178	1226	1228

Table 2. Experimental Density (ρ_{exp}), Refractive Index (n_{exp}), and Speed of Sound (u_{exp}) and values obtained from theoretical models (u_{Sch}, u_{Nom}, u_{Jacob} & n_{L-L}, n_{D-G}, n_{Eykman}) and Isentropic Compressibility (k_s) of Binary Liquid Mixtures of 1-Butyl-3- methylimidazolium Tetrafluoroborate + 1-Pentanol T = (298.15 to 313.15) K

x_1	ρ_{exp}/kg·m^{-3}	n_{exp}	u_{exp}/m·sec^{-1}	u_{Sch}/m·sec^{-}	u_{Nom}/m·sec^{-}	u_{Jacob}/m·sec^{-}	n_{L-L}	n_{D-G}	n_{Eykman}	k_s/TPa^{-1}
					298.15K					
0.1045	889.12	1.4083	1287.2	307.6	1267.2	1297.1	1.4080	1.4074	1.4087	395.47
0.2036	903.24	1.4093	1312.5	332.2	1291.2	1304.1	1.4089	1.4082	1.4093	382.74
0.3044	951.23	1.4117	1350.2	1370.2	1331.4	1321.5	1.4113	1.4093	1.4099	372.48
0.4062	978.12	1.4127	1386.2	401.5	1361.5	1341.2	1.4126	1.4099	1.4113	364.36
0.4946	1004.5	1.4143	1420.5	440.2	1401.2	1358.5	1.4141	1.4121	1.4127	358.83
0.6071	1021.34	1.4151	1425.2	461.2	1411.4	1401.2	1.4149	1.4132	1.4139 .	353.01
0.6973	1056.15	1.4163	1465.7	467.5	1481.2	1445.5	1.4151	1.4136	1.4146	349.19
0.7830	1098.23	1.4189	1501.2	488.8	1500.1	1496.2	1.4182	1.4156	1.4171	345.71
0.9106	1102.13	1.4202	1557.2	525.4	1537.5	1522.1	1.4191	1.4172	1.4183	342.15

					303.15K					
0.1045	882.12	1.4081	1296.1	1301.2	1271.5	1290.2	1.4076	1.4074	1.4084	406.17
0.2036	893.12	1.4089	1333.4	1357.4	1297.1	1330.3	1.4083	1.4079	1.4088	392.47
0.3044	947.12	1.4111	1371.2	1381.2	1335.4	1362.3	1.4094	1.4083	1.4089	381.43
0.4062	974.13	1.4122	1400.6	1421.5	1389.7	1381.5	1.4099	1.4091	1.4107	372.67
0.4946	1000.50	1.4131	1406.5	1431.2	1400.2	1396.7	1.4111	1.4101	1.4113	366.80
0.6071	1018.60	1.4146	1437.2	1451.4	1411.5	1407.5	1.4136	1.4117	1.4123	360.47
0.6973	1051.04	1.4158	1472.5	1492.5	1461.3	1467.9	1.4148	1.4132	1.4137	356.20
0.7830	1093.15	1.4173	1501.2	1521.8	1489.3	1491.2	1.4167	1.4146	1.4172	352.62
0.9106	1098.21	1.4182	1536.3	1539.3	1517.8	1527.7	1.4178	1.4163	1.4177	348.60
					308.15K					
0.1045	872.20	1.4078	1270.2	1296.5	1251.4	1281.3	1.4074	1.4073	1.4082	417.36
0.2036	890.12	1.4086	1306.4	1322.4	1283.2	1336.4	1.4089	1.4082	1.4088	402.64
0.3044	936.04	1.4096	1341.2	1366.5	1317.5	1342.2	1.4091	1.4099	1.4097	390.76
0.4062	971.02	1.4111	1370.2	1390.2	1347.4	1367.5	1.4078	1.4107	1.4120	381.33
0.4946	997.30	1.4118	1391.6	1413.7	1368.2	1376.4	1.4112	1.4111	1.4109	374.84
0.6071	1011.41	1.4131	1421.6	1441.5	1392.2	1393.2	1.4123	1.4129	1.4121	368.10
0.6973	1034.12	1.4137	1452.8	1468.5	1411.3	1417.3	1.4129	1.4130	1.4133	363.45
0.7830	1046.17	1.4140	1489.2	1489.2	1427.5	1421.2	1.4138	1.4131	1.4144	359.34
0.9106	1088.04	1.4162	1521.2	1521.2	1459.4	1489.4	1.4154	1.4152	1.4172	355.04
					313.15K					
0.1045	861.12	1.4074	1276.1	1276.1	1236.4	1276.2	1.4074	1.4070	1.4080	428.90
0.2036	889.16	1.4082	1310.2	1310.2	1270.2	1286.4	1.4079	1.4076	1.4088	413.10
0.3044	932.12	1.4091	1347.5	1347.5	1301.4	1301.2	1.4092	1.4081	1.4093	400.33
0.4062	969.13	1.4098	1372.3	1372.3	1327.2	1333.4	1.4096	1.4099	1.4112	390.18
0.4946	994.02	1.4101	1394.2	1394.2	1347.5	1351.5	1.4101	1.4107	1.4117	383.16
0.6071	995.14	1.4111	1420.4	1420.4	1381.9	1389.2	1.4117	1.4123	1.4123	375.88
0.6973	1006.12	1.4123	1451.4	1451.4	1411.2	1411.3	1.4117	1.4134	1.4136	370.85
0.7830	1036.11	1.4132	1496.5	1496.5	1449.5	1437.2	1.4130	1.4133	1.4141	366.50
0.9106	1083.12	1.4141	1530.2	1530.2	1489.3	1491.4	1.4142	1.4149	1.4162	361.70

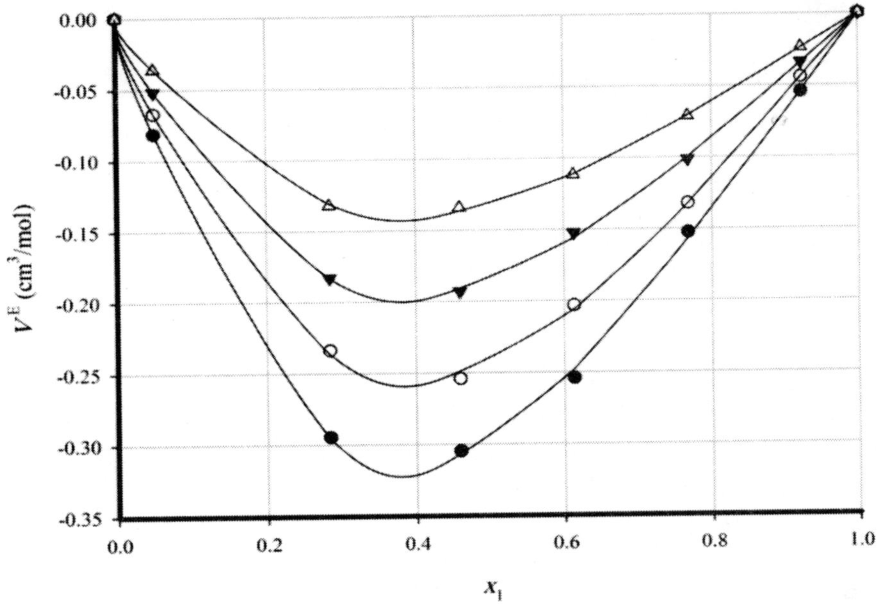

Figure 1 Excess molar volumes, V^E, as a function of x_1 for {x [Bmim][BF4] + (1 − x) 1-pentanol} binary mixtures, at T = 298K (●),303K (o), 308K (▼) and 313K (Δ).

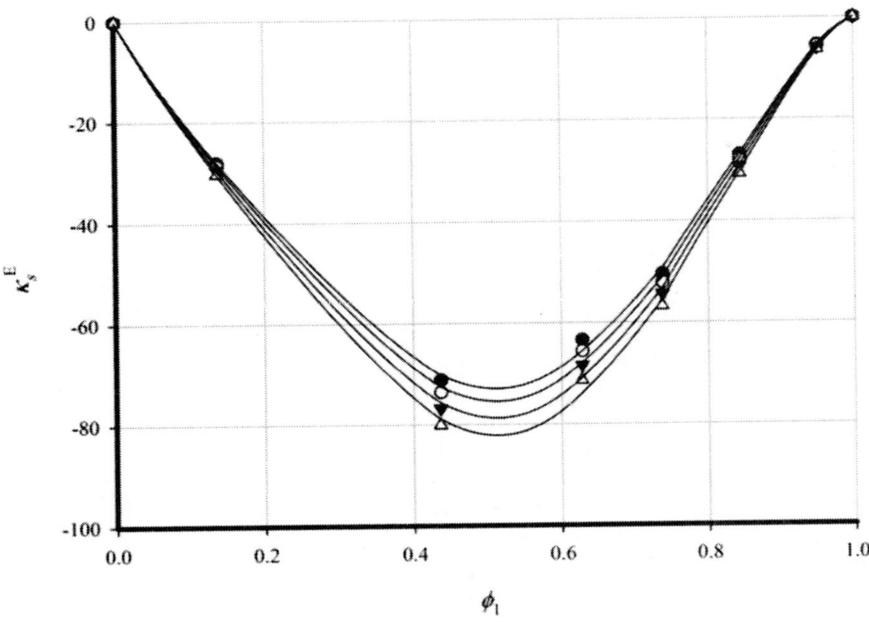

Figure 2 Excess isentropic compressibility, k_s^E as a function of f_1 for {x [Bmim][BF4] + (1 − x) 1-pentanol } binary mixtures, at T = 298K (●),303K (o), 308K (▼), 313K (Δ).

5.   Acknowledgements

The authors are very thankful to the department of chemistry, for their cooperation and help.

6.   References

1.   H. Shekaari, S. M. Sedighehnaz, Fluid Phase Equilib. 291 (2010) 201–207.

2.   J.-Y. Wang, F.-Y. Zhao, Y. Min Liu, X.-L. Wang, Y.-Q. Hu, Fluid Phase Equilib. 305 (2011) 114–120.

3.   P. F. Requejo, E. J. Gonzalez, E. A. Macedo, A. J. Dominguez, Chem. Thermodyn. 74 (2014) 193-200.

4.   A. B. Pereiro, A. Rodiguez, J. Chem. Eng. Data 52 (2007) 600–608.

5.   U. Domanska, A. Pobudkowska, A. Wisniewska, J. Solution Chem. 35 (2006) 311- 334.

6.   O. Redlich, A. T. Kister, Ind. Eng. Chem. 40 (1948) 345-348.

7.   W. Schaffs. Molekularakustich; Springer-Verlag, Berlin 1963, (Chapters. XI and XII).

8.   B. Jacobson, Acta. Chem. Scand. 8 (1952) 1485-1498. [36] B. Jacobson, J. Chem. Phys. 20 (1952) 927- 928.

9.   O. Nomoto, J. Phys. Soc. 13 (1958) 1528-1532.

10.   L. Lorentz, Weid. Ann. 11 (1880) 70-75.

11.   J. H. Gladstone, T. P. Dale, Philos. Trans. 153 (1863) 317-343.

12.   J. F. Eykman, Reel. Trao. Chim Pays-Bas 14 (1895) 185-188.

13.   T. M. Letcher, U. Domanska, E. Mwenesongole, Fluid Phase Equilib. 149 (1998) 323– 337.

14.   G. C. Benson, O. Kiyohara, J. Chem. Thermodyn. 11 (1979) 1061-1064.

15.   M. S. AlTuwaim, K. H. A. E. Alkhaldi, A. S. Al–Jimaz, A. A. Mohammad, J. Chem. Eng. Data 59 (2014) 1955–1963.

DRD2 TaqI A Polymorphism in Eastern Uttar Pradesh Population

Amrita Chaudhary, Upendra Yadav, Pradeep Kumar, Vandana Rai*

Human Molecular Genetics Laboratory, Department of Biotechnology, VBS Purvanchal University, Jaunpur-222003, India
**E-mail: raivandana@rediffmail.com*

ABSTRACT

Dopamine receptor D2 (DRD2) encoded by DRD2 gene, is located on chromosome 11q22-23. Dopamine plays the central role in motivation, cognition, and reward seeking behaviour. Its dysfunction is implicated in numerous neurological and psychiatric disorders including drug abuse, schizophrenia, ADHD etc. The TaqI A polymorphism is localized 9.8 kb downstream from DRD2 gene in exon 8 of protein kinase gene (ANKK1). It is a SNP demonstrated to cause Glutamate to Lysine substitution at 713 amino acid residue in putative binding domain of ANKK1. Due to the central role of dopamine in reward seeking behavior, DRD2 TaqI A loci is a suitable candidate for investigation of molecular basis of addiction. The aim of the present study is to evaluate the frequency of DRD2 TaqI A polymorphism in Eastern Uttar Pradesh population. 3ml blood samples were collected from 50 individuals randomly selected from Eastern UP. Written informed consent along with profile detail was taken from each subject prior to blood sample collection. DRD2 TaqI A polymorphism analysis was done by PCR-RFLP method.

Genomic DNA was extracted from each collected blood samples and amplified using DRD2 Taq1 region specific primers. PCR amplification produced 310bp long amplicon which was digested with Taq 1 enzyme for polymorphism analysis. In case of A2 allele, Taq1 enzyme cleaved 310bp long fragment into two fragments of 180bp and 130bp. In case of A1 allele, a C to T substitution demolished the restriction site of Taq1, so amplicon of A1 allele remained uncut. In total 50 sample analyzed in present study, A2/A2, A2/A1 and A1/A1 genotype were found in 12, 32 and 06 samples respectively. The genotypic frequencies of mutant homozygous (A1/A1) is 0.12, heterozygous (A2/A1) is 0.64 and normal homozygous (A2/A2) is 0.24. The allelic frequency of A1 is 0.44 and of A2 is 0.56. In conclusion, the results of present study suggests that in TaqI A polymorphism of DRD2 gene, the frequency of allele A2 is higher than that of A1 allele in population of Eastern Uttar Pradesh.

Keywords: Dopamine D2 receptor, gene polymorphism, dopamine, PCR-RFLP, psychiatric disorders.

1. Introduction

One of the most important system intervening reward mechanisms is considered to be dopaminergic pathways. Dopaminergic neurons are present in VTA of midbrain, projected into nucleus accumbens and ventral striatum [1] All the genes, involved in regulating the assembly of this system in brain is of great interest and can be a suitable candidate for investigation of molecular basis of addiction and several other psychiatric disorders [2]. Among these, the gene of interest that effect the dopaminergic neurotransmission is the Dopamine D2 receptor (DRD2) gene that is located at chromosome 11q22-23 encoding a G- Protein coupled receptor (Gi -inhibitory G protein) in post synaptic neurons [3] performing dual function of inhibitory auto receptor and a post synaptic receptors [4].

Several polymorphisms are reported in DRD2 gene (Taq1 B, Taq1D, -141 Ins/Del, Ser-Cys(S311C) but Taq1 A polymorphism is well studied in different psychiatric disorders including schizophrenia [5], depression [6], bipolar disorder [7], ADHD [8], and PTSD [9] and drug abuse [3]. TaqI A is SNP (rs1800497) located 9.8 kb downstream of DRD2 gene within exon 8 of functionally unrelated neighbouring gene, Ankyrin repeat and kinase domain containing-1(ANKK1). It causes Glutamate to Lysine substitution at 713 amino acid residue in putative binding domain of ANKK1 [10] with two alleles attributed as A1 and A2. This polymorphism leads to alteration of the activity of promoter region of DRD2 gene and also the expression of D2-type receptors [11]. Individuals with A1A1 genotype have approximately 49% reduced number of dopamine receptors than to those without A1. Less number of DRD2 receptors in nucleus accumbens and striatum increases craving for alcohol. Hence, the aim of present study is to determine the frequency of DRD2 TaqIA polymorphism in Eastern Uttar Pradesh population.

2.   Materials and Methods

All 50 participants were recruited from Eastern Uttar Pradesh (Jaunpur) population, informed written consent was taken from each participants. Prior blood sample collection clearance certificate was taken from the Institutional Ethics Committee of VBS Purvanchal University, Jaunpur.

3.   Genotyping

3 ml blood was drawn from each individual and genomic DNA was isolated by the method of Bartlett and White [12]. Polymerase chain reaction (PCR) based genotyping was done by using gene specific primers according to the method of Grandy et al. [13]. The reaction conditions were enlisted in table 1. Restriction Taq1 enzyme digested products were separated on 2% agarose gel with 100 bp marker.

Table 1. Representing gene, PCR primers, annealing temperature, time, and restriction enzyme used.

Gene	SNP	Primers	Annealing temp/time	Amplicon size	Restriction enzyme/ method used
DRD2	Taq1A	Forward: 5'- CGTCGACGGCTGGCCAAGTTGTCTA-3' Reverse: 5'-CCGTCGACCCTTCCTGAGTGTCATCA- 3'	62°C/1 mins	310-bp	Taq1/RFLP

4.   Statistical Analysis

Allele frequency was determined by gene counting method.

5.   Results and Discussion

PCR amplification produced 310 bp long amplicon, which after digestion with TaqI produced 180bp and 130 bp long fragments in case of normal C allele (A2) and mutant T allele (A1) remain uncut after TaqI digestion (Fig. 1 and 2).

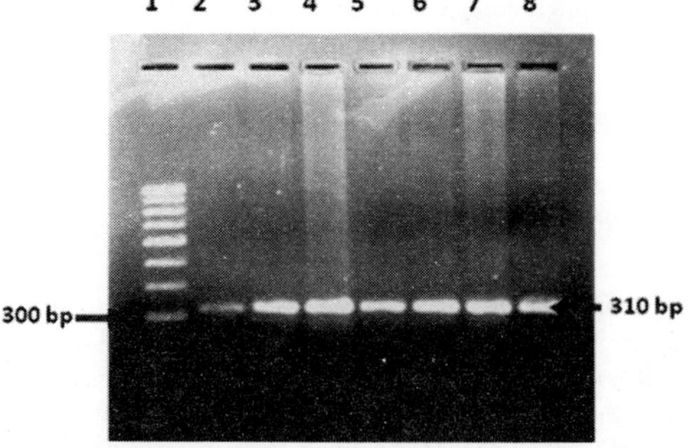

Figure 1. Agarose gel showing amplicon of 310 bp and 100-bp ladder in lane 1

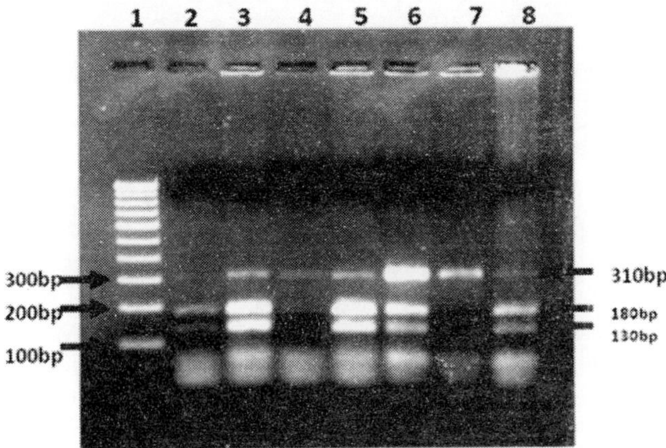

Figure 2. Restriction digestion of amplicon by TaqI with 100 bp marker in lane 1.

In total 50 samples analyzed, normal homozygous genotype was found in 12, heterozygous genotype was observed in 32 and mutant homozygous genotype was observed in 6 individuals. The C and T allele were found as 0.56 and 0.44 respectively (Table 2).

Table 2. Genotype and allele frequency distribution in studied subjects.

DRD2 gene SNP	Genotype Number (%)			Allele Number (Frequency)	
	CC	CT	TT	C	T
Taq1A(rs1800497)	12 (24%)	32 (64%)	6(12%)	56(0.56)	44 (0.44)

Four alleles (genetic variants) are reported at Taq1A locus referred to as A1 A2, A3 and A4. Where A2 is the most common form and A3 and A4 are the rare variants [14]. DRD2gene Taq1A polymorphism was very well studied in world's different populations [3, 5, 9, 15, 16] as well as in different Indian regions [17-27]. Various studies reported presence of A1 allele is significantly higher in certain drug of abuse such as alcoholism and other behavioural characteristics as well [28]. Here our report suggests that there is higher frequency of A2 allele in Jaunpur population. Our study is co-related with numerous studies from India where they also reported higher frequency of A2 allele in control population. Juyal et al. [26] studied South and North Indian population, worked on Parkinsons disease reported frequency of A2 allele to be 0.66 and A1 allele to be 0.33 in their control group. One other study of Kumudini et al. [29] studied South Indian population also found nearly the same result. They reported 0.68, A2 allele frequency and 0.31 A1 allele frequencies. However, few reports are also available that shows the higher frequency of A1 allele in control group. The report of Vijayan et al. [25] indicates the A2 allelic frequency is 0.34 and A1 allele is 0.65. Various international studies also report the higher prevalence of A2 allele in their control group. Alfimova et al. [5] stated A2 allele frequency to be of 0.80 and A1 allele to be of 0.19 in Moscow population. Another study on PTSD of Voisey et al. [15] of Australia studied control Caucasians reported A2 allele frequency 0.82 and A1 allelic frequency 0.17. Despite contradictory results were indicated by a study of China by Lee et al. [16] worked on Tourette syndrome explored control group and reported 0.47 A2 allele frequency and 0.52 A1 allele frequency. Hence, these findings showing the variations in the allelic frequency suggest that prevalence of higher A2 allelic frequency can be population specific.

6.   References

1.   Matosic, A., Marusic, S., Vidrih, B., Kovak-Mufic, A., Cicin-Sain, L.: Neurobiological bases of alcohol addiction. Acta Clin Croat 55(1), 134-50 (2016).

2.   Ma, Y., Yuan, W., Jiang, X, Cui, W.Y., Li, M.D.: Updated findings of the association and functional studies of DRD2/ANKK1 variants with addictions. Mol Neurobiol 51(1), 281-99 (2015).

3.   Panduro, A., Ramos-Lopez, O., Campollo, O., Zepeda-Carrillo, E.A., Gonzalez-Aldaco, K., Torres-Valadez, R., Roman, S.: High frequency of the DRD2/ANKK1 A1 allele in Mexican Native Amerindians and Mestizos and its association with alcohol consumption. Drug Alcohol Depend 172, 66-72 (2017).

4.   Tunbridge, E. M., Narajos, M., Harrison, C. H., Beresford, C., Cipriani, A., & Harrison, P. J.: Which dopamine polymorphisms are functional? Systematic review and meta-analysis of COMT, DAT, DBH, DDC, DRD1–5, MAOA, MAOB, TH, VMAT1, and VMAT2. Biological Psychiatry. (2019). doi:10.1016/j.biopsych.2019.05.014

5.   Alfimova, M. V., Golimbet, V. E., Korovaitseva, G. I., Lezheiko, T. V., Tikhonov, D. V., Ganisheva, T. K., Berezin, N.B., Snegireva, A.A., Shemyakina, T. K.: The role of the interaction between the NMDA and dopamine receptor genes in impaired recognition of emotional expression in schizophrenia. Neurosci. Behavior. Physiol. 49(1), 153–158 (2019).

6.   Hayden, E. P., Klein, D. N., Dougherty, L. R., Olino, T. M., Laptook, R. S., Dyson, M. W., Bufferd, S.J., Durbin, E., Sheikh, H.I., Singh, S. M.: The dopamine D2 receptor gene and depressive and anxious symptoms in childhood: associations and evidence for gene–environment correlation and gene–environment interaction. Psychiatric Genetics 20(6), 304–310 (2010).

7.   Hu, M.C., Lee, S.Y., Wang, T.Y., Chang, Y.H., Chen, S.L., Chen, S.H., Chu, C.H., Wang, C.L., Lee, I.H., Chen, P.S., Yang, Y.K., Lu, R.B.: Interaction of DRD2TaqI, COMT, and ALDH2 genes associated with bipolar II disorder comorbid with anxiety disorders in Han Chinese in Taiwan. Metab Brain Dis 30(3), 755-65 (2015).

8.   Sery, O., Drtilkova, I., Theiner, P., Pitelova, R., Staif, R., Znojil, V., Lochman, J., Didden, W.: Polymorphism of DRD2 gene and ADHD. Neuro Endocrinol Lett 27(1-2), 236-40 (2006).

9.   Xiao, Y., Liu, D., Liu, K., Wu, C., Zhang, H., Niu, Y., & Jiang, X.: Association of DRD2, 5-HTTLPR, and 5-HTTVNTR gene polymorphisms with posttraumatic stress disorder in tibetan adolescents: a case–control study. Biolog. Res. Nurs. 21(3), 286–295 (2019).

10.   Pan, Y.Q., Qiao, L., Xue, X.D., Fu, J.H.: Association between ANKK1 (rs1800497) polymorphism of DRD2 gene and attention deficit hyperactivity disorder: a meta-analysis. Neurosci Lett 590, 101-5 (2015).

11.   Marinho, V., Oliveira, T., Bandeira, J., Pinto, G.R., Gomes, A., Lima, V., Magalhaes, F., Rocha, K., Ayres, C., Carvalho, V., Velasques, B., Ribeiro, P., Orsini, M., Bastos, V.H., Gupta, D., Teixeira, S.: Genetic influence alters the brain synchronism in perception and timing. J Biomed Sci 25(1), 61 (2018).

12.   Bartlett, J.M., and White, A., Extraction of DNA from blood. In: Bartlett, J.M., Stirling, D., (eds.) Methods in Molecular Biology. PCR Protocols. 2nd ed., vol. 226. Totowa, NJ: Humana Press Inc. (2003).

13.   Grandy, D.K., Zhang, Y., Civelli, O.: PCR detection of the TaqA RFLP at the DRD2 locus. Hum Mol Genet 2(12), 2197 (1993).

14.   Blum, K., Cull, J. G., Braverman, E. R., & Comings D. E. : Reward deficiency syndrome. American Scientist 84(2), 132-145 (1996a).

15.   Voisey, J., Swagell, C.D., Hughes, I.P., Morris, C.P., van Daal, A,. Noble, E.P., Kann, B., Heslop, K.A., Young, R.M., Lawford, B.R.: The DRD2 gene 957C>T polymorphism is associated with posttraumatic stress disorder in war veterans. Depress Anxiety 26(1), 28-33 (2009).

16.   Lee, C.C., Chou, I.C., Tsai, C.H., Wang, T.R., Li, T.C., Tsai, F.J.: Dopamine receptor D2 gene polymorphisms are associated in Taiwanese children with Tourette syndrome. Pediatr Neurol 33(4), 272-6 (2005).

17.   Kaur, G., Chavan, B.S., Gupta, D., Sinhmar, V., Prasad, R., Tripathi, A., Garg, P.D., Gupta, R., Khurana, H., Gautam, S., Margoob, M.A., Aneja, J.: An association study of dopaminergic (DRD2) and serotoninergic (5-HT2) gene polymorphism and schizophrenia in a North Indian population. Asian J Psychiatry 39, 178-184 (2019).

18.   Roy, S., Pal, P., Ghosh, S., Bhattacharya, S., Das, S.K., Gangopadhyay, P.K., Bavdekar, A., Ray, K., Sengupta, M., Ray, J.: Potential Role of Brain-Derived Neurotrophic Factor and Dopamine Receptor D2 Gene Variants as Modifiers for the Susceptibility and Clinical Course of Wilson's Disease. Neuromolecular Med 20(3), 401-408 (2018).

19. Quraishi, R., Jain, R., Mishra, A.K., Ambekar, A.: Association of ankyrin repeats & kinase domain containing 1 (ANKK1) gene polymorphism with co-morbid alcohol & nicotine dependence: A pilot study from a tertiary care treatment centre in north India. Indian J Med Res 145(1), 33-38 (2017).

20. Suraj Singh, H., Ghosh, P.K., Saraswathy, K.N.: DRD2 and ANKK1 gene polymorphisms and alcohol dependence: a case-control study among a Mendelian population of East Asian ancestry. Alcohol Alcohol 48(4), 409-14 (2013).

21. Bhaskar, L.V., Thangaraj, K., Non, A.L., Singh, L., Rao, V.R.: Population-based case-control study of DRD2 gene polymorphisms and alcoholism. J Addict Dis 29(4), 475-80 (2010).

22. Prasad, P., Ambekar, A., Vaswani, M.: Dopamine D2 receptor polymorphisms and susceptibility to alcohol dependence in Indian males: a preliminary study. BMC Med Genet 11, 24 (2010).

23. Srivastava, V., Deshpande, S.N., Thelma, B.K.: Dopaminergic pathway gene polymorphisms and genetic susceptibility to schizophrenia among north Indians. Neuropsychobiology 61(2), 64–70 (2010).

24. Prasad, P., Kumar, K.M., Ammini, A.C., Gupta, A., Gupta, R., Thelma, B.K.: Association of dopaminergic pathway gene polymorphisms with chronic renal insufficiency among Asian Indians with type-2 diabetes. BMC Genet 9, 26 (2008).

25. Vijayan, N.N., Bhaskaran, S., Koshy, L.V., Natarajan, C., Srinivas, L., Nair, C.M., Allencherry, P.M., Banerjee, M.: Association of dopamine receptor polymorphisms with schizophrenia and antipsychotic response in a South Indian population. Behav Brain Funct 3, 34 (2007).

26. Juyal, R.C., Das, M., Punia, S., Behari, M., Nainwal, G., Singh, S., Swaminath, P.V., Govindappa, S.T., Jayaram, S., Muthane, U.B., Thelma, B.K.: Genetic susceptibility to parkinson's disease among south and north Indians: I. Role of polymorphisms in dopamine receptor and transporter genes and association of DRD4 120-bp duplication marker. Neurogenetics 7(4), 223-9 (2006).

27. Shaikh, K.J., Naveen, D., Sherrin, T., Murthy, A., Thennarasu, K., Anand, A., Benegal, V., Jain, S.: Polymorphisms at the DRD2 locus in early-onset alcohol dependence in the Indian population. Addict Biol 6(4), 331-335 (2001).

28. Blum, K., Sheridan, P.J., Wood, R.C., Braverman, E.R., Chen, T.J., Cull, J.G., Comings, D.E.: The D2 dopamine receptor gene as a determinant of reward deficiency syndrome. J R Soc Med 89(7), 396-400 (1996b).

29. Kumudini, N., Umai, A., Devi, Y.P., Naushad, S.M., Mridula, R., Borgohain, R., Kutala, V.K.: Impact of COMT H108L, MAOB int 13 A>G and DRD2 haplotype on the susceptibility to Parkinson's disease in South Indian subjects. Indian J Biochem Biophys 50(5), 436-41 (2013).

Elastic and Ultrasonic Investigations on Hafnium Based Compounds

Jyoti Bala[1,*] Arvind Kumar Tiwari[2] and Devraj Singh[3,4]

[1] University School of Information, Communication & Technology, Guru Gobind Singh Indraprastha University, New Delhi–110078, India
[2]Department of Physics, B.S.N.V.P.G.College Lucknow-226001, India
[3]Department of Applied Physics, Amity School of Engineering & Technology Delhi, Noida-201313, India
[4]Department of Physics, AIAS, Amity University Uttar Pradesh, Noida-201313, India
*E-mail: jyoti_pu@yahoo.com

ABSTRACT

We have investigated and evaluated the higher order elastic constants, ultrasonic and thermo-physical properties of hafnium based compounds HfX(X=Os, Ir and Pt) at 27°C temperature using Hiki approach. The second order elastic constants have been applied to calculate the mechanical properties such as Young's modulus, bulk modulus, Lame modulus, shear modulus, tetragonal modulus, Poisson's ratio, Zener anisotropy factor, Pugh's indicator etc. The chosen materials have shown the ductile nature. Further elastic constants have been applied to compute ultrasonic velocities for longitudinal and shear modes. We have also evaluated thermal conductiv ity, Debye velocity and thermal relaxation time at 27°C temperature. Finally ultrasonic attenuation has been estimated due to phonon-phonon interaction and thermoelastic relaxation mechanisms. We found that HfOs is strongest and most fit material for crystallographic study among other hafnium based compounds due to its high valued elastic constants and mechanical properties. The obtained results were discussed for the chosen materials for their future prospects.

Keywords: Elastic property, thermal property, ultrasonic property.

1.   Introduction

The halfnium compounds have wide applications in medical field due to their excellent mechanical and corrosion properties [1-2]. Most of the hafnium based compounds exhibit B2 crystalline structure. Various nvestigations have been performed on hafnium based compounds to carried out the study of electronic structure, structural phase stabilities in the B2 phase using ab-initio studies [3-9]. Out of which Iyigör et al. [10] explained structural, electronic, elastic and vibrational properties of HfX (X = Rh, Ru and Tc) compounds. Arıkana [11] carried out the elastic and phonon properties of HfOs using first-principles method. In the available literature, we did not find temperature and orientation dependent theoretical work on the thermal and ultrasonic properties of these compounds. Due to limited theoretical studies on these compounds we motivated to make new analysis on these materials. In present work we evaluate temperature dependent study on the elastic, ultrasonic and thermal properties of hafnium based compounds HfX(X=Rh, Pd, Ag) with respect to different orientations. Also, we investigated the mechanical and thermophysical properties of hafnium based compounds. Finally the ultrasonic attenuation for hafnium based compounds was computed at 27°C temperature by means of the computed parameters.

2.   Computational Approach

In present investigation, we have followed Hiki theoretical approach [12-13] to calculate higher order elastic constants outlined by Brugger's potential model. The obtained value of SOECs have been used to find out the mechanical constants such as bulk modulus (B), shear or rigidity modulus (G), Young's modulus (Y), Poisson's ratio (σ), Lame modulus (λ), Hardness (H), Pugh's indicator (B/G) and Zener's anisotropy factor (A)) at 27°C temperature using the expressions as given in literature [14]. In the cubic structured material, the ultrasonic velocities are function of SOECs and density[15]. The Debye average velocity and Debye temperature are related to constituent velocities as given in paper [16].

When wave was propagated through the specimen, there is a dissipation of energy in various forms like absorption, diffraction, scattering, etc. This ultrasonic attenuation has been originated due to multiple mechanisms such as electron-phonon interaction (e-p), phonon-phonon interactions (p-p) and thermo-elastic relaxation. But at high temperature region, the ultrasonic attenuation is caused mainly due to two mechanisms i.e. thermo-elastic relaxation and phonon-phonon interaction processes. The expressions to evaluate the ultrasonic attenuation have been given in literature [14]. The physical quantities Cv and E0 can be obtained from qD/T tables of AIP Handbook [17]. The minimum thermal conductivity of material has been obatained from literarture [18].

3.   Results and Discussion

The higher order elastic constants i.e. SOECs and TOECs lattice parameter for Hafnium based compounds HfX (X=Os, Ir and Pt) are 3.236 Å, 3.253 Å and 3.298 Å respectively are analysed at 27°C temperature and presented in Table 1. The electronic configurations of Hf, Os, Ir and Pt are [Xe] $4f^{14} 5d^2 6s^2$, [Xe] $4f^{14} 5d^6 6s^2$, [Xe] $4f^{14} 5d^7 6s^2$, [Xe] $4f^{14} 5d^7 6s^2$, [Xe] $4f^{14} 5d^9 6s^1$ respectively which represent that Os has unfilled d-sub shell vis-à-vis to other compounds. This represents that Os makes a stronger bond with hafnium rather than Rh, Pd and Ag. Table 1 also provides that HfOs has greater elastic moduli than other chosen hafnium compounds. The The order of the elastic constants are observed same as that for intermetallic, semi-metallic, polonoids and monopnticides compounds [19-22].

Table 1: SOECs for HFX at 300K (in the unit of 10^{11} Nm^{-2})

HFX	C_{11}	C_{12}	C_{44}	C_{111}	C_{112}	C_{123}	C_{144}	C_{166}	C_{456}
	36.97	4.53	10.69	-313.8	-230.2	-254.7	-59.3	-52.1	-202.8
HfOs	43.65 [a]	17.9 [a]	13.05 [a]	-	-	-	-	-	-
	36.61 [b]	15.2 [b]	10.56 [b]	-	-	-	-	-	-
HfIr	25.33	4.89	7.38	-174.1	-86.9	-97.8	-48.1	-49.2	-85.0
	25.57 [a]	20.2 [a]	9.07 [a]	-	-	-	-	-	-
HfPt	19.04	5.28	6.52	-126.1	-37.4	-43.0	-26.4	-29.2	-39.5
	19.36 [a]	8.27 [a]	5.63 [a]	-	-	-	-	-	-

[a]Ref. [23],[b]Ref. [24]

The Vickers hardness (H) describes the hardness of material/compound while Young's modulus represents the stiffness of the material. It can be observed from Table 2 that H has the largest value of 0.27 GPa for HfOs whereas HfPt has the lowest value among all these compounds. Table 2 also highlights the shear modulus and Young's modulus of HfPt being lowest amongst other hafnium based compounds. This makes HfPt the most soft (ductile) materials among the all these compounds.

Table 2: Mechanical properties of hafnium based compounds at room temperature

Materials	B	Y	G	G/B	Σ	A	H	ρ	λ
	$(10^{11}\,N/m^2)$	$(10^{11}\,N/m^2)$	$(10^{10}\,N/m^2)$		(Poisson ratio)		$(10^{10}\,N/m^2)$	$(10^3\,kg/m^3)$	$(10^{10}\,N/m^2)$
HfOs	15.2	30.2	12.9	0.82	0.17	0.66	0.27	18.07	65.83
	26.5 [a]	33.5 [a]	12.9 [a]		0.29 [a]		1.28 [a]		
HfIr	11.59	20.59	8.55	0.72	0.20	0.72	0.16	17.89	58.89
	25.5 [a]	15.96 [a]	5.72 [a]		0.39		3.0 [a]		
HfPt	9.77	16.32	6.68	0.67	0.22	0.94	0.12	17.20	53.17
	13.48 [a]	15.6 [a]	5.99 [a]		0.31 [a]		1.8 [a]		

Table 3. Ultrasonic velocities V_L, V_{s1}, V_{s2} ($10^3 ms^{-1}$), thermal conductivity k, specific heat per unit volume C_v, Energy density E_θ, acoustic coupling constant (D_L, D_S), thermal relaxation time τ_s, ultrasonic attenuation (all in in $10^{-16} Nps^2 m^{-1}$) and Debye temperature Θ_D (in K) at 27°C temperature along <110> direction

Material / Parameters	HfOs	HfIr	HfPt
V_1	4.17	3.54	3.29
V_{s1}	2.43	2.03	1.95
V_{s2}	2.99	2.39	2.00
V_D	2.92	2.40	2.18
Θ_D	339	278	248
$E_\theta \times 10^8\,(Jm^{-3}K^{-1})$	23.4	25.1	24.9
$C_v \times 10^6\,(Jm^{-3})$	11.5	11.6	11.2
$k\,(Wm^{-1}K^{-1})$	0.61	0.49	0.44
D_L	40.76	24.05	7.11
D_{s1}	33.67	14.78	4.07
D_{s2}	18.56	2.25	1.22
$\tau\,(ps)$	1.86	2.22	2.47
$(\alpha/f^2)_L$	1.78	2.22	0.94
$(\alpha/f^2)_{s1}$	3.72	3.62	1.30
$(\alpha/f^2)_{s2}$	1.09	0.34	0.36
$(\alpha/f^2)_{th}$	0.01	0.01	0.01
$(\alpha/f^2)_{total}$	6.62	6.20	2.61

The ductile nature of the materials has been confirmed by G/B ratio for these hafnium based compounds. The anisotropic value of these compounds is not equal to 1, this means that these hafnium based compounds in this work fall in the category of anisotropic material. We also benchmarked the obtained results with literature available and found same mechanical nature of chosen materials.

The resultant densities of materials Hf, Os, Ir and Pt are 13.2g cm^{-3}, 22.59g cm^{-3}, 22.56g cm^{-3} and 21.45g cm^{-3} respectively. The densities of HfOs, HfIr and HfPt in our case are 18.07g cm^{-3}, 17.89g cm^{-3} and 17.20g

cm^3 respectively. It also indicates that hafnium compounds become lighter after alloying. Due to the non-availability of experimental data for ultrasonic velocities and Debye average velocity, we compare our with other cubic type materials [25-26]. The similar order and nature of V_D was observed with these materials. The thermal relaxation time is of the order of picosecond which shows the intermetallic nature of materials [27-28]. Also, thermal conductivity of chosen compounds is found to decrease with the increase in molecular weight presented in Table 3. Hence HfOs material can be used as most thermal-conductive material. The similar order and nature of ultrasonic attenuation is found in other cubic type materials [29-30].

4.   Conclusion

On the basis of above results, analysis and discussion of the obtained results, we can conclude following points

- The elastic properties of HfOs are predominant over those of the other chosen materials.

- The hardness of the materials decreases with increase in the molecular weight of the materials.

- Alloying of hafnium helps in the reduction of density of materials Os, Ir and Pt.

- HfOs has the highest Debye average velocity, Debye temperature and the thermal conductivity. This also confirms that HfOs has good thermal performance.

- The thermal relaxation time can be derived in order of picosecond, which further confirms the intermetallic nature of the chosen materials.

- HfPt has least value of attenuation due to its lowest values of D_L, D_{s1} and D_{s2}.

These results help us to understand the applications of these materials for the as well as for the industrial uses.

5.   References

1.   H. Diez, C. Mas-Moruno, C., Neubauer, S., Kessler, ACS Appl. Mater. Interfaces , 8(4), (2016), 2517–2525.

2.   H. Okamoto, Hf-Is(rhenium –Osmium), J Phase Equilibria Diffus, 28, (2007), 593

3.   O. Levy, G.L.W. Hart and S. Curtarolo, Acta Mater. 58, (2010), 2887-2897

4.   V. N. Eremenko, L. S. Kriklya, V. G. Khoruzhaya, T. D. Shtepa,,Powder Metall 30, 9, (1991), 765-770

5.   J K Waterstrat, R.M., J. Ph. Equilib. Diffus., 35, (2014), 15–23

6.   Q. Guo, O.J. Kleppa, J. Alloys Compd. 266, (1998), 224-229 .

7.   Q. Guo, O.J. Kleppa, J. Alloys Compd. 321, (2001), 169-182

8.   N. Novakovic, N. Ivanovic, V. Koteski, Intermetallics, 14, (2006), 1403–1410.

9.   W. Xing, X. Chen, Li. D., Intermetallics, 28, (2012), 16–24

10.   A. Iyigör, M. Özduran, M. Ünsal, Philos. Mag. Lett. , 97, (2017), 110–117

11.   N. Arıkana, O. Örnekb, Z. Charific, H. Baazizc, J. Phys. Chem. Solids, 96-97, (2016), 121-127

12.   K Brugger, Phys. Rev., 133, (1964), A1611–A1612

13.   M. Born, J.E. Mayer, Z. Phys. 75, (1931), 1-18

14.   R. R. Yadav , D. K. Pandey, Acta Phys. Pol. A 107, (2005), 933.

15.   A Khan, C.P.Yadav, D K Pandey, D Singh, D. Singh, J. Pure Appl. Phys. 41, (2019), 1-8

16.   V Bhalla, D. Singh, Indian J Pure Appl Phys, 54, (2016), 40–45

17.   D E Gray, American Institute of Physics Handbook (McGraw Hill: New York) 1981

18.   Y. Shen, D.R. Clarke, P.P.A. Fuierer, Appl. Phys. Lett., 93, (2008), 102907–3

19.   S. K. Kor, G. Pandey, D. Singh, Indian J. Pure Appl. Phys. 39, (2001), 510–513

20.   D. Singh, V. Bhalla, J. Bala , S. Wadhwa, Z Naturforsch A, 72, (2017), 977-983

21.   D. Singh, A. Singh, R. Kumar, Proc. Natl. Acad. Sci India: Sect. A Phy. Sci. (2018), 1-7

22.   L. Xianfeng, X. Cunjuan, W. Mingliang, Metals, 7, (2017), 317

23.   Q. J. Liu, N. C. Zhang, F. S. Liu, Z. T. Liu, J. Alloys Comp. 589, (2014), 278-282

24.   D. Singh, S. Kaushik, S K Pandey, G Mishra, VNU J Sci Math Phys, 32, (2016), 43–53

25.   A. Khan, C. P. Yadav, D. K. Pandey, D. Singh and D. Singh, J. Pure Appl. Ultrasonic 41, (2019) 1-8.

26.   D Singh, D K Pandey, Pramana J. Phys., 72(2), 2009, 389-398

27.   V. Bhalla, D. Singh, Pramana J. Phys. 36, (2016), 1355-1367

28.   V Bhalla, D Singh, G Mishra, J Pure Appl Ultrason, 38, (2016), 23–27

29.   C.P. Yadav, D. K. Pandey and D.Singh. Z. Naturforsch. A (2019). (Article in Press).

30.   C Tripathy, D. Singh, R. Paikaray, Can. J. Phys., 96(5), 2018, 513-518.

Biomaterial from White Rot Fungas and its Enzymatic Studies

Nand Lal*, Neelam Pal, Anuradha Tiwari

Department of Chemistry, VSSD College, Kanpur-208002, India
*Email: drnandlal71@ rediffmail.com

ABSTRACT

Laccase is an oxidase enzyme. The extracellular secretion of laccase in the liquid culture growth medium of Pleurotus sajor- caju has been studied. Maximum activity appeared on the 5th day of inoculation of spores of fungal strain in the liquid culture medium. The activity of laccase detected by UV/Vis spectrophotometer using guiacol as substrate. The enzymatic characteristic like Km, pH and temperature optimum were reported for this enzyme and have been found to be 0.30mM, 4.7 and 58°C respectively.

Kewords: Laccase, pleorotus sajor-caju, enzymatic studies.

1.   Introduction

Laccase [E. C.10.3.2] are multicopper enzymes belonging to the group of blue oxidases[1-3], found in many plants, fungi and microorganism[4-7]. They catalyze the oxidation of phenolic compounds such as ortho- and para-diphenols to their corresponding quinones with the concomitant reduction of oxygen to water[4]. A general reaction scheme has been proposed as:

$$4RH + O_2 \rightarrow 4R + 2H_2O$$

Since laccase recycles on molecular oxygen as an electron acceptor and does not require any other co-substrate. It is the most promising enzyme of oxidoreductases group for industrial applications[3,8,9]. Phenol oxidases[6,7] and peroxidases (lignin and manganese peroxidases) are two oxidative enzymes (laccases) have the greatest attention. Laccase are used as bioremediation[10] agent to clean up herbicides, pesticides and certain explosive in soils. It is used in the biodegradation of lignin[4,11] wood, lignocellulosic compounds[12,13], biotransformation of many persistent environmental pollutants, like azodyes[14] and polycyclic aromatic hydrocarbons[15,16].

The biotechnological importance of laccase have increased after discovery that oxidizable reaction substrate range could be further extended in the presence of small readily oxidizable molecules called mediators[17,18]. They can be paired with an electron mediator to facilitate electron transfer to a solid electrode wire. The applications of laccase mediated systems have reviewed which comprise of pulp bleaching, textile biofinishing and environmental processes[20]. It is proposed that laccases play a role in the formation of lignin by promoting the oxidative coupling of lignols, a family of naturally occurring phenols[21]. Laccases have been examined as the cathode in enzymatic biofuel, cells as medical diagnostic tools and in the design of biosensor. During the last few decades, laccases have turned out to be most promising enzymes for industrial uses[8,9], having applications in food, pulp and paper, textile dyeing / textile finishing, wine cork making, teeth whitening, many other industrial and synthetic uses[22,23]. Laccases are also used as catalysts for the manufacture of anti-cancer drugs and even as ingredients in cosmetics. This communication, reports production of laccase from special type of fungal strain with different substrate specificities.

2.   **Material and Methods**

Peptone (bacteriological) was from Qualigens, Mumbai, yeast extract powder type was from Himedia Laboratory Pvt. Ltd. Mumbai, agar- agar (bacteriological grade) was from India Drugs and Pharmaceuticals Ltd. Hyderabad. All other chemicals used in these investigations were either from CDH (Delhi) or Loba Chemie (Mumbai) and were used without further purifications. The fungal strain was from procured from Tamil Nadu Agriculture University, Coimbatore and was maintained on agar slants with medium composition as reported by Tien and Kirk[24] which consisted of glucose 10g, malt extract 10g, peptone 2g, yeast extract 2g, asparagines 1g, KH_2PO_4 2g, $MgSO_4.7H_2O$ 1g, thimine-HCl 1mg and agar 20g per litre of double distilled water.

The liquid culture growth medium reported by Tien & Kirk was used for screening of fungal strain for the production of extracellular laccase. This medium consisted of 10 ml of trace element solution, 5ml of basal solution, 2 ml of ammonium tartarate solution, 5ml of 10% sucrose solution and 2g of coir dust into 250ml culture flask. The composition of trace element solution was $MgSO_4$ 3g, $MnSO_4$ 0.5g, NaCl 1.0g, $FeSO_4.7H_2O$ 0.1g, $CoCl_2$ 0.1g, $ZnSO4.7 H_2O$ 0.1g, $CuSO_4$ 0.1g, $AlK(SO_4)_2.12H_2O$ 10mg, H_3BO_3 10mg, $Na_2MoO_4.2H_2O$ 10mg and nitrilotriacetate 1.5g per litre of double distilled water and composition of basal medium per litre was KH_2PO_4 20g, $MgSO_4$ 5g, and $CaCl_2$ 1g. The sterilized growth medium was inoculated with five days old mycelia approx. 10mg wet weight under aseptic condition and the fungal culture was grown under stationary culture condition at 21°C in BOD incubator. In order to monitor the production of laccase in the liquid culture medium, 2ml aliquots of growth medium were withdrawn at a regular time intervals of 24 hrs and filtered through sterilized millipore filter(0.22μm) and were assayed for the activity of laccase using the following method.

3.   **Assay Method**

The filtered extract was analyzed for the activity of laccase using UV/Vis spectrophotometer Hitachi (Japan) model U-2000 was fitted with electronic temperature control unit. The least count of absorbance measurement was 0.001 unit. The enzyme assay solution 1ml contained 10 mM guiacol in 40 mM sodium phosphate buffer pH 2.0 maintained at 25°C. The enzymatic reaction was initiated by adding 0.2ml of the culture filtrate. The reaction was monitored by measuring absorbance change at 470 nm with time. The enzymatic activity was calculated using molar extinction coefficient vale of 2.66×104 $M^{-1}cm^{-1}$. One enzyme unit is the amount of enzyme that produces 1μ mole of the product per minute. Each assay was done in triplicate.

4.   **Secretion of Laccase and Optimization of the Conditions**

Extracellular secretion of laccase in the liquid culture medium by Pleurotus sajor-caju was determined by plotting the enzyme unit/ml of the growth medium against the number of days after inoculation of the fungal mycelium. Each point on the curve is an average of the three measurements. On the 5th day of inoculation of the fungal mycelia, the maximum activity of laccase appeared in the liquid culture medium. The culture flasks were taken out the BOD and mycelia were removed by filtration through four layers of cheese cloth. The filtered solution was passed through sterilized Millipore membrane filter unit (0.22 μm) and concentrated by freeze drying. The concentrated solution was kept in the fridge at 4°C which remained fully active for a month.

The enzymatic characteristics like Km, pH and temperature optimum were determined using guiacol as the substrate for assessing the experimental conditions suitable for biotechnological applications of this enzyme. The enzyme assay solution and assay methods were same as mentioned above. The steady state velocity of the enzyme catalyzed reaction was determined at different substrate concentrations. The Km value was determined from the double reciprocal plot following the standard procedure25. For determine the pH optimum of the enzyme steady state velocity of the enzyme catalyzed reaction was measured at a fixed saturating concentration of the substrate at a fixed pH and varying the temperature of the reaction medium.

5.   Results and Discussion

Figure 1 shows secretion of laccase in the liquid culture medium in which Pleurotus sajor –caju was grown. It is obvious that maximum activity appears on the 5th day after inoculation of the fungal mycelia. The peak value of the laccase is 0.20 enzyme unit/ml indicating that Pleurotus sajor –caju is reasonably good source of extracellular laccase. In order to finding out the conditions under which the enzyme will exhibit its maximum activity pH and temperature optimum of the enzyme were determined. Fig. 2 shows the variation of enzyme activity with pH which indicate that the pH optimum for the enzyme is 4.7 and it as appreciable activity in the pH range 3.0 to 7.0. The laccase enzyme of reported fungal strain is suitable for biotechnological applications in the pH range acidic to neutral. The variation of activity of laccase produced by Pleurotus sajor- caju with temperature is shown in fig. 3, indicates that the temperature optimum of this laccase is 58°C and it has reasonable activity in the temperature range 30°C to 65°C. Thus this enzyme is suitable for practical applications because temperature of the most of the industrial waste water is near 30°C or above.

Figure 4 shows the Michaelis- Menten behavior of the laccase produced by Pleurotus sajor- caju using guiacol as substrate. The double reciprocal plot given in the Fig. 4 shows that the laccase obey Michaelis - Menten equation and has Km values of 0.30 mM. The organic substrate oxidation by laccase is a one electron reaction generating a free radical which may take part in a polymerization reaction giving an insoluble product. During the course of monitoring steady state enzyme kinetics of Pleurotus sajor –caju laccase, one interesting observation found that the guiacol a phenolic compound taking as substrate converted into insoluble products and were got precipitated and removed from aqueous phase. Thus Pleurotus sajor-caju laccase has potential for removing phenolic compounds from the waste waters containing these compounds.

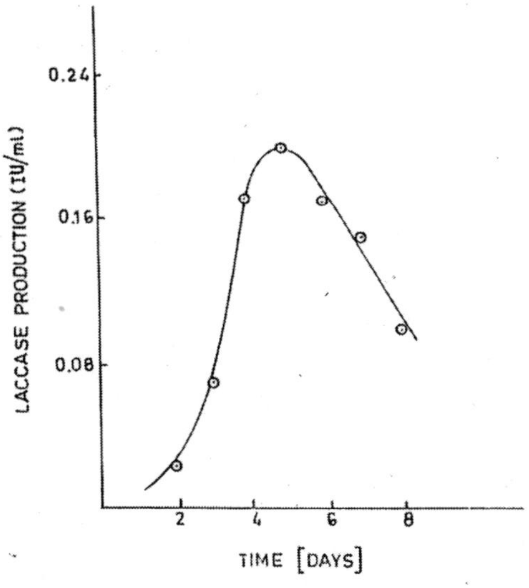

Figure 1 Production of laccase by Pleurotus sajor – caju. 3 ml assay solution contains: 0.6 of phosphate buffer pH 6.2, 0.2 M, 0.2 ml of 90 mM guaiacol ; 0.2 ml of filtered filtrate and 2.0 ml of quartz double distilled water, temperature 57.50ºC.

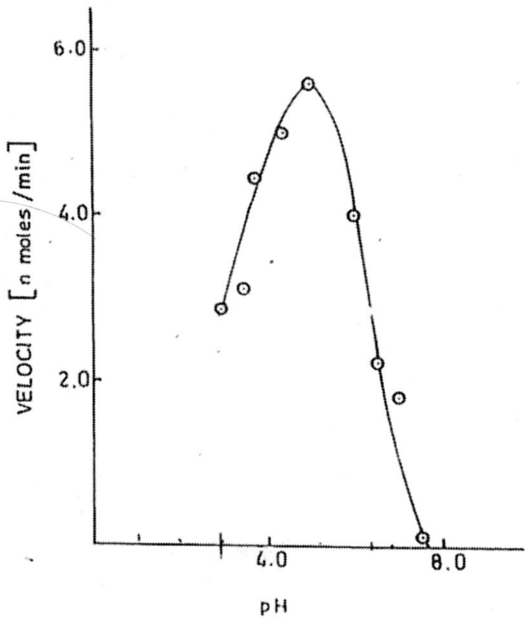

Figure 2 Activity – pH profile of Pleurotus sajor – caju laccase : pH varied and all other parameters are same as in legend to the figure 1.

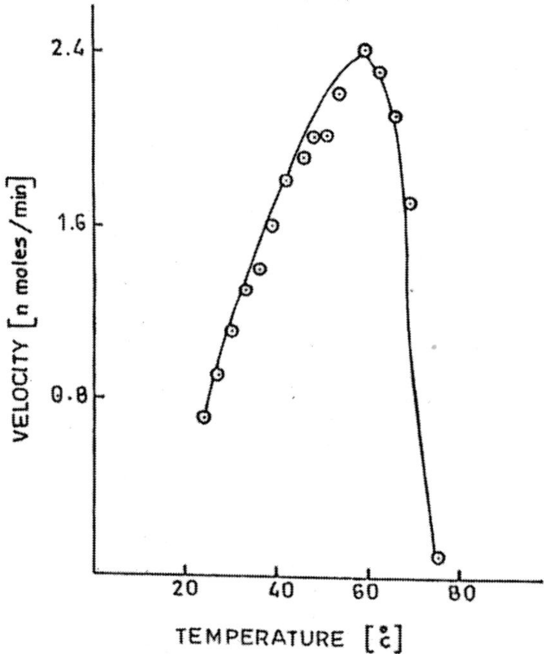

Figure 3 Temperature - activity profile of Pleurotus sajor – caju laccase: Temperature varied and all other parameters are same as in legend to the figure 1.

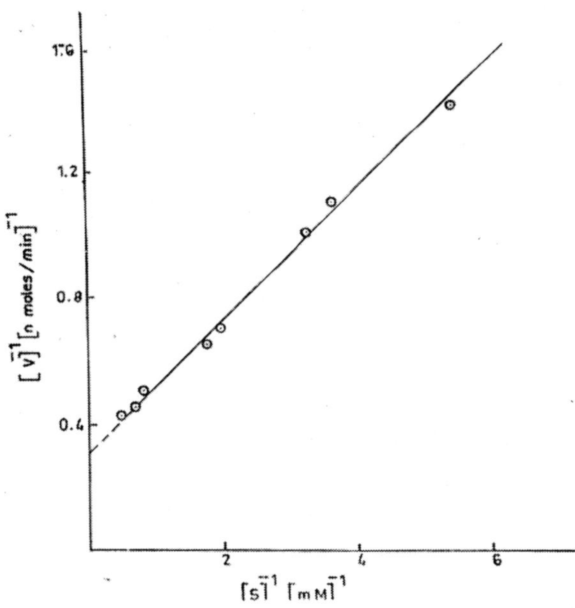

Figure 4 Double reciprocal plot of Pleaurotus sajor – caju laccase Guaiacol concentrations varied. All other parameters are same as in legend to the figure1.

6. Conclusion

The laccase enzyme produced from reported fungal strain has ability for biotechnological applications in acidic to neutral range. This laccase enzyme can apply up to higher temperature range, because temperature optimum of this enzyme is very high. Thus reported laccase enzyme can be used for removal of phenolic compounds from industrial waste water.

7. Acknowledgement

Author is thankful to Dr. K. D. S. Yadav, Emeritus Professor, Department of Chemistry, D. D. U. Gorakhpur University, Gorakhpur for valuable guidance and providing necessary facilities and also the department of Environment and forests, Govt. of India, New Delhi for financial support.

8. References

1. Messerchmidt A. Multi-copper oxidases. Singapore: World Scientific, 1997.
2. Yadav M, Yadav KDS. Kuhad KC, Singh A(eds). New Delhi: International Publishing house Pvt. Ltd. 2007.
3. Wandrey C, Liese A, Kihumbu D. Industrial biocatalysis: Past, present and future. Org Proc Res Dev, 4(4) 285-290 (2000).
4. Zofia Olempska-Beer. Chemical and Technical Assesment, 61st JECIA. FAO (2004).
5. Mariana Mansur et. al., Mycologia 95(6) 1013-1020 (2003).
6. Thurston CF. Microbiology.140 19-26 (1994).
7. Leonowicz A, et. al. J. Basic Microbiol. 41 185-217 (2009).

10. Suresh PS, et. al., J. Mol.Graph. Model 26(5) 845-849 (2008).

11. Bourbonnais R, Paice M G. FEBS Lett. 267 99-102 (1990).

12. Delgado G, et. al., Kuwahara M, Shimadam Eds. Biotechnology in pulp and paper industry. Tokyo: UNI Publishers. 209-214 (1992).

13. Klibansky M et. al., Acta Biotechnological. 13 69-76 (1993).

14. Michael M et. al., Appl. Environ. Microbiol. 71(5) 2600-2607 (2005).

15. Alcadle M et. al., J. Biomol. Screen, 7(6) 547-553 (2002).

16. Hunsa, P et al., African Journal Biotechnology. 8(21) 5897-5900 (2009).

17. Acunzo DF, Gallic C, J. Eur. Biochem. 270 3634-3640 (2003).

18. Morozova O V , Shumakovich G P, Shleev S V, et. al., A review. Appl. Biochem. Microbiol. 43(5) 523-535 (2007).

19. Wheeldon, I R et. al., Proceedings of the National Academy of Sciences of the USA, 105(40)15275-15280 (2008).

20. Rochefort D, Leech D, Bourbonnais R. Green Chem. 6 14-24 (2004).

21. Edwards I, et al. Chemical Reviews.96 2563-2606 (1996).

22. Coniglio A , Gallic C, Gentili P, J. Mol. Catal. B: Enzyme, 50(1) 40-49 (2008).

23. Xu Feng. Industrial Biotechnology (Mary Ann. Liebert, Inc.) 1(1)38-50 (2005).

24. Tien, M and Kirk TK, Methods in Enzymol. 161 2239 (1988).

25. Engel P C. Enzyme Kinetics, Chapman & Hall, London (1997).

Effect of Mg^{2+} ion on luminescence properties of Na$_2$Ca$_{2-x}$Mg$_x$(SO$_4$)$_3$: RE^{3+} (RE^{3+} : Ce, Dy)

S.P. Puppalwar*, P.C. Dhabale, A.S. Puppalwar

Department of Physics, Kamla Nehru Mahavidyalaya, Nagpur 440009, India
*E-mail: suresh.puppalwar@gmail.com

ABSTRACT

Synthesis, optical properties and effect of Mg^{2+} ion on Na$_2$CaMg(SO$_4$)$_3$ phosphors are reported here. Rare earths Ce and Dy doped Na$_2$Ca$_{2-x}$Mg$_x$(SO$_4$)$_3$ phosphors are prepared by wet-chemical method. Powder X-ray diffraction and scanning electron microscopy techniques and luminescent properties are used to characterize the prepared phosphors at room temperature. The influence of Ce^{3+} and Dy^{3+} on photoluminescence (PL) of Na$_2$CaMg(SO$_4$)$_3$ phosphor was also discussed. The changes in concentration of Mg^{2+} in the host affect the photoluminescence characteristics of Na$_2$Ca$_{2-x}$Mg$_x$(SO$_4$)$_3$: RE^{3+}.

Keywords: Na$_2$Ca$_2$-xMg$_x$(SO$_4$)$_3$, rare earths Ce and Dy, Photoluminescence, XRD, SEM.

1. Introduction

In recent years, the rare earth ions are mostly used as activators in the field of luminescent materials. It is well known that rare earth ions which are doped into solid host materials can give rise to sharp emissions in the visible spectral range. Light-emitting diodes (LEDs) are a vital solid-state light source for the next generation lighting industry and display systems due to their unique properties including but not limited to eco-friendliness, energy savings, and long persistence [1]. The white light in white LEDs is the combination of a phosphor layer with UV or blue LEDs, which are usually defined as phosphor converted WLEDs. Therefore at present, researchers pay much attention to the design and development of tricolor phosphors which can be excited by UV or blue LEDs. The most popular material that fluorescence when struck by a charged particle or high energy photons are sodium sulphates [2-5] doped with different rare earth. The sulphates are attractive mineral class and include very interesting and an important specimen. Some sulphate minerals class is soluble and several are fluorescent material. Recently, Puppalwar and co-workers [6-8] have reported several phosphors on rare earth (RE) ions doped mixed sulphate and they have shown how these ions can exist in different valence states as result to irradiation which can induce valence changes conversion and back conversion during heating, this change has been claimed to play an important role [9,10]. Other than Sulphates and Halosulphates [11], some investigators are going in progress on mixed sulphates based materials [12-15].

In the present work, the incorporation of Ce^{3+} and Dy^{3+} in mixed sulphates Na$_2$CaMg(SO$_4$)$_3$ via wet chemical synthesis method is reported. Here Ce^{3+} and Dy^{3+} activated MCMS phosphors gave excellent and wide range tunable emission under UV excitation, and therefore MCMS might be promising as a host material for use in solid state lighting and display fields. We have made experiments along these lines and come up with the effect of Mg on PL intensity in MCMS phosphors.

2. Experimental

Na$_2$CaMg(SO$_4$)$_3$: RE^{3+} (RE^{3+}: Dy, Ce) phosphors were prepared by the wet chemical method. All the starting materials Na$_2$SO$_4$, CaSO$_4$, MgSO$_4$ and (RE^{3+}: Dy, Ce Tb) were analytical grade (AR grade of 99.99% purity-LOBA). Two steps are necessary for synthesizing the samples. Initially, stoichiometric amounts of Na$_2$SO$_4$,

$CaSO_4$ and $MgSO_4$ were taken in separate beakers and dissolved in double distilled de-ionized water so that their transparent solutions were obtained. These transparent solutions were then mixed together. Dy_2O_3 (AR grade of 99.99% purity – E. Merck) dissolved in dilute nitric acid in a separate beaker was also added to obtain $Na_2CaMg(SO_4)_2$: Dy. The concentrations of Dy were taken as y = 0.2, 0.5, 1, 1.5 mol%. All the salts completely dissolved in water to get a homogeneous transparent solution and thus get reacted. The materials were prepared according to the chemical formula $Na_2Ca_{(2-x)}Mg_x(SO_4)_3$:$yDy^{3+}$. In this formula, the x value indicates the varying value of $CaSO_4$ and $MgSO_4$ in (0.1<x<1) and the y value indicates the concentration of impurity in 0.2–1.5mol%. The compound $Na_2CaMg(SO_4)_2$:Dy in its powder form is obtained by evaporating with constant stirring continuously at 80°C about 8 hrs. Then, the dried sample was calcined at 700°C for 2 hr in carbon atmosphere, where the redox reaction occurs. The resultant powder is crushed to fine particles in a mortar pestle. This powder is used as a phosphor in further study. The similar procedure was adopted for the preparation of $Na_2CaMg (SO_4)_3$: Ce^{3+} phosphor.

The prepared samples, which were characterized for their phase purity and crystallinity by X-ray diffraction (XRD) using a PAN analytical diffractometer (Cu–Kα radiation) at a scanning step of 0.01°, continue time 20 s, in the 2θ range 10–80°. The photoluminescence (PL) emission and excitation spectra of the samples were recorded by using a fluorescence spectrophotometer (Shimadzu, RF 5301 PC). The same amount of sample was used in each case. Emission and excitation spectra were recorded using a spectral slit width of 1.5 nm. All PL characteristics were taken at room temperature.

3.   Results and Discussion

3.1   Phase identification and morphology

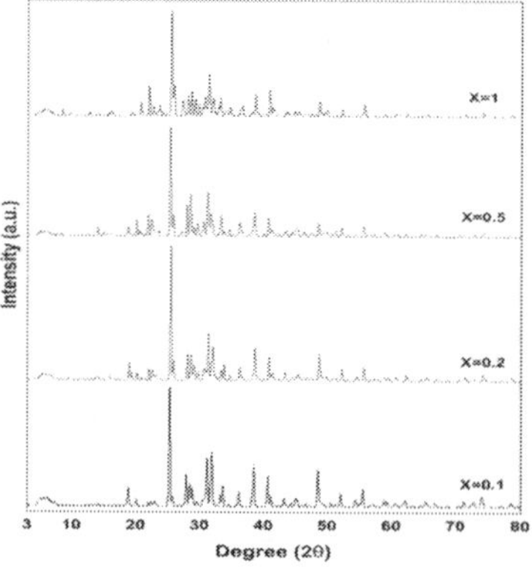

Figure 1. XRD pattern of $Na_2Ca_{2-x}Mg_x(SO_4)_3$ host, (0.1 ≤ X ≤1) phosphors

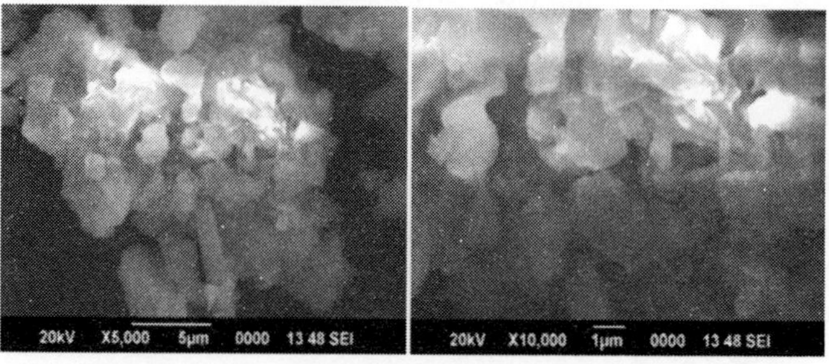

Figure 2. SEM images of $Na_2CaMg(SO_4)_3$ phosphor

The composition and phase purity of the prepared powder samples were examined by XRD. Fig.1 shows the XRD patterns of the different content of Mg substituted NCMS samples. The results for all NCMS samples with different content of Mg are similar. No other phase or impurity can be detected, indicating that there is no significant effect of different content of Mg^{2+} ions other than intensity, on the Na$_2$CaMg(SO$_4$)$_3$ host without inducing significant changes in the crystal structure.

The morphology aspects of the samples were investigated by SEM. Fig. 2 shows both the representative low and high-magnification SEM micrograph of the sample. These images show that the powder sample has non-uniform shapes and sizes. This non-uniformity of shape and size is due to the non-uniform distribution of temperature and mass flow during the annealing process.

3.2   PL properties of Na$_2$CaMg (SO$_4$)$_3$: Dy^{3+}

The PL excitation and emission spectrum of NCMS: Dy^{3+} sample is shown in Fig 3. The excitation spectrum in the range between 300-400nm consists of the f-f shell transition of Dy^{3+}. The figure shows several peaks at 322, 348, 362 and 386nm correspond to the transition from ground state $^6H_{15/2}$ to the excited state $^6P_{7/2}$, $^4G_{11/2}$, $^4I_{15/2}$, and $^4F_{9/2}$ of Dy^{3+}. Since high intense and sharp excitation peak was observed at 348nm, emission spectrum has been measured at 348 nm excitation. The emission for the Dy^{3+} ions in NCMS sample has three bands: 483(blue), 575nm (yellow) and 674 nm (Red). They are assigned due to $^4F_{9/2} \rightarrow {}^6H_{15/2}$, $^4F_{9/2} \rightarrow {}^6H_{13/2}$, $^4F_{9/2} \rightarrow {}^6H_{11/2}$ electronic transition. It is known that Dy^{3+} emission around 483nm ($^4F_{9/2} \rightarrow {}^6H_{15/2}$) due to magnetic dipole moment and 575nm ($^4F_{9/2} \rightarrow {}^6H_{13/2}$) due to electric dipole moment. The transition $^4F_{9/2} \rightarrow {}^6H_{13/2}$ is predominant only when Dy^{3+} ions located at low symmetry sites with no inversion center. With increasing Dy^{3+} concentration in NCMS, the emission intensity of the peaks increases and reaches maximum at 0.5 mol%, as shown in Fig.4.

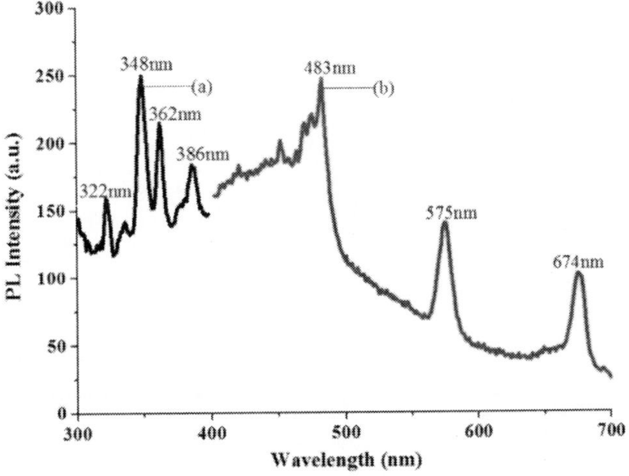

Figure 3. Excitation and Emission spectra of Na$_2$CaMg (SO$_4$)$_3$: 0.005Dy^{3+}.
(a) Excitation (λ_{emi} = 483nm). (b) Emission (λ_{ext} = 348 nm).

When the concentration of Dy^{3+} ion exceeds this level the emission intensity decreases due to concentration quenching. The concentration quenching of Dy^{3+} in phosphors is mainly caused by cross-relaxation, i.e. energy transfers from one Dy^{3+} ion to another neighbor Dy^{3+} ion by transitions. Here, the Dy^{3+} ion may enter into the host lattice to suitable for Na$^+$, Ca^{2+}, Mg^{2+} or it may be locate on surfaces of the crystals. As the ionic radii of Dy^{3+} (91.2pm) is much larger than Mg^{2+} (72pm) and near to Ca^{2+} (99pm) and Na$^+$ (102pm). Therefore

Dy^{3+} ion might be easily replaces the calcium of host atom to occupy statistically cation position in the unit cell. Hence most of Dy^{3+} occupies the group of Ca^{2+}; it creates lower symmetry of local environment around Dy^{3+} ions.

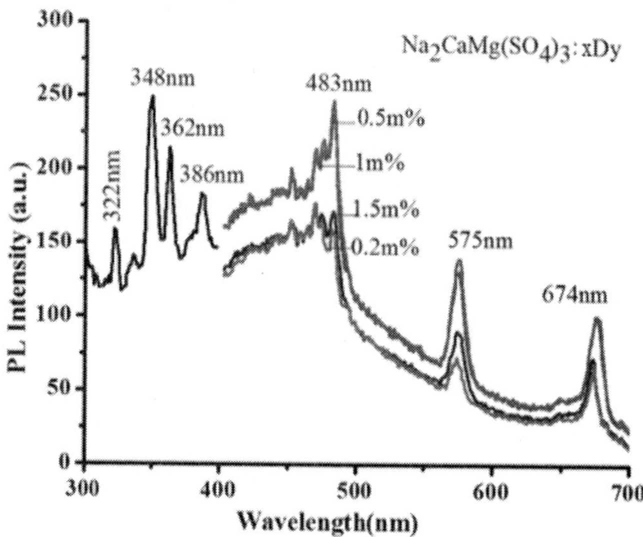

Figure 4. PL spectra of NCMS: xDy phosphor monitored at 348nm excitation.

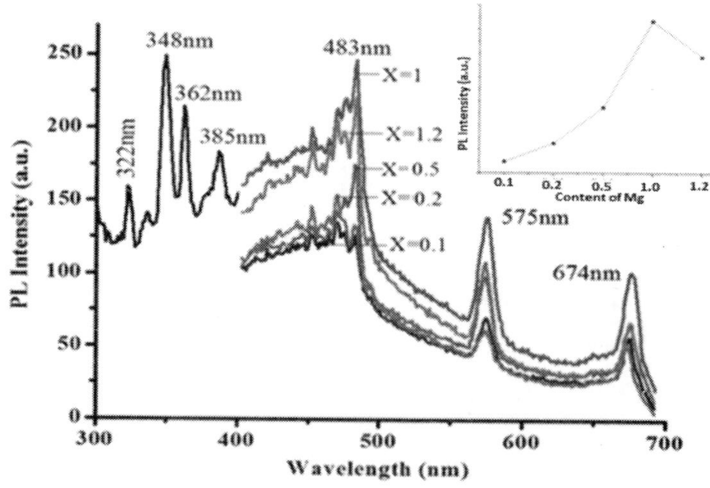

Figure 5. PL spectra of Na$_2$Ca$_{2-x}$Mg$_x$(SO4)3: Dy (0.5m %) with varying content of Mg. Inset shows the effect of variation of Mg content on phosphor.

Figure 5 shows PL emission spectra of NCMS: $Dy^{3+}_{(0.5m\%)}$ samples with varying values of Mg^{2+} ($x = 0.1 \leq x \leq 1.2$) ion and effect of Mg on the emission intensity was investigated. With increasing content of Mg (x), the peak intensity increases and maximum intensity was observed for x = 1. The entire peak profile is same and the PL characterics of the material is better for x = 1 than other values of x in the sample. The effect of Mg content on NCMS: Dy^{3+} is shown in inset.

3.3   PL properties of Na$_2$CaMg(SO$_4$)$_3$: Ce^{3+}

The excitation and emission spectra of NCMS: Ce at 300 K is shown in Fig 6. There are two principal centers in excitation spectra; one of them is at around 252 nm and another at around 292 nm. The emission spectra of Ce^{3+} doped NCMS for different concentrations of Ce^{3+} excited at 292 nm. Two resolved peaks in emission spectra are observed at 310 and 330 nm, assigned to the 5d-4f transition of Ce^{3+} ions, which is the characteristic of Ce^{3+} ion and could be attributed to 5d-4f (^{2}F$_{5/2}$, ^{2}F$_{5/2}$) transitions. The fluorescence intensity increases up to 0.5 mol% concentration of Ce^{3+} ion beyond which, the fluorescence intensity tends to quench. It is also noticed that the peak positions of the emission bands are not changed. The strong PL emission of Ce^{3+} ion is observed in NCMS: Ce^{3+} (0.5 mol%) and it may be useful for scintillation applications.

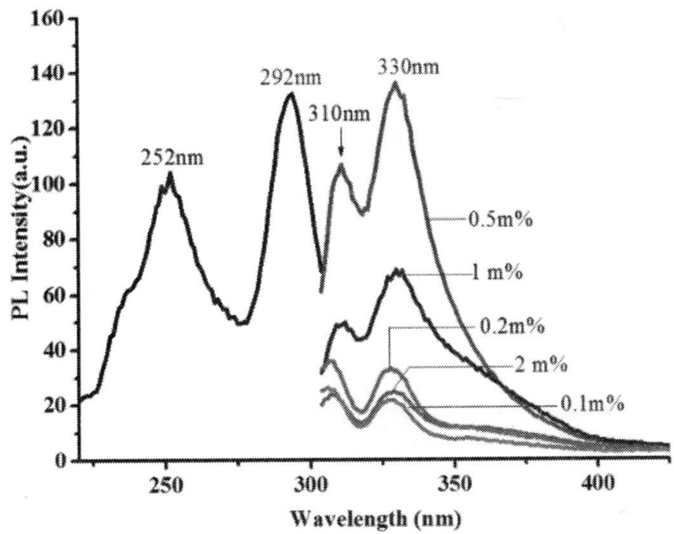

Figure 6. PL excitation and emission spectra of NCMS:xCe monitored at 292 nm excitation. (λ_{emi}=330 nm).

Figure 7 shows PL of a series of NCMS: Ce^{3+} (0.5m %) sample with varying values of Mg^{2+} (x = 0.1 ≤ x ≤ 1) ion and effect of Mg^{2+} on the emission intensity was investigated. It is observed that there no any change in peak profile but only peak intensity increases with increase in (x) value of Mg2+ and the maximum intensity was observed for x = 1, shown in Fig. 7. The PL characteristics of the material is better for x = 1 than other values of x in the sample.

4.   Conclusion

Ce and Dy doped Na$_2$CaMg(SO$_4$)$_3$ samples have been synthesized by wet chemical method. The emission spectra of Na$_2$CaMg(SO$_4$)$_3$: Dy^{3+} gives an intense peaks at 483nm (blue), 575nm (yellow) and 674nm (red). The low symmetry location of Dy^{3+} results in predominance emission of ^{4}F$_{9/2}$→^{6}H$_{15/2}$ transition. The Ce^{3+} doped samples show typical Ce^{3+} emission and the ^{4}f → ^{5}d excitation bands of Ce^{3+} are also observed. The PL spectrum of Na$_2$CaMg(SO$_4$)$_3$:Ce^{3+} excited at 292nm shows emission at 310 and 330nm for near UV region. This material can be applied to fluorescent lamps, solid state lightening devices, nuclear physics, X-ray and neutron diffraction etc.

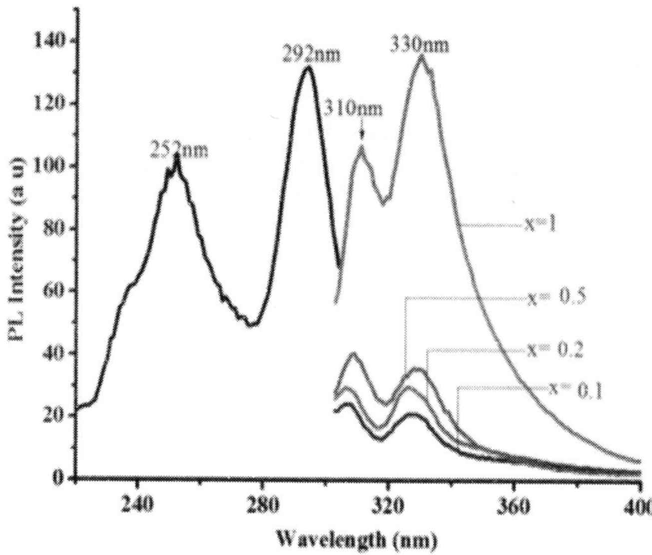

Figure 7. PL spectra of $Na_2Ca_{2-x}Mg_x(SO_4)_3$:$Ce_{(0.5m\%)}$ monitored at 292nm excitation.

5. Acknowledgement

Author SPP is thankful to management of the Institution KNM, Nagpur for providing useful facilities of the instrumentation, SHIMADZU Spectrofluorophotometer (RF-5301 PC).

6. References

1. Ye S, Xiao F, Pan YX, Ma YY, Zhang QY. Phosphors in phosphor converted white light-emittin diode. Mat Sci Eng R(71)1–34, (2010).

2. Manik U, Gedam SC, Dhoble SJ, The characterization and mechanism of energy transfer in $Na_2Mg(SO_4)_2$: Ce phosphor co-doped by Dy, Mn, Tb. J. Lumin (136), 191-195(2013).

3. Taode ST, Ingle NB, Omanwar SK. Characterization and Photoluminescence study of Dy^{3+} doped Na_2SO_4 phosphor prepare by Re-crystallization method, IOSR J. App. Phy. (IOSR-JAPs), 2278-4861 (2015).

4. Gaikwad S, Mistry R R, Barve R., Patil RR, Moharil SV. Luminescence of Cu^+ in Na_2SO_4, Indian J. pure and Appl. Phy, (51) 235-240 (2013).

5. Gd-doped natural thenardite: Eu photoluminescence properties of europium, Guzaliaya J. Tuerxun A, Aizitialli A, Aierken S, Guange Puxue, Yu Guang Pu Fen Xi, 32(6) 1496-9 (2012).

6. Shinde N, Dhoble NS, Gedam SC, Dhoble SJ. PL enhancement in Na_3SO_4Cl: X ($X=Ce^{3+}$, Eu^{3+}, Dy^{3+}) material, Luminescence 30(6) 898 (2015).

7. Deshmukh PB, Puppalwar SP, Dhoble NS, Dhoble SJ. Optical properties of $CaA(SO_4)_2$ Br: RE (RE= Dy, Eu, Ce) novel phosphor, Luminescence DOI: 10.1002/bio.2591 (2014),

8. Deshmukh PB, Puppalwar SP, Dhoble NS, Dhoble SJ. Luminescent properties of $MAl(SO_4)_2$ Br: Eu^{3+} (M = Sr or Mg) red phosphor for near-UV light emitting diode, (30) 118-121 (2015).

9. Salah N, Sahare PD,.Kumar P, TL and PL in $BaSr(SO_4)_2$:Eu mixed sulphate, Physica status solidi (a), 203(5) (2006)897-905.

10. Moharil SV, Bodade SV, Sahare PD, Dhopte SM, Muthud PL, Luminescence in LiNa (SO_4): Eu phosphor, Radiation effects and defects in solid, 127(2) 177-182 (1993).

11. Poddar A, Gedam SC, Dhoble SJ, Development of Orange–Red emitting phosphor and studies of TL characteristics of $KMgSO_4F$ material, J. Lumin (149) 245 (2014).

12. Kore BP, Dhoble SJ, PL and TL proportion of DY $^{3+}$/ Eu^{2+} activated $Na_{21}Mg$ $(SO_4)_{10}$ cl_3 phosphor, J. Lumin, (143) 337-342 (2013).

13. Vidya YS, Lakshminarasappa BN, Preparation, characterization and Luminescence properties of orthorhombic sodium sulphate , Physics Research International, Article ID (7) 631-641 (2013).

14. Gedam SC, Dhoble SJ, Moharil SV, Luminescence in Ce^{3+} doped mixed sulphate fluoride phosphors $NaMgSO_4F$ and Na_3SO_4F. J.Appl phy 37(1) 73-78 (2007).

15. Choubey SR, Gedam SC, Dhoble SJ, PL and TL study of $NaMgSO_4F$: X(X=Dy or Ce) fluoride phosphor by SSD method, J. Lumin (142) 48 (2013).

Advances in Ultrasonic Gauging and Imaging of Tubes and Pipes

N.Pavan Kumar[1, 2*], V.H.Patankar[1,2]

[1]Homi Bhabha National Institute (HBNI), Mumbai, Maharashtra, 400094
[2]Bhabha Atomic Research Centre (BARC), Mumbai, Maharashtra, 400085
*E-mail: npavan@barc.gov.in

ABSTRACT

Various tubular objects are utilized for strategic and critical applications in nuclear, aviation, space and petrochemical industries. Major tubular objects employed in these industries are tubes, pipes and vessels, which are inspected for planar and volumetric defects such as cracks, voids, inclusions, porosities and notches. Accurate measurement of Inner Diameter (ID), Outer Diameter (OD) and Wall Thickness (WT) is also an important requirement of tubes/pipes. Ultrasonic testing is a very popular and safe NDT technique to perform flaw detection, sizing and characterization of tubes /pipes. In recent years, various semi-automated and automated Ultrasonic Imaging and Gauging Systems have been designed and developed by various researchers and manufactures suitable for tubes/pipes.

Internal Rotary Inspection System (IRIS) is one of the advanced inspection tools suitable for inspection of heat exchanger tubes [4]. Very accurate Ultrasonic-Zirconium Tube meter has also been developed by Lithuania for inspection of coolant channels of RBMK nuclear reactors [6]. Similarly, completely automated CIGAR system (Channel Inspection and Gauging Apparatus for Reactors) has been developed by Canada for inspection of pressure tubes of CANDU reactors [1]. BARC has developed Channel Inspection System suitable for gauging and flaw detection of pressure tubes of PHWR [2]. Ultrasonic Pipe Inspection and Gauging (PIG) apparatus is one of the most useful gadgets available for inspection of petrochemical pipes. One of such systems is from Germany for inspection of oil pipelines [3]. This paper provides details of various advanced Ultrasonic gauging and imaging inspection systems developed by national and international researchers and manufactures for tubes/pipes.

Keywords: Ultrasonic, NDT, Flaw detection, Pipe Inspection, PIG, Tube Inspection, Gauging, Ultrasonic Imaging.

1. Introduction

Tubes and Pipes play an extremely important role in strategic and critical applications like aviation, warships, missiles, atomic energy, space technology, aerospace, petrochemical industries and other strategic fields. Usually tubes and pipes work under the condition of high temperature and high pressure. But during the pre-fabrication, fabrication, In-service and post-service stages it is mandatory to carry out flaw detection & gauging of tubes/pipes. To provide high level of safety, reliability and quality assurance, there is a need to inspect flaws as well as to measure ID, OD and WT of tubes/pipes. Some of the advanced Ultrasonic gauging and imaging inspection systems suitable for tubes and pipes have been elaborated in next sections.

2. Advanced Ultrasonic Testing Systems for Tubes

Technique of Ultrasonic Testing of tubes has matured over a few decades and it also caters to gauge the metallic tubes [5]. Similarly, Ultrasonic systems are available which provide imaging of tubes for flaw detection [5]. In this paper, it has been discussed about advanced ultrasonic Imaging and Gauging systems for tubes, developed by national and international designers and developers.

IRIS is one of the widely used advanced ultrasonic inspection tools for the internal inspection of tubes using water immersion technique [4]. The operating principle is mainly based on the pulse-echo immersion technique with a mirror reflector to inspect thin walled tubes, from ID side. Schematic diagram for transducer assembly is as shown in Fig 1.0. A transducer excited by a high frequency pulser produces ultrasonic waves that propagate into water. A mirror reflects the waves to produce a normal incident beam on the ID of the tube. Echoes, reflected back from each metal- water interface, are digitized and processed to extract the time of flight and amplitude data of the front wall echo and back wall echoes. Further processing is applied to calculate the tube ID, OD, and WT. During the inspection, B-scan (as shown in Fig 2.0) and images are also recorded in real time, for analysis. IRIS is able to measure tube of diameter range from 100 mm to 1000 mm, length up to 750 m and wall thickness up to 40 mm. IRIS has limitation, tubes need to be cleaned before inspection. Results can also get affected by dirty /low-pressure couplant water, bonded scales, loose debris and electrical interference.

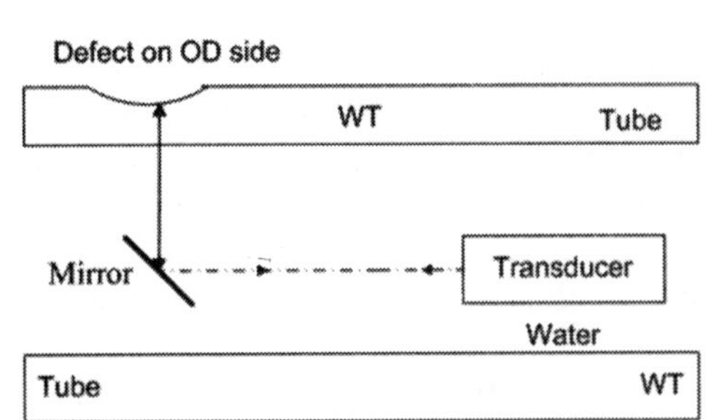

Figure 1. Schematic diagram for transducer assembly of IRIS

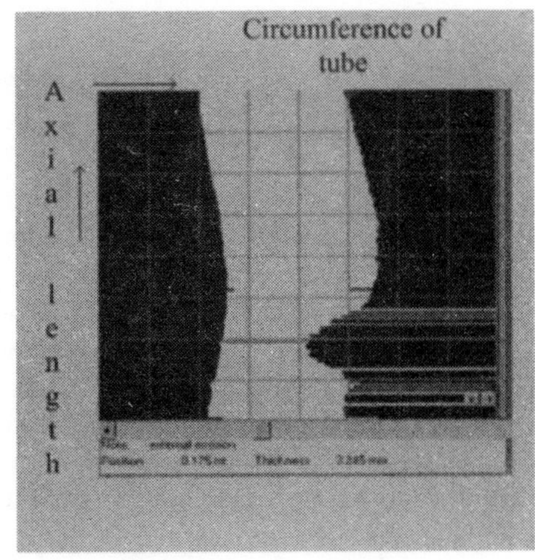

Figure 2. Typical B-Scan image of a thin Walled tube acquired by IRIS

AECL Canada has developed completely automated CIGAR (Channel Inspection and Gauging Apparatus for Reactors) for pressure tubes of CANDU reactors *[1]*. The CIGAR tool has six ultrasonic transducers used for defect detection, sizing and characterization. There are two normal incidence transducers, one of them is of 10MHz and another of 20MHz as shown in Fig 3.0. The normal incidence transducers are always operated in pulse-echo mode. Four numbers of angled beam shear wave transducers operate at a frequency of 10MHz. These transducers are operated either in pulse-echo or T-R mode and are orientated around the 20MHz normal incidence transducer so that any point on the pressure tube will be inspected from above as well as from the front, back and each side via full-skip method. Typical B-scan image acquired for the pressure tubes of CANDU reactor is shown in Fig 4.0. Another inspection system developed by AECL is known as BRANDE, which is available with the same ultrasonic transducer configuration as CIGAR but records B-scan image over the entire length of the pressure tube and at a higher resolution compared to CIGAR.

Lithuania has developed Ultrasonic-Zirconium Tube meter for inspection of coolant channels of RBMK nuclear reactors [6]. This system is mainly used for the measurement of wall thickness, inner diameter and outer diameter of Zirconium tubes. The operating principle is mainly based on the measurement of precise time of flight (TOF) in liquids and solids. If the transmit and receive ultrasonic waves are located on this line, inner diameter and wall thickness can be determined. For compensation of a non-uniform temperature (40-80° C) of water inside a tube, the reference channel is used, for applying correction factor to the change of acoustic velocity with reference to temperature. Ultrasonic-Zirconium Tube Meter is capable of measurement of wall thickness with an accuracy of 50 microns.

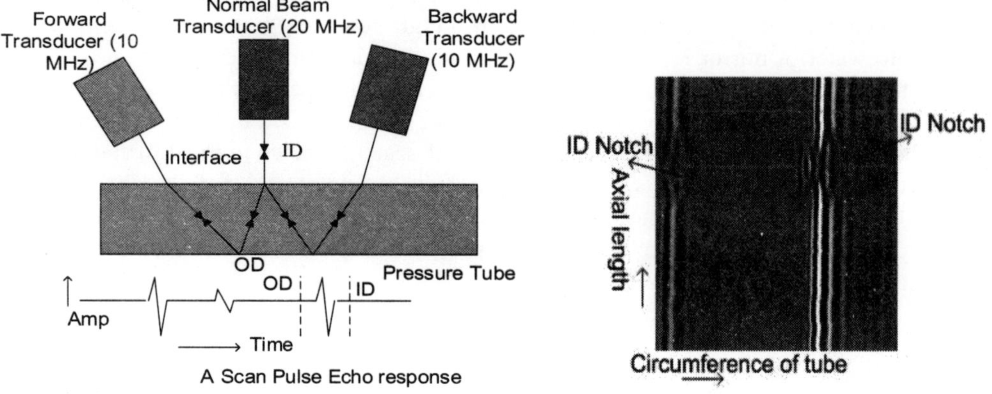

Figure 3. Inspection Setup for BRANDE system   **Figure 4.** Typical B scan image acquired for Pressure tube of CANDU reactor

BARC has developed BARCIS (BARC Channel Inspection System) for Reactors, which performs gauging and flaw detection of pressure tubes of PHWR [2]. BARCIS has been developed for In-Service- Inspection (ISI) of coolant channels of PHWR. The inspection is carried out from one end of the channel with the reactor in the shutdown condition and coolant pumps in operation. BARCIS Inspection Head is provided with dedicated angle beam immersion ultrasonic transducers – one for axial scan and other for circumferential scan. These are line focused transducers having frequency of 10MHz. The axial scan transducer angulated to have a 45 degree beam inside the tube material and, moves along the tube axis, where the transducer is sensitive to flaws extending mainly in circumferential direction. The circumferential transducer uses offset method to produce a 45 degree shear beam inside the Zircaloy tube and it moves along with the circumference which are sensitive to flaws extending along the tube axis. Angle beam Transducer is used for axial and circumferential scan of pressure tube as shown in Fig 5.0. Flaw (0.5 Skip OD flaw and 1.5 skip flaw) location and size are determined by using DAC (Distance Amplitude Curve) and echo amplitude. Normal beam Transducer as shown in Fig. 6. Difference in Time of Flight (TOF) value corresponds to the flaw depth and the displacement of the transducer provides the length or width of the flaw. Ultrasonic Imaging is also carried out for detection of zirconium hydride blisters inside pressure tubes. BARCIS is capable of inspecting an average of two coolant channels per day.

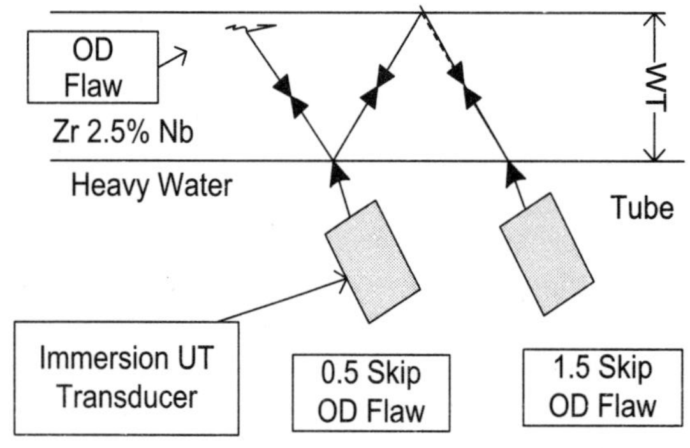

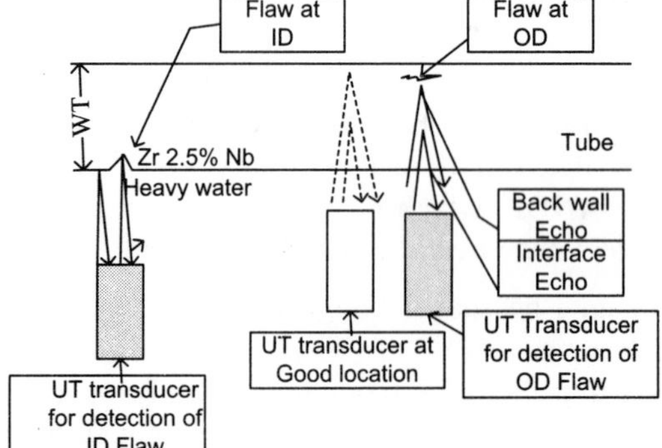

Figure 5. Angle beam technique for flaw detection of tube   **Figure 6.** Time of Flight Difference for flaw detection in tube

A novel intelligent compensation ultrasonic system has been developed by China for wall-thickness and diameter measurement of the zirconium alloy cladding tube. The measurement precision of diameter and wall thickness is improved by using novel intelligent compensation technique for ultrasonic system embedded with Artificial Neural Network (ANN) [9]. Another inspection system is available from China for detection of circumferential defects of boiler tubes using Ultrasonic Guided Wave technique. Ultrasonic Testing Systems are available for measurement of wall thicknesses of more than 0.7 mm and diameters of more than 18.75 mm for welded tubes from Western Instruments, Canada. The measurement precision of diameter is 2.5% in a pressure tube. Karl Deutsch has developed Ultrasonic Inspection Systems for Tubes for diameter of range from 20 mm up to 610 mm using contact and immersion techniques. Ultrasonic inspection of Tubes without transducer rotation has been developed by Kinetic Inc., Canada, for improvement in inspection speed. Quasi-Tomographic approach using ultrasonics is also available for flaw characterization of tubes. Another System TRUSTIE has been proven to be a valuable tool for inspecting the unique design configuration of CANDU steam generator (SG) tubes.

3.   Advanced Ultrasonic Testing Systems for Pipes

3.1   Pipe; External Inspection [3]

An Ultrasonic External Pipe Inspection system (Ultrasonic PIG) has been developed by Germany. Ultrasonic Transducer is operated in contact mode. The Ultrasonic waves are transmitted in the pipeline. Part of the waves are reflected by the inside wall of the pipe and thus the echoes are received. The principle of the setup is explained by means of Fig 7.0. An extension of the method and the transducer enables the recognition of different pipes if the sound velocities of these pipes differ. Results of External Pipe Inspection System gets affected due to offset of mechanized head during motion and loss of contact. Inspections are carried out for gas pipelines also. It is known, that pigging of ultrasound through the wall in the gas environment can succeed in high-pressure condition. However, a certain minimum pressure must be maintained during the inspection.

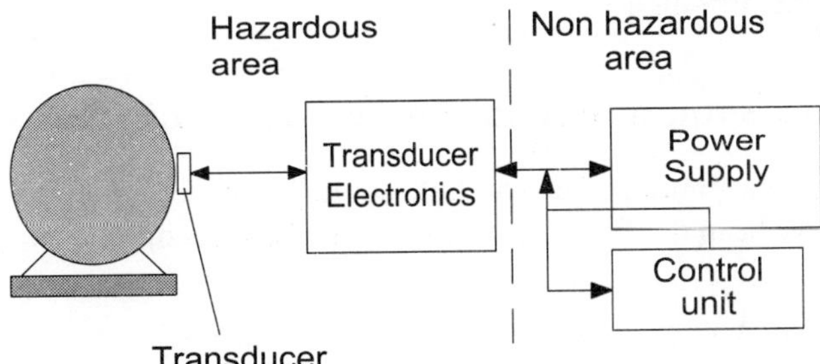

Figure 7. Typical Ultrasonic PIG instrument set up for External Pipe Inspection and Gauging

3.2   Pipe; Internal Inspection [7]

An automated Ultrasonic internal pipe inspection system of China is operated which is based on non-contact technique (i.e. immersion technique). The pipeline characteristics will not get affected due to immersion technique of the measurement. Ultrasonic internal pipe inspection tool consists of housing batteries, Transducer electronics, data storage and Ultrasonic Transducers as shown in Fig 8.0. Normal Beam Transducers are used to measure the wall thickness, corrosion measurement and crack detection. The position of pipe inspection system is monitored by means of encoder and GPS device. Major challenge of the inspection tool is in collection and storing large amount of data and major R&D efforts are put into designing electronics to handle it. Measurement accuracy improves with the advancement of electronics, mechanical design and digital processing algorithms etc.

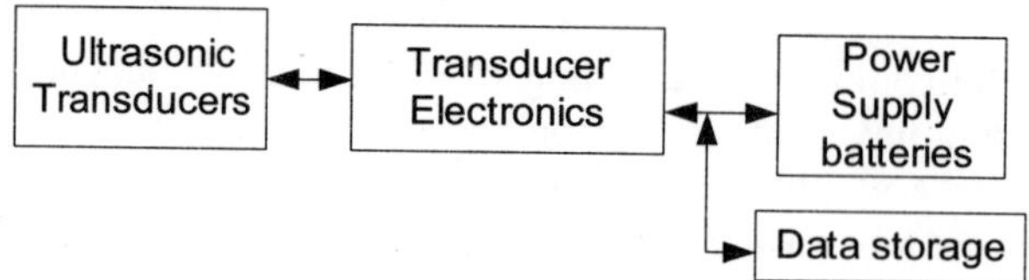

Figure 8. Typical PIG instrument set up for Internal Pipe Inspection and Gauging

Various researchers and manufacturers have developed advanced Ultrasonic Imaging and Gauging Systems for pipes. The major manufacturers of automated ultrasonic inspection systems for pipelines are: Olympus Corporation – Canada, APPLUS+RTD – Netherlands, DACON inspection services – Norway, Girard Industries –USA, Phoenix Inspection Systems Ltd. – England JIREH Industries – Canada, IMG Ultrasuoni – Italy and LinScan- UAE. Some of the Advanced Ultrasonic Imaging and Gauging Systems developed by various manufactures and researchers for pipes have been elaborated as below:

American Petroleum Institute (API), USA has developed Advanced UT Rotary System for inspection of steel tubes and pipes, including accurate measurement of WT, ID, OD and longitudinal and transversal defects in pipe [10]. Ultrasonic Crack Detection System by Tokyo, Japan on Multi-Diameter PIG Robots is available for crack and corrosion Detection as well as inspection of multi diameter pipelines. It has used ultrasonic transducers with relative software filtering techniques and is used to improve the measurement accuracy. China has developed Measurement System for the Wall Thickness of Pipe for accurate measurement of wall thickness with high speed (25 m/min). The operating principle is based on the measurement of Time of Flight values. An Ultrasonic Testing system has been developed for detection of creep damage in welded steel pipes by Kaunas University of Technology, Lithuania. It is able to detect defects with an accuracy in microns. An Ultrasonic inspection system has been developed for flaw detection of long-range gas pipelines using ultrasonic guided waves by South Korea. Karl Deutsch, Germany has developed an Automated Ultrasonic Pipe Weld Inspection system which is available for wall thickness measurement and flaw detection using contact and immersion testing techniques.

4.   New Trend of Ultrasonic Inspection Technologies for Tubes and Pipes [8]

With the advent of technology and science of Ultrasonic Testing, new trends of advanced ultrasonic inspection technologies have been developed. Some of the new trends of ultrasonic inspection technologies are described as below:

1.   Combined numerical simulation analyses with ultrasonic inspection are major research contents.

2.   Robotic vehicles play an important role in future ultrasonic testing systems for pipes due to their cost, safety and accessibility to areas where manual inspection is not possible.

3.   Signal processing and wavelet transforms have been developed to improve quality of image and sizing accuracy.

4.   Phased array Ultrasonic Testing has been used to improve the scan speed and sizing accuracy.

5.   Conclusions

In this paper, various advanced ultrasonic gauging and imaging systems developed by various researchers and manufacturers have been discussed suitable for tubes/pipes, including testing methodologies, features and limitations etc. In the last, the latest trends for the better future of tube/pipe inspections have also described.

6.   Acknowledgement

Authors are grateful to Mrs. Anita Behere, Outstanding Scientist and Head, Electronics Division, BARC, for her guidance and support.

7.   References

1.   Timothy Lardner, Graeme West, Gordon Dobie, Anthony Gachagan, "Automated sizing and classification of defects in CANDU pressure tubes", Nuclear Engineering and Design, V.No 325, pp no: 25-32, 2017.

2.   Gurpartap Singh, A. M. Kadu, H. M. Bapat, Amit K. Haruray, Manojit Bandyopadhyay, D. N. Badodkar, "Localization & Characterization of Flaws in Pressure Tubes by UltrasonicTechnique during In-Service Inspection of Indian PHWRs", National Seminar & Exhibition on NDE, Pune, December 2014, Vol.20 No.6.

3.   Peter Holstein, Hans-Joachim Munch, Santerzur Horst-Meyer, "Ultrasonic PIG Detection at Pipelines", Pigging Products and Service Association (PPSA) Seminar, Germany, November 2010.

4.   Joseph. A, Sharma, Govind. K, Jayakumar. T, "Ultrasonic Internal Rotary Inspection System (IRIS) for heat exchanger and steam generator tubes", Journal of Pure and Applied Ultrasonics; CODEN JPAUEW, v. 31(1), 2009, p. 24-30.

5.   Patankar V.H, Joshi V.M., Lande B.K, "Development of an Automated - Ultrasonic System for Inspection and Gauging of Tubes/Pipes", NDE-2006 Conference, Hyderabad, Dec-2006

6.   R. Kazys, L. Maieika, R. Sliteris, A. VladiSauskas, A. VoleiSis and K. Kundrotas, "Ultrasonic measurement of zirconium tubes used in channel- type nuclear reactors", NDT&E International journal, Vol. 29, 1995, pp. 37-49.

7.   Qingshan Feng, Rui Li, Baohua Nie, Shucong Liu, Lianyu Zhao and Hong Zhang, "Literature Review: Theory and Application of In-Line Inspection Technologies for Oil and Gas Pipeline Girth Weld Defection", MDPI Sensors Journal, Dec 2016.

8.   Michael Moles and Ed Ginzel, "Phased Arrays for Small Diameter, Thin-Walled Piping Inspections", WCNDT, Durban, South Africa, April 2012.

9.   Xiang Xiao, Bin Gao, Gui Yun Tian,"Novel Ultrasound System With Intelligent Compensation for High Precision Measurement of Thin Wall Tube" IEEE sensors journal, vol. 18, August 2018.

10.   Zhongqing You, John Venczel and Dudley Boden, "Advanced NDE for Pipes and Tubes as per API Specifications", National Seminar & Exhibition on Non-Destructive Evaluation, NDE-2009, USA, 2009.

Effect of Particle Size, Shape Upon Rheological Properties of Methanol based Nanofluids at 303K

Nandkishor N. Padole[1*], Omprakash P. Chimankar[2], N. R. Pawar[3] and Vilas Tabhane[4]

[1*]Department of Physics, Shri Sai College Of Engineering & Technology, Bhadrawati, 441907, India
[2]Department of Physics, RTM Nagpur University, Nagpur, 440033, India
[3]Department of Physics, ACS college Maregaon, 445303, India
[4]Department of Physics, S. P. University, Ganeshkhind, Pune, 411007, India
*Email: nandupadole12@gmail.com

ABSTRACT

The past decade has seen the rapid development in the study of acoustical and thermal properties of nanofluids for potential applications. Most of the researcher has focused their attention on the thermal conductivity of these fluids. However, rheological properties of nanofluids are also important which affects the acoustical and thermal properties of nanofluids. In this paper, results on density and viscosity in methanol based nanofluids at low concentration (0.002M-0.01M) are presented. The purpose of present study was to identify effect of particle size, shape on rheological properties of nanofluids at 303K. The experimental results show that the viscosity and density increases with an increase of particle volume fraction. Also it is observed that nanoparticles with higher surface area exhibit lower density and viscosities. The changes in density and viscosity occur as a result of interfacial forces, surface area and particle shape and size distribution.

Keywords: **Nanofluids, TEM, viscosity, density.**

1. Introduction

Nanofluids are composites consisting of solid nanoparticles with sizes varying generally from 1 to 100 nm dispersed into a liquids such as water, methanol, ethylene glycol and propylene glycol etc.[1]. Nanofluids are of great significance because of their enhanced acoustical and rheological properties. Results like these have drawn much interest from the industrial and science communities to explore the rheological properties of nanofluids[2].

Rheological properties of nanofluids are strongly related to the nanofluids microstructure[3]. It is depends upon the particle concentration, particle shape and size, particle distribution and the extent of particle-particle interactions. Also agglomeritio and clustering of nanoparticles can lead to an undesirable changes in nanofluids. Therefore, a proper understanding of nanofluids is a prerequisite for effective utilization of nanofluids for various applications. Rheological properties of nanofluids provide information on the nature of interactions in the constituent. Many literature provides extensive data on the density and viscosity of liquids and liquid mixtures but a combined study of viscosity and density of nanofluids is quite scarce. Therefore results of effect of particle size on viscosity and density of methanol based SnO_2, $CaCO_3$, CaF_2, ZnS and silver nanofluids are presented.

2. Experimental

2.1. Materials

Aniline, ammonium persulphate, ammonium hydroxide, Stannic chloride and hydrochloric acid were used for the synthesis of SnO_2 nanoparticles. In the preparation of CaF_2, we used calcium chloride dehydrate

($CaCl_2 \cdot 2H_2O$, Merk-99.9%), nitric acid (conc. HNO_3, Merk-99.99%), ammonium fluoride (NH_4F, Merk-99.50%), bismuth nitrate (Bi $(NO_3)_3 \cdot 5H_2O$, Merk-99.50%), and ethanol as raw materials. The synthesis of ZnS nanoparticles was carried out by chemical method using Zinc Acetate [$Zn(CH_3COO)_2$], DMF [H-CO-N($CH_3)_2$] and Na_2S as source materials. The silver nanoparticle were synthesized by thermal decomposition method at 700°C. Reducing agent NH2CONH2 is added to the mixture of AgNO3 in order to form the silver nanoparticle. All the reagents were of analytical grade and used without further purification.

2.2   Methods

2.2.1. Preparation of Samples

Nanofluids preparation is not as simple as mixing some solid nanoparticles in a base fluid[4]. There are two techniques mainly used for synthesizing nanofluids: single step method and two step method.

In a single step method[5] both preparation of nanoparticles and synthesis of nanofluids are done in a combined process. This method has advantages such as stability increase and minimized agglomeration. There are some disadvantages like the fact that only low pressure fluids are suitable for this process hence limiting the scope of utilization.

In two step method[6] nanoparticles are initially prepared and then dispersed into the fluid by some techniques like ultrasound[7]. Nowadays, availability of nanoparticles from commercial sources makes this method fairly attractive to the researchers and different industries. Most of the researches utilized two step dispersion method and ultrasonic vibrations for proper mixtures.

In present work, methanol based nanofluids with molar fractions of 0.002, 0.004, 0.006, 0.008 and 0.01 were prepared using two step methods. Nanofluids with a required molar concentration was prepared by dispersing a specified amount of nanoparticles in methanol under stirring process to get a uniform dispersion of nanofluids.

3.   Results and Discussion

The SEM images of synthesized SnO_2, $CaCO_3$, CaF_2 and ZnS particles are shown in Figs. 1(a), 1(b), 1(c) and 1(d) respectively. It can be seen from the images that the particles size are in the range of nanometer. SnO_2, $CaCO_3$, CaF_2 nanoparticles are spherical in shape while ZnS nanoparticles are elongated in shape.

3.1   Effect of particle size on rheological properties

All researchers and most of the investigations available in the literature on the viscosity and density of nanofluids, regarding the effect of volume fraction agree upon the fact that viscosity and density of nanofluids increases with increasing the volume fractions. Das et al. [8], Putra et al. [9], Prasher et al.[10] and Chevalier et al. [11] showed that viscosity of nanofluids increased with increasing the particle concentration.

There are very few results available in literature about particle size and shape effect on rheological properties of nanofluids. However, viscosity of nanofluids has a strong dependence with nanoparticle shape. Timofeeva et al. [12] report that elongate particles like platelets and cylinders result in higher viscosity at the same volume fraction. Nguyen et al. [13] studied particle size effect for Al_2O_3/water nanofluids and observed that particle size effects are more significant for high particle volume percentage. They found that viscosity of nanofluids decrease with increasing the diameter of the particle.

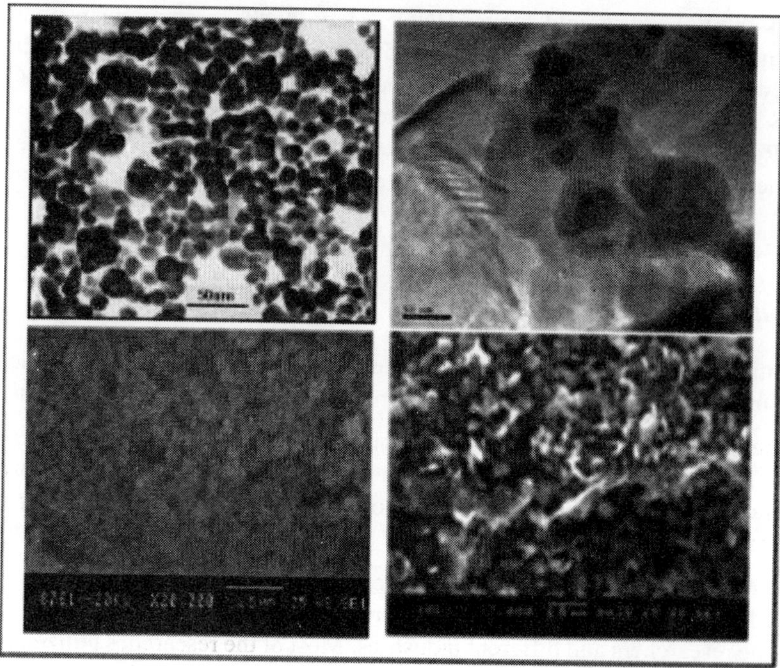

Figure 1. SEM images of SnO$_2$, CaCO$_3$, CaF$_2$ and ZnS.

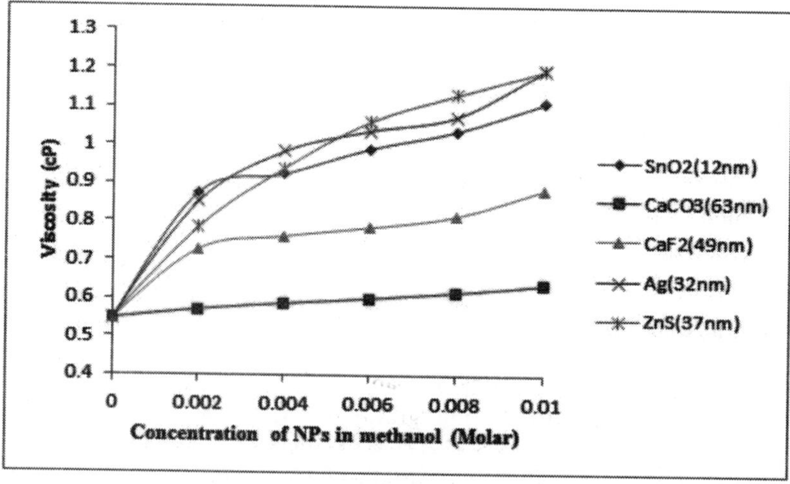

Figure 2. Variation of viscosity of SnO$_2$, CaCO$_3$, CaF$_2$, ZnS and silver nanofluids of different particle size at 303K

Figure 2 shows that viscosity of nanofluids increased with increase in molar concentration. For methanol based SnO$_2$ nanofluids, the viscosities were 0.8742cP, 0.9224cP, 0.989cP, 1.0353cP and 1.1087cP higher than that of methanol based CaCO$_3$ nanofluids which is 0.5704cP, 0.5862cP, 0.5998cP, 0.6155cP and 0.6357cP respectively. Experimental investigation revealed that viscosity of all prepared nanofluids depends on the particle size, particle size distribution and shape of nanoparticles. In present system, it is observed that the viscosity of methanol based calcium carbonate nanofluids is lowest among all the studied nanofluids because of its larger particle size and the viscosity of nanofluids increases with reducing particle size. The distinguish feature of this dispersed system is that the area of contact between the dispersed particles and the methanol is relatively large and it increases with reducing particle size. Hence viscosity of nanofluids increases with decrease in particle size. But in case of methanol based zinc sulphide nanofluids, even though particle size is large still it shows higher viscosity. This can be explained on the basis of particle size distribution and shape of dispersed nanoparticles. All the particles used for the preparation of nanofluids have spherical shape but ZnS nanoparticles have elongated shape and hence due to elongated shape ZnS nanofluids have larger viscosity among all nanofluids [14]. Also in case of methanol based silver nanofluids, due to its narrow particle size distribution it provides less free space to move around and eventually makes the sample more viscous[15]

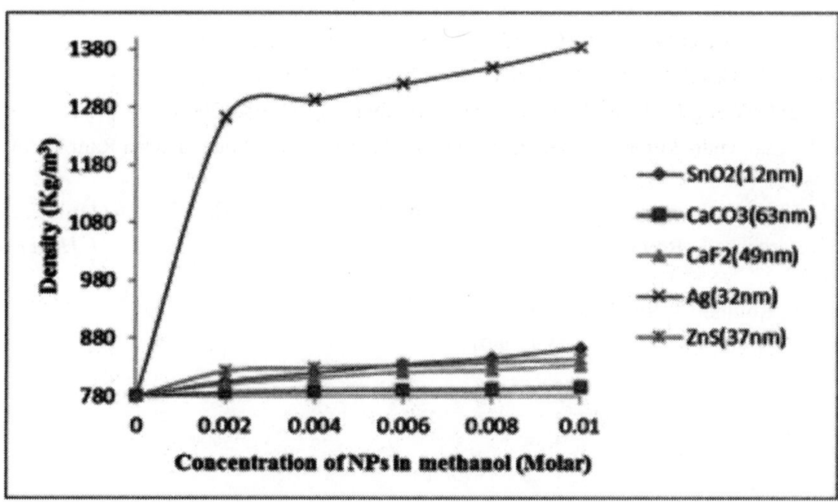

Figure 3. Variation of density of SnO_2, $CaCO_3$, CaF_2, ZnS and silver nanofluids of different particle size at 303K

It is observed that the density of methanol based nanofluids becomes size dependent and increased with decrease in particle size as shown in Fig. 3. The density of nanofluids is higher than the base fluids. The experimental value of density of methanol based calcium carbonate nanofluids having particle size 63 nm is minimum and it is 795.2 kg/m³ for 0.01M concentration, where as the density of methanol based tin oxide nanofluids having particle size 12 nm is maximum and it is 863.88 kg/m³ for 0.01M concentration. The increase in density of methanol based nanofluids is due to dispersion of high density nanoparticles in the base fluids. Again the number of particles per unit area is greater for smaller size particles as compared to bigger size particles.

4.   Conclusion

The viscosity and density of methanol based SnO_2, $CaCO_3$, CaF_2, ZnS and silver nanofluids was measured using capillary tube viscometers and density bottle respectively. The results show that the viscosity of nanofluids decreases with increasing particle diameter. The particle shape and size distribution also influence the viscosityof nanofluids. Elongated size ZnS nanoparticles shows higher viscosity than spherical size SnO_2, $CaCO_3$, CaF_2, and silver nanoparticles at the same concentration.The density of nanofluids increases somewhat with increasing concentration. Silver nanoparticles shows highest density among all studied nanofluids because of dispersion of high density nanoparticles in methanol.

5. References

1. Nalle P. B; Navpute A; Jadhav S. P; Shinde B. R; Shinde S, U; Jadhav K, M; *International Symposium on Ultrasonics-* (2015)

2. Namburu P. K; Fairbanks, A. K; Kulkarni D. P; Dandekar A; Das D. K; *IET Micro & Nano Letters* 2, 3 (2007)

3. Kim S; Kim C; Lee W. H; and Park S. R; *Journal of Applied Physics*, 110, 034316, (2011)

4. Mahbubul I. M; Saidur R; Amalina M, A; *International Journal of Heat and Mass Transfer,* 55, 874, (2012)

5. Eastman J; Choi S; Li S; Yu W; Thompson L;*Appl. Phys. Lett.*, 78 (6), 718, (2001)

6. Paul G; Philip J; Raj B; Das P. K; Manna I; *Int. J. Heat Mass Transfer*, 54 (15), 3783, (2011)

7. Chimankar O P, Padole N N, Pawar N R and Tabhane V. A., , Journal of Pure and Applied Ultrasonics **(39)**, 79, (2017)

8. Das S. K; Putra N; Roetzel W; *Int. J. Heat Mass Transfer*, 46 (5), 851(2003)

9. Putra N; Roetzel W; Das S. K; *Heat Mass Transfer*, 39 (8), 775,(2003)

10. Prasher R; Song D; Wang J; Phelan P; *Appl. Phys. Lett.*, 89 (13),133108, (2006)

11. Giridhar mishra, satyendra kumar verma, Devraj Singh, Pramod kumar Yadava, Raja Ram Yadav, Open Journal of acoustics, No.1, 9-14, (2011)

12. Timofeeva E. V; Yu W; France D. M; Singh D; Routbort J. L; *Nanoscale Res. Lett.*, 6 (1), 182, (2011)

13. Nguyen C; Desgranges F; Roy G; Galanis N; Mare T;Boucher S; Anguemintsa H; *Int. J. Heat Fluid Flow*, 28 (6), 1492, (2007)

14. Timofeeva E. V; Routbort J; Singh D;J. *Appl. Phys.*, 106(1), (2009)

15. Goharshadi E. K; *Phys. Chem. Res*, 1(1), (2009)

Decoloration of Synthetic Textile Swiss Pink Dye Using a Potent Bacterial Isolate

Shweta Singh, Roshan Lal Gautam, and Ram Naraian*

Department of Biotechnology, Faculty of Science, Mushroom Training & Research Centre (MTRC),
Veer Bahadur Singh Purvanchal University, Jaunpur-222003, India
*E-mail: ramnarain_itrc@rediffmail.com

ABSTRACT

As nature is known to be rich with diversified biodiversity of microorganisms, we have isolated a novel bacterium bearing strong and efficient potency of dye decoloration. The dye decoloration efficiency of bacterial isolate was tested under submerged liquid media containing synthetic textile swiss pink dye. The bacterium very efficiently decolourized as well as degraded the textile dye in liquid media. The highest and completedye decoloration was achieved within 360 minutes of incubation under submerged conditions. Decoloration of synthetic textile swiss pink dye was also efficiently conducted using culture extract of bacterial isolate. The decoloration of swiss pink from culture extract was achieved within only 260 minutes, which was faster in comparison to bacterial decoloration. However, other bacterium tested in this study found not capable to degrade swiss-pink dye under both solid and liquid conditions. Based on the result obtained in the present study it can be concluded that bacterial degradation of swiss pink dye is very cost-effective and environment-friendly, which can be recommended for the degradation and decoloration of textile industry effluentscontaining carcinogenic dyes in large amountsthrough industrial effluent treatment plant (ETP).

Keywords: Decoloration, textile effluent, swiss pink dye, dye degradation, bioremediation

1. Introduction

Textile industries are the crown of India's economy but they areconsistently becoming problematic day by day becauseof their threating discharges of untreated densely colored industrial effluents,which contains huge amount of dyestuffs.Such,synthetic dyestuffs of high coloring pigmentare extremely carcinogenic for living organisms of natural ecosystem especially water bodies.In addition, discharge of untreated textile dyes effluent in aqueous ecosystems also leads to reduction in sunlight penetration and negatively influences the level of dissolved oxygen,photosynthetic activity and several vital qualities of water. Discharge of textile industries contains a mixture of a large amount of coloring dyes and a very dark color, which creates serious environmental threats by damaging natural ecosystem. Therefore, direct discharge of textile industry effluents cannot be recommended, though the government has declared a standard governing policy regarding the discharge of effluents after their complete biological and non-biological treatments. Persistenceof untreated textile dyecontaining wastewater causes severe environmental dangerand the overall integrity of biome becomes disturbed, having an unpredictable health troubles globally[1,2]. The presence of −N=N− bond synthetic azo dyes makes them recalcitrant and carcinogenic in nature [3]. Several studies have been indicated that the involvement of various microorganisms produced extracellular reductive and oxidative enzymes such asazoreductase, laccase, tyrosinase, lignin, and manganese peroxidases degraded azo dyes [4,5].

Primarily degradation and decoloration of textile dye effluents are achieved by physical and chemical procedures, those are indeed not ecofriendly. In the recent past, many bioremediation techniques based on microbial members have been employed for the ecofriendly and cost-effective treatment of textile dyes and effluents. A few decades beforeseveral bioremediation techniques based on microbial cells,microorganisms (bacteria, fungi, and yeast) as well as their enzymes also have vast capabilities of dye degradation for successful bioremediation of textile dyes [6],and through their enzymes have been investigated for the treatment of industrial effluentsthat have an attractive potential in degrading highly complex dyes. This microbiological decolorization of dyes has recently received much attention as it is a cost-effective method for dye degradation[7].Consequently, degradation metabolites generated as result of dye decolorization found less toxic compared to untreated effluents [8], and the resultant effluent was able to release in open environment without any harming effect.For the textile effluent decolorization from a group of microorganisms like bacteria, fungi, actinomycetes,algae, etc. have been attempted [7,8,9,10,11,12], butamong of them, bacteria and fungi, the best potential to degrade dyes with diverse mechanism of color removal. However, from theviewpointoflarge scale treatments, bacteria got more attention because of their ease of applicability in comparison to others. Hence the current study was undertaken with the isolation, purification,screening, and characterization of potent isolate along with the excellent capacity of dye degradation in short time.

2.   Materials and Methods

2.1   Sampling

The untreated textile effluent samples were collected from different small dyeing industries located in Bhadoi, Uttar Pradesh (Latitude:25°25'12:00N; Longitude:82°34' 12:00E), India. The samples were collected in sterile plastic bottles and transported to the laboratory in icebox. All sample were processed within 1 h and stored at 4° C for further studies.

2.2   Isolation andpurification of bacteria

Several dye decolorizing bacteria were isolated from textile dye effluent by serial dilution and plating appropriate dilutions on modified nutrient agar plates. Plates were incubated at 37°C for 24 hours. The morphologically distinct bacterial isolates showing clear zone around their colonies due to the decoloration of dye were selected for further studies and rescreened. The pure cultures were stored on nutrient agar slopes at 5°C in refrigerators.

2.3   Maintenance of bacteria

Bacterial isolates were maintained in to nutrient agar (Peptone0.5%,beef extract 0.3%, NaCl 0.5%, agar 1.5%, pH 7) slants. For the storage purpose slants were stored in refrigerators at 5°C and culture were revived after fortnightly.

2.4   Textile dye

The famous carpet industry textile 'swiss pink' dye was used in the present study.It was purchased from the local dye market,of famous 'Carpet City' Bhadohi, U.P.,India.Liquid preparations of swiss pink dye of specific concentration were employed for dye decoloration studies.

2.5   Decoloration of swiss pink dye

Decoloration of swiss pink textile dye was conducted in liquid media under submerged conditions employingnewly isolated potent bacterial isolate. For this at specific concentration (0.05g/50ml) of swiss pink were inoculated by the inoculums of bacterial culture.All experimental sets were conducted in 200 ml sized Erlenmeyer conical flasks containing 100 ml broth in at least triplicates (n=3). After inoculation all experimental sets were incubated at 37°C in BOD incubators to perform dye degradation. The experimental sets were under consistent monitoring and to analyze the decoloration. The samples from each set were taken after regular intervals viz., 60,120,180,240,300& 360 minutes.

2.6   Determination of decoloration

The percent (%) decoloration ofswiss pink was calculated as follows:

$$\text{Decolouration (\%)} = \frac{100(Abs_{t0} - Abs_{tf})}{Abs_{t0}}$$

Where, Abs_{t0} = Absorbance at initial time of culture.

Abs_{tf} = Absorbance at the final time of culture.

2.7   Preparation of crude enzyme extract:

Pregrown culture of bacterial isolate was homogenized and centrifuged at 1000g for 5min. Thus obtained supernatant was used as crude enzyme extract for the dye decoloration studies.

2.8   Statistical analysis

Each experiment was performed in triplicate (n=3) and the standard deviation (SD) was calculated using Microsoft Excel, and results presented as mean ± SD value.

3.   Results and Discussion

3.1   Biochemical characterization of dye decolorizing bacteria

The promising isolate thatwas able to successfully decolorize swiss pink dye was subjected for various biochemical and physiological tests to characterize the isolate according to Bergey's Manual [13]. This bacterial strain was further employed in decoloration studies of swiss pink dye. The results are shown Table 1.

Table 1 Morphological and biochemical characterization of the bacterial isolate

Morphological & Biochemical traits	Results
Gram's Reaction	+ve
Shape	cocci
Motility	-ve
Endospore	-ve
Oxidase Test	+ve
IndoleTest	-ve
Methyl Red	+ve
Vogesproskauer	-ve
Citrate Utilization	+ve
Nitrate Reduction	+ve

Urease Test	-ve
Glucose fermentaion	+ve
Lactose fermentation	-ve
Sucrose fermentation	+ve
Casein Test	-ve
Gelatin hydrolysis Test	-ve

+ Positive; - Negative

n= 3(All experiment performed in triplet)

3.2   Effect of isolated bacteria on dye decoloration under submerged conditions

Decoloration of textile swiss pink dye was performed in submerged fermentation conditions in a medium having dissolved dye inoculated with novel bacterial isolate. Investigations of dye decoloration were monitored with simultaneous intervals of 60 minutes. A gradual decrease in the color of dye was observed in each set. The calculated increases in percentage of dye decoloration with respect to time can be presented as 50%, 58%, 66%, 78%, 89%, and 100% during 60,120,180,240,300 and 360min correspondingly (Fig. 1(a)). In consequence, it was observed that up to 360 min of bacterial treatment resulted complete decoloration of swiss pink dye and turned its color from pink to absolutely colorless.Khan and Abdul[14] reported decoloration of Reactive Black 5 dye up to 93% after 120 h incubation with isolated strain of Pseudomonas entomophila BS1.Similarly, Hossen et al [15] also reported decolorization of NSB-G approximately 90% after 96 h of cultivation at 37°C and pH 8.0 by the bacterial isolate.Therefore, in comparison to the findings of other studies, the bacteria isolated in my study have better capability for swiss pink dye decoloration only within 360 minutes of incubations.

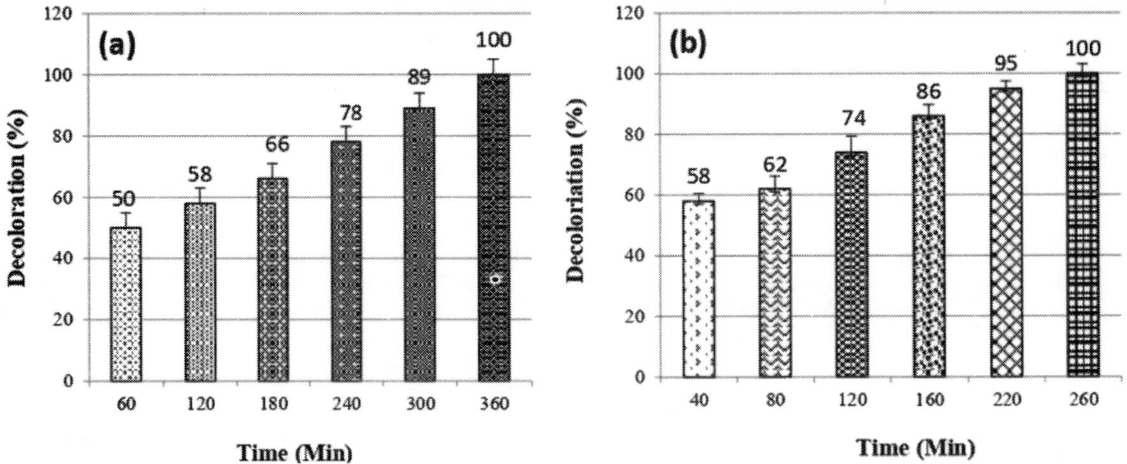

Figure 1. Percent decoloration ofswiss pink (0.05g/50ml)dye through bacterialisolate: (a)directby bacteria (b) by bacterial crude enzyme extract.

3.3   Effect of crude enzyme extract on dye decoloration

The impact of enzyme extract on decoloration of textile dye (swiss pink) was studied at a concentration of 0.05g/50ml dye. The investigations of dye decoloration were monitored with simultaneous intervals of 40 min. A gradual decrease in the color of dye was observed. The calculated increases in percentage of dye decoloration with respect to time can be presented as 58%, 62%, 74%, 86%, 95%and 100% during 40,80,120,160,220 and 260 minutes corresponding (Fig. 1.b). In consequence, it was observedthat treatments with crude enzyme were observed highly effective and showed decoloration up to 100% of 0.05g/50ml dye within 260 min and turned its color from pink to absolutely colorless.Hashemet al [16] observed that decoloration of 200 mg L−1 Remazol black B dye reached 100% in 32 h by P. aeruginosa KY284155. Similarly, Ladeet al [17]reported that two bacterial strain *P. rettgeri* strain HSL1 and *Pseudomonas sp*. SUK1 have capability to decolorize two azo dyes DR 78 (36 and 42 h) and RO 16 (24 and 18 h) completely. In present time-course study revealed that the decoloration of swiss pink textile dye by isolated bacterial crude enzyme saturated (100%) within 260 min of incubation, which shows high efficacy in comparison to other's studies.

4.　Conclusion

Based on the finding of the present study it can be concluded that the bacterial isolated was potentially able to decolorize the swiss pink textile dye in a very short time of 5 hours under optimized condition.However, the culture filtrate for bacterial culture showed a very faster dye decoloration within only 260min of treatment, which was faster in comparison to direct bacterial treatments.Therefore,the present bacterial isolate can be exploited for the bioremediation of swiss pink dye and textile industry effluent at large scale.

5.　Acknowledgments

The authors wish to acknowledge Hon'ble Vice-Chancellor, Veer Bahadur Singh Purvanchal University, Jaunpur, India for their consistent encouragement and providing the facilities.

6.　Reference

1.　Solis, M., Solis, A., Perez, H.I., Manjarrez, N., Flores, M.: Microbial decoloration of azo dyes: a review. Process Biochemistry 47, 1723–1748 (2012).

2.　Sarkar, S., Banerjee, A., Halder, U., Biswas, R., Bandopadhyay, R.: Degradation of Synthetic Azo Dyes of Textile Industry a Sustainable Approach Using Microbial Enzymes. Water Conserv Science Engineering 2, 121–131(2017).

3.　Saratale, R. G, Saratale, G. D, Chang, J. S, Govindwar, S. P.: Bacterial decolorization and degradation of azo dyes: a review. Journal of Taiwan Institute Chemical Engineering 42,138–157 (2011).

4.　Karim, M. E., Dhar, K., Hossain, M. T.: Decolorization of textile reactive dyes by bacterial monoculture and consortium screened from textile dyeing effluent. Journal of Genetic Engineering and Biotechnology 16(2), 375–380 (2018).

5.　Naraian, R., Kumari, S., Gautam, R. L.: Biodecolorization of brilliant green carpet industry dye using three distinct Pleurotus spp. Environmental Sustainability 1, 141–148 (2018).

6.　Kumari,S. ,Naraian.R.: Decolorization of synthetic brilliant green carpet industry dye through fungal co-culture technology. Journal of Environmental Management 180, 172-179 (2016).

7.　Patil, P. S., Phugare,S. S., Jadhav, S. B., Jadhav, J. P.: Communal action of microbial cultures for Red HE3B degradation. Journal of Hazardous material 181(1-3), 263–27 (2010).

8.　Imran, M.., Crowley, D. E., Khalid, A., Hussain, S., Mumtaz, M. W., Arshad ,M.,: Microbial biotechnology for decolorization of textile wastewaters. Enviromental Science Biotechnology 14,73–92 (2015).

9.　Fu, Y., Viraraghavan,T.: Fungal decolorization of dye wastewater:A review. Bioresource Technology 79(3), 251–62 (2001).

10.   Mohan, S. V., Rao, C.N., Prasad, K., Karthikeyan.,J.,: Treatment of stimulated reactive yellow 22 (azo) dye effluent using Spirogyra sp. Waste Manage. 22(6), 575-82 (2002).

11.   Park, C., Lee, Y., Kim, T., Lee, M., Lee, B., Lee, J., Kim, S.: Enzymatic decolorization of various dyes by Trametes versicolor KCTC 16781. Korean Journal of Biotechnology and Bioengineering 18,398–403 (2003).

12.   Satiroglu, N., Yalcinkaya, Y., Denizli, A., Arica, Y .M., Bektas, S., Genc.O., : Application of NaOH treated Polyporus versicolor for removal of divalent ions of group 11B elements from synthetic waste water. Process Biochemistry 38, 65–7 (2002).

13.   Wang, H., Su, Q .J., Zheng, W. X., Tian, X. Y., Xiong, J., T. L., Zheng.: Bacterialdecolorization and degradation of the reactive dye Reactive red 180 by Citrobacter sp. CKS. International Biodeterioration & Biodegradation 63, 395–399 (2009).

14.   Sarima, M. K, Kukrejaa, K., Shahb, I., Choudhary, C. K.: Biosorption of direct textile dye Congo red by Bacillus subtilis. Bioremediation Journal 10:1-11 (2019).

15.   Holt, J. G., Krieg, N. R., Sneath, P. H. A., Williams, S. T.: Bergey's Manual of Determinative Bacteriology. Ninth ed., Williams and Wilkins, Baltimore, Maryland, USA.175-189 (1994).

16.   Hossen, Z. M., Hussain, E. M., Hakim, , A., Islam , K., Uddin, N. M., Azad, K. A.: Biodegradation of reactive textile dye Novacron Super Black G by free cells of newly isolated Alcaligenes faecalis AZ26 and Bacillus spp obtained from textile effluents. Heliyon 5(6),1-11 (2019).

17.   Hashem, A. R., Samir, R., Essam, M. T., Ali, E. A., Amin, A. M.: Optimization and enhancement of textile reactive Remazol black Bdecolorization and detoxification by environmentally isolated pH tolerant Pseudomonas aeruginosa KY284155. AMB Express 8(1),1-12 (2018).

18.   Khan, S., Abdul, M.: Degradation of Reactive Black 5 dye by a newly isolated bacterium Pseudomonas entomophila BS1. Canadian Journal of Microbiology 62(3), 220–232 (2015).

19.   Lade, H., Kadam, A., Paul, D., Govindwar, S.: Biodegradation and detoxification of textile azo dyes by bacterial consortium under sequential microaerophilic/aerobic processes. Experimental and Clinical Sciences Journal 14,158-174 (2015).

Bio-polymer Electrolytes Based on CS-NaI-IL: Structural, Thermal and Electrical Transport Properties Study

A. L. Saroj

Department of Physics, Institute of Science, BHU, Varanasi, India
E-mail: al.saroj@bhu.ac.in

ABSTRACT

Bio-polymers have drawn much attention for developing solid polymer electrolytes due to the presence of functional groups with the side chains of backbone and film forming ability. Present study is focused on the effect of ionic liquid (IL), 1-ethyl-3-methylimidazolium methyl sulfate [EMIM][MeSO$_4$] on structural, thermal and ion transport properties of Chitosan (CS)-NaI based bio-polymeric films. CS-NaI-xwt% IL with x= 20, 30, 40 based bio-polymeric films were prepared using solution-casting method. ATR-FTIR analysis shows the interaction/complexation between the functional groups of CS with the dopant salt, NaI and cations of IL, [EMIM]$^+$. TGA results show that onset decomposition temperature ($T_{d, onset}$) decreased with increasing IL in [CS-NaI] based films. AC conductivity and dc conductivity studies were carried out to understand the ion transport mechanism for prepared IL based BPE films.

Keywords: Biopolymer, Ionic Liquid, ATR-FTIR, TGA.

1.   Introduction

In last few decades bio-polymer electrolytes (BPEs) have drawn much attention due to their potential applications, chemical stability, thin film forming ability, leak-proof, light weight and design flexibility [1]. Polymers are divided into two categories; synthetic and natural polymer. A vast number of synthetic polymers, such as polyethylene oxide (PEO), polymethyl methacrylate (PMMA), polyvinyl alcohol (PVA), poly acrylonitrile (PAN) and polyvinyl pyrrolidone (PVP) etc. have been synthesized for electrolyte applications [2-5]. Synthetic polymer based polymer electrolytes have several advantageous properties, like high energy density, flexibility, high operating temperatures and safety, leakage free, etc. But, low room temperature ionic conductivity and environmental pollution issues limits their performance in the development of electrochemical devices [2]. Several renewable resources based biopolymers, such as cellulose, chitosan, starch, and agarose are suitable to be used as host polymer in polymer electrolytes. Bio-polymer electrolytes based on these bio-polymers can undergo biodegradation as well as show the high room temperature ionic conductivity and compatible with the dopant salts due to presence of different functional groups. The various fascinating properties of biopolymer electrolytes such as ease of fabrication into a thin film with a large surface area to provide a high energy density, the ability to provide a wide range of ionic salt doping compositions, good electrode-electrolyte contact, high ionic conductivity, wide electrochemical stability, solvent free and leakage free, etc. made them suitable for electrolyte applications in electrochemical devices, like batteries, fuel cells, super capacitors, DSSCs [6], etc. On the basis of sources and origins, biopolymer electrolytes can be classified in different types such as (i) Synthetic bio-polymer based bio-polymer electrolytes (ii) naturally occurring bio-polymer based bio-polymer electrolytes. Some naturally abundant bio-polymers such as cellulose, Chitosan (CS) and starch are widely used in research. In order to enhance the room temperature ionic conductivity several methods were adopted like use of plasticizers (such as EC, PC, low molecular weight PEG, Ionic liquid) for developing the gel bio-polymer electrolytes, blending of two bio-polymers, use of ceramic fillers (like SiO$_2$, Al$_2$O$_3$, ZnO, etc.). CS is one of the important bio-polymer derived from

Chitin which is most abundant polysaccharide generally obtained from crustacean shells, fungi and insect. CS is a co-biopolymer of glucosamine and N-acetyl glucosamine with different polar functional groups like NH_2 (primary Amine), O-H (Hydroxyl group) and C-O-C (glucosamine/ether). Presence of theses functional groups with the side chains of CS make them suitable for bio-medical applications, food packaging [1], etc. The chemical structures of chitosan and chitin are shown in Fig. 1. Ionic liquids (ILs) have drawn a wide recognition for developing the electrochemical devices because of their unique properties such as negligible vapor pressure, high thermal and chemical stability, non-volatile nature, high room temperature ionic conductivity [7, 8]. Due to these important properties of ILs, they are replacing the volatile, toxic, flammable and less chemically stable organic plasticizers (i.e. EC, PC and low molecular weight PEG. In this chapter CS-NaI-IL based new bio-polymer electrolytes have been studied in terms of structural (ATR-FTIR and XRD), thermal (TGA), electrical transport properties (dc conductivity and ac conductivity).

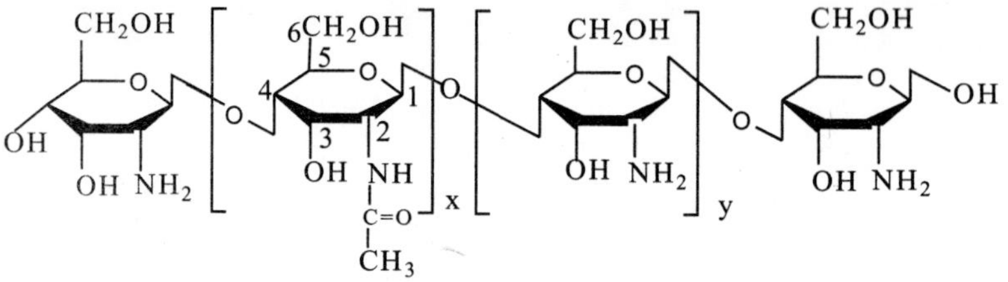

Chemical structure of chitin (if x > 50%) and chitosan (if y > 50%)

Figure 1 Transformation of chitin to Chitosan and similarities in their chemical structures.

2.   Experimental Details

Chitosan (CS) is insoluble in water but it is soluble in organic acids such as lactic acid, acetic acid and formic acid. In the present work diluted acetic acid solution was used as solvent. For the preparation of CS-NaI-IL based bio-polymer electrolytes, 1.5 g CS (obtained from Merck, Germany) was mixed in 150 ml diluted acetic acid solution (98% triply distilled water+2% acetic acid (procured from Merck, Germany)) at 50°C. Then desired wt% of NaI and IL, 1-ethyl-3-methylimidazolium methyl sulfate [EMIM][MeSO$_4$] (procured from Alfa SR, purity $\geq$ 98%) were added with mixture. The mixture was stirred for 72 hrs at 50°C and finally viscous slurry were obtained and poured into Poly-propylene Petri dishes and left to dry at 40°C in oven. The dried flexible films have been obtained with thickness ~100μm. All the films were then kept in desiccators (filled with dried silica gel) for further measurements.

3.   Results and Discussion

3.1   ATR-FT-IR analysis

Attenuated total reflection-Fourier transform infrared (ATR-FTIR) spectroscopy was performed by using Perkin Elmer Frontier spectrometer in the frequency range of 400cm^{-1} to 4000cm^{-1} with the resolution of 1cm^{-1}. ATR-FTIR measurement was performed for knowing the interactions between function groups of CS and cations of dissociate salt and IL. Scheme- 1 shows the possibility of interactions with interacting sites/positions of CS as C2, C3 and C6. In these sites, C6 is more effective because it is outside from the ring of CS. Fig. 2 shows the ATR-FTIR spectra of CS-NaI-IL based bio-polymeric films. From Fig. 2 it has been observed that CS related vibrational band frequencies are appeared at (1104-1130)cm^{-1}, (1413-1475) cm^{-1}, 1564 cm^{-1}, 1686 cm^{-1} and 3423 cm^{-1} associated with C-O-C symmetric and asymmetric stretching, C-N stretching, NH_2 (Amine), C=O-NHR (Carboxamide) and O-H (hydroxyl group) [9]. From Table 1 it has been observed that with the loading of NaI and IL in CS system these vibrational bands have been found to changes/shifts due to the complexation/interactions between the bio-polymer-salt and IL.

Table 1: Vibrational band frequencies (cm⁻¹) associated with the functional group of CS and CS complexed with salt/IL.

Vibrational band frequencies (cm⁻¹)			Assignments
CS	**[CS+40NAI]**	**[CS+40NAI]+40IL**	
1107	1054	1109	(C-O-C) Symmetric Stretching
1345	1390	1470	C-N stretching
1563	1558	1563	NH_2 (Amine)
1600	1660	1684	C=O-NHR (Carbonyl)
3423	3530	3535	(O-H) Related vibration

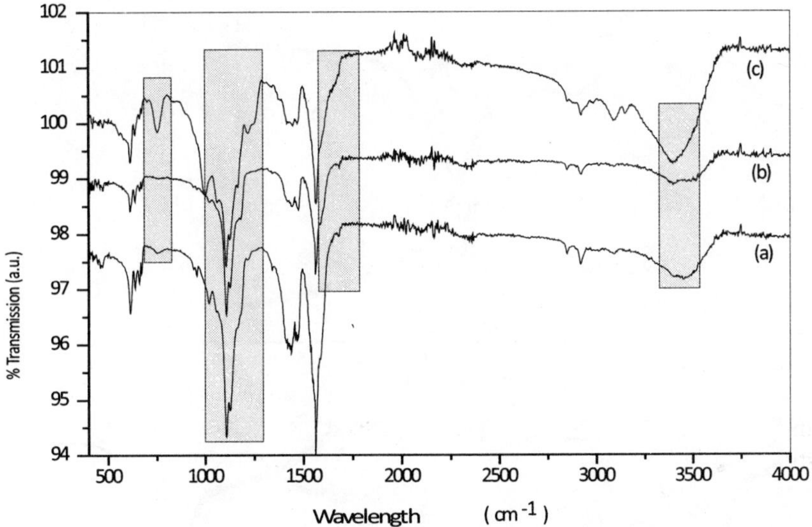

Fig. 2 FTIR spectra of (a-c) [CS-40NaI]-xwt%IL (x=20, 30, 40), respectively based bio-polymeric films.

Scheme 1: Possible interaction of functional groups of CS with cation and anion of salt and IL

3.2   Thermo-gravimetric analysis (TGA)

To investigate the decomposition of CS-NaI-IL based films TGA (supported by DTGA) measurement was performed by using Mettler Toledo TGA/DSC-I at the heating rate 10°/min in the presence of N_2 as inert atmosphere from 30°C to 600°C. Figs. 3 show the TGA (supported by DTGA) thermograms of CS-NaI-IL based bio-polymer electrolyte films. From Figs. 3 (a-c) it has been observed that CS-NaI-IL based films decompose in multi steps. First step of TGA thermograms (weight loss ~16% and ~17%) is observed at ~194°C, associated with the evaporation of absorbed water/moisture and second step observed at ~248 to 256 °C is associated with decomposition of the basic unit of polysaccharides [10]. Third step in TGA thermogram is started at ~300°C, related to the decomposition of CS-NaI-IL complexed. From Figs. 3(a-c) it is also observed that decomposition peak area appeared at ~300°C increases with increasing IL content in CS-NaI based films.

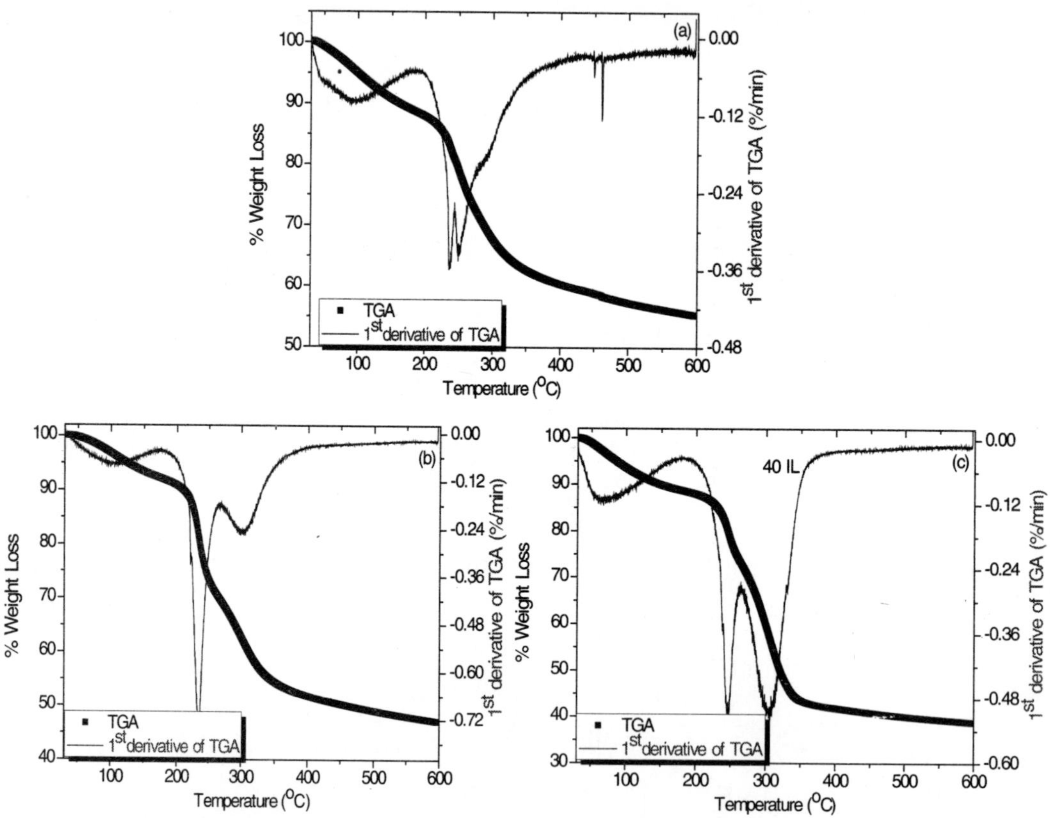

Figs. 3 TGA thermograms of (a-c) [CS-40NaI]-xwt%IL (x=20, 30, 40), respectively based bio-polymer electrolyte films.

3.3   AC and DC conductivity study

In order to understand the ion transport mechanism in terms of ac conductivity and dc/bulk conductivity study, electrochemical impedance spectroscopy has been done by using HIOKI-3536 LCR meter in the frequency rage 20Hz to 8MHz with 100mV signal voltage. For the data collection, the film of suitable shape was sandwiched between the two stainless electrodes assembled in WayneKerr sample holder. Fig. 4(a) shows the ac conductivity spectra for CS-NaI-40wt%IL based film. From Fig. 4(a) it has been found that ac conductivity vs. frequency plot follows the Jonscher's power law (JPL) stated as where is the dc/bulk conductivity (independent of frequency), A is a constant and is the power law exponent (n<1).

The complex impedance $Z^*(\omega)$ (= $Z' - j\,Z''$; where Z' (ohm) is real and the Z'' (ohm) is the imaginary (Z'') part of complex impedance) is defined as ratio of voltage V(t) to current I(t) in the time domain on applying a sinusoidal signal of low amplitude across a solid electrolyte. Fig. 4(b) shows the Cole-Cole plot (or Nyquist plot) for CS-NaI-40wt%IL based bio-polymer electrolyte film, which is used to calculate the dc/bulk ionic conductivity (defined as, where l (cm) is the thickness, A (cm^2) is the electrode–electrolyte contact area and R_b is the bulk resistance). The dc/bulk conductivity is found to be ~3.93×10^{-5} S/cm for 40wt%IL loaded sample.

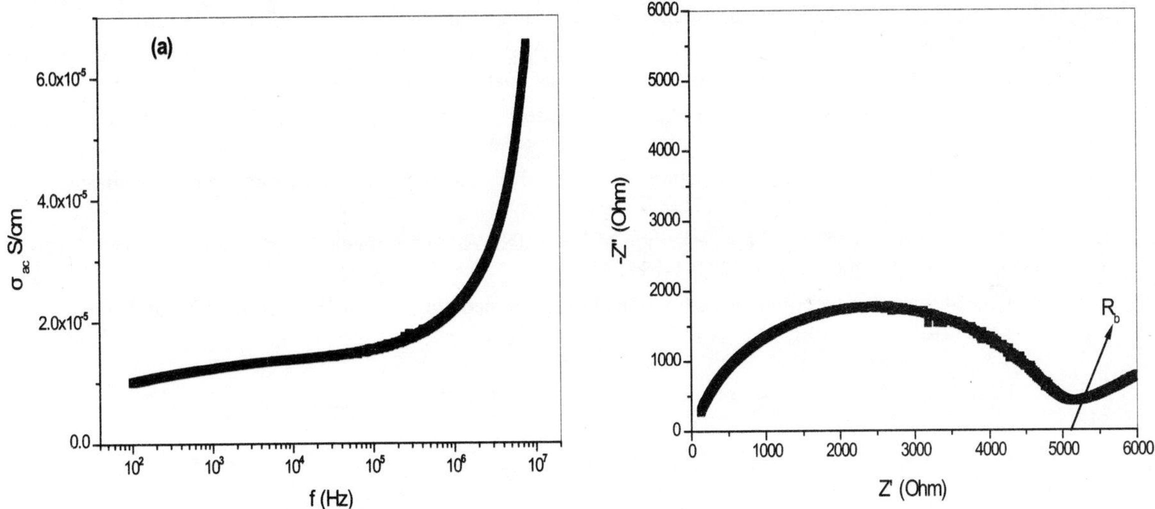

Figs: 4 (a) AC conductivity vs. frequency plot and (b) Nyquist plot for CS-NaI-40wt% IL based bio-polymeric film at room temperature.

4. Conclusion

1. CS-NaI-IL based bio-polymeric films were synthesized successfully by using solution casting technique.

2. ATR-FTIR analysis reveals the interaction/complexation between the function groups of Chitosan with the cations/anions of dopant salt/IL.

3. TGA results show that CS-NaI-IL based films decomposes in multi steps and it is also evident that thermal stability decreases with increasing IL content. TGA (supported by DTGA) thermograms also exhibits the complexation between CS-NaI and IL.

4. AC conductivity spectra for CS-NaI-IL based bio-polymer electrolyte films follows the JPL and 40wt%IL loaded sample shows optimum dc conductivity ~3.93×10^{-5} S/cm.

5. Acknowledgements

The author ALS is thankful to SERB, India for providing financial assistance through Major research project EEQ/2018/000862.

6. References

1. Ma J., Sahai Y., Chitosan biopolymer for fuel cell applications, Carbohydrate Polymers 92, 955– 975 (2013).

2. Gray F. M., Solid Polymer Electrolytes: Fundamentals and Technological Applications, VCH, New York, 1991.

3. Saroj A. L., Singh R. K., Thermal, dielectric and conductivity studies on PVA/Ionic liquid [EMIM][EtSO$_4$] based polymer electrolytes, J. Phys. Chem. Solids 73, 162-168 (2012).

4. Chaurasia S. K., Singh R. K., Chandra S., Structural and transport studies on polymeric membranes of PEO containing ionic liquid, EMIM-TY: Evidence of complexation, Solid State Ionics 183, 32-39 (2011).

5. Saroj A. L., Krisnamoorthi S., Singh R. K., Structural, thermal and electrical transport behaviour of polymer electrolytes based on PVA and imidazolium based ionic liquid, J. Non-Cryst. Solids 473, 87–95 (2017).

6. Low F. W., Lai C. W., Recent developments of graphene-TiO2 composite nanomaterials as efficient photo electrodes in dye-sensitized solar cells: A review, Renewable and Sustainable Energy Reviews 82, 103–125 (2018).

7. Goodenough J. B., Park K. S., The Li-ion rechargeable battery: a perspective. J. Am. Chem. Soc. 135, 1167–1176 (2013).

8. Hasa I., Hassoun J., Passerini S., Nanostructured Na-ion and Li-ion anodes for battery application: a comparative overview, Nano Res. 10, 3942–3969 (2017).

9. Wang W., Yu W., Preparation and characterization of CS-g-PNIPAAm microgels & application in a water vapour permeable fabric, Carbohydr. Polym. 127, 11-18 (2015).

10. Kunl M. et al., Structure and thermal properties of a chitosan coated polyethylene bilayer film, Polym Degrad Stab. 97, 1232-1240 (2012).

Synthesis of Boron Nitride Nanofluids and Study of its Ultrasonic Characterization

R. D. Chavhan[1], N. R. Pawar[2,*], O. P. Chimankar[2] and S. J. Dhoble[2]

[1]Department of Physics, RTM Nagpur University, Nagpur- 440 033, India
[2]Department of Physics, Arts, Commerce and Science College, Maregaon - 445 303, India
*E-mail: pawarsir1@gmail.com

ABSTRACT

Boronnitride (BN) nanofluids were synthesized by two step method. In this method BN nanopowder was initially prepared and the powder was dispersed in methanol base fluid. The nanofluid exhibits much greater properties as compared to base fluid. BN nanoparticles possess high thermal conductivity, and are a good conductor of heat. They are also a good electrical insulator, and have high-temperature lubricity features. Boron nitride nanoparticles are graded as an irritant and could possibly causes serious eye irritation, and allergy or asthma symptoms or breathing difficulties if inhaled. Boron nitride nanoparticles should be sealed in vacuum and stored in cool and dry room so as to avoid damp reunion as it would affect its dispersion performance and other usage effects [1-3].

BN nanoparticles were synthesized via sol-gel method by using 6.18g boric acid (H_3BO_3, Merck) dissolved in 200 ml distilled water. The solution is kept at 100^0C. The 6.30g melamine $C_3H_6N_6$ Merck is now added to the solution. The material prepared is placed upto 48 hours in room temperature. $B_4N_3O_2H$ is obtained after filtering and drying the solution. This is the precursor of BN. Then it is heated at 500^0C temperature for three hours without any gas flow. After that, material heated under nitrogen gas flow. Nitrogen gas flow is allowed for one hour with 800°C. The sample so obtained was grinded to get it in powdered form [4-6]. The prepared sample was characterized by X- ray diffraction (XRD), FTIR and Scanning electron microscopy (SEM). Average particle size has been estimated by using Debye-Scherrer formula [7-8]. It was found to be 70 nm. Nanofluids of BN in methanol base fluid were prepared and their acoustical studies were made such that different types of interactions could be assessed. Thermo-acoustical parameters of this nanofluids system were computed from ultrasonic velocities, densities and viscosities at temperatures 293K, 298K, 303K, 308K and 313K at fixed frequency 5MHz over the entire range of concentrations. The obtained results of present investigation have been discussed in the light of interactions between the nanoparticles and the molecules of methanol based fluids.

Keywords: Nanofluids; ultrasonic characterization; XRD; FTIR; SEM.

1. Introduction

Boron nitride nanoparticles possess high thermal conductivity, and are a good conductor of heat. They are also a good electrical insulator, and have high-temperature lubricity features. Boron nitride nanoparticles are graded as an irritant and could possibly causes serious eye irritation, and allergy or asthma symptoms or breathing difficulties if inhaled. Boron nitride nanoparticles should be sealed in vacuum and stored in cool and dry room so as to avoid damp reunion as it would affect its dispersion performance and other usage effects. BN nanoparticles have been synthesized by sol-gel method. The prepared sample was characterized by X- ray diffraction (XRD), FTIR and Scanning electron microscopy (SEM). Thermo-acoustical parameters of SC nanofluid were computed from ultrasonic velocities, densities and viscosities at temperatures 293K, 298K, 303K, 308K and 313K at fixed frequency 5MHz over the entire range of concentrations [9-11].

2. Preparation of BN Nanofluids

Boron Nitride is synthesized by using 6.18g·boric acid (H_3BO_3, Merck) dissolved in 200 ml distilled water. The solution is kept at 100°C. The 6.30g melamine $C_3H_6N_6$ Merck is now added to the solution. The material prepared is placed upto 48 hours in room temperature. $B_4N_3O_2H$ is obtained after filtering and drying the solution. This is the precursor of BN. Then it is heated at 500°C temperature for three hours without any gas flow. After that, material heated under nitrogen gas flow. Nitrogen gas flow is allowed for one hour with

800°C. The sample so obtained was grinded to get it in powdered form. The BN nanopowder was initially prepared and the powder was dispersed in methanol base fluid.

3.   Spectroscopic Characterization of BN Nanoparticles

Figure 1 shows the XRD pattern of BN nanoparticles. It is seen that the materials is well crystalline in nature and well agreed with standard JCPDS file number 034-0421 shown in figure 2. The estimate size of SiC nanoparticles using Debye Scherrer formula is found about 70 nm.

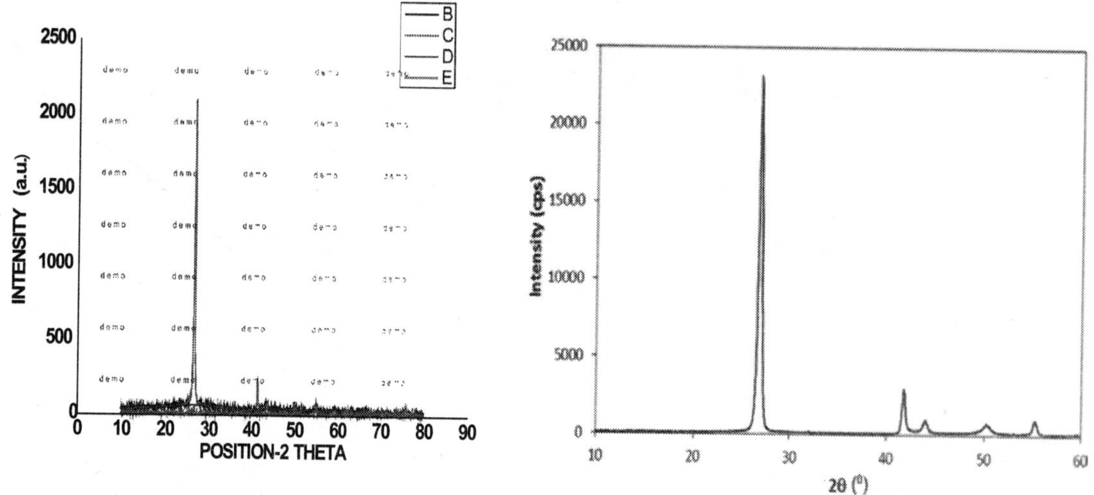

Figure 1 XRD pattern of BN Nanoparticles **Figure 2** XRD pattern of BN nanoparticles JCPDS file

FTIR analysis indicated the vibrations of metal oxygen (M–O) groups. FTIR spectroscopy shows the degradation phases and absorption in different regions which indicates structural relationship between them. From figure 3 it is seen that the inorganic groups is gradually decomposed at 1340.58 cm^{-1} and 767.23 cm^{-1}. SEM study is carried out to observe the overall surface morphology and crystallite sizes of the prepared nanomaterials shown in figure 4.

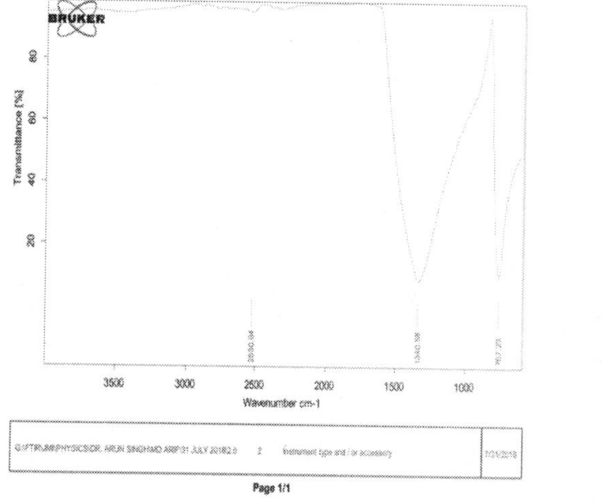

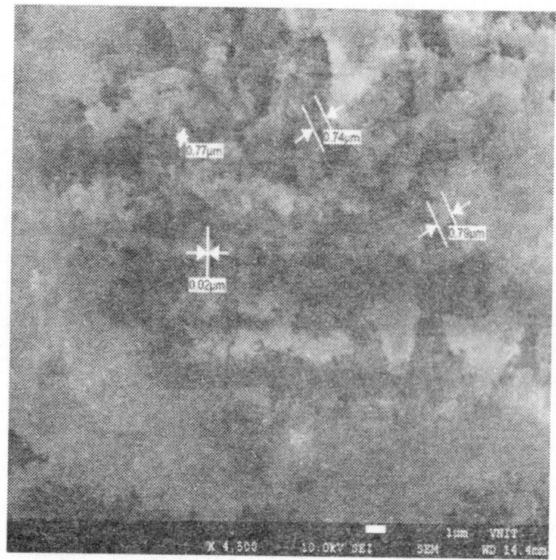

Figure 3. FTIR analysis of BN nanoparticles **Figure 4** SEM of BN nanoparticles

4.   Results and Discussion

The experimentally measured values of ultrasonic velocity, adiabatic compressibility, density and viscosity are represented graphically in Figs. 5-8.

Ultrasonic velocity gets increases with increasing the molar concentration of the BN nanoparticles in methanol this shows that the physical parameters of the sample changes by increasing the molar concentration. Nanoparticles suspensions do not settle which provides a long self- life which imparts ultrasonic velocity to them variation with molar concentration is represented in the figure 5. The cause behind this increase of ultrasonic velocity with increase in molar concentration (x) is due to strong interaction between nanosize particle and micro sized fluid molecule and also the Brownian motion of nanoparticles in nanofluids. Ultrasonic velocity can be interpreted as the nanosize BN particles have more surfaces to volume ratio and which can absorb more methanol molecules on its surface, which enhances the ultrasonic velocity.

The variation of adiabatic compressibility versus molar concentration of BN nanoparticles in methanol based nanofluids shows that adiabatic compressibility (βa) decreases with increase in molar concentration. The surface area of the material is increased by the reduction in particle size. Due to this higher percentage of the BN Nanoparticles can interact with surrounding fluids. It may due to decrease in interspacing of BN nanoparticles in nanofluids with increase in molar concentration. The variation of adiabatic compressibility with molar concentration is given in figure 6.

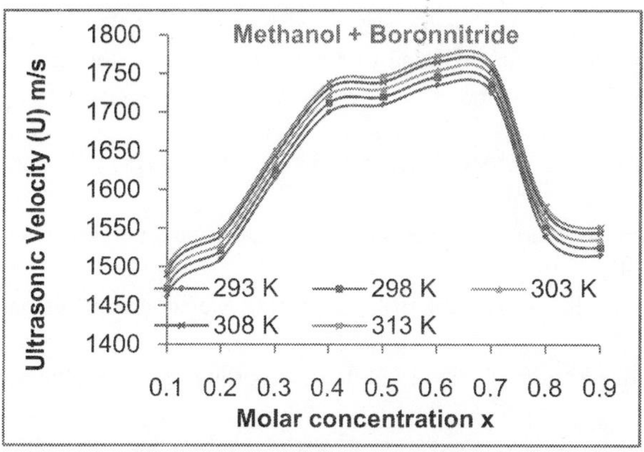

Figure 5 Variation of u versus x

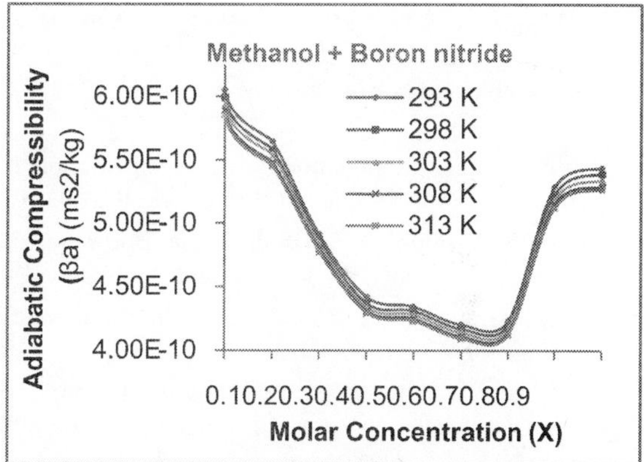

Figure 6 Variation of β_a versus x

Figure 7 shows the variation of density with molar concentration of BN nanoparticles in methanol. Densities of the nanosuspension are calculated by measuring the weight of the nanofluid using 25 ml of specific gravity bottle and also by using the standard value of density of water. Nanofluids of BN have more density than methanol. Increase in density indicates the close packing between the BN nanoparticles in methanol base fluid.

The plot of viscosity (η) versus molar concentrations clearly shows that viscosity slightly increases with increase in molar concentration of BN nanoparticles in methanol based nanofluids. As the motion of nanoparticles becomes more rapid when the temperature of the medium was raised which lowers the viscosity of the medium as the size of the particles was reduced. Hence viscosity of nanofluids decreases with increase in temperature. The viscosity of BN nanoparticle strongly depends on structure of BN nanoparticles and consequently interactions between the BN nanoparticles and molecules of the fluid.

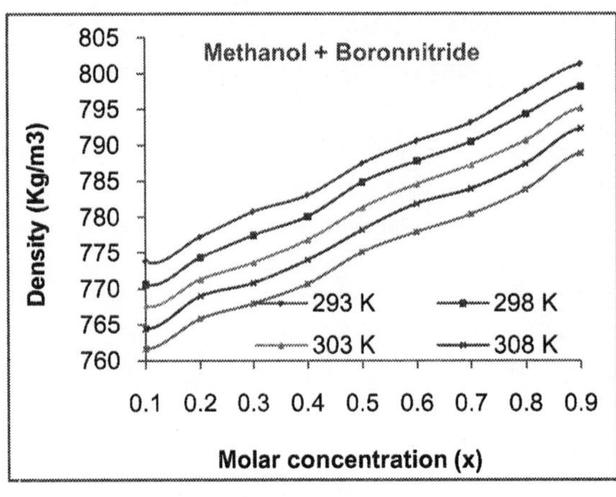

Figure 7 Variation of ρ versus x

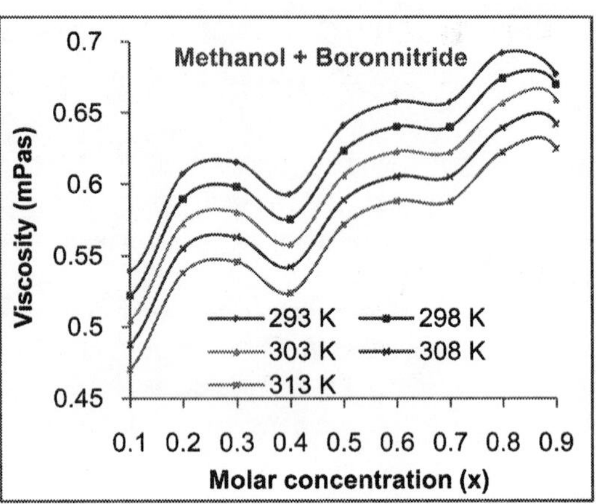

Figure 8 Variation of η versus x

5.   References

1.   D.H. Kumar, H.E. Patel, V.R.R. Kumar, T. Sundararajan, T. Pradeep and S.K. Das, Model for heat conduction of nanofluids, Physical Review Letters, 94 (14), 1-3.

2.   S. Rajagopalan, S. J. Sharma and V.Y. Nanotkar, Ultrasonic characterization of silver nanoparticles, Journal of Metastable and Nanocrystalline Materials, 23, 271-274 (2005).

3.   C. Peng, J. Zhang, Z. Xiong, B. Zhao, P. Liu, Fabrication of porous hollow γ-Al2O3 nanofibers by facile electro spinning and its application for water remediation, Microporous and Mesoporous Materials, 215, (2015) 133-142, 2002, pp. 1896-1899. doi:10.1557/JMR.2002.0281

4.   L. M. S. Ansaloni, E. M. B. de Sousa, Boron nitride nanostructured: synthesis, characterization and potential use in cosmetics, Materials Sciences and Applications, 4 (2013) 27066 (7 pp.)

5.   J. Y. Huang and Y. T. Zhu, Advances in the Synthesis and characterization of boron nitride, Defect and diffusion forum, 186-187, (2000) 1-32..

6.   Y. Chen, M. Conway J. S. Williams and J. Zou, Large-quantity production of high-yield boron nitride nanotubes, Journal of Materials Research, 17 (2002) 1896-1899.

7.   R D Chavhan, Abhranil Banerjee, Mrunal Pawar, O P Chimankar and N R Pawar, Synthesis and ultrasonic characterization of boron nitride nano suspension in organic base fluids, J Pure Appl Ultrason 41 (2019) 80-83.

8.   R D Chavhan, Abhranil Banerjee, Mrunal Pawar, O P Chimankar, S. J. Dhoble and N R Pawar, Synthesis and ultrasonic characterization of silicon carbide nano suspension in organic base fluids, JETIR, 6, (2019) 309-318.

9.   Tourino A.; Casas L.M.; Marino G.; Iglesias M.; Orge B.; Tojo J.: Liquid phase behaviour and thermodynamics of acetone + methanol + n-alkane (C9-C12) mixtures. Fluid Phase Equilib. 206 (2003) 61-85

10.   R. Kiruba, M. Gopalakrishnan, T. Mahalingam, A.K.S. Jeevaraj, Ultrasonic studies on zinc oxide nanofluids, Journal of Nanofluids, 1(2012) 97-100.

11.   A. G. Murugkar and A. P. Maharolkar, Investigation on some thermo physical properties of methanol and nitrobenzene binary mixtures, RJCABP, 1, 39- 43 (2014).

Ultrasonic Absorption and Thermoacoustic Study of Some DNA in Aqueous Solution by Non Destructive Technique

P. D. Bageshwar[1], N. R. Pawar[2,*] and O. P. Chimankar[3]

[1]Department of Physics, Mungsaji Maharaj Mahavidyalaya, Darwha – 445 304, India
[3]Department of Physics, Arts, Commerce and Science College, Maregaon – 445 303, India
[2]Department of Physics, RTM Nagpur University, Nagpur- 440 033, India
* E-mail: pawarsir1@gmail.com

ABSTRACT

Ultrasonic absorption of DNA in double distilled water by non destructive technique is essentials for utilizing them in biomedical technology. In biological sciences nitrogenous bases are increasingly termed nucleobases because of their role in nucleic acids their flat shape is particularly important when considering their roles as the building blocks of DNA. The present paper reports the ultrasonic absorption and thermo-acoustic study of some DNA in double distilled water by nondestructive technique at different molar concentrations, temperatures and at frequency 3 MHz of the ultrasonic transducer. The non-linear and complex behavior of investigated aqueous solution of DNA in medium helps to detect phase separation and strength of intermolecular interactions between the components in the medium.

Keywords: Aqueous solution of DNA; ultrasonic absorption; thermoacoustic parameters: structural relaxation process, etc

1.   Introduction

Ultrasonic wave velocity in a medium provides valuable information about the physical properties of the medium [1-3]. It also provides important information about various inter and intra-molecular processes such as relaxation of the medium or the existence of isomeric states or the exchange of energy between various molecular degrees of freedom [4-6]. Ultrasonic parameters are extensively being used to study molecular interactions in pure liquids binary liquid mixtures and ionic interactions in single and mixed salt solutions of bio-liquids [7-8]. The experimental investigations have shown that derived parameters provide a better insight into molecular processes. Aqueous of Adenine of DNA is used for this study.

2.   Results and Discussion

Figure1 contains the plot of ultrasonic velocity versus molar concentration of adenine in aqueous solution at different temperatures. It is observed that ultrasonic velocity increases with increase in molar concentration of thymine and there is complex formation at molar concentration 0.06 due to molecular aggregation. The association in the constituent molecules may involve due to hydrogen bonding or due to dipole-induced dipole interaction between the constituent molecules. Amino group in thymine are act as hydrogen bond acceptor or donor, hence association may be possible through hydrogen bonding. Figure 2 shows the variation of density with molar concentration of adenine in aqueous solution. It is observed that density increases with increase in concentration of thymine in aqueous solution. Increase in density decreases the volume indicating association in component molecules. It may be increase due to structural reorganization.

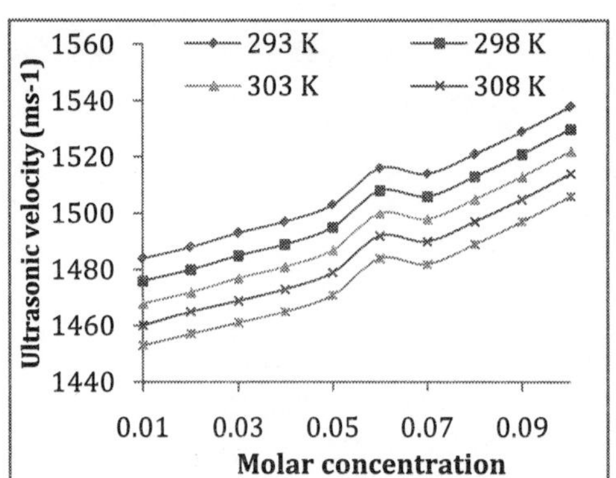

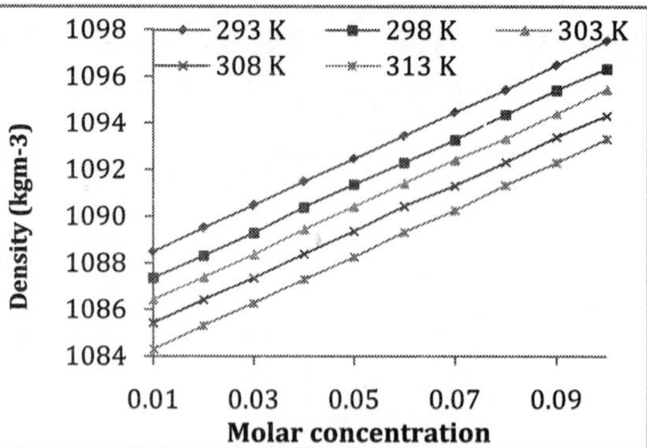

Figure 1 Ultrasonic velocity of aqueous adenine   **Figure 2** Density of aqueous adenine

Figure 3 contains the plots of adiabatic compressibility versus molar concentration. It is observed that adiabatic compressibility decreases with increase in molar concentration indicating strong molecular interaction in the component molecules of thymine in aqueous solution, shows associating tendency of constituents. The observed decrease of adiabatic compressibility with molar concentration indicates the enhancement of degree of association in the constituents. Hence the intermolecular distance decreases with increase in molar concentration. It is primarily the compressibility that changes with structure which leads to change in ultrasonic velocity. Figure 4 contains the plot of acoustic impedence (Z) versus molar concentration. It is observed that, the values of acoustic impedance increases with increase in the molar concentration of component thymine molecules in aqueous solution. It is in good agreement with the theoretical requirements because ultrasonic velocity increases with increase in molar concentration.

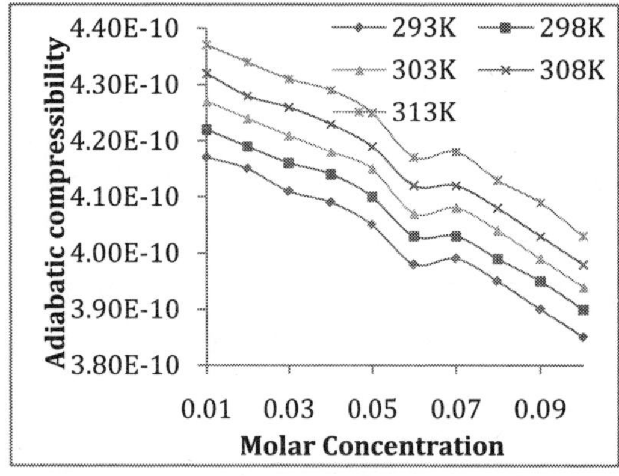

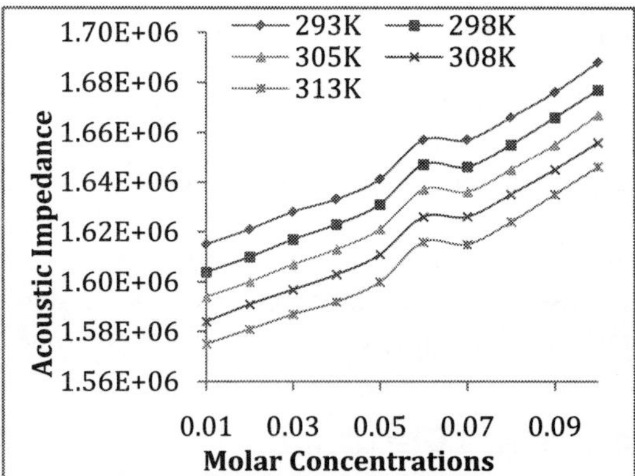

Figure 3 βa of aqueous adenine   **Figure 4** Acoustic impedance of aqueous adenine

Figure 5.5.18 contains the plot of experimental ultrasonic absorption (α/f^2) versus molar concentration at different temperatures 293K, 298K, 303K, 308K and 313K (table 5.5.6). It is observed that the ultrasonic absorption (α/f^2) increases with increase in the molar concentration of adenine in distilled water. It is clearly seen that smaller the temperature, greater the ultrasonic absorption. It is also observed that ultrasonic absorption (α/f^2) increases with increase in the molar concentration of adenine in distilled water, indicating more stability of adenine molecules. Adenine molecule has four resonating structure which increases the relaxation time, iecrease in relaxation time increases the ultrasonic absorption. The propagation of ultrasonic wave through binary liquid mixture disrupts thermal and structural equilibrium of the solution and produces energy transfer between different modes of the molecules. In this system structural relaxation plays a predominant role over thermal relaxation process. The increase in ultrasonic absorption with increase in molar concentrations is due to the possible structural relaxation process in this binary liquid mixture. The non-linear variation of ultrasonic absorption with molar concentration strongly supports the presence of strong intermolecular interaction through hydrogen bonding in the component molecules of this binary system. From the Graph it is clear that, the remarkable peak is observed at molar concentration 0.07. This shows that, the constituent's molecules are more stable hence absorbs more ultrasonic energy.

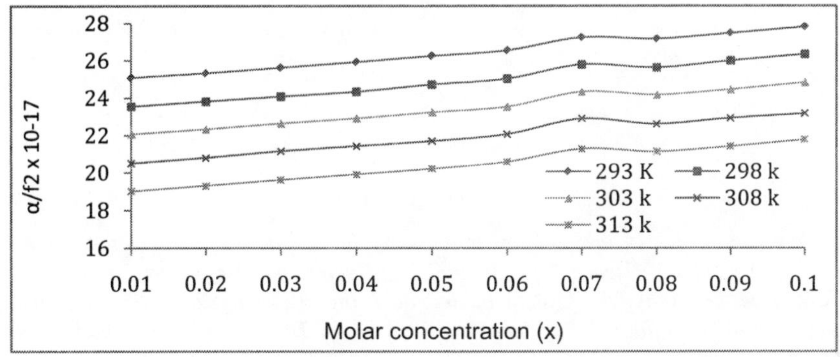

Figure 5 α/f^2 of ultrasonic absorption of aqueous adenine for 3 MHz

3. Conclusion

1. The observed molecular association may be due to the formation hydrogen bond or due to interstitial accommodation or due to induction or due to London dispersion forces in the constituent molecules.

2. Decrease in adiabatic compressibility with increase in molar concentration is due to molecular aggregation.

3. Thermo-acoustic parameters indicate the strength of molecular interactions.

4. References

1. Sk Md Nayeema and D. Krishna Raob, Ultrasonic Investigations of Molecular Interaction in Binary Mixtures of Benzyl Benzoate with Isomers of Butanol Int JP Research and Review, 2014, 3, 2 65-78.

2. N.R. Pawar and O.P. Chimankar, Comparative study of ultrasonic absorption and relaxation behavior of polar solute and non-polar solvent J Pure Appl Ultrason, 2012, 34, 49-52.

3. Kumar J., Kumar V., Kailesh and Shrivastava S. K., Temperature dependent anharmonic properties of calcium oxide crystal, J. Pure Appl. Ultrason., 2013, 35, 68

4. Singh D., Kaushik S., Tripathi S., Bhalla V. and Gupta A. K. Temperature dependent elastic and ultrasonic properties of berkelium monopnictides, Arab. J. Sci.Eng., 2014, 39, 485.

5. Rita Mehra, Meenakshi Pancholi and Avneesh K Gaur, Ultrasonic and thermodynamic studies in ternary liquid system of toluene+1-dodecanol+cyclohexane at 298, 308 and 318 K Arch Appl Sci Research, 2013, 5, 1, 124-133.

6. Pawar N. R., Ph.D thesis Summary on Investigation of Ultrasonic wave absorption in some Bio-liquids, J Pure Appl Ultrason, 2014, 36, 69-70.

7. A. Ali and A. K. Nain, Ultrasonic study of molecular interaction in binary liquid mixtures at 30°C, Pram J Phys 2002, 58, 4, 695-701.

8. T. Sumathi and M. Varalakshmi, Ultrasonic velocity, density, viscosity measurement of methionine in aqueous electrolytic solution at 303K, .Ras J Che, 2010, 3,3, 550-555.

Ultrasonic Absorption and Thermoacoustic Study of Some RNA in Aqueous Solution by Non Destructive Technique

Deoram V. Nandanwar[1] P. D. Bageshwar[2], N. R. Pawar[3,*] and O. P. Chimankar[4]

[1]Department of Physics, Shri M. M. College of Science Nagpur- 440 024, India
[2]Department of Physics, Mungsaji Maharaj Mahavidyalaya, Darwha – 445 304, India
[3]Department of Physics, Arts, Commerce and Science College, Maregaon – 445 303, India
[4]Department of Physics, RTM Nagpur University, Nagpur- 440 033, India
* E-mail: pawarsir1@gmail.com

ABSTRACT

Ultrasonic absorption of RNA in double distilled water by non destructive technique is essentials for utilizing them in biomedical technology. In biological sciences nitrogenous bases are increasingly termed nucleobases because of their role in nucleic acids their flat shape is particularly important when considering their roles as the building blocks of RNA [1-4]. The present paper reports the ultrasonic absorption and thermo-acoustic study of some RNA in double distilled water by nondestructive technique at different molar concentrations, temperatures and at frequency 3 MHz of the ultrasonic transducer. The non-linear and complex behavior of investigated aqueous solution of RNA in medium helps to detect phase separation and strength of intermolecular interactions between the components in the medium [5-6].

Keywords: Aqueous solution of RNA; ultrasonic absorption; thermoacoustic parameters: structural relaxation process, etc

1.   Introduction

In the biological sciences nitrogenous bases are increasingly termed as nucleobases because of their role in nucleic acids their flat shape is particularly important when considering their roles as the building blocks of RNA. There are five nitrogenous bases and all are non-polar. Purines are Adenine and Guanine, while Pyrimidines are Cytosine, Thymine and Uracil. These are used in the construction of nucleotides which in turn build up the nucleic acids like RNA. The present study deals with the experimental measurements of ultrasonic velocity, absorption, density and viscosity of nitrogenous bases in aqueous solution. The various thermo-acoustical and derived parameters and ultrasonic absorption were study. Adenine, Guanine, Cytosine, Thymine and Uracil are RNA. This study play very important role for determination of strength of intermolecular interactions between the components in the medium

2.   Results and Discussion

The plot of ultrasonic velocity (u) versus molar concentration of aqueous solution of uracil, shows that, ultrasonic velocity increases with increase in molar concentration except peak at 0.06 due to molecular aggregation indicating association in the component molecules. The association in the constituent molecules may involve due to hydrogen bonding or due to dipole-induced dipole interactions between the constituents. The variation of velocity with molar concentration is uracil in aqueous solution is given in figure1. The plot of ultrasonic velocity (u) versus molar concentration of aqueous solution of thymine, shows that, the ultrasonic velocity increases with increase in molar concentration except peak at 0.06 due to molecular aggregation, indicating association in the component molecules.The association in the constituent molecules may involve due to hydrogen bonding or due to dipole-induced dipole interactions between the constituent in binary mixture [7-11]. The variation of ultrasonic velocity with molar concentration is given in figure 2.

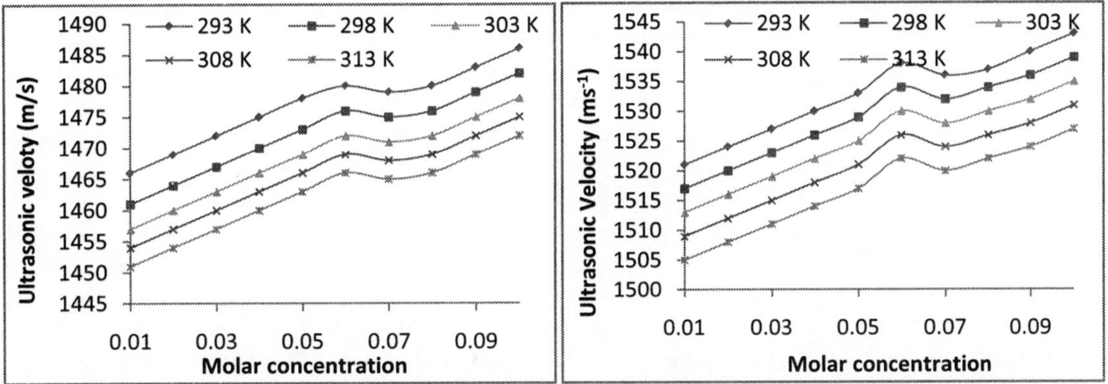

Fig. 1 Ultrasonic velocity of aqueous uracil

Fig. 2 Ultrasonic velocity of aqueous thymine

The variation of adiabatic compressibility versus molar concentration of aqueous solution of uracil shows that adiabatic compressibility (β_a) decreases with increase in molar concentration with a remarkable dip at 0.06. It is observed that adiabatic compressibility decreases with increase in molar concentration indicating strong molecular interaction in the component molecules, shows associating tendency of constituents. Hence the intermolecular distance decreases with increase in molar concentration. It is primarily the compressibility that changes with structure which leads to change in ultrasonic velocity. The variation of adiabatic compressibility with molar concentration is given in Fig. 3. The variation of adiabatic compressibility versus molar concentration of aqueous solution of thymine shows that adiabatic compressibility (β_a) decreases with increase in molar concentration with a remarkable dip at 0.06. Decrease in adiabatic compressibility with increase in molar concentrations indicating associating tendency of the constituents. Hence the intermolecular distance decreases with increase in molar concentration. It is primarily the compressibility that changes with structure which leads to change in ultrasonic velocity. The variation of adiabatic compressibility with molar concentration is given in Fig. 4.

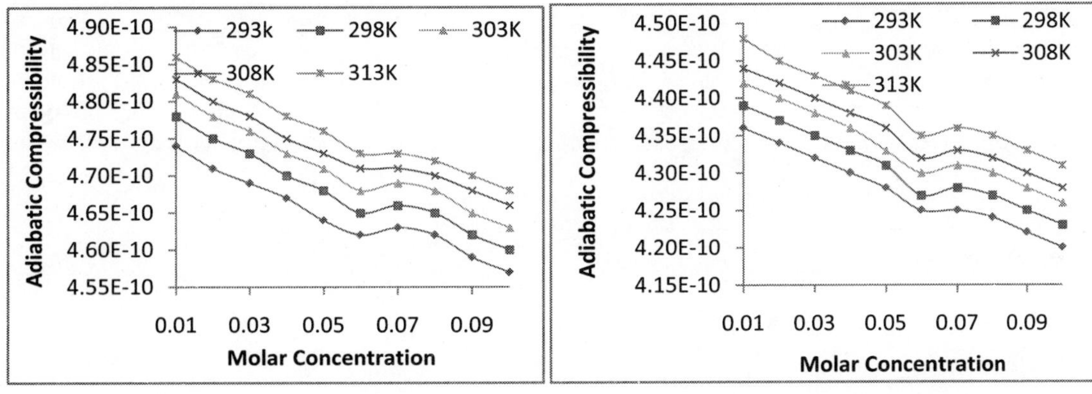

Fig. 3 βa of aqueous uracil

Fig. 4 βa of aqueous thymine

Figure 5 contains the plot of experimental ultrasonic absorption (α/f^2) of uracil versus molar concentration at different frequencies 2 MHz, 4 MHz, 6 MHz and 8 MHz. It is observed that the ultrasonic absorption

(α/f^2) increases with increase in the molar concentration of uracil in distilled water. It is clearly seen that smaller the frequency, less is the ultrasonic absorption. It is also observed that ultrasonic absorption (α/f^2) increases with increase in the molar concentration of uracil in distilled water, indicating more stability of uracil molecules. Uracil molecule has four resonating structure which increases the relaxation time. Increase in relaxation time increases the ultrasonic absorption in this binary liquid system. The non-linear variation of ultrasonic absorption in each curve with molar concentration strongly supports the presence of intermolecular interactions through hydrogen bonding. The hydrogen bonding exists between oxygen atom of uracil and hydroxyl group of water in the molecules of the constituents in this binary system. From the Graph it is clear that, the remarkable peak is observed at molar concentration 0.07. This shows that, the constituent's molecules are more stable hence absorbs more ultrasonic energy. Figure 6 contains the plot of experimental ultrasonic absorption (α/f^2) versus molar concentration at temperatures 293K, 298K, 303K, 308K and 313K (table 5.4.6). It is observed that the ultrasonic absorption (α/f^2) decreases with increase in the molar concentration of thymine in distilled water. It is clearly seen that smaller the temperature, greater the ultrasonic absorption. It is also observed that ultrasonic absorption (α/f^2) increases with increase in the molar concentration of thymine in distilled water, indicating more stability of thymine molecules. Thymine molecule has two resonating structure which increases the relaxation time, more the relaxation time more will be the ultrasonic absorption. The non-linear variation of ultrasonic absorption in each curve with molar concentration strongly supports the presence of strong intermolecular interaction through hydrogen bonding and dipole-induced dipole interactions. In this system structural relaxation plays a predominant role over thermal relaxation process. The increase in ultrasonic absorption with increase in molar concentration is due to the possible structural relaxation process in this binary system. From the Graph it is clear that, the remarkable peak is observed at molar concentration 0.07. This shows that, the constituent's molecules are more stable hence absorbs more ultrasonic energy.

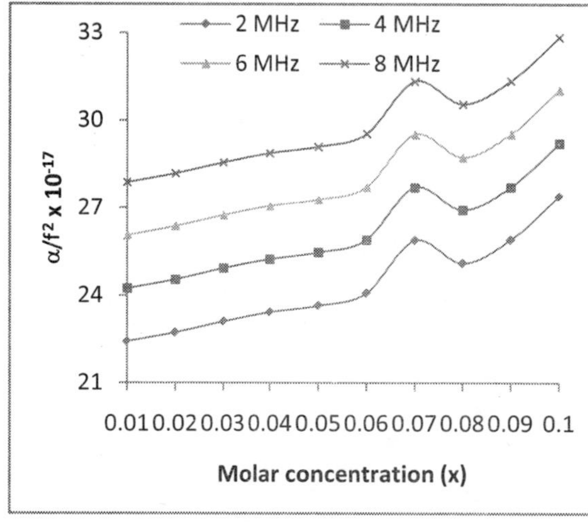

Fig. 5 α/f^2 of aqueous uracil at various frequencies

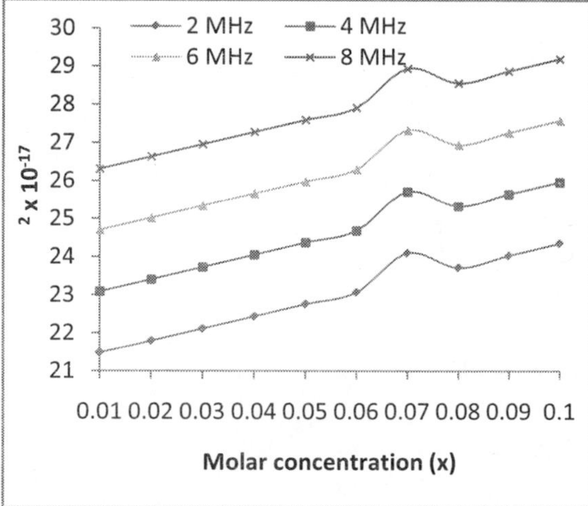

Fig. 6 α/f^2 of aqueous thymine at various frequencies

3.   References

1.   Sk Md Nayeema and D. Krishna Raob, Ultrasonic Investigations of Molecular Interaction in Binary Mixtures of Benzyl Benzoate with Isomers of Butanol Int JP Research and Review, 2014, 3, 2 65-78.

2.   N.R. Pawar and O.P. Chimankar, Comparative study of ultrasonic absorption and relaxation behavior of polar solute and non-polar solvent J Pure Appl Ultrason , 2012, 34, 49-52.

3. Kumar J., Kumar V., Kailesh and Shrivastava S. K., Temperature dependent anharmonic properties of calcium oxide crystal, J. Pure Appl. Ultrason., 2013, 35, 68

4. Singh D., Kaushik S., Tripathi S., Bhalla V. and Gupta A. K. Temperature dependent elastic and ultrasonic properties of berkelium monopnictides, Arab. J. Sci.Eng., 2014, 39, 485.

5. Rita Mehra, Meenakshi Pancholi and Avneesh K Gaur, Ultrasonic and thermodynamic studies in ternary liquid system of toluene+1-dodecanol+cyclohexane at 298, 308 and 318 K Arch Appl Sci Research, 2013, 5, 1, 124-133.

6. Pawar N. R., Ph.D thesis Summary on Investigation of Ultrasonic wave absorption in some Bio-liquids, J Pure Appl Ultrason, 2014, 36, 69-70.

7. Sunanda S.Aswale Shashikant R. Aswale, Rajesh S.Hajare, Journal of Chemical and Pharmaceutical Research, 4(5): 2671-2677, 2012.

8. V.N.Maruya, Diwinder Kaur Arora, Er. Avadhesh Kumar Maruya, R.A.Goutam., World of Sciences Journal ISSN 2307-3071, 2013 (02).

9. Kauzman W &Eyring H, J Am Chem. Soc, 62, 1940, 3113.

10. Kiyohara O & Benson G C, J Chem. Thermodyn, 11, 1979, 861.

11. S.Thirumaran, P.Inbum, Indian Journal of Pure and Applied Physics., Vol 49, p.p 451- 459, 2011.

Study of Acoustic and Thermodynamic Properties of Gallic Acid in Ethanol at Temperature 298K-313K

G.M. Jamankar[1,*], M.S. Deshpande[2,**], N.R. Pawar[2]

[1]Department of physics, Vidya Niketan College, Chandrapur Dist. Chandrapur (M.S) INDIA
[2]Department of physics, ACS College MaregaonDist.Yavatmal (M.S.), INDIA
Email: *gm_jamankar@rediffmail.com; **mil2des@yahoo.com

ABSTRACT

The properties of tannins are based on their chemical structures having two or three phenolicHydroxyl groups on a phenyl ring, in a molecule of moderately large size. Ultrasonic velocity (u), density (ρ) and viscosity (η) for binary liquid mixture of gallic acid in ethanol have been measured at temperature range 298K-313K over the entire molar concentration range 0.1M-0.9M and some thermo-acoustical parameters like adiabatic compressibility, acoustic impedance (Z), Gibb's free energy (ΔG), Classi cal absorption (α/f²) are computed. The non-linear variations of these resulting acoustical parameters with different concentration of the solute explained on the basis of structural changes occurring in a solution. Ultrasonic parameter measurements expose the thermodynamic properties of the liquid mixture.

Keywords: Tannins, Gallic acid, adiabatic compressibility, Gibb's energy, acoustic impedance.

1. Introduction

Ultrasonic investigation of liquid mixture containing components is of significant importance in understanding intermolecular interaction between the component molecules as that finds application in several industrial and technological processes. The rapid development of ultrasonic techniques and the introduction of new materials for producing powerful ultrasonic vibrations have opened up wide fields of research and technical applications in medicine and industry. Ultrasonic techniques and FTIR analysis having significant importance in understanding intermolecular interaction between the component molecules as that finds application in several industrial and technological processes(1-2). Here the attempts have been made for experimental investigations of derived parameters such as the ultrasonic velocity, adiabatic compressibility (βa), density, and viscosity of pure binary liquid Gallic acid in ethanolatvarious molarconcentrationsintherangeof0.1molto0.9 molfortheultrasoundfrequency2MHzat 298K, 303Kand 308K and313K.

2. Materials and Methods

The liquid mixture of various concentrations in mole fraction was prepared by taking AR grade chemicals. The study was carried out for the temperatures 298K-313K at fixed frequency 2 MHz and temperature of the liquid mixture was kept constant within an accuracy of ±0.1K by using thermostat. The experimental temperature was maintained constant by circulating water with the help of thermostatic water bath. Viscosity measurements were taken using Ostwald's viscometer with an accuracy of ±0.1Kg/m³. The density of the solution was determined accurately using 10ml specific gravity bottle and electronic balance and accuracy in the density measurement is ±1×10⁻⁵gm/cm³. An average of triple measurements was taken into account.

3. Result and Discussion

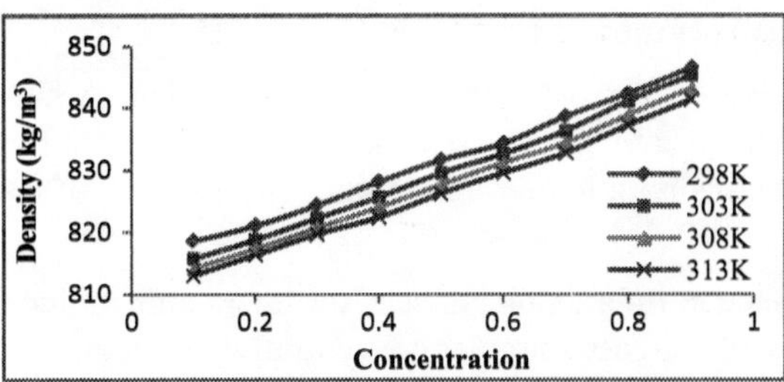

(a) Variation of Density with molar concentration of ethanol.

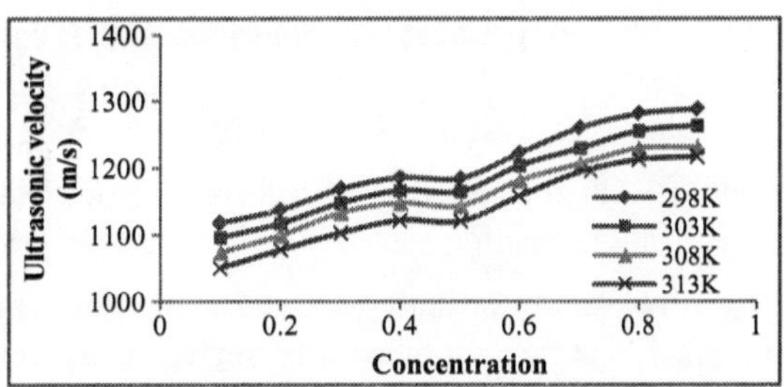

(b) Variation of Ultrasonic velocity with molar concentration of ethanol.

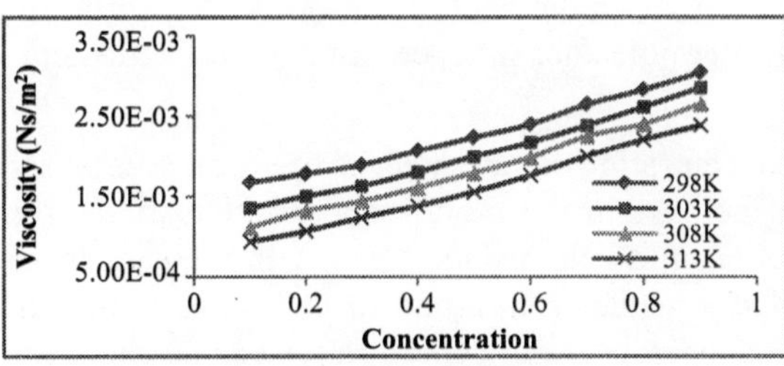

(c) Variation of Viscosity with molar concentration of ethanol.

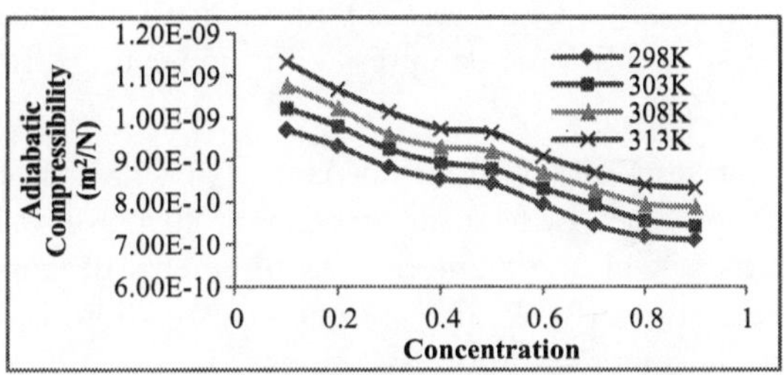

(d) Variation of Adiabatic compressibility with molar concentration of ethanol.

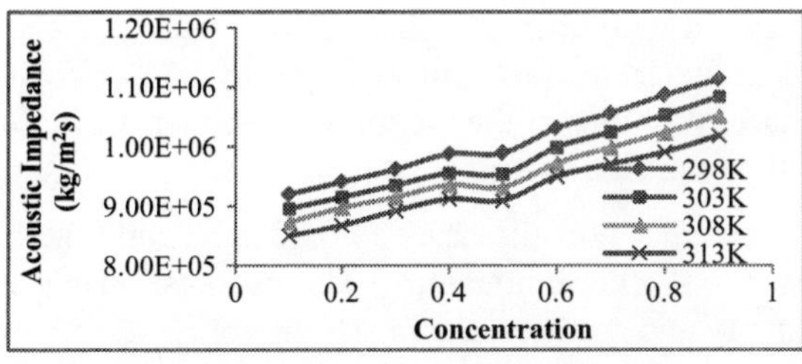

(e) Variation of Acoustic impedance with molar concentration of ethanol.

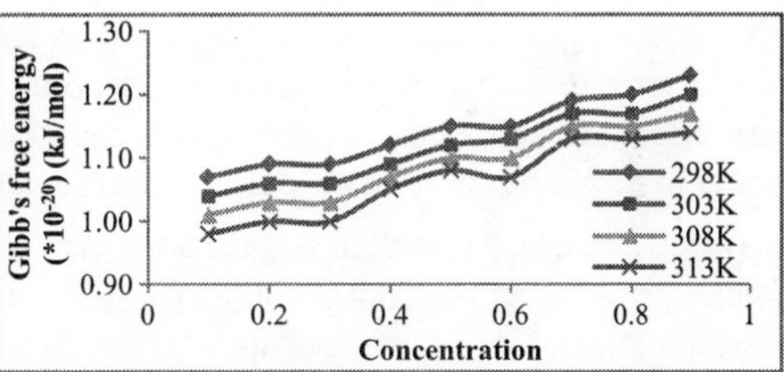

(f) Variation of Gibb's free energy with molar concentration of ethanol.

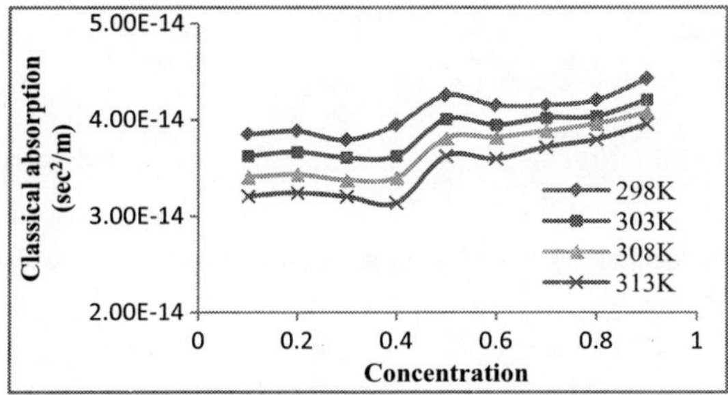

(g)Variation of Classical absorption with molar concentration of ethanol.

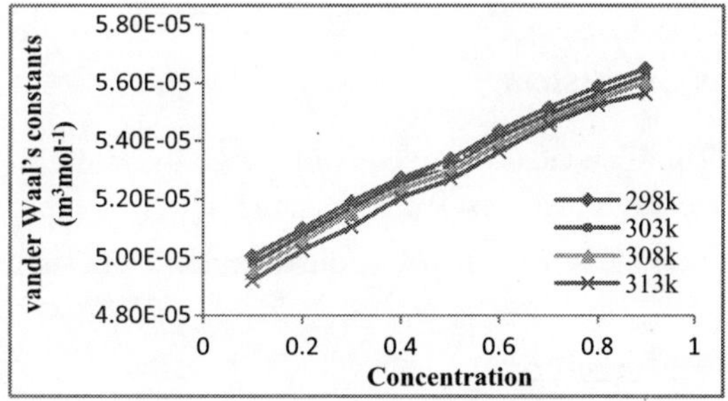

(h)Variation of vander Waal's Constant with molar concentration of ethanol.

In fig. (a) It is observed that density increases with increase in concentration of Gallic acid in Ethanol. Increase in density decreases the volume indicating association in component molecules. Measurement of density is very important tool for determination of adiabatic compressibility.

In fig.(b) The ultrasonic velocity shows non-linear variation for different composition which shows the presence of intermolecular interaction between molecules and structural changes occurring in binary solution(3-4). It is observed that ultrasonic velocity increases with increase in molar concentration of Gallic acid in Ethanol indicating association in the component molecules.

The viscosity gives information about the strength of molecular interaction between the interacting molecules. In fig.(c) it is observed that viscosity slightly increases with increase in molar concentration of Gallic acid in Ethanol and decreases with increase in temprature. Measurements of viscosity in binary mixture yield some reliable information in the study of molecular interaction.

Adiabatic compressibility is a measure of intermolecular association or dissociation or repulsion. Adiabatic compressibility (β_a) decreases with increase in concentration of Gallic acid in Ethanol as shown in fig (d). Decrease in adiabatic compressibility indicating strong intermolecular interaction between Gallic acid and Ethanol(5-6).

The variation of acoustic impedance (Z) with molar concentration represented in fig. 5(e). It is observed that, the values of acoustic impedance increases with increase in the molar concentration. It is in good agreement with the theoretical requirements because ultrasonic velocity increases with increase in molar concentrations (7). In the present investigation, acoustic impedance is found to be almost reciprocal of adiabatic compressibility. The increase in acoustic impedance with molar concentration can be explained on the basis of intermolecular interaction between component molecules, which decreases the intermolecular distance, making relative fewer gaps between the component molecules. This also indicates significant interactions in this binary liquid system(8).

Gibb's free energy (ΔG) is the free energy which is associated with chemical changes occurring in the given medium. Gibb's free energy versus concentration shows in fig.(f), it shows nonlinear behaviour for different concentration and temperature. Gibb's free energy measures mobility of the medium(9). Higher the mobility of the medium, higher will be the entropy and lower will be the free energy.

From fig(g) it is clear that Classical absorption (α/f^2) show that non- linearity for different concentration. It shows dip at 0.4M concentration and peak at 0.5M for all the temperature. The decrease in classical absorption indicates that less absorption of ultrasonic energy and the decrease in stability of mixture.

Infig. (h) it is observed that vander Waal's constant increases with increase in concentration of gallic acid in ethanol. This is because of the association of a closed packing of the interacting molecules inside the shell. The change in vander Waal's constant would be due to a change in intermolecular geometry(10).

4.   Conclusion

1. The acoustical parameters in the Gallicacidwithethanol suggeststhestrong molecular interactions in the unlike molecules of the system.

2. Nonlinear behavior of Acoustic parameters suggests the formation of complex in the mixture.

5.   References

1.   Cezaryn M. Kinart, WojciectKinart, and Anetacwiklinska, J.Chem.Eng. Data 47(1), 76-78(2002).
2.   Eben Henry Archibaild and WillianUre,J.Chem.soc.Trans, 125, 726-731(1924).

3. Londge M.G.,Kendre B. V. International Journal research in chemistry and environment 3, 106-112(2013).

4. V.Venkatalakshmi, P.Venkateswarlu, K.S.Reddy, International Journal of innovative research in science and engineering and technology,3 17556-17566(1994).

5. S.Prabhakar and K.Rajagopal, Pure Applied Ultrasonic, 27, 41-48(2005).

6. K. Sarvanakumar, R. Baskaran and T.R.Kubendran, Journal of Applied Sciences 10(15), 1616-1621(2010).

7. David G. Roux And Daneel Ferreira Pure &Appl.Chem., 54(12), 2465-2478 (1982).

8. Takuo Okuda and Hideyuki Ito Molecules16, 2191-2217(2011).

9. S, Anuradha, S, Prema and K.Rajagopal, Pure Applied Ultrasonic, 27, 49-54(2005).

10. K.Narendra, P. Narayanamurthy, CH.Shrinivasu, Asian Journal of Applied Sciences 4(5), 535-541(2011).

Temperature Dependent Structural Transition in Manganese Oxide and its Electrochemical Study

Avinash Kumar Singh[1,2], Tarun Kumar Dhiman[1], GBVS Lakshmi[1] and Pratima R. Solanki[1*]

[1] Special Centre for Nanoscience, JNU, New Delhi-110067, India
[2] School of Physical Sciences, JNU, New Delhi-110067, India
*Email: pratimarsolanki@gmail.com

ABSTRACT

Nanostructured manganese oxide has excellent properties. Due to the structural flexibility and redox activities manganese oxide has wide applications in catalysis, electric field-effect transistor, molecular sieves and nanobiosensor etc. In this study, we report phase transformation of manganese oxide NPs upon calcination at different temperatures, which were synthesized by co-precipitation method. These nanoparticles were calcined at 350°C and 650°C and lead to the formation of a constant phase of MnO_2 at 350°C. Further, at 650°C calcination, MnO_2 altered phaseS transition into Mn_2O_3. These two different phases of manganese oxide NPs were characterized by X- Ray diffraction, Raman spectroscopy, Fourier transform Infrared spectroscopy, UV- vis absorption spectroscopy, and field effect scanning electron microscopy to study phase, crystallinity, structure, absorption and morphology. The average crystallite size of MnO_2 Nps calcined at 350°C were obtained between 20-30 nm, while for 650°C calcined Mn_2O_3 NPs the average crystallite size were found between 30-45 nm. SEM studies confirmed the nanoparticular morphology of the material along with average particle sizes in the range of 50-100 nm. Maximum UV-Vis absorbance of MnO_2 was observed around 300 nm. In this study, we also report the electrochemical properties of these nanoparticle calcined at 350 °C and 650 °C, films were prepared on ITO coated glass substrates.

Keywords: MnO_2 nanostructure, nanobiosensor, field effect-transistor.

1. Introduction

Manganese oxide is a semiconductor nanomaterial owing to multiple properties like smaller in size, large surface to volume ratio, one-dimensional nanostructure, paramagnetic behaviour, etc. Therefore, it finds widely important applications such as; in wastewater treatment, as a catalyst, in sensors and biosensors, in nanocomposites, in supercapacitors, and in alkaline rechargeable batteries [1-4]. Manganese oxide can exist in a verity of stoichiometric forms as stable oxides like MnO, MnO_2, Mn_2O_3, Mn_3O_4, and Mn_5O_8 [5-7]. Out of which, particularly MnO and MnO_2 exhibit great role in the fabrication of the lithium ion batteries due to its low cost, environmental friendly and other special properties [3, 8]. A hydrous form of manganese oxides (MnO_2) has application as a scavenger for trace metals and other anions such as phosphate and chromate in marine and fresh water [9]. However, Mn_2O_3 attained higher oxidation state and acts as an environmental friendly catalyst to remove nitrogen oxide and carbon monoxide (CO) from waste gases [7]. These oxides have a specific property of changing their phases with increasing calcination temperature. Thermal decomposition studies showed that MnO_2 continuously gets converted into lower oxides under suitable conditions of temperature and oxygen partial pressure. MnO_2 decomposes to Mn_2O_3 at above 600 °C and this decomposed oxide converts into Mn_3O_4 upon further calcination above at 1000 °C [10, 11]. In this paper, we report phase transition property of manganese oxide prepared using the co-precipitation method and the electrochemical properties of these manganese oxides in two different phases after calcining. A high DPV peak current (in ampere) was observed in both the cases before and after the phase transformation which is its specific exciting property as compared to other oxide materials.

2.   Material and Methods

2.1   Reagents

Manganese acetate tetrahydrate (99.99%) and sodium hydroxide (98%) were purchased from Sigma-Aldrich and Fisher Scientific used for the preparation of manganese oxide nanomaterials. ITO coated glass substrate (Baltracom 247 ITO, 1.1mm thick, sheet resistance 25 Ω sq^{-1}, transmittance 90%) were procured from Balzers, UK.

2.2   Synthesis of manganese oxide nanomaterial

Manganese oxide nanomaterials have been synthesized using co-precipitation method. Manganese acetate tetrahydrate (0.1M) and sodium hydroxide (0.25M) were used as the precursor and reducing agent, respectively. Sodium hydroxide was added drop by drop into manganese acetate at constant stirring at 300 rpm till the pH of the solution reached to pH~12. After that, the precipitate was filtered out using Whatman filter paper and neutralised to pH~7 and dried in an oven at 80°C for overnight. The obtained dried powder was firstly ground to fine powder and calcined at 350°C and part of which was further calcined at 650°C for 4 h to obtain black powders in two phases of MnO_2 (350°C) and Mn_2O_3 (650°C).

2.3   Characterization techniques

Phase and structure of synthesized nanomaterial were examined by X-ray diffraction (XRD) spectra using XRD, Rigaku MiniFlex 600 X-Ray Diffractometer with CuKα radiation at λ=1.54Å; operating at 40 kV and 15 mA of the samples from 20°-80° at a scan rate of 3° per minute with step size 0.02°. Raman spectra were recorded using Enspectr R 532 in the range of 250-1250 cm^{-1} with 532 nm excitation wavelength. The morphology, shape & structure of the materials were explored by MIRA II KMH-TESCAN field emission scanning electron microscope (FE-SEM) operated at 25 keV. For this study, manganese oxide nanomaterials were ultrasonically dispersed in absolute isopropyl alcohol and dropped onto the ITO coated glass. Fourier transform infrared (FTIR) spectroscopy was used to study the proper formation of material and attached functional groups within the manganese oxide materials. Electrochemical study was performed using an electrochemical analyser (Autolab-AUT).

3.   Results and Discussion

3.1   Structural Studies

XRD spectra were recorded at room temperature to determine the crystal structure and phase purity of manganese oxide. XRD patterns of manganese oxides calcined at 350°C and 650°C are shown in fig.1 (a). The diffraction peaks for Mn_2O_3 (650°C) were found at 2θ = 22.7°C, 32.5°C, 37.97°C, 44.96°C, 49.06°C, 54.93°C, 60.4°C, 63.89°C, 65.67°C, 67.3°C and 69.01°C are indexed as (211), (222), (400), (332), (134), (125), (611), (145), (622), (136), (444), (046) and (721) represent cubic structure of Mn2O3. However, the diffraction peaks for MnO2 (350°C) at 2θ = 37.02°C, 42.02°C and 56.81°C are indexed as (100), (101) and (102) ascribed the hexagonal structure of MnO2.

Raman spectra of MnO_2 (350°C) and Mn_2O_3 (650°C) recorded at 532 nm of wavelength. Raman spectra of MnO_2 (350°C) showed three peaks around 276, 335 and 637 nm. Peaks at 276 and 335nm showed bending vibration of Mn-O bond and another peak around 637nm show stretching vibration in manganese oxide bond. While three peaks were observed for Mn2O3 (650°C). First two peaks at 295 and 345nm ascribed bending vibration of Mn-O and other one indicated, stretching vibration at 633 nm [12, 13].

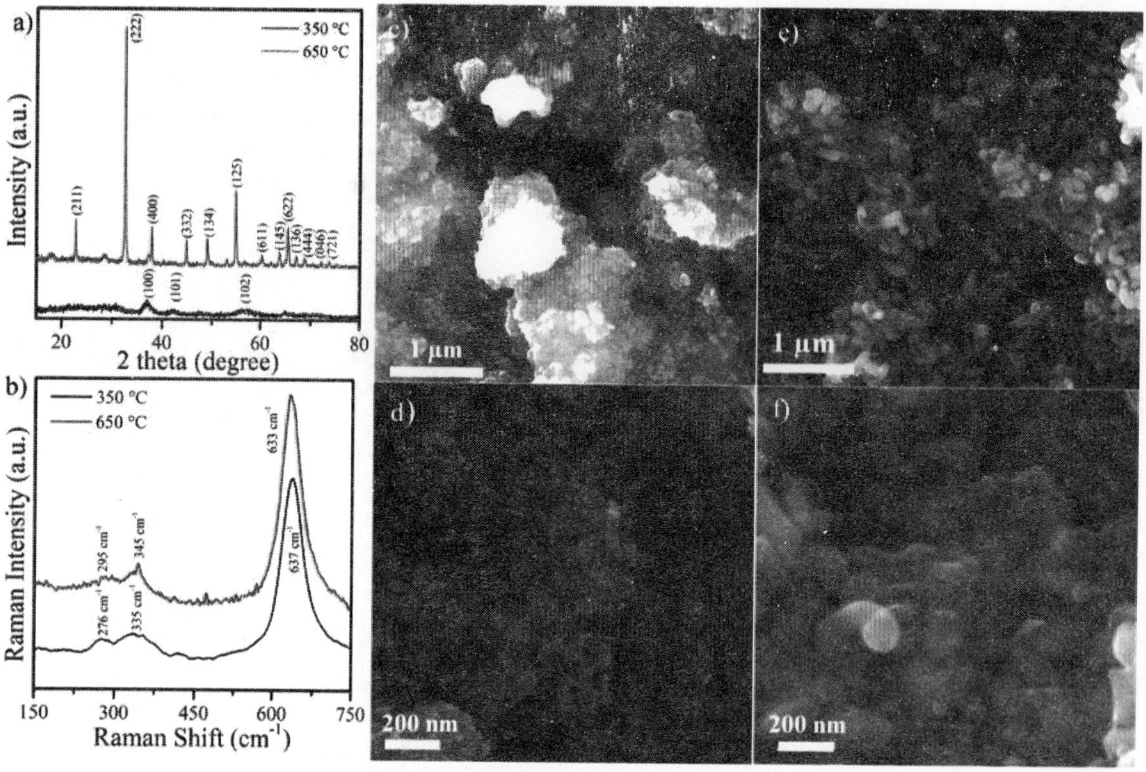

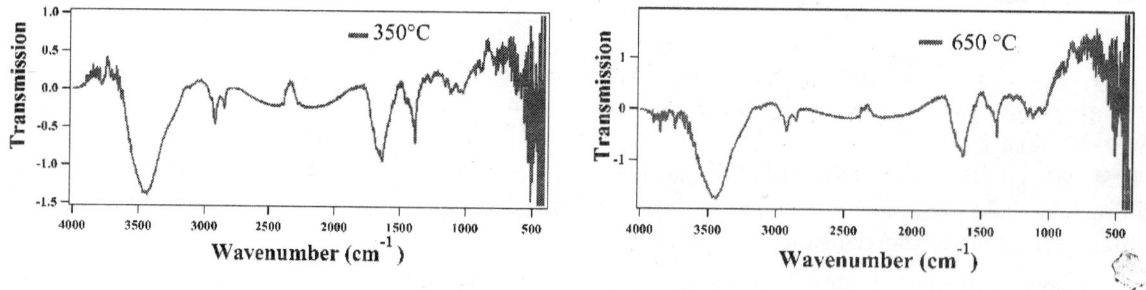

Figure 1. (a) XRD patterns (b) Raman spectra of MnO_2 (350°C) and Mn_2O_3 (650°C) (c), (d) FE-SEM images of MnO_2 (350°C) and (e), (f) FE-SEM images of Mn_2O_3 (650°C).

FE-SEM study was used to observe the shape and morphology of MnO_2 (350°C) and Mn_2O_3 (650°C). MnO_2 (350°C) showed the spherical shape of the nanomaterial with ~ 50 nm average size while Mn_2O_3 (650°C) described rod shaped structure with nearly 250 – 300 nm in length and the range of width was observed in between 100 – 120 nm.

3.2   FTIR study of Manganese oxide nanomaterial

Figure 2. FTIR spectra of MnO_2 (350°C) and Mn_2O_3 (650°C).

The FTIR spectra of MnO_2 (350°C) and Mn_2O_3 (650°C) were carried out in the wavenumber between 400 – 4000 cm^{-1} as shown in figure 2. Mn-O peaks can be assigned in the region between 400 – 800 cm^{-1} in both cases [14, 15]. In case of MnO_2 (350°C), the peaks around at 588 and 780 cm^{-1} can be ascribed to Mn-O bond among MnO_2 structure. The absorption peaks at 1025, 1120 and 1385 cm^{-1} matched to the O-H bending mode connected with Mn atom. Another peak around 1630 cm^{-1} which was also correspond to bending mode of water Mn-OH [16]. The broadest peak at 3440 cm^{-1} shows stretching vibration of a hydroxyl group (O-H) of manganese oxide. Similarly, in case of Mn_2O_3 (650°C) shows little bit shifted peaks in the region between 800 to 1500 cm^{-1} corresponding to O-H bending and other peaks are almost similar.

3.3   Electrochemical Studies of manganese oxide

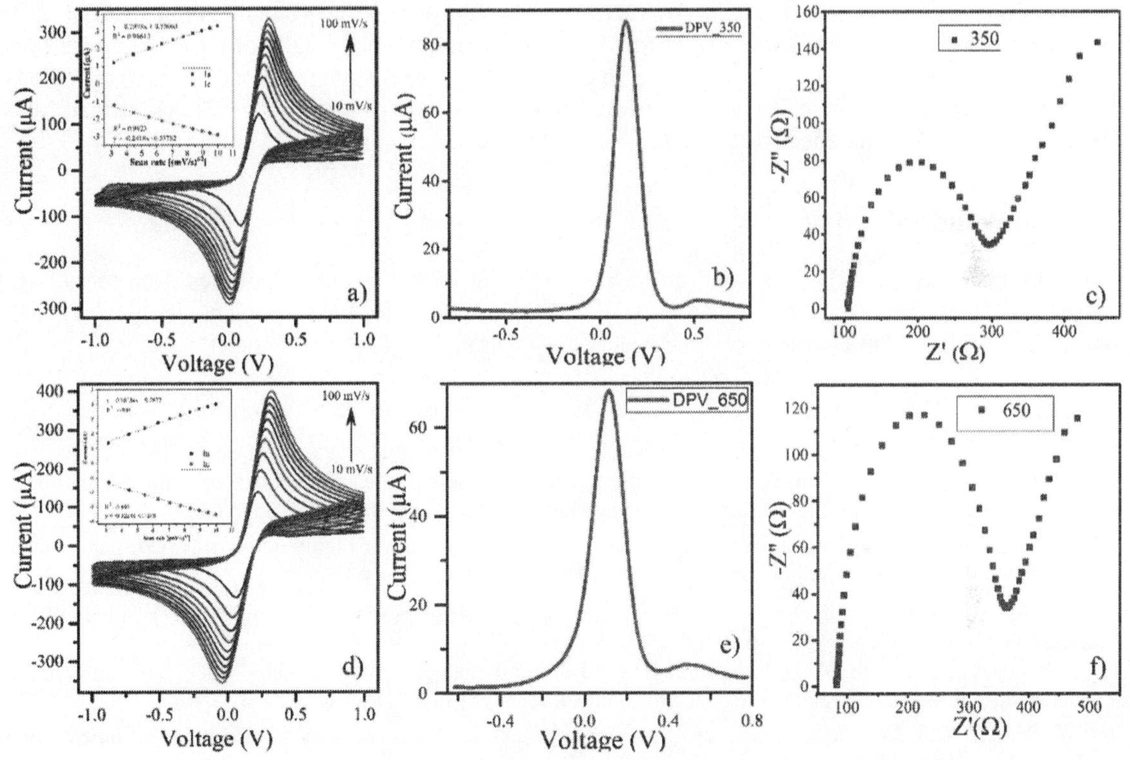

Figure 3. **(a)** Cyclic voltammetry curve of MnO_2 (350°C)/ITO at different scan rates **(b)** DPV plot of MnO_2 (350°C)/ITO **(c)** EIS plot of MnO_2 (350°C)/ITO **(d)** Cyclic voltammetry curve of Mn_2O_3 (650°C)/ITO at different scan rate **(e)** DPV plot of Mn_2O_3 (650°C)/ITO **(f)** EIS plot of Mn_2O_3 (650°C)/ITO.

Figure 3 shows the electrochemical characterization of synthesized MnO_2 (350°C) and Mn_2O_3 (650°C). The cyclic voltammetry (CV) curves of MnO_2(350°C)/ITO and Mn_2O_3(650°C)/ITO electrodes at different scan rates from 10-100 mV/S in 0.1M PBS containing [0.5 mM $Fe(CN)_6$]$^{-3/-4}$ are shown in (a) and (d). It has been observed that the magnitude of oxidation and reduction peak current and voltage are increasing with scan rate, resulting in the homogeneous electron transfer of the electrodes. The anodic (Ia) and cathodic (Ic) peak currents of MnO_2 (350°C)/ITO and Mn_2O_3 (650°C)/ITO electrodes exhibited a linear relationship (linear regression coefficient 0.99) with the square root of the scan rate, indicating a facile charge transfer kinetics. The DPV curves of MnO_2 (350°C) and Mn_2O_3 (650°C) were shown in (b) and (e) respectively, showing the high peak current obtained in the case of MnO_2 as compared to Mn_2O_3 with fairly high current of tens of μA.

The R_{ct} values of MnO_2 (350°C) and Mn_2O_3 (650°C) were obtained from the EIS curves given in (c) and (f) and the values obtained as 107 and 250.4 Ω respectively.

4.   Conclusion

Here, we have synthesized manganese oxide nanomaterial using co-precipitation process. These synthesized nanomaterials were initially calcined at 350 °C which converted into MnO_2 phase having hexagonal structure and these MnO_2 phase were further calcined at 650 °C, formed Mn_2O_3 phase and crystal structure change from hexagonal to cubic. These phase transitions were confirmed by using XRD, FESEM, Raman and FTIR characterization technique. The FESEM shown the conversion of spherical nanomaterial (MnO_2) at 350 °C into rod shaped nanomaterial (Mn_2O_3) at 650 °C. Cyclic voltammetry results of these nanomaterials in electrochemical study shown the proper increase in current with increasing the scan rate from 10 mV/s to 100 mV/s. The DPV results show the peak current was higher in the case of MnO_2 (350°C) than that of Mn_2O_3 (650 °C). The R_{ct} values obtained were comparable with values as 107 and 250.4 Ω respectively.

5.   Acknowledgement

Authors are thankful to AIRF (JNU) and SCNS for providing instrumentation facilities. One of us (AKS) thanks to UGC for financial support. **One of us (GBVSL)** thanks DST for Women Scientist project. Financial support was obtained from Department of Biotechnology, Through Indo Russia Project.

6.   References

1.   S. Shanmugam, A. Gedanken, Easy single-step route to manganese oxide nanoparticles embedded in carbon and their magnetic properties, The Journal of Physical Chemistry C, 112 (2008) 15752-15758.

2.   X. Han, F. Zhang, Q. Meng, J. Sun, Preparation and characterization of highly activated MnO_2 nanostructure, Journal of the American Ceramic Society, 93 (2010) 1183-1186.

3.   X. Liu, C. Chen, Y. Zhao, B. Jia, A review on the synthesis of manganese oxide nanomaterials and their applications on lithium-ion batteries, Journal of Nanomaterials, 2013 (2013).

4.   P. Ragupathy, H. Vasan, N. Munichandraiah, Synthesis and characterization of nano-MnO_2 for electrochemical supercapacitor studies, Journal of the Electrochemical Society, 155 (2008) A34-A40.

5.   W. Wei, X. Cui, W. Chen, D.G. Ivey, Manganese oxide-based materials as electrochemical supercapacitor electrodes, Chemical society reviews, 40 (2011) 1697-1721.

6.   X. Chen, C. Wang, F. Ye, Q. Zhu, G. Du, Y. Zhong, X. Peng, J. Jiang, Phase transition of manganese (oxyhydr) oxides nanofibers and their applications to lithium ion batteries and separation membranes, CrystEngComm, 14 (2012) 3142-3148.

7.   R. Najjar, R. Awad, A. Abdel-Gaber, Physical Properties of Mn_2O_3 Nanoparticles Synthesized by Co-precipitation Method at Different pH Values, Journal of Superconductivity and Novel Magnetism, (2019) 1-8.

8.   C. Julien, A. Mauger, Nanostructured MnO_2 as electrode materials for energy storage, Nanomaterials, 7 (2017) 396.

9.   S. Shakeel Iqubal, Nanosized MnO_2: preparation, characterisation and its redox activity, International Journal of Nanoparticles, 2 (2009) 321-328.

10.   G. Mukherjee, S. Vaidya, C. Karunakaran, High pressure and high temperature studies on manganese oxides, Phase Transitions, 75 (2002) 557-566.

11.   K. Terayama, M. Ikeda, Study on thermal decomposition of MnO_2 and Mn_2O_3 by thermal analysis, Transactions of the Japan institute of metals, 24 (1983) 754-758.

12.   T. Gao, M. Glerup, F. Krumeich, R. Nesper, H. Fjellvåg, P. Norby, Microstructures and spectroscopic properties of cryptomelane-type manganese dioxide nanofibers, The Journal of Physical Chemistry C, 112 (2008) 13134-13140.

13. H.R. Barai, A.N. Banerjee, N. Hamnabard, S.W. Joo, Synthesis of amorphous manganese oxide nanoparticles–to–crystalline nanorods through a simple wet-chemical technique using K+ ions as a 'growth director' and their morphology-controlled high performance supercapacitor applications, RSC Advances, 6 (2016) 78887-78908.

14. L. Kang, M. Zhang, Z.-H. Liu, K. Ooi, IR spectra of manganese oxides with either layered or tunnel structures, Spectrochimica Acta Part A: Molecular and Biomolecular Spectroscopy, 67 (2007) 864-869.

15. Q. Feng, Y. Miyai, H. Kanoh, K. Ooi, Lithium (1+) extraction/insertion with spinel-type lithium manganese oxides. Characterization of redox-type and ion-exchange-type sites, Langmuir, 8 (1992) 1861-1867.

16. M. Mylarappa, V.V. Lakshmi, K.V. Mahesh, H. Nagaswarupa, N. Raghavendra, A facile hydrothermal recovery of nano sealed MnO_2 particle from waste batteries: An advanced material for electrochemical and environmental applications, in: IOP Conference Series: Materials Science and Engineering, IOP Publishing, 2016, pp. 012178.

A Survey on Machine Learning Methods for Phishing Detection

Pravin Kumar Pandey[1*], Sandip Kumar Singh[2,] Deep Prakash Singh Senger

[1]Department of Computer Science & Engineering, UNSIET, VBS Purvanchal University, Jaunpur-211001, India
[2] Department of Mechanical Engineering, UNSIET, VBS Purvanchal University, Jaunpur-211001, India
*E-mail: pravin108786@gmail.com

ABSTRACT

Phishing is an electronically connected criminal activity in which the attacker steals the user's personal information like username, countersign, credit/debit card number, password, pin, legitimacy, confidential patient record, CVV number, etc. to benefit financially. Email-based phishing is the most common and traditional way of phishing scams, in which the phisher will send a suspicious email with an embedded URL and ask the user to click the URL. When the user clicks on the link, the link will be redirected to a spoofed site that looks the same to the original site to steal their credentials and displays some error message. Later the phishers use those credentials for malicious purposes. To overcome these scams, many anti-phishing tools have developed. Among that the machine learning-based approaches can give better results. This paper is an extensive survey of the various machine learning-based anti-phishing approaches that detect the phishing URL's from the URLs with URLs features.

Keywords: Phishing, anti-phishing, machine learning, phishtank, legitimate, suspicious.

1.   Introduction

Phishing is one kind of deceitful activity through which the attacker steals user personal information. Phishing is popular with cybercriminals, as it is so far easier to trick someone into clicking a malicious link in a seemingly legitimate email than trying to break through a computer's defenses. Although some phishing emails are poorly written and fake, sophisticated cybercriminals employ the technique of professional marketers to identify the most effective types of message [1].

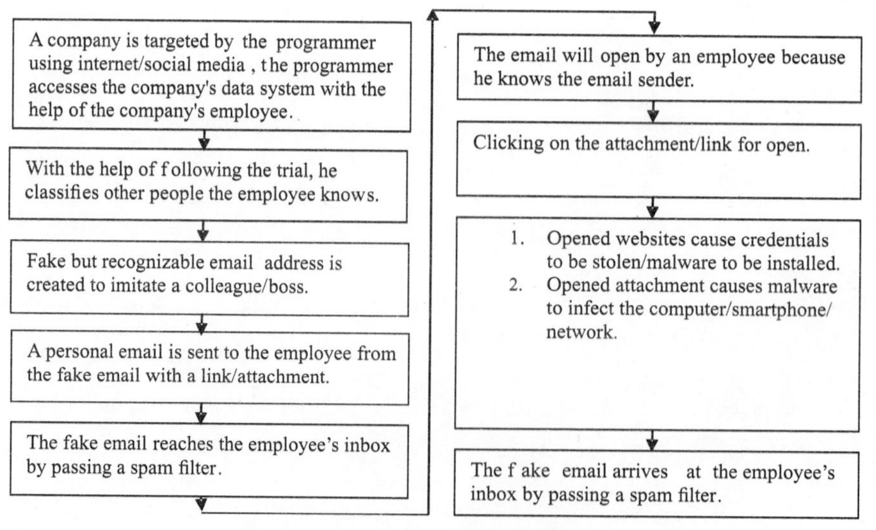

Figure 1 Phishing working procedure

1.1   Motivation for Phishing

1.1.1 Financial gain: E-mail spoofing is also called spear phishing which is used for fraud that targets a specific organization, seeking unauthorized access to confidential data.

1.1.2 Theft the login credentials: Typically the networked login credentials of prominent high-street banking organizations and successive access to funds ready to transfer and seizure the home address mobile, number and other personal information.

1.1.3 Theft the bank credentials: More recently, the increase in networked share trading businesses have portended that a customer's trading attention gives an uncomplicated direction for global money transfers.

1.1.4 Malware distribution: Although outdated, but malware families are still used to spreading malware and infecting online user computers with the help of email attachments. This type of infection depends on the consumer pressing on the email attachment. A present methodology that uses email as a dispersal implement is to put links to malicious websites.

1.1.5 Distribution of Botnet and Ddos agent: Illegitimate person uses phishing hustles to install special bot and DDoS instrumentalities on unsuspecting computers and append them to their distribution networks.

2.   Machine Learning

Machine learning [2] is defined as the complex computation process of automatic pattern recognition and intelligent decision making based on training sample data. Learning models use statistical functions or rules to describe the dependencies among data and causalities and correlations between input and output. Learning is the process of building a scientific model after discovering knowledge from a sample data set or data sets. Generally, the machine learning technique used for classification and prediction, based on the known qualities already, which has been written from the training data. To detect phishing machine learning can be broadly classified into two categories: supervised and unsupervised learning, which can be further explained in detail in the further section.

2.1   Types of machine learning

2.1.1 Supervised machine learning

2.1.1.1 Support Vector Machine: Support Vector Machine is a supervised machine learning algorithm that can be used for both classification or regression. SVM with the maximizing margin (i.e. the distance between the closest data point and the hyperplane) yields an improved outcome.

2.1.1.2 Neural Network: Neural Network is used for the prediction and models that are encouraged by the function or structure of biological neural networks and neural network is a class of pattern matching that is commonly used for classification and regression problems.

2.1.1.3 Naïve Bayes: Bayesian methods are those that exceptionally apply Bayes' theorem for problems such as classification and regression.

2.1.1.4 Random Forest: Random Forest is ensemble methods are models composed of numerous uncertain models that are individually trained and whose predictions are integrated in some way to make the comprehensive prediction.

2.1.1.5 Decision Tree: Decision Tree is a supervised learning algorithm (known outcome) that is frequently used in classification problems. Whatever is output by the decision tree will be visible in binary tree format. The decision tree keeps such rules with which it can easily predict the target variable.

2.1.2 Unsupervised machine learning

2.1.2.1 k Nearest Neighbor: k Nearest Neighbor is an instance-based learning model which is based on a decision problem with instances and the k-nearest neighbor classification algorithm is a non-parametric classification algorithm.

2.1.2.2 k Means: K-Means clustering is an unsupervised machine learning algorithm, as the name implications, finds an immovable number (k) of clusters in a set of data. A *"cluster"* refers to a group of data points grouped because of their identical features. When using a k-Means algorithm, a cluster is defined by a "k" also known as *"centroid"*, which is a point either imaginary or real location representing at the center of a cluster.

3.   Survey-Based Table

Sn.	Title, Author, Publication/ Reference, Year	Description	Classifier	Dataset	Features
1.	A novel lightweight URL phishing detection system using SVM and similarity index, Mouad Zouina *et al.*, SPRINGER [3], 2017.	This paper presents a novel lightweight phishing detection approach completely based on the URL (uniform resource locator) and also in this paper the targeted websites of the phishing attack are vital therefore all the retained 1000 phishing website records must contain their respective target.	SVM, Naive Bayes, PSO-SVM.	Alexa and phishtank.	URL size, number of hyphens, number of dots, number of numeric characters, IP address, similarity index.
2.	Classifying Phishing URLs Using Recurrent Neural Networks, Alejandro Correa *et al.*, IEEE [4], 2017.	In this paper, we explored the use of URLs as input for machine learning models applied for phishing site prediction. In this way, we compared a feature-engineering approach followed by a Random Forest classifier against a novel method based on recurrent neural networks.	LSTM, RF.	Common crawl, phishtank.	The domain exists in alexa rank, subdomain length, URL length, path length, URL entropy, length ratio, '@' and '-' count, punctuation count, other TLDs count, IP, suspicious words count, euclidean distance, kolmogorov-smirnov statistic, kullback-leibler divergence.
3.	Comparing writing style feature-based classification methods for estimating user reputations in social media, Suh *et al.*, SPRINGER [5], 2016.	This paper proposed a research framework to design and examine an automatic system that estimates user reputations of social media into good and bad classes by adopting writing styles. Using the most popular Web forum in South Korea, Daum Agora.	C4.5, NN, SVM, NB and RS-C4.5, RS-NN, RS-SVM, RS-NB.	Web forum in South Korea, Daum Agora.	Lexical, syntactic, structural, content-specific.
4.	MASPHID: A Model to Assist Screen Reader Users for Detecting Phishing Sites Using Aural and Visual Similarity measures, Gunikhan Sonowal *et al.*, ACM [6], 2016.	This paper proposes a model titled "MASPHID" (Model for Assisting Screen Reader users in Phishing Detection) to assist persons with visual impairments in detecting phishing sites that are aurally similar but visually dissimilar.	Support Vector Machine.	Phishtank.	Page rank, alexa rank, age, DNS records, abnormal URL, long URL, prefix suffix, sub-domains, Http/Https, and IP address.

5.	Particle Swarm Optimization Trained Class Association Rule Mining: Application to Phishing Detection, Kshitij Tayal *et al.*, ACM [7], 2016.	This paper presents a new algorithm called Particle Swarm Optimization trained Classification Association Rule Mining (PSOCARM) for associative classification that generates class association rules (CARs) from the transactional database by formulating a combinatorial global optimization problem, without having to specify minimal support and confidence, unlike other conventional associative classifiers.	CBA, CMAR, PRM, CPAR, FOIL, PSOCARM.	Phishtank.	Foreign anchor, nil anchor, IP address, dots in page address, dots in URL, slash in page address, slash in URL, foreign anchor in identity set, URL"s having @ symbol, server form handler (SFH), foreign request, foreign request URLs in identity set, cookie, SSL certificate, search engine, whois" lookup, blacklist.
6.	A novel approach to protect against phishing attacks at client side using auto-updated white-list, Ankit Kumar Jain *et al.*, SPRINGER [8], 2016.	In this paper, we proposed a novel approach to protect against phishing attacks using an auto-updated white-list of legitimate sites accessed by the individual user.	CANTINA, CANTINA+, phishnet, DNS-based black-list, automated individual white-list, visual signature.	Phishtank, alxa, stuffgate, online payment service provider.	URL address, webpage feature, DNS-IP mapping, hyperlink features such as number of the webpage that contains no hyperlinks/null links, number of points to the foreign domain (>=threshold).
7.	Intelligent phishing URL detection using association rule mining, S. Carolin Jeeva *et al.*, SPRINGER [9], 2016.	This paper focuses on discerning the significant features that discriminate between legitimate and phishing URLs.	Predictive Apriori algorithm, Apriori algorithm.	Phishtank, yahoo, google's top 1000, alexa's, netcraft's, millersmiles's top most visited sites.	Features such as length of the host URL, number of slashes in URL, dots in hostname of the URL, number of terms in the hostname of the URL, special characters, IP address, unicode in URL, transport layer security, subdomain, certain keyword in the URL top-level domain, number of dots in the path of the URL, hyphen in the hostname of the URL, URL length.
8.	A phish detector using lightweight search features. Gaurav Varshney *et al.*, ELESVIER [10], 2016.	In this paper advances, search engine based anti-phishing research and presents the lightest possible phishing detection system named the lightweight phish detector (LPD). The LPD can run on client browsers for phishing detection.	Lightweight phish detector.	Phishtank, alexa.	URL Domain.
9.	Spammer Classification using Ensemble Methods over Structural social network features, Sajid Yousuf Bhat *et al.*, IEEE [11], 2014.	In this paper, we evaluate the performance of some ensemble learning methods using community-based structural features extracted from an interaction network for the task of spammer detection in an online social network.	J48 (Decision Tree), IBk (k-NN), Naïve Bayes.	Facebook.	Community-based feature.

4.   **Discussion and Conclusion**

Machine learning is one of the phishing detection technique that used to detect the phishing based on four different types of features which have been collected from URLs such as **structured based features, web-based features, email-based features,** and **third-party features**. Machine learning provides two types of algorithm to detect phishing such as supervised and unsupervised. Observing the above table we find that both machine learning algorithms are used to detect phishing from web/emails/URLs. It is also observed that respective machine learning algorithms/classifiers calculate the accuracy rate for respect measurement of effectiveness.

In this paper, the literature review describes machine learning algorithms, which are responsible to detect the phishing from the URLs and corresponding accuracy rate. There are so many solutions to phishing obstacles available today, but phishing problems are not just scientific/mechanical problems only. The phishers always try to arise with more advance and unique approaches for attacking online users. Online users should initiate regular susceptibility scrutiny to determine and plug deficiency. Therefore, there is always a need to develop a preventive approach against the new phishing attacks.

5.   References

1.   Lininger, R, and R. D. Vines. *Phishing: Cutting the identity theft line.* John Wiley & Sons, 2005.

2.   Buczak, A. L., and E Guven. A survey of data mining and machine learning methods for cyber security intrusion detection. *IEEE Communications Surveys & Tutorials* 18.2 (2015): 1153-1176.

3.   Zouina, Mouad, and Benaceur Outtaj. A novel lightweight URL phishing detection system using SVM and similarity index. *Human-centric Computing and Information Sciences* 7.1 (2017): 17.

4.   Bahnsen, A. C., et al. Classifying phishing URLs using recurrent neural networks. *2017 APWG Symposium on Electronic Crime Research (eCrime).* IEEE, 2017.

5.   Suh, J. H. Comparing writing style feature-based classification methods for estimating user reputations in social media. *Springer Plus* 5.1 (2016): 261.

6.   Sonowal, G. and K. S. Kuppusamy. Masphid: a model to assist screen reader users for detecting phishing sites using aural and visual similarity measures. *Proceedings of the International Conference on Informatics and Analytics.* ACM, 2016.

7.   Tayal, K., and V. Ravi. Particle swarm optimization trained class association rule mining: Application to phishing detection. *Proceedings of the International Conference on Informatics and Analytics.* ACM, 2016.

8.   Jain, A. K., and B. B. Gupta. A novel approach to protect against phishing attacks at client side using auto-updated white-list. *EURASIP Journal on Information Security* 2016.1 (2016): 9.

9.   Jeeva, S. C., and E. B. Rajsingh. Intelligent phishing url detection using association rule mining. *Human-centric Computing and Information Sciences* 6.1 (2016): 10.

10.   Varshney, G., M. Misra, and P. K. Atrey. A phish detector using lightweight search features. *Computers & Security* 62 (2016): 213-228.

11.   Bhat, S.Y., M.A., and A. A. Mirza. Spammer classification using ensemble methods over structural social network features. *Proceedings of the 2014 IEEE/WIC/ACM International Joint Conferences on Web Intelligence (WI) and Intelligent Agent Technologies (IAT)-Volume 02.* IEEE Computer Society, 2014.

Thermo-acoustical Investigation of Nitrogenous Urea at Different Concentration and Temperature

Paritosh L. Mishra[1*], Ajay B. Lad[2], Urvashi P. Manik[3]

[2]Department of Physics, Amolakchand Mahavidyalaya, Yavatmal-445002, India
[1,3]Department of Physics, Sardar Patel Mahavidyalaya, Chandrapur-442401, India.
*E-mail: paritoshlmishra@gmail.com

ABSTRACT

The present paper reports the ultrasonic characterization of nitrogen contained aqueous Urea at different concentration and temperature. Ultrasonic velocity (U) and density (ρ) measurement were carried out by 2MHz frequency interferometer at 298.15K and 303.15K temperature respectively. Using the experimental values thermodynamic parameter such as adiabatic compressibility (β), intermolecular free length (L_f), acoustic impedance (Z), isothermal compressibility (k_T), relative association (R_A), surface tension (σ) and relaxation strength (r) have been estimated using the standard relations. The thermodynamic and acoustical studies clarify the nature of interaction between binary solutions. The variation in ultrasonic velocity and other parameters play a significant role in understanding the solute-solvent interaction between the constituent molecules. These studies have application in pure and applied research in the field of bio-medical industrial process as well as in agriculture field. This study will also lead to better understanding of Nitrogen contained Urea for possible application to be used as life saving medicine and fertilizers. Therefore the proposed study is worthwhile and interesting from number of aspects.

Keywords: fertilizer, urea, density, velocity, adiabatic compressibility, free length.

1.   Introduction

Today, ultrasonic field have received the status of an important inquest to study the properties of science, industries, metallurgy, medicine and also in agriculture.[1-2] The ultrasonic velocity has been measured in order to understand the nature of molecular interactions in pure, binary and ternary mixtures.[3-5] Acoustical parameters are computed from the experimentally determine values of ultrasonic velocity (U) and density (ρ). Such studies as a function of concentration and temperature are useful in gaining insight into the structure and bonding of associated molecular compounds and other molecular processes. Though a number of investigations were carried out in mixture having Urea as one of the components at a constant frequency are reported.[6-9]

Knowledge of thermodynamic and acoustical properties is of great importance in studying the physico-chemical behavior and molecular interaction between various essential molecules in a living organism and plants and co-solutes are very important. Urea is highly active compound in a variety of biological functions in our body and has been referred as protein denaturing agent. Urea provides a significant role in the metabolism of compounds having nitrogen by animals and the light amount of substance contain nitrogen. Further urea is one of the essential basic materials for the chemical industry as well as in fertilizers for agriculture.

Thus for clear observations, we report in this paper, the effect of urea on water, we study the various parameters of molecular interaction in aqueous urea solutions through ultrasonic measurements. The ultrasonic sound velocity (U) and density (ρ) measurements [10-11] and their aligned parameters such as adiabatic compressibility (β), intermolecular free length (L_f), acoustic impedance (Z), Isothermal compressibility

(k_T), Relative association (R_A), surface tension (σ) and relaxation strength (r) find the wide applications in characterizing the physic-chemical behavior of solution mixture.

2. Experimental

AR grade Urea (99.8%), was obtained from Himedia, Mumbai. Chemicals were used without further purification. The concentration of urea in water was changed by weight.

Ultrasonic velocity was measured by single crystal interferometer operating at frequency 2 MHz. The source of ultrasonic waves was a quartz crystal excited by a radio frequency oscillator placed at the bottom of a double jacketed metallic cylinder container. The cell was filled with the desired solution and water at constant temperature was circulated in the outer jacket. The cell was allowed to equilibrate for 30min. prior to making the measurements.

The densities of the solutions were determined accurately using 10ml specific gravity bottle and electronic balance. An average of triple measurements was taken into account. The experimental temperature was maintained constant by circulating water with the help of thermostatic water bath

3. Defining Relations

For the derivation of several acoustical and thermo-dynamical parameters the following defining relations reported in the literature are used:

(I)   Adiabatic Compressibility:$(\beta) = 1/(U^2\rho)$

(II)   Intermolecular free length:$(L_f) = K(\beta)^{1/2}$

(III)   Isothermal Compressibility:$(k_{T1}) = 1.33*10^{-8}/(6.4*10^{-4}U^{3/2}\rho)^{3/2}$

(IV)   Isothermal Compressibility:$(k_{T2}) = 17.1*10^{-4}/(T^{4/9}U^2\rho^{1/3})$

(V)   Acoustic Impedance:$(Z) = U\rho$

(VI)   Relative Association:$(R_A) = (\rho/\rho_0)(U_0/U)^{1/3}$

(VII)   Surface Tension:$(\sigma) = (6.3*10^{-4})\rho U^{3/2}$

(VIII)   Relaxation Strength:$(r) = 1 - \left(\dfrac{U}{U\infty}\right)^2$

Isothermal Compressibility values have been computed using the McGowan's[12] Expression, using the arbitrary constant in the denominator of McGowan's expression by a temperature term. Pandey et al.[13] suggested a relation for the evaluation of isothermal compressibility.

4. Results and Discussion

In the present study the studies on aqueous urea were carried out. The variation in the various physical parameters as a function of concentration as well as temperature in case of urea dissolved in water can be explained. The measured values of ultrasonic velocity (U) and density (ρ) at different concentration and temperature of aqueous urea and the values of derived parameters are tabulated in the table.

Increase in ultrasonic velocity (U) with concentration at two different temperatures shown in fig. (a) Of aqueous urea solution indicates that the presence of solute-solvent interactions.[14] The increase in ultrasonic velocity with rise in concentration for the present system confirms the greater molecular association. Urea (H_2N-CO-NH_2) molecules contain $-NH_2$, $-CO_2$ groups which are hydrophilic groups. So interaction between solute and water molecules complete through hydrophilic hydration. As the temperature is increased several water molecules from the hydration co-sphere relaxes.[15] This result in more and more number of monomeric water molecules. These forms closed packed structure and behaves as a stiff material medium for the propagation of ultrasonic wave. Hence ultrasonic velocity increases with rise in temperature.

Table: The values of various physical parameters as a function of concentration of System (Urea + Water) at temperature 298.15K and 303.15K

Concentration (mol kg^{-1})		0.00	0.02	0.04	0.06	0.08	0.10	0.12	0.14	0.16	0.18	0.20
U (ms^{-1})	298.15K	1498.101	1498.955	1499.340	1499.862	1500.284	1500.850	1501.750	1502.599	1503.101	1503.676	1504.284
	303.15K	1507.284	1507.512	1507.862	1508.441	1509.599	1510.668	1511.340	1511.922	1512.503	1513.668	1514.251
ρ (kgm^{-3})	298.15K	997.0	997.122	997.537	997.679	998.014	998.247	998.460	998.774	999.058	999.250	999.443
	303.15K	995.6	995.874	996.127	996.604	997.050	997.618	997.750	998.258	998.673	998.988	999.647
$\beta * 10^{-10}$ (m^{2}N^{-1})	298.15K	4.469	4.463	4.459	4.456	4.452	4.447	4.440	4.434	4.430	4.426	4.421
	303.15K	4.421	4.418	4.415	4.410	4.401	4.392	4.388	4.382	4.377	4.369	4.363
$L_f * 10^{-11}$ (m)	298.15K	4.348	4.345	4.343	4.342	4.339	4.337	4.333	4.331	4.329	4.327	4.325
	303.15K	4.364	4.363	4.361	4.359	4.354	4.350	4.348	4.345	4.342	4.338	4.335
$K_{T1} * 10^{-12}$ (m^{2}N^{-1})	298.15K	59.10	59.01	58.94	58.88	58.82	58.74	58.65	58.54	58.48	58.41	58.34
	303.15K	58.41	58.37	58.32	58.23	58.09	57.94	57.87	57.78	57.69	57.57	57.46
$K_{T2} * 10^{-12}$ (m^{2}N^{-1})	298.15K	60.62	60.55	60.51	60.46	60.42	60.37	60.29	60.22	60.17	60.12	60.07
	303.15K	59.47	59.44	59.41	59.36	59.26	59.16	59.11	59.05	58.99	58.90	58.84
$Z * 10^6$ (Rayls)	298.15K	1.493607	1.494640	1.495647	1.496381	1.497304	1.498219	1.499437	1.500757	1.501685	1.502549	1.503446
	303.15K	1.500652	1.501292	1.502022	1.503318	1.505146	1.507069	1.507940	1.509288	1.510496	1.512136	1.513717
R_A	298.15K	1	0.999932	1.000253	1.000289	1.000531	1.000639	1.000652	1.000779	1.000952	1.001017	1.001075
	303.15K	1	1.000225	1.000401	1.000752	1.000944	1.001278	1.001262	1.001643	1.001932	1.001990	1.002523
σ (Kg/m^2 sec)	298.15K	36420.62	36456.21	36485.46	36509.71	36537.37	36566.59	36607.28	36649.86	36678.65	36706.77	36736.12
	303.15K	36704.39	36722.82	36744.96	36785.06	36842.59	36902.74	36932.24	36972.36	37009.09	37063.52	37109.41
r	298.15K	0.1233	0.1223	0.1219	0.1212	0.1208	0.1200	0.1190	0.1180	0.1174	0.1168	0.1160
	303.15K	0.1125	0.1122	0.1118	0.1111	0.1098	0.1085	0.1078	0.1070	0.1064	0.1050	0.1043

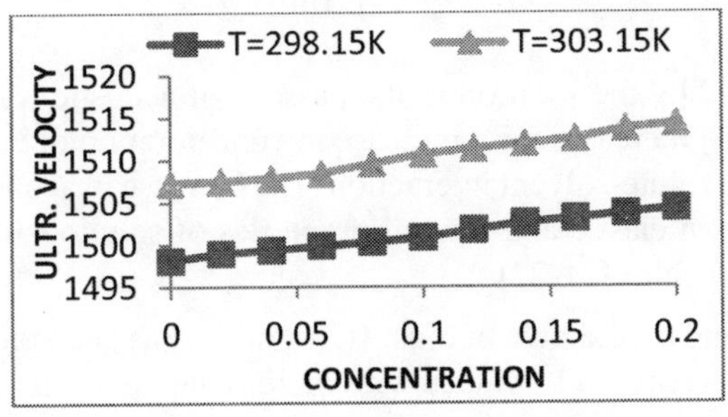

Fig. 1(a)

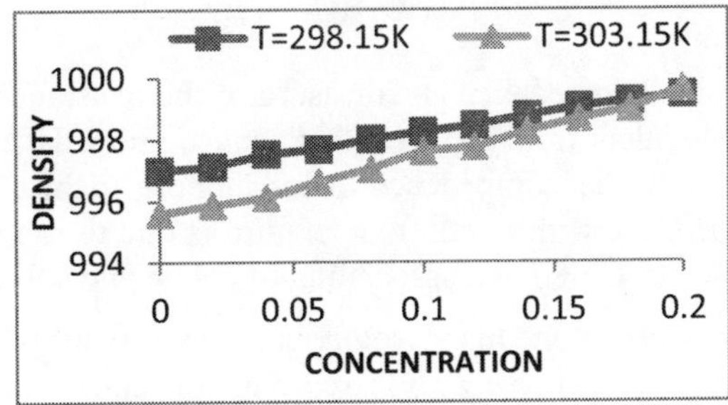

Fig. 1(b)

The increase in density(ρ) with increase in concentration of urea (shown in Fig. 1(b)) is due to association occurs between the solute and solvent molecules and decrease with rise in temperature shows decrease in intermolecular forces due to increasing thermal energy of the system.[16]

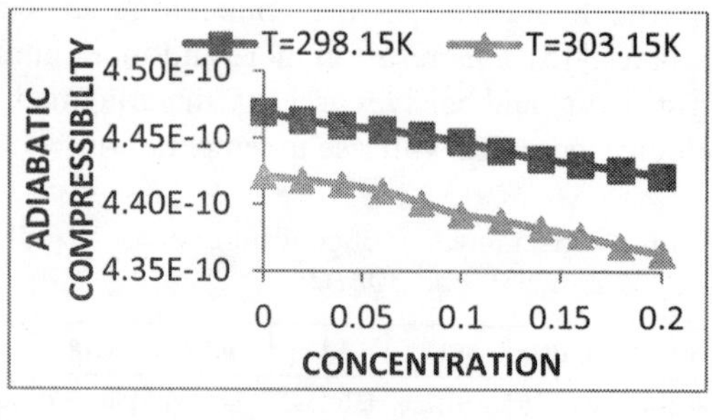
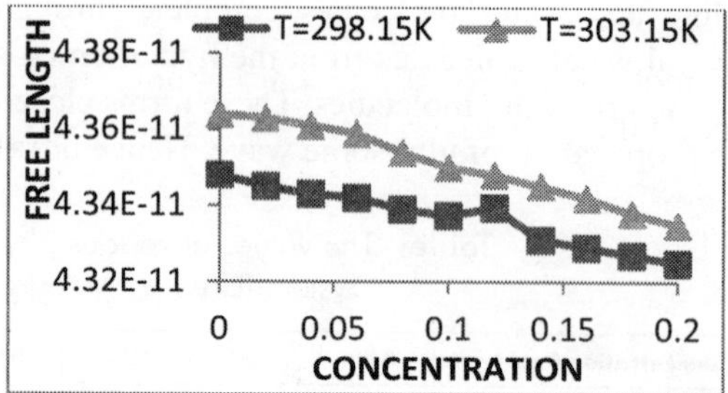

Fig. 1(c)

Fig. 1(d)

Figure 1(c) Shows the variation of adiabatic compressibility with concentration of urea at couple of temperature (298.15K and 303.15K) respectively. The decrease in adiabatic compressibility with increase in concentration of urea confirms molecular association in the present system.[17] Further, with the increase of temperature the mean distance between the molecules tend to increase with a corresponding decrease in compressibility.[18]

As free length is the average distance between the surfaces of two neighboring molecules, which is called intermolecular free length.[19] The decrease in free length values, with rise in concentration of urea (shown in Fig. 1(d)) Suggest that the distance between the molecules of the mixture decreases and thereby increasing the potential energy of the interaction between the molecules which leads to observed increase in the value of ultrasonic velocity (U).[20]

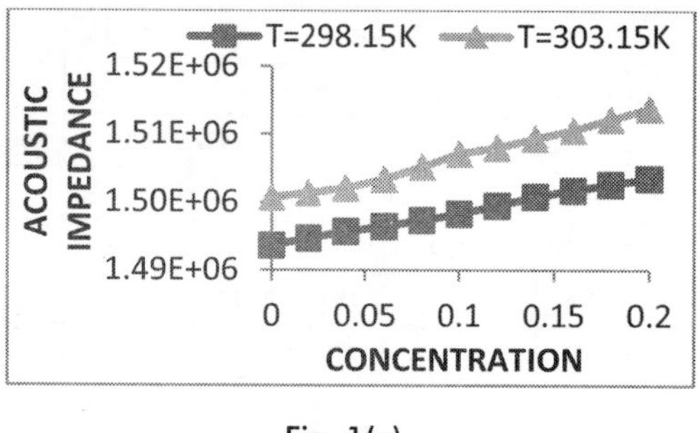
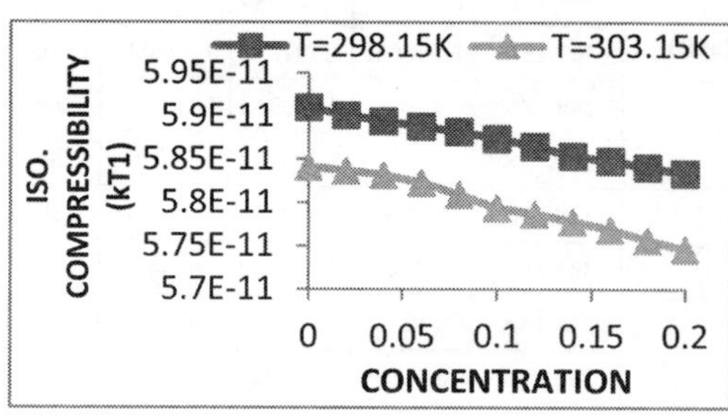

Fig. 1(e)

Fig. 1(f)

Acoustic impedance is a measure of the resistance offered by the solution to the passage of acoustic wave. It is evident from Fig. 1(e) that acoustic impedance values increases with increase in concentration of urea. The increase in impedance values supports to the effective solute-solvent interaction. The increase in acoustic impedance with rise in temperature is due to ion change in elastic and inertial properties of solution. This indicates the greater association of solute and solvent molecules.[21-22]

The overall trend in the isothermal compressibility's (k_{T1} and k_{T2}), shown in Figs. 1(f) and 1(g) has been found that to be decrease with increase in concentration. The decrease in k_T values with increase in concentration seems to be the result of corresponding decrease in free volume.[23] Surface tension is directly proportional to the density and velocity, it shows the result as that of velocity, confirming significant associative interaction in the solution[24] as shown in Fig. 1(h).

Relative association (R_A) is depend upon two factors: (1) The breaking of solvent structure on addition of solute to it and (2) the salvation of solutes that are simultaneously present. As shown in Fig. (i), the increase of R_A with concentration suggests that close association of component of molecules and there exist intermolecular interactions. Furthermore as temperature increases the value of R_A also increases which support that increase in molecular interaction of the system.[25-26]

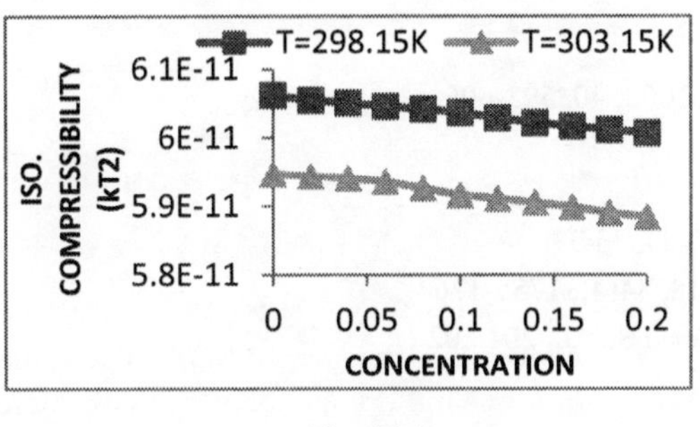

Fig. 1(g)

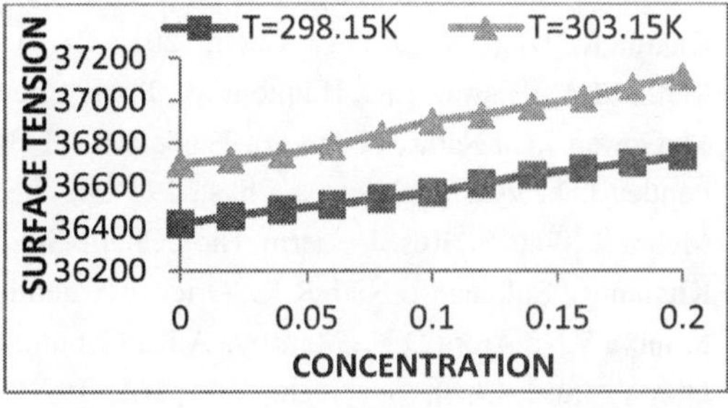

Fig. 1(h)

Relaxation strength is directly related with adiabatic compressibility and isothermal compressibility and totally depends on the factor [1]. Here U be the ultrasonic velocity of solution and is constant, has value 1600 m/sec. the decrease in values of relaxation strength with increase in concentration indicates solute- solvent interaction in the system (shown in Fig. 1(j)). Which suggest the greater association between urea and water. [27]

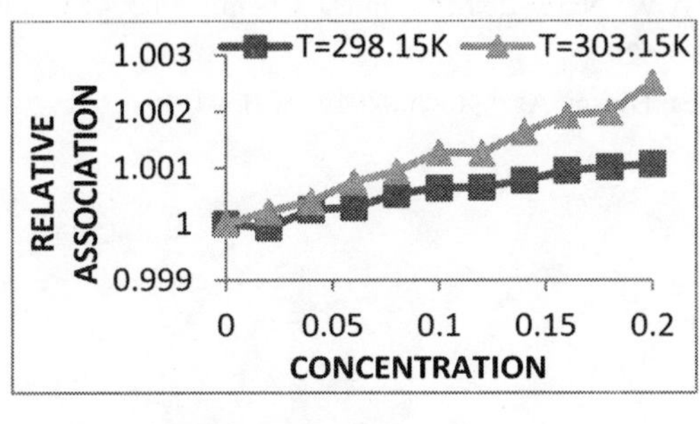

Fig. 1(i)

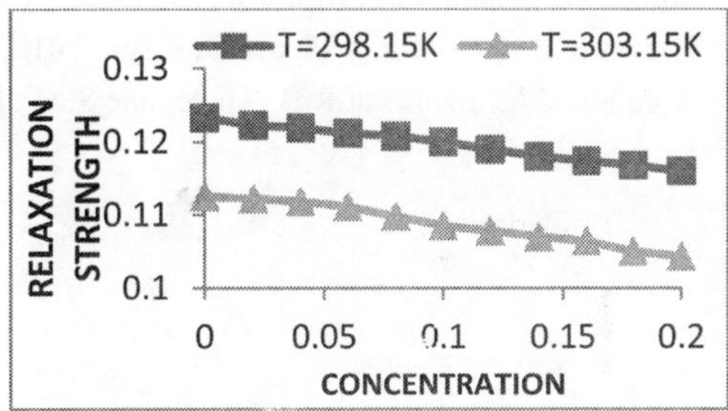

Fig. 1(j)

5. Conclusion

Ultrasonic and volumetric measurements were carried out on aqueous urea for various concentrations (0.02-0.2 mol-kg^{-1}) at 298.15K and 303.15K temperatures. In the light of above experimental values of ultrasonic velocity, density and their allied thermo-acoustical parameters, it may be concluded that there exist of solute-solvent interaction in the present system. The increase in the value of U, Z, R_A, L_f, σ and decrease in the value of rest parameters with rise in temperature confirms the presence of solute-solvent interaction in the system.

6. References

1.   Jahagirdar D.V., Arbad B.R., Mirgane S.R., Lande M.K., Shankarwar A.G., J. Mol. Liq., 1998, 75(1), 33-43.

2.   Nain A., Pal R., Sharma R., J. Mol. Liq., 2012, 165,154-160.

3.   Pitzer K.S., Thermodynamics 3rd edition Mc-Graw-Hill., NY, 1995, ISBN 0-07-05022,1-8.

4.   Srinivasulu V., Naidu P.R., J. Pure Appl. Ultrason., 1995, 17, 14-28.

5.   Praharaj M.K., Satapathy A., Mishra S., Mishra P.R., J. Chem Pharm. Res., 2012, 4(4), 1910-1920.

6.   Malasane P.R., Res. J. Chem. Sci., 2013, 3(8), 73-77.

7.   Parmar M.L., Dhiman D.K., Thakur R.C.,Ind. J. Chem., 2002, 41A, 2032.

8.   Korolev V.P., J. Struc. Chem., 2008, 49(4), 660-667.

9.   Mehra R., Vats S., Arch. Phys. Res., 2010, 1(3), 15-22.

10.   Khatun R., Islam N., Orient J. Chem., 2012, 28(1), 165-187.

11.   Matin M.A., Biswas T.K., Huque E.M., Phys. Chem. Liq., 2002, 40, 593-605.

12.   McGowan J.C., Nature (London), 1966, 210, 43, 36.

13.   Pandey J.D., Vyas, Pramana, J. Phys., 1994, 43, 36.

14.   Mehra R., Vats S., Res. J. Pharm. Biol. Chem. Sci., 2012, 3(1), 26-33.

15.   Khatun R., Sultana R., Nath R.K., Orient J. Chemistry, 2018, 34(4), 1755-1764.

16.   Maurya V.N., Arora D.K., Mauruya A.K., Gautam R.A.,World Sci. J., 2013,02.

17.   Dhir V., Int. J. Chem. Sci. Tech., 2011, 1(2), 19-38.

18.   Iqbal M., Vernall R.E., Can. J. Chem.,1989, 67(4), 727-735.

19.   Thirumaran S., Inbum P., Ind. J. Pure and Appl. Phys., 2011, 49, 451-459.

20.   Mishra P.L., Manik U.P., Int. J. Sci. and Res., 2015, 215-217.

21.   Giratkar V.A., Lanjewar R.B., Gadegone S.M., Patil K.C., Der. Pharma. Chemica., 2017, 9(13), 46-54.

22.   Patil K.C., Dudhe C.M., Der. Pharma. Chem., 2015, (12), 219-226.

23.   Basharat R., J. Chem. And Pharm. Res., 2012, 4(1), 160-169.

24.   Ravichandran S., Ramnathan K., Int. J. Appl. Biol. Pharma. Tech., 2010, 1(2), 695-702.

25.   Idrees M., Siddiqui M., Agrawal P.B., Doshi A.G., Raut A.W., Narwade M.L., Ind. J. Chem., 2003, 42A, 526-530.

26.   Mehra R., Vats S., Int. J. Pharm Bio. Sci., 2010, 1(4), 523-529.

27.   Giratkar V.A., Lanjewar R.B., Gadegone S.M., Int, J. Res. Biosci. Agri. Tech., 2017, 5(3), 41-45.

Assessment of Plant Growth Promoting activity of Bacteria Isolated from the Rhizospheric region of Carrot (Daucus carota)

S. Sonam[1,*], S.P. Tiwari[2], R. Sharma[1]

[1]Department of Biotechnology, V.B.S. Purvanchal University, Jaunpur, UP-222003
[2]Department of Microbiology, V.B.S. Purvanchal University, Jaunpur, UP-222003
*E-mail: sonamshwetamicro@gmail.com

ABSTRACT

Plant Growth Promoting Rhizobacteria (PGPR) is group of bacteria that can increase the plant growth by using various mechanisms. This can be include direct (Nitrogen fixation, Phosphate solubilization, Siderophore production and Phytohormones production) or indirect (bio control agents, HCN production, antibiotic production, production of lytic enzymes and induced systemic resistance) mechanisms of plant growth promotion. These bacteria can act as efficient biofertilizers for increasing the productivity of several crops. PGPR as biofertilizers are well recognized as efficient soil bacteria for sustainable agriculture. The current work aimed to study the plant growth promoting attributes of the bacteria isolated from the rhizospheric soil of carrot. Soil samples were taken from different carrot grown fields. Among all the 28 bacterial isolates, 10 bacteria were isolated from the orange carrot, 9 bacteria were isolated from the red carrot and 9 bacteria were isolated from the black carrot. Isolated bacterial cultures were showing the multiple plant growth promoting attributes.

Keywords: Rhizosphere, PGPR, biofertilizers, Daucus carota.

1.   Introduction

Beneficial bacteria residing in rhizospheric region of plants and promote the growth and productivity of plants are referred as Plant Growth Promoting Rhizobacteria (Kloepper et al., 1980). These microbes can be grouped under two categories on the basis of their relationship with host plant such as extracellular (ePGPR) and intracellular (iPGPR) (Bhattacharyya et al., 2012). Growth promotion and enhancement of productivity is due to two different mechanisms of these microbes. In direct mechanisms microbes supply nutrients, produce growth promoters while in indirect mechanisms it suppresses the pathogenic microbial forms, capable to establish infection in host plants. Application of PGPR is a modern and ecofriendly approach in agriculture as an alternative of chemical fertilizer and pestisides. Carrot (Daucus carota L., 2n = 18) is a annual plant of the Umbelliferae (or Apiaceae) family. The most important characteristics of carrot is the massive accumulation of carotenoids that in the root, which is responsible for its characteristic color in most cultivars. β-carotene is a deoxygenated carotenoid and it is a parent molecule for synthesis of a group of oxygenated carotenoids called 'ketocarotenoids', which impart a distinct pink to red colour to tissues in which they are accumulated, such as the flesh of salmon, shells of shrimp and other crustaceans, and feathers of birds such as flamingoes and quails (Guerin et al., 2003). An important ketocarotenoids is astaxanthin which is of particular interest because of its many fold applications in various industries (food and pharmaceutical) (Guerin et al., 2003). Astaxanthin used as colorant mainly obtained through chemical synthesis procedure (Hussein et al., 2006) but various other biological sources such as algal and microbes has been investigated for its production (Yokoyama et al., 1994, Dufossé, 2006). The present investigation has been carried out for isolation of PGPR from carrot rhizosphere and evaluation of their PGPR traits.

2. Material and Methods

2.1 Sampling

Samples were collected from various carrot grown fields of District Jaunpur. The root adhering samples was collected from rhizospheric region of the healthy carrot plants for which portions of the carrot plant along with roots and soil down to a depth of 15-30 cm was carefully dig out with the help of narrow bladed sampling tool. For each plant the adhering soil was removed with the help of a brush. For each field, all the collected subsamples were pooled and mixed well. The samples were grinded and sieve through 9 mesh per square inch sieve. Three Samples (orange, red and black carrot) were taken from Muftiganj, Sipah and Khetasarai respectively.

2.2 Isolation of rhizospheric bacteria

Four selective media were used for the isolation of different types of bacteria from soil samples (Crystal Violet Agar, Methyl Red Agar, N-free Jensen's Agar and NBRI-P media). For the isolation of rhizospheric bacteria, one gram of rhizospheric soil from each sample was added to 9 ml of sterile water. Ten fold dilutions were made and spread on to different media. Plates were incubated for 3 days at 28-30°C. After incubation bacterial colonies were selected randomly on the basis of their appearance & color. Then purification of the selected cultures was done by using streak plate method on the respective media, used for isolation. Bacterial cultures were maintained on the respective slants and stored at 4°C.

2.3 Characterization of isolates

Isolates were initially characterized by morphological and staining characteristics. Gram staining was done as Gram, 1884.

2.4 Determination of plant growth promoting activities

2.4.1 Siderophore production Petri plates were poured with CAS media (Chrome azoural S agar) and Siderophore production was observed by inoculating the bacterial isolates (Schwyn and Neilands, 1987).

2.4.2 Phosphate solubilization The isolates were point inoculated on the plates containing Pikovskya's medium and incubated at 30°C for 3 days. The plates were then examined for the formation of clear zone (Pikovaskya, 1948).

2.4.3 Potassium solubilization Isolates were point inoculated on Aleksandrov agar plates and incubated for 3 days at 37°C. After incubation plates were observed for the formation of zone (Sugumaran and Janarthanam 2007).

2.4.4 Cellulase production Detection of cellulase producing bacteria is done by using CMC media. Cultures were point inoculated on CMC media plates and incubated for 3 days at 37°C. After 3 days incubation plates were flooded with 1% congo red solution for 15 min. After removing congo red plates were again flooded with 1 M NaCl solution for 15 min and plates were observed for formation of a clear zone around the colonies (Apun *et al.*, 2000).

2.4.5 Pectinase Production Bacterial isolates were point inoculated on plates with basal media for pectinase and incubated for 3 days. After incubation plates were observed for the formation of zone (Reda *et al.*, 2008).

3. Results

3.1 Isolation of PGPR

Three different varieties of carrots were used for isolation of PGPR and total twenty eight strains were isolated from the rhizosphere of three different carrot varieties grown in fields of District Jaunpur and named on the basis of media used for isolation.

3.2   Characterization of PGPR

Staining procedure used for initial characterization of isolates. The presence of mainly spherical and rod shaped bacteria were recorded. Among all isolates mostly Gram positive strains and a few Gram negative strains were obtained.

3.2.1 Result of Siderophore production: Among all 28 isolates 19 isolates gave positive result for Siderophore production. Zone size ranging from 9 mm to 8 mm was observed in J-O-1, NBRI-R-1 and MR-B-1 from orange carrot, red carrot and black carrot respectively (Fig-1).

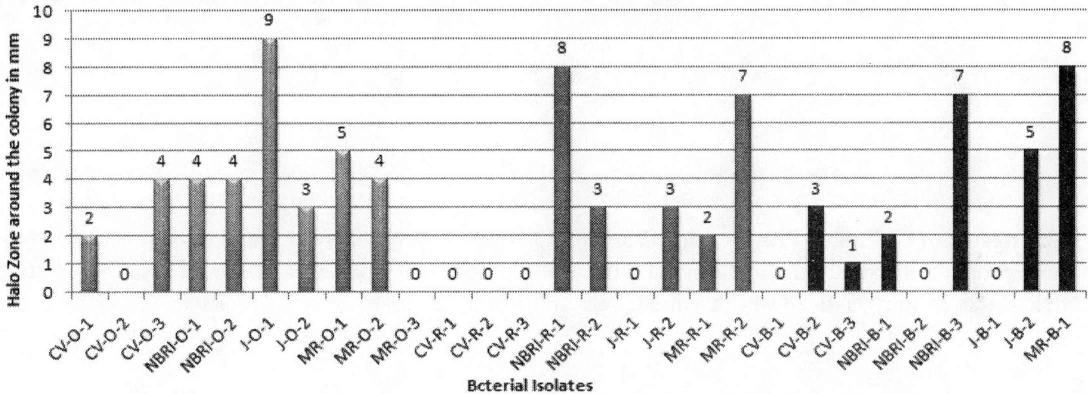

Fig. 1 Graph showing the result of Siderophore Production

3.2.2 Result of Phosphate solubilization: Among all the isolates 18 cultures gave positive result for phosphate solubilization. Out of which maximum solubilization zone was observed in NBRI-O-2 (17 mm) followed by NBRI-R-2 (12 mm) (Fig-2).

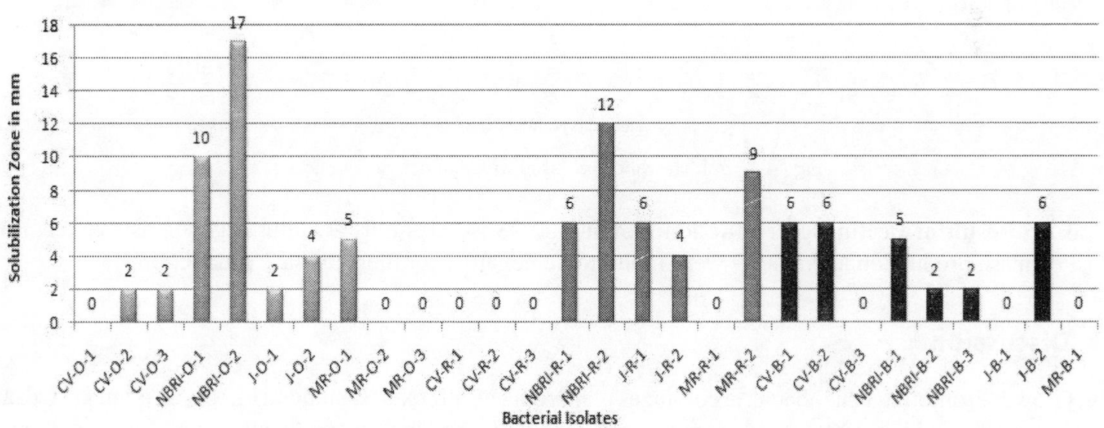

Fig. 2 Graph showing the result of Phosphate Solubilization

3.2.3 Result of Potassium solubilization: Out of all 17 isolates were found to be positive for the Potassium solubilization assay. Solubilization zone ranging from 17 mm to 13 mm was observed in J-O-1, MR-B-1 (17 mm), J-O-2 (16 mm) and J-R-1, NBRI-B-1 (13 mm) (Fig-3).

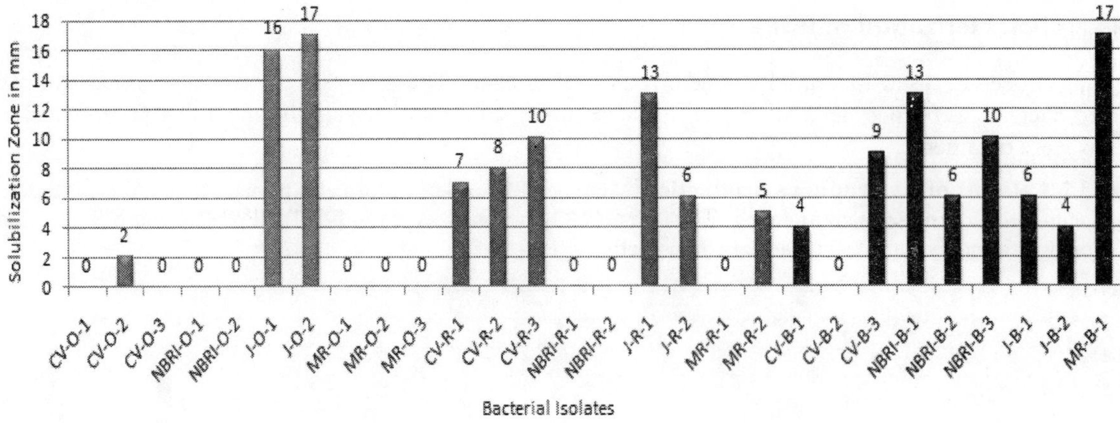

Fig. 3 Graph showing the result of Potassium solubilization

3.2.4 Result of Cellulase Production: From all 28 isolates, only 10 were found to be positive for Cellulase production. Solubilization zone ranging from 22 mm to 13 mm was observed in J-B-1 (22 mm), NBRI-O-2 (18 mm), J-B-2 (14 mm) and CV-B-1 (13 mm) (Fig-4).

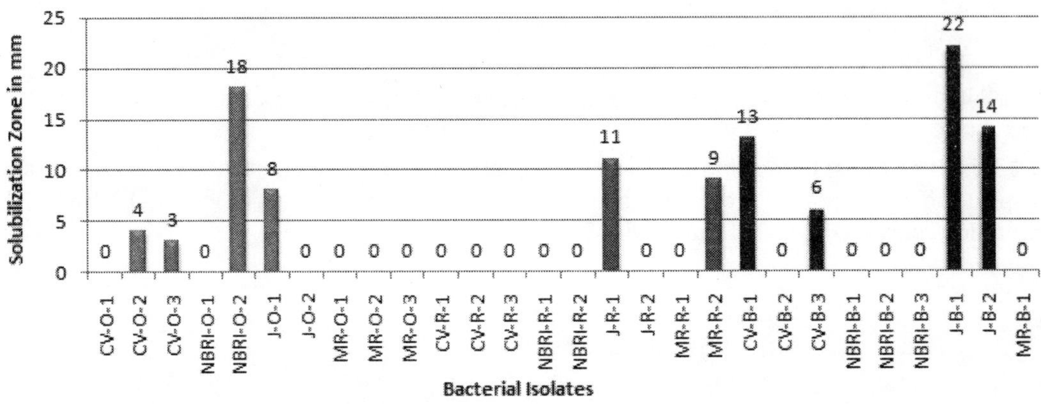

Fig. 4 Graph showing the result of Cellulase Production

3.2.5 Result of Pectinase Production: Among all 28 isolates only 9 cultures gave positive result for Pectinase production and rest 19 were found to be negative for the pectinase production.

4. Discussion

Plant Growth Promoting Rhizobacteria colonizes plant roots PGPR exert beneficial effects on plant growth and development by a wide variety of mechanisms including direct and indirect mechanisms. Nutrient availability is one of the most important aspects of PGPR for the growth promotion of plants. Phosphorus is one of the major nutrients, after the nitrogen is essential for plant growth and productivity of plants. Most of phosphorus in soil is present in the form of insoluble phosphates and cannot be utilized by the plants. The ability of bacteria to solubilize mineral phosphates has been of interest to agricultural microbiologists as it can enhance the availability of phosphorus and iron for plant growth (Verma *et al.*, 2001). In the present investigation 18 isolates gave positive result for phosphate solubilization. The results obtained are in accordance to earlier reports which suggests that in comparison to non-rhizospheric soil, a considerably higher concentration of phosphate-solubilizing bacteria is commonly found in the rhizosphere (Raghu and MacRae, 1966). As a vital element, iron is needed by all the living organisms from unicellular to multicellular for their numerous cellular processes. The Siderophore have ability to chelate the iron molecules and make it available for plant growth. Among all isolated cultures, 19 isolates were found capable to produce the Siderophore. Potassium is one of the mass nutrients essential for plant growth and development. Microbes play an important role in natural K cycles. Many studies have shown that soil contains a variety of KSB (Friedrich *et al.*, 2004). Some microbes decompose silicate minerals. They transform solid K in the soil into available K that can be directly absorbed by plants and they secrete active substances that promote plant growth. Out of all 28 isolates, 17 gave positive result for potassium solubilization. Cellulases are the enzymes responsible for the cleavage of the β–1, 4–glycosidic linkages in cellulose. They are members of the glycoside hydrolase families of enzymes that hydrolyze oligosaccharides and polysaccharides. Among all 28 isolates, only 10 were able to produce the cellulase. Pectinases are the enzymes which breaks pectic substances. It has a wide range of applications in food, agriculture and environmental sectors. In present observation total 9 isolates were found to be positive pectinase production. The present research focuses on the isolation and efficiency assessment of isolates for their Growth promotion attributes. The growth of plant can directly be correlated with the metabolite production in the plant. Probably the rhizospheric microbes might be playing important role in production of carotenoids (Loganathan *et al.*, 2014). Evaluation of their role in pigment production and their characterization process is in progress.

5.   Acknowledgments

One of the authors Shweta Sonam acknowledges the support provided by the Deptt. of Microbiology, V.B.S.P.U. Jaunpur.

6.   References

1.   Akihiro Yokoyama, Production of Astaxanthin and 4-Ketozeaxanthin by the Marine Bacterium, Agrobacterium aurantiacum. Biosci. Biotech. Biochem., 58, 1842-1844, (1994).

2.   Bhattacharyya, Plant growth-promoting rhizobacteria (PGPR) Emergence in agriculture. World J. Microbiol. Biotechnol. 28, 1327–1350 (2012).

3.   Friedrich S. Chemical and microbiological solubilization of silicates. Acta Biotechnol, 11, 187–196 (2004).

4.   Gram. C., General Bacteriology, ASM Press, Washington D.C., Ueber die isolirte Färbung der Schizomyceten in Schnitt-und Trockenpräparaten. Fortschritte der Medcin, (2), 185-189 (1884).

5.   Guerin, Haematococcus astaxanthin: applications for human health and nutrition. Trends Biotech. 21, 210–216 (2003).

6.   Hussein, Astaxanthin, a carotenoid with potential in human health and nutrition. J Nat Prod 69, 443–449 (2006).

7.   J.W. Kloepper, Effect of rhizosphere colonization by plant growth promoting rhizobacteria on potato plant development and yield Phytopathology 70, 1078-1082 (1980).

8.   K. Apun, Screening and isolation of a cellulolytic and amylolytic Bacillus from sago pith waste. Journal of General and Applied Microbiology, 46, 263–267 (2000).

9.   L. Dufossé, Microbial Production of Food Grade Pigments. Food Technol. Biotechnol. (3) 44, 313–321 (2006).

10.   M. Loganathan, Plant growth promoting rhizobacteria (PGPR) induces resistance against Fusarium wilt and improves lycopene content and texture in tomato. African journal of microbiology research, (11) 8, 1105-1111 (2014).

11.   Raghu K., Occurrence of phosphate-dissolving microorganisms in the rhizosphere of rice plants and in submerged soils. J. Appl. Bacteriol. 29, 582-586 (1966).

12. Reda, "Production of Bacterial Pectinase(s) from Agro-Industrial Wastes Under Solid State. Journal of Applied Sciences Research, (4) 12, 1708-1721, (2008).

13. Schwyn, Universal chemical assay for the detection and determination of siderophores. Anal. Biochem 160, 47-56 (1987).

14. Sugumaran P, Solubilization of potassium containing minerals by bacteria and their effect on plant growth. World J. Agric. Sci. (3) 3, 350–355 (2007).

15. Verma SC, Evaluation of plant growth promoting and colonization ability of endophytic diazotrophs from deep water rice. J. Biotechnol. 91, 127-141 (2001).

Optimization of Surface Sterilization Process for Isolation and Cultivation of Bacterial Endophytes from Allium Sativum

P. Srivastava[1,*], S.P. Tiwari[2], R. Sharma[1]

[1]Department of Biotechnology, VBS Purvanchal University, Jaunpur, UP-222003
[2]Department of Microbiology, VBS Purvanchal University, Jaunpur, UP-222003
*Email id: pratimamicro@gmail.com

ABSTRACT

In recent year, bacterial endophytes gained attention as they have beneficial effect on plant and have ability to produce bioactive metabolites that have various biomedical applications. Study hypothesize that only 0.001-1% of all plant associated bacteria are cultivable. The isolation procedure is critical step when working with endophytic microorganism. Endophytes isolation protocol initiated with combined surface sterilization process followed by crushing or thin slice cutting plant tissue then plating on specific media. In the present investigation surface sterilization protocol for isolation of endophytes from leaf and bulb of Allium sativum were optimized by using ethanol and sodium hypochlorite. The procedure of the surface sterilizations vary for each plant part, species, age and surface properties of the plant. The present investigation aimed to optimize surface sterilization process as well as culturing of these bacteria on different specific media because after successful isolation many endophytic bacteria exhibited reduced re-growth capacity. In our laboratory total 37 bacteria were isolated out of which 9 bacteria were isolated from leaf and 28 bacteria were isolated from bulb of Allium sativum.

Keywords- Endophytes, Surface sterilization, Allium sativum

1. Introduction

Endophytic bacteria can be defined as those bacteria that colonize the internal tissue of the plant showing no sign of infection or negative effect on their host (Holliday, 1989; Schulz and Boyle, 2006). The term "endophyte" is derived from the Greek words "endon" meaning within and "phyton" meaning plant (De Bary 1866). These endophytes residing inside the plants are commonly known to improve plant growth and act as source of novel bioactive compounds (Ryan et al., 2008). In contrast to pathogens which invade the plant and impart harmful effect, the endophytes play beneficial role in the growth promotion of plant either by direct or indirect methods (Lodewyckx et al., 2002). Endophytes may reside in almost every internal part of plant tissues like of the roots, stem, leaf, fruit and seed (Hallmann et al., 1997 a & b). The endophyte population varies depending upon the tissue; plant developmental stage and the surrounding environment such as season (Kuklinsky-Sobral et al., 2004). Recent researches are mainly focused on plant microbes association and their role in production of valuable metabolites. One of the major problems facing by medical and pharmaceutical sciences is increasing drug resistance among the pathogens hence, researcher across the globe focus on an alternative to drug resistance and plant may play an important role in this context. Microorganism associated with medicinal plant act as reservoir of bioactive metabolites (Yu et al., 2010). Therefore, in the present investigation endophytic bacteria associated with Allium sativum were isolated because of its well known medicinal properties. It has antidiabetic, hypocholesterolemic, antilipidemic, fibrinolytic and anticancer activity (Bayan et al., 2014). In comparison to rhizospheric bacteria, endophytic bacteria are difficult to isolate and cultivate because they are more closely associated and dependent on the plant, therefore different procedures have been adopted for proper surface sterilization of plant parts for isolation of endophytic bacteria. The most commonly used isolation procedure is combination of ethanol and sodium hypochlorite at particular concentration at definite time period for surface sterilization of plant parts. Perhaps this will be the first comprehensive report from India on optimization of surface sterilization process for isolation of bacterial endophytes from Allium sativum. The present study is carried out to with an aim to optimize effectiveness of surface sterilizing agent for isolation of endophytic bacteria from Allium sativum.

2. Materials and Methods

2.1 Collection of samples

For isolation of bacterial endophytes healthy *Allium sativum* plant were collected from different *Allium sativum* grown field of district Jaunpur UP. These plants were uprooted from field, placed in clean sterile plastic bag and brought to laboratory and used for experimental purpose. For the isolation of endophytes from *Allium sativum* plant intact bulb and fresh leaves were used.

2.2 Isolation of Endophytic bacteria

2.2.1 Pretreatment

In the laboratory selected *Allium sativum* plants were thoroughly washed under running tap water then washed several times with sterile distilled water to remove adhering soil to remove majority of rhizospheric and phyllospheric bacteria.

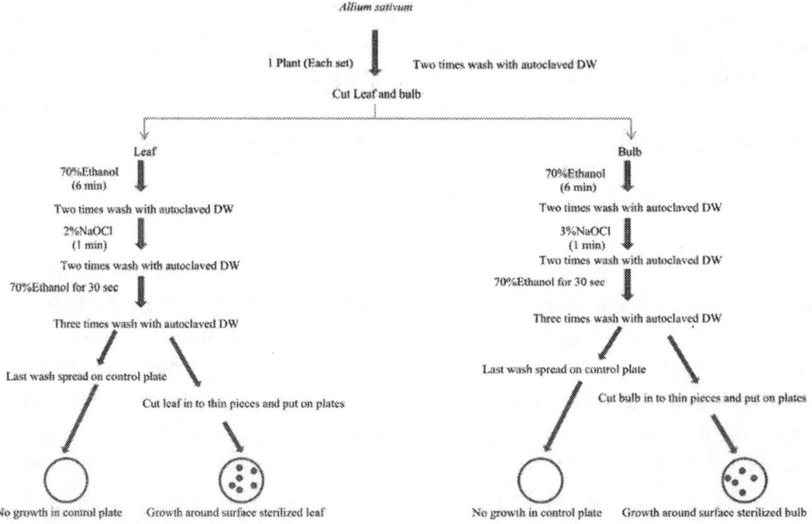

Figure 1. Flow chart of surface sterilization of leaf and buld of allium sativum

2.2.2 Surface sterilization

Surface sterilization is initial and critical step for isolation of endophytic bacteria. Sterilizing agent generally kills microorganism either by oxidizing or reducing properties of the compounds being used. For sterilization of explants, ethanol (70%, 80% & 90%) and NaOCl (2%, 3% & 4%) were used. For proper sterilization of explants first concentration of individual sterilizing agent were optimized. After optimization of concentration of individual agent then combination of 70% ethanol with 2% and 3% of NaOCl were used to optimize time duration for treatment of these sterilizing agent. To check the effectiveness of surface sterilization process final wash were spread on nutrient agar plate as control and incubated at 30^0C for 48-72 hrs and observed for possible microbial growth (McInroy and Kloepper 1994). Samples were used for isolation of endophytes when no growth appears on control plate of final wash. All the experiments were carried out in triplicate.

2.2.3 Isolation and morphological characterization of Endophytic bacteria

For isolation of endophytic bacteria surface sterilized leaf and bulb were cut into 1cm pieces followed by thin slices and placed on plates containing nutrient agar media (Carroll 1995; Boyle *et al.*, 2001). The choice of growth medium is crucial as it directly affects the number and the type of endophytic bacteria.

3. Result

Endophytic bacteria were selected on the basis of different colony morphology and differential staining. Out of 37 bacteria 9 bacteria were isolated from leaf and 28 bacteria were isolated from bulb of *Allium sativum*. Most of the endophytic bacteria isolated from leaf are Gram positive while Gram negative from bulb of *Allium sativum* were observed.

Surface sterilization is the most crucial aspect of endophytic bacteria isolation because if the surface is not sterilized properly the isolates will be contaminated with bacteria residing outside parts of plant while over sterilized resulting in to killing of endophytic bacteria. It is important to select a sterilizing agent for proper sterilization of plant surface. In the present investigation for surface sterilization different concentrations of ethanol (70%, 80% and 90%), Sodium hypochorite (2%, 3% & 4%) and combination of both (70% ethanol and 2%, 3% Sodium hypochorite) for different time intervals were used. The result obtained suggested that in comparison of 70% ethanol, 80% and 90% ethanol were more effective to remove surface bacteria for 4 minutes but treatment of 80% and 90% ethanol decreased the appearance of endophytic bacteria with increasing time and concentrations as shown in Table 1.

Table 1. Effect of concentration of ethanol (70%, 80% & 90%) on growth and contamination of endophytic bacteria on nutrient agar

Ethanol		Control (Last wash spreading)			Treatment					
70%	Time	C1	C2	C3	G	C	G	C	G	C
	4 min	+++	+++	+++	+++	++	+++	++	+++	++
	6 min	++	++	++	++	+	++	+	++	+
	8 min	+	+	+	++	+	++	+	++	+
80%	4 min	++	++	++	++	+	++	+	++	+
	6 min	++	++	++	+	+	+	+	+	+
	8 min	+	+	+	-	+	-	+	-	+
90%	4 min	+	+	+	+	-	+	-	+	-
	6 min	-	-	-	-	-	-	-	-	-
	8 min	-	-	-	-	-	-	-	-	-

C1-C3: Control plate obtained after culturing of last wash of material after surface sterilization.
Treatment: Sample of plant material after surface sterilization kept on nutrient agar plate where G represent growth of endophytes and C represent growth of contaminant as unusual growth of microbes. G: Represents Growth of endophytes of treated sample, C: Represents Contamination of treated sample. (+++) represents highest growth, (++) represents moderate growth and (+) represents low growth, (-) represent no growth

Sodium hypochlorite is very effective sterilizing agent because hypochlorite (OCl⁻) is strong oxidizing agent that denature by aggregating the proteins of bacteria. On the other hand when sodium hypochorite concentrations (2%, 3% & 4%) were used for surface sterilization, 2% and 3% concentrations were found to be effective for surface sterilization because 4% NaOCl concentration was found to be inhibitory for growth of endophytic bacteria as shown in Table 2.

Table 2. Effect of concentration of NaOCl (2%, 3% & 4%) on growth and contamination of endophytic bacteria on nutrient agar

Sodium hypochlorite		Control (Last wash spreading)			Treatment					
2%	Time	C1	C2	C3	G	C	G	C	G	C
	2 min	++	++	++	++	+	++	+	++	+
	4 min	++	++	++	+	+	+	+	+	+
	6 min	+++	+++	+++	+	+	+	+	+	+
3%	2 min	++	++	++	++	+	++	+	++	+
	4 min	++	++	++	+	+	+	+	+	+
	6 min	++	++	++	+	+	+	+	+	+
4%	2 min	++	++	++	+	+	+	+	+	-
	4 min	++	++	++	+	+	+	-	+	-
	6 min	+++	+++	+++	+	+	+	-	+	-

Different combination of ethanol and sodium hypochlorite solution were also used for surface sterilization at different time intervals. Combination of 70% ethanol for 6minute treatment, 2% sodium hypochlorite solution for 1minute treatment and followed by 70% ethanol for 30 second were found to be effective for sterilizing the surface of Allium sativum leaf while 70% ethanol and 3% NaOCl keeping the same time period were found to be effective for sterilizing the surface of Allium sativum bulb. Similarly, 70% ethanol for 6 minute treatment followed by 2% sodium hypochlorite for 4minute treatment and 70% ethanol for 8 minute treatment followed by 2% sodium hypochlorite for 4minute treatment were found to be effective for sterilizing the surface of Allium sativum bulb but exhibited reduced growth of endophytic bacteria on nutrient agar plate. Therefore, combination of 70% ethanol for 6minute treatment, 3% sodium hypochlorite solution for 1minute treatment and followed by 70% ethanol for 30 second were found to be most effective for sterilizing the surface of Allium sativum bulb.

4.   Discussion

Present investigation was conducted to optimize surface sterilization process of *Allium sativum* leaves and bulb for isolation of bacterial endophytes. In India only a few reports were available on isolation of endophytic bacteria and fungi from medicinal plants (Anjum and Chandra 2015). There is no report on endophytic bacteria from *Allium sativum* from India although existence of fungal endophytes with antimicrobial activity has been reported in *Allium sativum* (Shentu *et al.,* 2014). For isolation of endophytic bacteria *Allium sativum* must be surface sterilized before inoculating them on nutrient agar medium. Chemical disinfectant ethanol (70%) and sodium hyochlorite (2% &3%) gave significant result when used in combination as compared to individual treatment. Akinsanya *et al.* (2015) isolated bacterial endophyte from leaf and root of *Aloe vera* by using 90% ethanol (5min) and 3% sodium hypochlorite (2min) followed by 75% ethanol (5min) that exhibiting antimicrobial activity against *Bacillus cereus* and *Candida albicans.* In the present study when 90%

ethanol was used for surface sterilization the growth of endophytes isolates significantly reduced. Reports are available for use of ethanol and sodium hyochlorite for surface sterilization of Rambutan fruit (Suhandono *et al.*, 2016), *Hypericum perforatum* and *Ziziphora capitata* (Egamberdieva *et al.*, 2017) by using 70% ethanol and 5% sodium hypochlorite. *Burkholderia stabilis* (Kim *et al.*, 2019) and *Bacillus velezensis* LDO2 (Chen *et al.*, 2019) were isolated from ginseng root and peanut respectively by using a particular concentration of sodium hypochlorite and ethanol. Our results are in accordance to the earlier reports and several endophyte isolate were obtained from *Allium sativum* by using the combined disinfectants on the other hand the application of 4% sodium hypochlorite in the present investigation inhibited the appearance of endophytes. Our results also reveal that different combinations should be applied for disinfecting leaves and bulb of *Allium sativum*. *Allium sativum* was used in the present investigation because of its many fold medicinal property and investigation of endophytes from this plant is important for exploration of new antibiotics of plant origin. Further investigation regarding characterization of isolates, their bioactive compounds, and their antimicrobial activity is in progress.

5. Conclusion

Effective surface sterilization are not seen when 70% ethanol, 2% sodium hypochlorite and 3% sodium hypochlorite are use individually at different time intervals. The combination of 70% ethanol (6min), 2% sodium hyochlorite (1min) and 70% ethanol (30 sec) is best for surface sterilization of leaf and 70% ethanol (6min), 3% sodium hyochlorite (1min) and ethanol (30 sec) for bulb of *Allium sativum*. In present investigation most of endophytic bacteria isolated from leaf are Gram positive while Gram negative were observed from bulb of *Allium sativum*. Endophytes isolated from *Allium sativum* in future can be used to asses antimicrobial activity. Bioactive compound produced by potent isolates that exhibit wide spectrum of activity and molecular identification of the potential isolates is in under progress. In future, isolation of endophytic bacteria from *Allium sativum* will be promising source for producing novel antibiotics.

6. Acknowledgement

One of the authors Ms. Pratima Srivastava is thankful to Department of Science and Technology (DST), Government of India New Delhi for providing financial assistance under DST Women Scientist A (WOS-A) scheme, as a Principal investigator (File No. SR/WOS-A/LS-11/2018). Thanks are also due to Prof. Rajesh Sharma (mentor); Prof. Vandana Rai, HOD Department of Biotechnology and Dr. S.P Tiwari, Associate Professor, Department of Microbiology for providing laboratory facilities and support.

7. References

1. Akinsanya, M.A. Diversity, antimicrobial and antioxidant activities of culturable bacterial endophyte communities. in Aloe vera. FEMS Microbiol. Letters. 362, (2015).

2. Anjum, N. Endophytic bacteria: optimization of isolation procedure from various medicinal plants and their preliminary characterization. Asian. J. Pharm.Clin. Res. 8(4), 233-238 (2015).

3. Bayan, L. Garlic: a review of potential therapeutic effects. Avicenna Journal of Phytomedicine (AJP).4(1), 1-14 (2014).

4. Boyle, C., Gotz, M., Dammann-Tugend, U., Schulz, B. Endophyte-host interaction III. Local vs. systemic colonization.Symbiosis 31(4), 259-281 (2001).

5. Carroll, G.C. Forest endophytes: pattern and process. Can. J. Bot. 73 (S1), 1316-1324 (1995).

6. Chen, L. Antimicrobial, plant growth-promoting and genomic properties of the peanut endophyte Bacillus velezensis LDO2. Microbiol. Res. 218, 41–48 (2019).

7. De Bary A. Morphology and physiology of fungi, lichens, and myxomycetes. hofmeister's. Handbook of Physiological Botany. Leipzig, Germany: Springer-Verlag (1866).

8. Egamberdieva, D. Antimicrobial Activity of Medicinal Plant Correlates with the Proportion of Antagonistic Endophytes. Front. Microbiol.199 (8), 1-11(2017).

9. Hallmann, J. Application of the Scholander pressure bomb to studies on endophytic bacteria of plants. Can. J. Microbiol. 43, 41 1-416 (1997a).

10. Hallmann, J. Interactions between Meloidogyne incognita and endophytic bacteria in cotton and cucumber. Soi.l Biol. Biochem. (1997b).

11. Holliday, P, (1989) A Dictionary of Plant Pathology. Cambridge University Press, Cambridge.

12. Kim, H. Antimicrobial potential of metabolites extracted from ginseng bacterial endophyte Burkholderia stasbilis against ginseng pathogens. Biological control.128, 24-30 (2019).

13. Kuklinsky-Sobral, J. Isolation and characterization of soyabean associated bacteria and their potential for plant growth promotion. Environ. Microbiol. 12, 1244-1251 (2004).

14. Lodewyckx, C. Endophytic bacteria and their potential applications. Crit. Rev. Plant. Sci. 21, 583–606 (2002).

15. McInroy, J.A., Kloepper, J.W. Studies on indigenous endophytic bacteria of sweet corn and cotton. In: O' Gara F, Dowing DN, Boesten B (eds) Molecular ecology of rhizosphere microorganisms. pp 19-28 VCH, Weinheim, Germany (1994).

16. Ryan, R.P. Bacterial endophytes: recent development and applications. FEMS Microbiol. Lett. 278, 1-9 (2008).

17. Schulz, B., Boyle, C. What are endophytes? Microbial Root Endophytes (Schulz BJE, Boyle CJC & Sieber TN, eds), pp.1–13. Springer-Verlag, Berlin (2006).

18. Shentu, X. Antifungal activity of the metabolite of the endophytic fungus Trichoderma brevicompactum from garlic. Brazilian. J. Microbio. 45(1), 248-254(2014).

19. Suhandono, S. Isolation and Molecular Identification of Endophytic Bacteria From Rambutan Fruits (Nephelium lappaceum L.) Cultivar Binjai. HAYATI J of Biosciences.23, 39-44 (2016).

20. Yu, H. Recent development and future prospect of antimicrobial metabolites produced by endophytes. Microbiol. Res. 165, 437-449 (2010).

Effect of Four Different Oil Seed Cakes on Yield and Lignocellulolytic Enzymes During Cultivation of Oyster Mushroom Pleurotus Florida

Roshan Lal Gautam, Shweta Singh, Manish Kumar Gupta and Ram Naraian*

Department of Biotechnology, Mushroom Training and Research Centre (MTRC), Faculty of Science,
Veer Bahadur Singh Purvanchal University, Jaunpur-222003, India
*Email: ramnarain_itrc@rediffmail.com

ABSTRACT

Oyster mushroom Pleurotus florida was cultivated on wheat straw (WS) as basal substrate supplemented with four different oil seed cakes such as groundnut seed cake (GSC), mahuaa seed cake (MSC), neem seed cake (NSC) and mustard cake (MC). The highest fruit body yield (2,514 g) was recorded in the sets of 2% (w/w) GSC supplemented substrate followed by 1,343, 1,243 and 1,062 g in the sets of 2% (w/w) MSC, NSC and MC respectively. The biological efficiency (BE) was also remarkably influenced of oil seed cakes. The order of BE achieved in response to oil seed cake supplementation in descending order as; 251.4 % > 134.3 % > 124.3 % > 106.2 % in GSC > MSC > NSC > MC. The mustard cake supplementation resulted the lowest yield and BE in comparison to other cakes. The enzyme profiling of cellulase, xylanase, laccase and manganese peroxidase (MnP) in all cultivation phases viz., complete mycelial run (CMR), pin head initiation (PHI), flush I, flush II and flush III were variably influenced. The supplementation of oil seed cakes also remarkably influenced to the duration of different cultivation phase. The GSC was found to be most superior to other tested cakes. Therefore, based on the results of present study the use of oil seed cake at 2 % (w/w) is recommended for oyster mushroom cultivation.

Keywords: *Pleurotus florida*, substrate, supplements, cultivation, yield, biological efficiency.

1.   Introduction

Pleurotus florida is an edible fleshy mushroom, commonly called as oyster mushroom, which is a second most cultivated mushroom, constituting approximately 19% of the world's mushroom output [1]. The increasing population of the world's and its decrease in per capita arable land, along with rapid urbanization and industrialization, climate change, and a demand for quality and functional foods, such as mushrooms, these are secondary agriculture and novel crops [2]. It is a diverse genus belonging to white-rot basidiomycete fungi and well known for their complexity of the enzymatic system and prominent lignocellulolytic property [3]. The white-rot fungi *P. florida* have potential to produces extracellular enzymes such as cellulase, xylanase, laccase and manganese peroxidase (MnP). The genus *Pleurotus* well-known for conversion of substrate into edible and fleshy mushrooms [4]. Mushrooms not only convert lignocellulosic waste materials into human food, but also can produce notable nutriceutical products, which have many health benefits [5]. Various oil seed cakes including ground nut, mustard, neem seed, mahuaa seed, cotton seed, and sunflower seed are used as supplements in mushroom cultivation. These supplement cakes boost up for mushroom growth and development.

Bioconversion of lignocellulosic wastes is performed by *Pleurotus* spp. cultivation which produces enzymes such as hemicellulases, cellulases and ligninases [6]. The enzymes secreted by *Pleurotus florida*, degrade complex material into simple unit. So, these enzymes have a potential role in mushroom growth and development [7]. The activities of enzymes laccase and cellulase produced by *Lentinus edodes* for important in mycelial growth and fruit body development of mushroom [8]. The level of extracellular enzyme activity varies substantially during the three flush cultivation stages of oyster mushrooms [9]. The addition of oil seed cakes affects the secretion of the mushroom enzymes with an increased degradation of the substrate polymers, finally resulting in an increased production of fruiting bodies [10].

In the present study, effect of different oil seed cakes on different parameters of oyster mushroom *P. florida* cultivation phases, yield or biological efficiency, and enzyme profile of lignocellulolytic enzyme was investigated.

2. Material and Methods

2.1 Mushroom strain

The strain of *P. florida* was obtained from Mushroom Training and Research Center (MTRC), Department of Biotechnology, Faculty of Science, Veer Bahadur Singh Purvanchal University, Jaunpur, Uttar Pradesh, India.

2.2 Maintenance of culture

Fungal culture was maintained in slants containing potato dextrose agar medium (potato 200 g, dextrose 20 g, and agar 20 g/L). The cultured slants were preserved in refrigerators at 5°C and fungal culture was maintained by regular sub-culturing every fortnightly.

2.3 Basal substrate and supplements

The wheat straw was used as basal substrate and oil seed cake such as groundnut seed cake (GSC), mahuaa seed cake (MSC), mustard cake (MC) and neem seed cake were employed as supplements.

2.4 Preparation of substrate

The sundried wheat straw substrate soaked in water containing 0.5% (w/v) bavistin plus 2% (v/v) formalin to sterilized substrate chemically. Then the wet wheat straw was spread over sterilized polythene sheet for squeezing extra water.

2.5 Supplementation

Different concentration (2, 3 and 5 % w/w) of oil seed cakes were weighed and properly mixed to wheat straw prior spawning.

2.6 Spawn preparation

The spawn of *P. florida* was prepared using water soaked boiled wheat grains, these grains were then mixed with calcium carbonate (4% w/w) and calcium sulfate (2% w/w). After filling grains in cotton plugging polythene bags. The bags were autoclaved at 20 lb for 45 min. The cooled at 20°C till complete cooling of grains with mycelia bags were incubated in BOD incubator (NSW, India).

2.7 Cultivation and harvesting

Cultivation of oyster mushroom was performed in polythene bags of (18 × 22 inc.) spawned with layer wise manner. After complete mycelial run polythenes torned apart and subjected for regular irrigation though sprinkling of fresh water, after the development of primordia into matured fruit body, these were harvested with gentle handling and weighed to record yield flush wise separately.

2.8   Yield and biological efficiency

The yield of fruit bodies was calculated with respect to weight of substrate and weight of fruit body per bag. The biological efficiency (BE) was calculated as % BE with respect to Kg fresh mushroom Kg^{-1} dry substrate used [11] as per to the formula given below.

$$\% \text{ Biological efficiency (\%BE)} = \frac{\text{Fresh weight of mushroom}}{\text{Dry weight of substrate}} \times 100$$

2.9   Enzyme assay

2.9.1. Cellulase activity

The activity of cellulase was determined by using 1 mL of 1% (w/v) carboxymethyl cellulose in 50 mM sodium acetate buffer pH 5.3 with 1 mL of extracellular crude enzyme extract of *P. florida* and incubated at 50°C for 15 min [12]. The reaction was terminated using Rochelle salt (sodium-potassium tartrate) solution. The absorbance was recorded spectrophotometrically at 540 nm.

2.9.2. Xylanase activity

Xylanase activity was used standard method [13], assay mixture contained 0.5 ml enzyme extract to 0.5 ml of 0.25 % (w/v) xylan (HiMedia) solution to 1 ml of 100 mM of phosphate buffer and 3.0 ml DNS reagent and incubated at 22°C. Using Rochelle salt solution for stopped reaction and intensity of color was measured.

2.9.3. Laccase activity

The laccase activity was used substrate guiaicol [14]. 5 ml of the reaction mixture containing 3.9 ml acetate buffer (10 mM, pH 5.0), 1 ml guaiacol (1.76 mM) and 0.1 ml enzyme extract were incubated at 25°C for 2 hour, the addition of 0.5 ml dimethylsulfoxide for stopped reaction. Thereafter, the absorbance was read at 450 nm.

2.9.4. Manganese peroxidase (MnP) activity

Activity of manganese peroxidase (MnP) was measured spectrophotometrically with 3 mM phenol sulfonpthalein as substrate. The reaction mixture contained 0.2 ml buffer enzyme preparation, 2 mM H_2O_2 and phenol sulfonpthalein, incubated at 22°C for 5 min. For stopped reaction using 2 M NaOH [15].

3.   Results and Discussion

3.1   Effect of different oil seed cakes on distinct cultivation phases

Effect of four different oil seed cakes on the cultivation phases (CMR, PHI, flush I, flush II and flush III) of oyster mushroom P. florida was evaluated. The fastest complete mycelial run took place within 13 days in response to 2% GSC, while 2% MC supplementation resulted most delayed CMR. In addition, GSC supplementation most efficiently influenced all phases including PHI, flush I, flush II and flush III as 16, 23, 35, and 39 days respectively. Therefore, the GSC was most efficient oil seed cake which have remarkably influenced to all cultivation phases of oyster mushroom P. florida (**Table 1**). Kalmis and Sargin [16] also reported starting of primordia on day 22nd of cultivation. In our study, the first pin head initiation in P. florida was noted on 16, 19 and 23 days with supplementation of GSC, MSC and NSC respectively. While, pin head initiation was started in supplements MC on 30 day. Ragunathan et al. [17] observed primordial initiation on the 22nd day in Pleurotus sajor-caju and Pleurotus platypus and on 27th day in Pleurotus citrinopileatus.

Table 1. Effect of different oil seed cake on different cultivation phases of Pleurotus florida

Mushroom Cultivation Phases	In days			
	NSC	MSC	GSC	MC
CMR	19±0.70	15±1.30	13±0.70	25±2.0
PHI	23±1.14	19±1.14	16±0.89	30±1.30
Flush I	31±1.48	28±1.48	23±1.14	40±1.64
Flush II	42±0.89	40±1.14	35±1.64	54±1.41
Flush III	47±1.58	44±2.44	39±0.70	59±1.67

CMR = Complete mycelial run, PHI = Pin head initiation, ± = Standard deviation (n=8)

3.2   Effect of different oil seed cakes on enzyme activity in different cultivation phases

The enzyme activity of cellulase, xylanase, laccase and MnP were studied during different cultivation phases (CMR, PHI, flush I, flush II and flush III) of oyster mushroom P. florida. The highest activity of laccase (4.30 U/ml) was recorded in the phase of CMR while the lowest (1.71 U/ml) in flush I phase. The highest cellulase activity (1.87 U/ml) was found in flush II phase that was followed by 1.51, 1.35, 0.90 and 0.82 U/ml in phase of CMR, PHI, flush I and flush III respectively. The lowest cellulase activity (0.82 U/ml) was recorded in flush III stage. In addition, the highest MnP activity was observed as (1.70 U/ml) in the phase of flush I and lowest (0.67 U/ml) in the phase of flush III. Xylanase activity was recorded highest (0.83 U/ml) in PHI and lowest (0.57 U/ml) in flush I phase. The highest enzyme activities of cellulase, xylanase, laccase and MnP can be represented as: 1.87, 0.83, 4.30 and 1.70 U/ml during the phases of flush II, PHI, CMR and flush I respectively (Table 2). Similar observations regarding enzymes in different phases were also resulted in several studies [6,9].

Table 2. Enzyme activities of lignocellulolytic enzymes during different cultivation phases of *Pleurotus florida*

Mushroom Cultivation Phases	Lignocellulolytic enzymes (U/ml)			
	Cellulase	Xylanase	Laccase	MnP
CMR	1.51±0.02	0.69±0.03	4.30±0.03	1.25±0.06
PHI	1.35±0.01	0.83±0.06	1.85±0.05	0.76±0.01
Flush I	0.90±0.03	0.57±0.06	1.71±0.04	1.70±0.03
Flush II	1.87±0.04	0.63±0.01	3.12±0.02	1.23±0.03
Flush III	0.82±0.05	0.67±0.02	2.35±0.04	0.67±0.02

CMR = Complete mycelial run, PHI = Pin head initiation, ± = Standard deviation (n=8)

3.3   The effect of oil seed cakes on fruit body yield

The oil seed cakes tested in the study remarkably influenced the fruit body yield of oyster mushroom P. florida. The highest 2,514 g of yield was obtained in the set of 2% (w/w) GSC supplementation which was followed by 1,343 g in the set of 2% (w/w) MSC. The MC represented its lowest 1,062 g of yield. Therefore, comparing the effect of oil seed cakes it was obvious the GSC was the superior in reference to other oil seed cakes tested (**Fig 1a).** Similar results were also reported in the study of oyster mushrooms by Zhang et al.

[18]. In addition, Rizki and Tamai [19] was reported fruit bodies obtained in the second and third flushes were comparatively lower to amounts of mushroom produced in first flush.

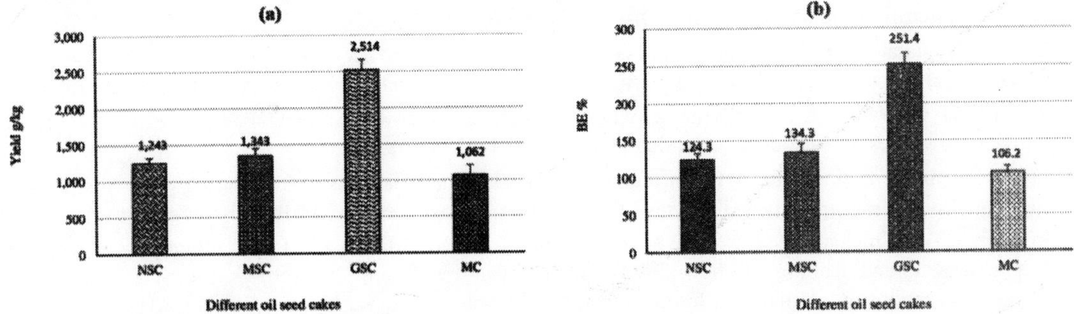

Figure 1. The effect of different oil seed cakes on: **(a)** yield and **(b)** biological efficiency (BE%) of Pleurotus florida

3.4   The effect of oil seed cakes on the biological efficiency (BE %)

As observed the oil seed cake supplementation with wheat straw resulted in a remarkable effect on the biological efficiency of oyster mushroom of P. florida. The highest 251.4% BE was recorded in 2% (w/w) supplementation of GSC, while it was followed to 143.3, 124.3 and 106.2% in the sets of MSC, NSC and MC supplemented at the rate of 2% (w/w), as compared the GSC was found to be the best oil seed cake in comparison to other these oil seed cakes (NSC, MSC and MC) test in study (Fig 1b). Betterley [20] suggested that with supplementation, the biological efficiency was obtained 90.0%. In comparison to several studies, we have found the higher biological efficiency (251.4%) of P. florida in GSC supplementation.

4.   Conclusion

Based on the results of the present study it can be concluded that the GSC was superior oil seed cake in comparison to other by providing better yield, biological efficiency. The also positively influenced to different cultivation phases and lignocellulolytic enzyme secretion. Therefore, the use of GSC in the cultivation of oyster mushroom is recorded for the better yield and biological efficiency with better quality of mushroom along with no harming effect to consumer.

5.   Acknowledgements

Authors are thankful to Hon'ble Vice-Chancellor, V. B. S. Purvanchal University, Jaunpur, Uttar Pradesh, India, for frequent encouragement and providing the facilities.

6.   References

1.   Zied, D. C., Pardo-Gimenez, A., de Oliveira, G. A., Carrasco, J., Zeraik, M. L.: Study of waste products as supplements in the production and quality of Pleurotus ostreatus var. Florida. Indian Journal of Microbiology 59(3), 328–335 (2019).

2.   Gupta, S., Summuna, B., Gupta, M., Annepu, S. K.: Edible mushrooms: cultivation, bioactive molecules, and health benefits. In: Merillon, J. M., Ramawat, K. G. (eds.) Bioactive Molecules in Food, Reference Series in Phytochemistry. Springer Nature Switzerland AG. pp 1815-1847 (2019).

3.   Naraian, R., Singh, M. P., Ram, S.: Supplementation of basal substrate to boost up substrate strength and oyster mushroom yield: an overview of substrates and supplements. International Journal of Current Microbiology and Applied Sciences 5(5), 543-553 (2016).

4.   Mandeel, Q. A., Al-Laith, A. A., Mohamed, S. A.: Cultivation of oyster mushrooms (Pleurotus spp.) on various lignocellulosic wastes. World Journal of Microbiology & Biotechnology 21(4), 601–607 (2005).

5.   Girmay, Z., Gorems, W., Birhanu, G., Zewdie, S.: Growth and yield performance of Pleurotus ostreatus (Jacq. Fr.) Kumm (oyster mushroom) on different substrates. AMB Express 6(1), 1-7 (2016).

6.   Kurt, S., Buyukalaca, S.: Yield performances and changes in enzyme activities of Pleurotus spp. (P. ostreatus and P. sajor-caju) cultivated on different agricultural wastes. Bioresource Technology 101, 3164–3169 (2010).

7.   Kuforiji, O. O., Fasidi, I. O.: Enzyme activities of Pleurotus tuber-regium (Fries) Singer, cultivated on selected agricultural wastes. Bioresource Technology 99(10), 4275–4278 (2008).

8.   Ohga, S., Royse, D. J.: Transcriptional regulation of laccase and cellulase genes during growth and fruiting of Lentinula edodes on supplemented sawdust. FEMS Microbiology Letters 201(1), 111–115 (2001).

9.   Elisashvili, V., Chichua, D., Kachlishvili, E., Tsiklauri, N., Khardziani, T.: Lignocellulolytic enzyme activity during growth and fruiting of the edible and medicinal mushroom Pleurotus ostreatus (Jacq.:Fr.) Kumm. (Agaricomycetideae). International Journal of Medicinal Mushrooms 5, 193–198 (2003).

10.   Bano, Z., Shashirekha, M. N., Rajarathnam, S.: Improvement of the bioconversion and biotransformation efficiencies of the oyster mushroom (Pleurotus sajor-caju) by supplementation of its rice straw substrate with oil seed cakes. Enzyme and Microbial Technology 15(11), 985-989 (1993).

11.   Naraian, R., Narayan, O. P., Srivastava, J.: Differential response of oyster shell powder on enzyme profile and nutritional value of oyster mushroom Pleurotus florida PF05. BioMed Research International 1-7 (2014).

12.   Casimir, S. J., Davis, S., Fiechter, A., Gysin, B., Murray, E., Perrolaz, J. J., Zimmermann, W. S.: Pulp bleaching with thermostable xylanase of Thermomonospora fusca. US Patent, (1996).

13.   Miller, G. L.: Use of dinitrosalicylic acid reagent for determination of reducing sugar. Analytical Chemistry 31, 426-428 (1959).

14.   Sandhu, D. K., Arora, D. S.: Laccase production by Polyporus sanguineus under different nutritional and environmental conditions. Experientia 41(3), 355-356 (1985).

15.   Glenn, J. K.: Gold, M. H.: Purification and characterization of an extracellular Mn (II)-dependent peroxidase from the lignin degrading basidiomycete Phanerochaete chrysosporium. Archives of Biochemistry and Biophysics 242, 329-341 (1985).

16.   Kalmis, E., Sargin, S.: Cultivation of two Pleurotus species on wheat straw substrates containing olive mill waste water. International Biodeterioration and Biodegradation 53(1), 43–47 (2004).

17.   Ragunathan, R., Gurusamy, R., Palaniswamy, M., Swaminathan, K.: Cultivation of Pleurotus spp. on various agro-residues. Food Chemistry 55, 139–144 (1996).

18.   Zhang, R., Li, X., Fadel, J. G.: Oyster mushroom cultivation with rice and wheat straw. Bioresources Technology 82, 277–284 (2002).

19.   Rizki, M., Tamai, Y.: Effects of different nitrogen rich substrates and their combination to the yield performance of oyster mushroom (Pleurotus ostreatus). World Journal of Microbiology and Biotechnology 27(7), 1695–1702 (2011).

20.   Betterley, D. A.: Supplementation rate; study and effect of supplementation at spawning on mushroom yield, size and quality. Spawnmate Newsletter 7, 1–4 (1988).

Synthesis of Copper Nanostructure Using Sonochemical Assisted Co-Precipitation Method and Their Antibacterial Study

Abhishek K. Bhardwaj[1], K. N. Uttam[2], Manish K. Gupta[3], Ram Naraian[3], and Ram Gopal[2,*]

[1]Department of Environmental Science, Veer Bahadur Singh Purvanchal University, Jaunpur-222003, (UP), India
[3]Department of Biotechnology, Veer Bahadur Singh Purvanchal University, Jaunpur-222003, (UP), India
*E-mail: profrgopal@gmail.com

ABSTRACT

Cupric oxide (CuO) and cuprous oxide (Cu_2O) nanoparticles (NPs) are two important oxide compounds of copper, with low cost preparation, potential of a catalyst, conductive ink or cooling fluid, antibacterial property and behaviors of p-type semiconductor. In this study, sonochemical co-precipitation method was opted for the synthesis of nanostructures of CuO and Cu_2O using the chemical reduction of copper sulfate with mixture of sodium borohydride and sodium hydroxide. The samples CuO and Cu_2O were prepared with variables of polyethylene glycol (PEG) concentrations as 2 ml, and 5ml respectively. The effect of different concentrations (2 ml, and 5 ml) of PEG after the exposure of constant ultrasonic power and time was studied on the morphology of the prepared CuO NPs using transmission electron microscopy (TEM). The TEM observations showed that the size of copper oxide nano sheets was increased with increasing PEG concentration during their synthesis. The larger size of Cu_2O sample nanostructure (nanoflower) treated with (5 mL PEG) was recorded with average width 150 nm, average lengths 80 nm and thickness about in between 10 to 12 nm. The optical properties of prepared nanoflowers were studied using UV-VIS spectroscopy. Fourier transforms infrared (FTIR) spectroscopy transmittance at wavenumber of 613 cm^{-1} can be attributed to the lattice vibration of the Cu_2O The remarkable antibacterial efficacy of CuO and Cu_2O NPs was observed against different pathogenic bacteria.

Keywords: Cupric oxide; Cuprous oxide; Antibacterial; Nanoparticles; Nano-sheet.

1. Introduction

Metal nanoparticles have gained considerable attention in recent years due to their unique properties and practical applications in the areas of information storage, catalysis, electronics, optics, water purification, catalytic and biomedical sciences [1,4,15]. Despite the preference of noble metals like Au and Ag in most of these applications, the high cost of these metals is a major constraint in their large scale production. The easily availability of copper, and having similar properties like of other expensive noble metals, has made it a better choice. The preparation of copper NPs has become a thrust area of study in material research as they are rightly considered as a possible replacement for gold and silver NPs [17, 23]. Various synthesis methods of copper NPs have been reported to control particle size and shape, including radiation, laser ablation [19], deposition [2, 6], supercritical technique, microwave reduction, sonochemical method [3], vacuum vapour deposition and micro-emulsion etc [8,11,12,18,26]. Earlier workers have prepared Cu_2O NPs by diversemethods but only few have potency to tailor specific structure. In recent scenario scientist are focused for the enhancing stability of copper NPs and develop low cost, environmental friendly techniques [7,21].

Cuprous oxide (Cu_2O) is an important metal-oxide p-type semiconductor with a direct small band gap of 2.17 eV [25], which makes it a promising material for the conversion of solar energy into electrical or chemical energy. Cu_2O nanostructure is useful for applications in gas sensing [22], CO oxidation [10], photo catalysis [5,9], photochemical evolution of H_2 from water [20], photocurrent generation [13,14,24].

In this manuscript simply copper nanostructures were synthesized using sonochemical method, which is the cost effective, environmental benign, single pot synthesis technique for the tailoring of nanostructure.

2.   Materials and Methods

Analytical grade copper sulfate pentahydrate ($CuSO_4.5H_2O$, 99.8%, pure), sodium hydroxide (NaOH, 99.0% pure), poly ethylene glycol (PEG-400) and double distilled water all from Merck as well as nutrient agar and nutrient broth (HiMedia Laboratories Pvt. Ltd) were used for synthesis.

2.1   Synthesis Process

In a typical synthesis of copper oxide nanoparticles, 100 ml of 0.02 M of copper sulfate pentahydrate ($CuSO_4.5H_2O$) was taken; different concentration of PEG was added. The mixture of copper sulphate was filled in burette and dropped into 0.2 M of aqueous solution sodium hydroxide (NaOH) at the rate of 1 ml/min. The pH of NaOH solution kept in a flask was adjusted approx 10 and was transferred in an ultrasonic bath operating at frequency 40 kHz for ultrasound irradiation. Blackish color precipitate was found which was separated using centrifuge machine and rinsed repeatedly for several times with double distilled water to remove the residual reactants. The precipitate was dried for 12 hrs using oven at 50°C and powder was homogenized using a pestle mortar. The complete processes of synthesis are illustrated in Fig. 1.

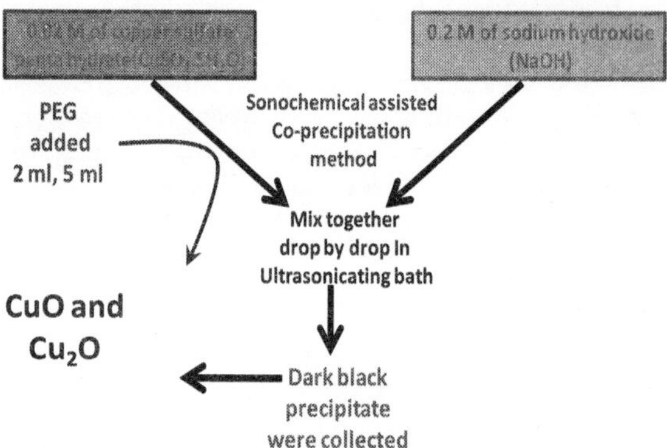

Figure 1 The schematic diagram of synthesis of Copper nanostructure

The sample CuO and Cu_2O were prepared the changing PEG concentration 2ml, and 5ml respectively. The effect of PEG concentration (2 ml and 5 ml) at constant ultrasonic power was studied on the morphology of the prepared Cu NPs.

3.   Characterization

Optical absorption spectra of synthesized copper NPs were recorded in the spectral region 300 - 800 nm using PerkinElmer Lambda 35 double beam UV-Visible spectrophotometer. In order to study on the surface moiety of copper NPs, infrared (IR) absorption spectra were recorded using FTIR spectrometer (ABB, Bomem Inc.) equipped with ATR unit in the spectral region 500 - 4000 cm^{-1} at a resolution of 4 cm^{-1}. High-resolution transmission electron microscope (Tecnai G2-20, FEI Company, Netherland) operating at 200 kV was used for the size and shape measurements of the prepared copper NPs. Samples for the transmission electron microscopy were prepared by putting a drop of colloidal solution on the carbon-coated copper grid and drying under the IR lamp.

4.   Results and Discussion

4.1   UV-VIS spectroscopy

UV–VIS absorption spectra of synthesized colloidal solutions of Cu NPs have been recorded using Perkin Elmer Lambda 35, double beam spectrophotometer in the range from 200 to 1000 nm (Fig. 2). The absorption band was found at 261 nm treatment of 2 ml PEG shownthe characteristic peak of CuO NPs. For another sample the peak is shifted to 323 nm which is characteristic peaks of Cu_2O NPs. This is due to increasing concentration of PEG which limits the supply of oxygen in synthesizing medium. The limited supply of oxygen restricts oxidation of copper and these consequences leads to reduce oxygen concentration in copper NPs with increasing amount of PEG. The peak broadening of Cu_2O shows that it can be due to the growth of copper nanostructure [16].

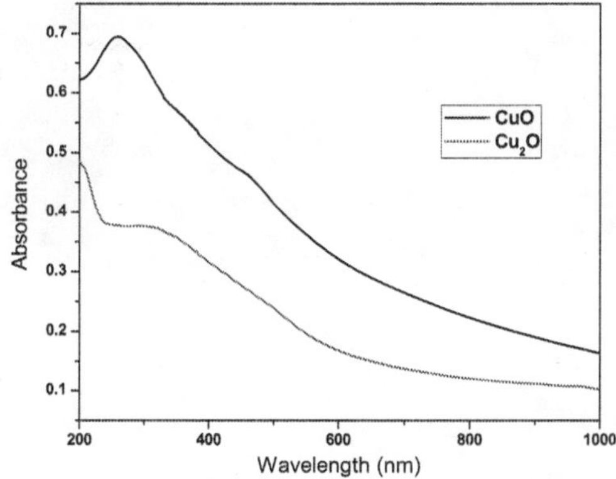

Figure. 2 UV-spectra of synthesized CuO and Cu_2O

4.2   ATR FTIR

IR spectrum of synthesized copper NPs was recorded using Bomem ATR-FTIR in the range 500–4000 cm^{-1} with a resolution of 4 cm^{-1} (Fig. 3). The band at wavenumber 518 cm^{-1} and 604 cm^{-1} were ascribed to CuO vibration and Cu_2O respectively. The CuO band is shifting towards higher wavenumber as the concentration of PEG increases. As PEG concentration increases level of oxygen decreases, which is responsible to formation of Cu_2O/Cu. In the all synthesized samples, the peak around 3435 cm^{-1} are due to the –OH bonds. FTIR spectra provides information about the nature of the copper oxide NPs is essential for verifying the type of the oxide. The study also confirms the formation and stabilization of Cu_2ONPs in the aqueous medium of PEG.

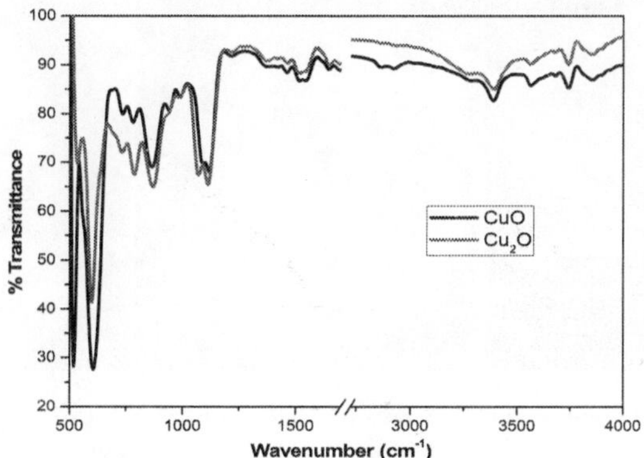

Figure 3. FTIR Spectra of CuO and Cu_2O

4.3   TEM Micrographs

High resolution transmission electron microscope Tecnai G2-20 operated at 200 kV was used to determine the particle size and shape of the synthesized Cu NPs. The TEM micrograph of the two samples of copperoxides NPs is shown in Fig. 4, almost of the copper sample were found in the form of nanoflowers. TEM image of sample C_1 shows small agglomerated nanorods [Fig. 4 (C1)]. Whereas the TEM image samples C_2 shows larger size of nanoflowers. TEM micrographs clearly reveal that the increasing concentration of PEG was responsible for the growth of copper nanosflowers and also form colloidal solution.

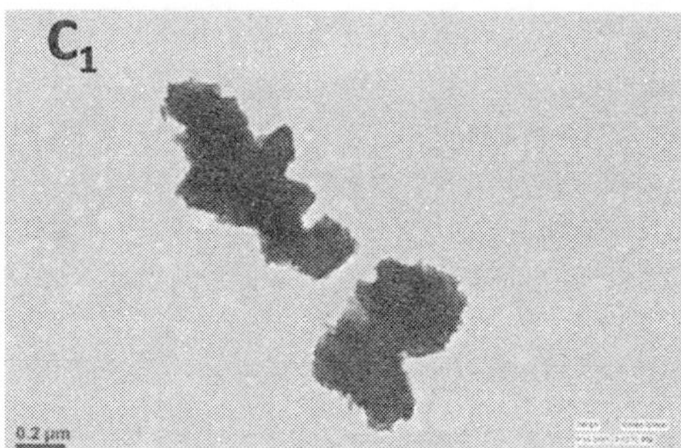
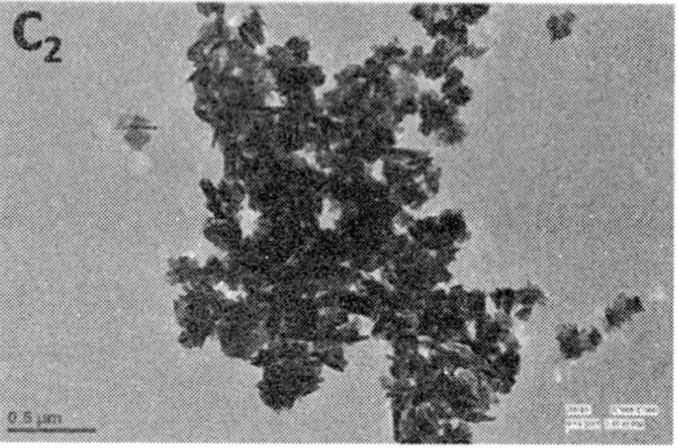

Fig.4 TEM of copper nanostructureCuOand Cu_2O

5.   Antibacterial Application

5.1   Zone of inhibition

Antibacterial study of synthesized copper nanosheets (50 ppm) was done against *E. coli, S. aureus* and *S. typhimurium* bacteria using disc diffusion method. The significant zone of inhibition diameter about 10, 8 and 16 mm were observed against *E. coli* (Gram negative), *S. aureus* (Gram positive) and *S. typhimurium* (Gram negative) respectively [Fig. 5]. No zone of inhibition was observed in control disc (loaded with distilled water). In all the experiments adequate aseptic measures were taken. For the disc diffusion method, 100 **µl** of *S. aureus* suspension of about 5×10^6 CFU ml^{-1} was spread over Mueller–Hinton agar plates using sterilized cotton swabs and 20 **µl** capacity disc placed on the bacterial lawns. The solutions are gradually diffused into the neighboring bacterial lawns and the area around the discs depleted of bacterial population was regarded as a measure of the antibacterial property of the copper solution.

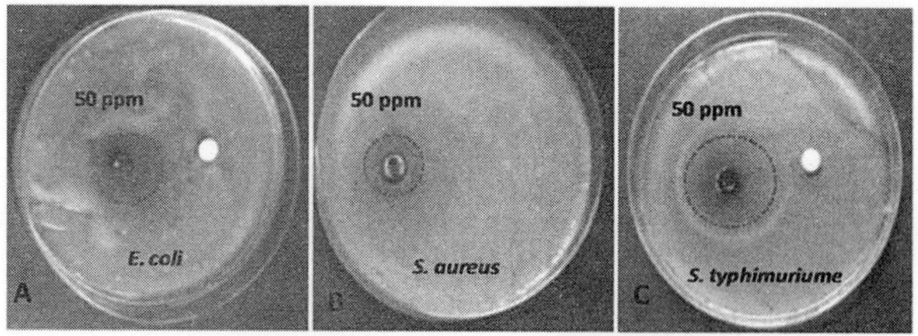

Figure 5 Zone of inhibition of synthesized copper NPs (50 ppm) against,
[A] E. coli [B] S. aureus and [C] S. typhimuriume

6. Conclusion

On the base of this study, copper oxide nanostructures were successfully synthesized by a sonochemical reduction method. Initially, presence of plasmon resonance of the highest concentration of PEG treated sample tells that the reaction was takes place oxygen resistant medium which formed copper nanostructures. It is observed that the size of nanosheets is increase with adding of PEG. The remarkable zone of inhibition has been observed against *E. coli,S. aureus* and *S. typhimurium*. Thesebacteria killing properties can be employed for the water decontamination, preservation of food and beverages.

7. Acknowledgement

The authors especially Dr. Abhishek K. Bhardwaj would like to thank VBS Purvanchal University for providing Purvanchal University Postdoctoral Fellowship (PUPDF) and facility from University of Allahabad, Prayagraj to carry out research.

8. Reference

1. Bhattacharya, D., and R. K. Gupta.: Nanotechnology and potential of microorganisms. Critical reviews in biotechnology 25:199-204 (2005)

2. De Jongh, P., D. Vanmaekelbergh, and J. Kelly.: Cu_2O: electrodeposition and characterization. Chemistry of materials 11:3512-3517 (1999).

3. Dhas, N. A., C. P. Raj, and A. Gedanken.: Synthesis, characterization, and properties of metallic copper nanoparticles. Chemistry of materials 10:1446-1452 (1998).

4. Dragieva, I., Z. Stoynov, and K. Klabunde.: Synthesis of nanoparticles by borohydride reduction and their applications. Scripta materialia 44:2187-2191 (2001).

5. Ho, J.-Y., and M. H. Huang.: Synthesis of submicrometer-sized Cu_2O crystals with morphological evolution from cubic to hexapod structures and their comparative photocatalytic activity. The Journal of Physical Chemistry C 113:14159-14164 (2009).

6. Huang, L., H. Wang, Z. Wang, A. Mitra, D. Zhao, and Y. Yan.: Cuprite nanowires by electrodeposition from lyotropic reverse hexagonal liquid crystalline phase. Chemistry of materials 14:876-880 (2002).

7. Iravani, S.: Green synthesis of metal nanoparticles using plants. Green Chemistry 13:2638-2650 (2011).

8. Joshi, S., S. Patil, V. Iyer, and S. Mahumuni.: Radiation induced synthesis and characterization of copper nanoparticles. Nanostructured materials 10:1135-1144 (1998).

9. Kuo, C.-H., C.-H. Chen, and M. H. Huang.: Seed-mediated synthesis of monodispersed Cu_2O nanocubes with five different size ranges from 40 to 420 nm. Advanced Functional Materials 17: (2007).

10. Kuo, C.-H., and M. H. Huang.: Facile synthesis of Cu_2O nanocrystals with systematic shape evolution from cubic to octahedral structures. The Journal of Physical Chemistry C 112:18355-18360 (2008).

11. Lisiecki, I., and M. P. Pileni.: Synthesis of copper metallic clusters using reverse micelles as microreactors. Journal of the American Chemical Society 115:3887-3896 (1993).

12. Liu, Z., and Y. Bando.: A novel method for preparing copper nanorods and nanowires. Advanced Materials 15:303-305 (2003).

13. McShane, C. M., and K.-S. Choi.: Photocurrent enhancement of n-type Cu_2O electrodes achieved by controlling dendritic branching growth. Journal of the American Chemical Society 131:2561-2569 (2009).

14. Ng, C. H. B., and W. Y. Fan.: Shape evolution of Cu_2O nanostructures via kinetic and thermodynamic controlled growth. The Journal of Physical Chemistry B 110:20801-20807 (2006).

15. Prabhu, S., and E. K. Poulose.: Silver nanoparticles: mechanism of antimicrobial action, synthesis, medical applications, and toxicity effects. International Nano Letters 2:32 (2012).

16. Salavati-Niasari, M., and F. Davar.: Synthesis of copper and copper (I) oxide nanoparticles by thermal decomposition of a new precursor. Materials Letters 63:441-443 (2009).

17. Songping, W., and M. Shuyuan.: Preparation of micron size copper powder with chemical reduction method. Materials Letters 60:2438-2442 (2006).

18. Sreeju, N., A. Rufus, and D. Philip.: Microwave-assisted rapid synthesis of copper nanoparticles with exceptional stability and their multifaceted applications. Journal of Molecular Liquids 221:1008-1021 (2016).

19. Swarnkar, R., and R. Gopal.: Controlled Synthesis of Cuprous Oxide Nanorings by Pulsed Laser Ablation of Copper Metal in Aqueous Media of Sodium Dodecyl Sulfate. Science of Advanced Materials 4:511-517 (2012).

20. Tang, B.-X., F. Wang, J.-H. Li, Y.-X. Xie, and M.-B. Zhang.: Reusable Cu2O/PPh3/TBAB system for the cross-couplings of aryl halides and heteroaryl halides with terminal alkynes. The Journal of organic chemistry 72:6294-6297 (2007).

21. Tang, S. L., R. L. Smith, and M. Poliakoff.: Principles of green chemistry: PRODUCTIVELY. Green Chemistry 7:761-762 (2005).

22. White, B., M. Yin, A. Hall, D. Le, S. Stolbov, T. Rahman, N. Turro, and S. O'Brien.: Complete CO oxidation over Cu_2O nanoparticles supported on silica gel. Nano letters 6:2095-2098 (2006).

23. Wu, S.-H., and D.-H. Chen.: Synthesis of high-concentration Cu nanoparticles in aqueous CTAB solutions. Journal of colloid and interface science 273:165-169 (2004).

24. Yang, Z., C.-K. Chiang, and H.-T. Chang.: Synthesis of fluorescent and photovoltaic Cu_2O nanocubes. Nanotechnology 19:025604 (2007).

25. Zhang, H., Q. Zhu, Y. Zhang, Y. Wang, L. Zhao, and B. Yu.: One☐Pot Synthesis and Hierarchical Assembly of Hollow Cu_2O Microspheres with Nanocrystals☐Composed Porous Multishell and Their Gas☐Sensing Properties. Advanced Functional Materials 17:2766-2771 (2007).

26. Ziegler, K. J., R. C. Doty, K. P. Johnston, and B. A. Korgel.: Synthesis of organic monolayer-stabilized copper nanocrystals in supercritical water. Journal of the American Chemical Society 123:7797-7803 (2001).

Comparison of Interaction Behaviour of Omeprazole and Rantidine with dil. HCl- An Ultrasonic Study

Monalisa Das[1,*], Smrutiprava Das[2]

[1]Govt. Women's College, Keonjhar, [2]Ravenshaw University, Cuttack
*E-mail: dr.monalisachem@gmail.com

ABSTRACT

Ultrasonic parameters have been used to predict different types of molecular association and their strengths involved in it. The density (ρ) and ultrasonic velocity (U) of omeprazole and rantidine in in dil. HCl are measured at room temperature over the entire range of composition. Using density and ultrasonic velocity the parameters such as adiabatic compressibility (β), inter molecular free length (L_f), acoustic impedance (Z), apparent molar compressibility (K_∞), and their excess parameters have also been calculated. These results have been explained on the basis of the intermolecular interactions present in the mixtures.

Keywords.** **Ultrasonic velocity, excess functions, omeprazole, rantidine, impedance

1.   Introduction

Gastric acid is secreted in the the stomach consists of HCl, KCl and NaCl. It plays a vital role in digestion of proteins by activating digestive enzymes that help in breaking down long chain of amino acids. It is produced in the lining of cells and other cells in the stomach produce bicarbonate that doesn't make the gastric acid too acidic. Such cells produce a viscous barrier to keep the stomach undamaged. Further a large amount of bicarbonate is produced by pancreas to neutralise the gastric acid completely for the functioning of digestive system. However protein denaturation occurs at highly acidic environment in the stomach. A typical adult human stomach will secrete about 1.5 liters of gastric acid daily[1]. The lowest pH of the gastric acid secreted is found to be 0.8[2] and it gets diluted in the stomach lumen to a pH varying from 1 and 3. In order to treat excess stomach acid H2 receptor blockers are used. Rantidine is one of the common antihistamine receptor blocker. Proton pump inhibitors (PPIs) also inhibit acid secretion available. These have pronounced effect on stomach acid production. these PPIs are given in inactive form. In acidic environment these inactive PPIs are protonated and converted to active form. These active forms of ppis are bonded covalently and irreversibly with gastric proton pump and deactivate it. Omeprazole is the common PPI. The use of PPI and H2 blocker is responsible for the lowering of pH that favours lowering of stomach acidity. However there is no proper evidence which clears the effectiveness of one drug over another[3,4] The objective of this study is to observe interaction of dil HCl with antihistamine receptor blocker and proton pump inhibitors and to determine their effectiveness on the basis of ultrasonic study. Ultrasonic study[5-7]and The excess thermo-acoustical parameters[8] helps to find out the nature and extent of strength of interaction. The study enables the determination of some useful acoustic or ultrasonic properties which are highly sensitive to molecular interactions in their solution mixtures. Ultrasonic parameters have been used to predict different types of molecular association and their strengths involved in it.

2.   Materials and method

Omeprazole and rantidine used in the study were purchased from local pharmaceutical company. HCl solution used anal r grade and water is double distilled. The sample solutions of omeprazole and rantidine were prepared at different molefractions of HCl. The sound velocity of different solutions was measured using ultrasonic interferometer (MITTAL enterprise, F-81) at frequency 2 MHz at 308.15K. The density was measured using densitometer. the different acoustical parameters and excess values were calculated using the following equations.

Various acoustical parameters such as adiabatic compressibility (β)[9,10] acoustic impedance (Z), inter molecular free length (L_f), apparent molar compressibility (K_ϕ) and corresponding excess values have been evaluated using the equations.

$$\beta = d^{-1} U^{-2} \quad Z = Ud \qquad L_f = K_j \beta^{1/2} \qquad\qquad (K_j \text{ is Jacobson constant} = 2.0965 \times 10^{-6})$$

$$K_\phi = 1000 \beta \ c^{-1} - \beta^0 \ d^{-1}\left(1000c^{-1} - M_2\right), \qquad \beta^0 \text{ is the adiabatic compressibility of the solvent.}$$

The excess properties Y^E are fitted to the polynomial equation of Redlich Kister [11]

$$Y^E = X_1 X_2 \Sigma A_i (X_1 - X_2)^i$$

3.   Result and Discussion

The structure of omeprazole and rantidine are given as

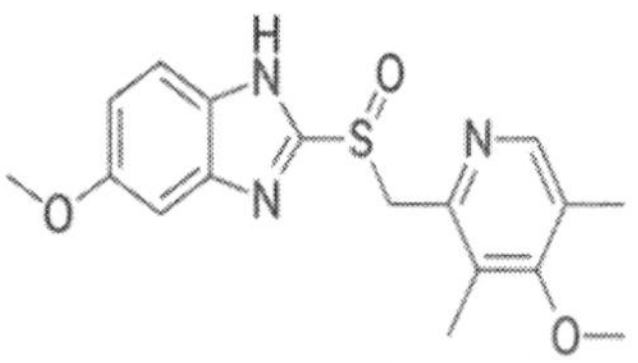

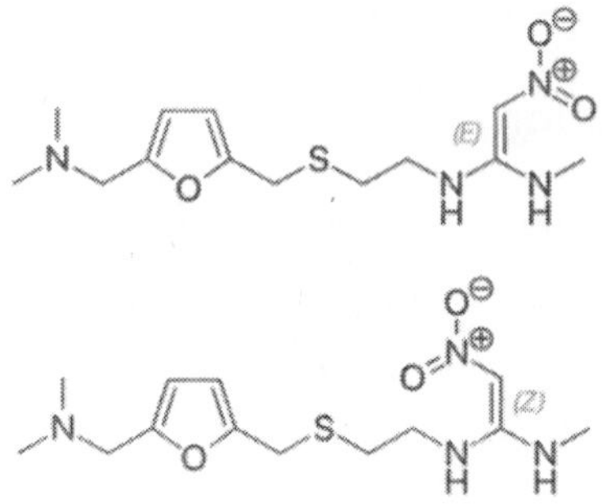

Fig. 1. Strucure of omeprazole   Fig. 2. Structure of rantidine

The calculated values of densies and the acoustic parameters of omeprazole and rantidine in HCl solution have been presented Table-1. In both the solutions the values of ρ and U increase with mole fraction of HCl. This increase is because of strong molecular interaction which leads to increase in cohesive forces that exist between the components **12**. In both cases β and Z values are positive but the increase is not regular in case of omeprazole while these values increase linearly for rantidine with molefraction of HCl. This suggests less packing between the components. The regular increase in L_f values in both systems indicates weak packing of omeprazole and rantidine with the medium at high molefraction of HCl. The variation of excess acoustical parameters are plotted against molefraction of HCl as shown in Figure, 3,4,5 6. The positive β^E values for omeprazole and rantidine indicate decreasing in dipole-dipole interaction. It also suggests the rupture of hydrogen bonds between the components. However OMZ system shows a minimum value at 0.03 molefraction of HCl. After attaining the minima these values increase which signify that the medium may be weakly packed. But the packing environment is lost at higher molefractions. It means omeprazole interactions less strongly with the medium. Positive excess velocity indicates the presence of dipole- induced dipole interaction in entire range of mole fraction of HCl which may be increase in interstitial accommodation of component molecules which results more excess velocity . It is also observed that Z^E decreases with increase in molefraction. These values are negative over the entire range of mole fraction of HCl indicating that interactions become weak with increase in mole fraction of HCl[13]. L_f^E values as calculated are positive which show weak dispersive force that indicates weak interaction components in the systems[14]. The values of K_ϕ^E increase with mole fraction. HigherK_ϕ^E values may reflect on the breakdown of associated cluster that creates less packing.

Table 1. Calculated values of density (ρ), ultrasonic velocity (U), adiabatic compressibility (β), intermolecular free length (L_f), acoustic impedance (Z), apparent molar compressibility (K_ϕ) of omeprazole and rantidine in different molefraction of HCl.

Mole Fraction (X_{org})	Density (ρ) x10³ (kgm⁻³)	Ultrasonic velocity (U) msec⁻¹	Adiabatic compressibility (β)x10⁻⁵ m²N⁻¹	Inter molecular free length (L_f) x10⁻³ m	Acoustic Impedance (Z)x10⁻³ kg m²s⁻¹	Apparent molar compressibility (K_ϕ)x10⁻¹⁰ m²N⁻¹
			Omeprazole in HCl			
0.1	1.0170	1564.6	2.4071	3.2503	1.5913	2.4071
0.2	1.0123	1576.5	2.4550	3.2826	1.5960	1.2275
0.3	1.0133	1568.0	2.4264	3.3283	1.5889	0.8088
0.4	1.0114	1579.3	2.4661	3.3263	1.5974	0.6165
0.4	1.0021	1582.0	2.4976	3.3290	1.5852	0.4995
0.5	1.0151	1592.7	2.4988	3.3312	1.6170	0.4165
0.6	1.0112	1602.7	2.5396	3.3387	1.6209	0.3628
0.7	1.0160	1631.6	2.6110	3.3391	1.6578	0.3275
0.8	1.0198	1643.1	2.6474	3.4087	1.6757	0.2942
0.9	1.0202	1678.2	2.7605	3.3481	1.7121	0.2751
			Rantidine in HCl			
0.1	1.0021	1531.2	2.3397	1.0134	1.5343	2.3397
0.2	1.0025	1565.5	2.4459	1.0135	1.5687	1.2226
0.3	1.0039	1571.2	2.4590	1.0388	1.5774	0.8197
0.4	1.0077	1578.6	2.4730	1.0418	1.5907	0.6183
0.4	1.0081	1581.4	2.4817	1.0438	1.5935	0.4963
0.5	1.0161	1588.2	2.4825	1.0467	1.6138	0.3567
0.6	1.0179	1592.5	2.4960	1.0460	1.6181	0.3114
0.7	1.0189	1592.5	2.4914	1.0524	1.6211	0.2804
0.8	1.0274	1603.5	2.5236	1.0661	1.6337	0.5900
0.9	1.0289	1625.9	2.5800	1.0678	1.6596	0.5331

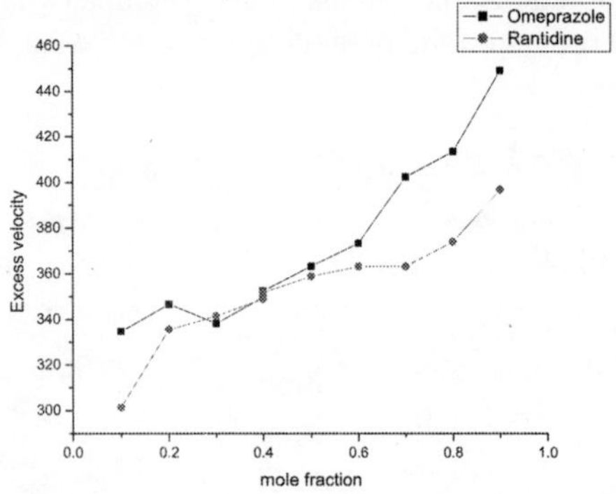

Fig 3 variation of excess velocity with molefraction of HCl compressibility

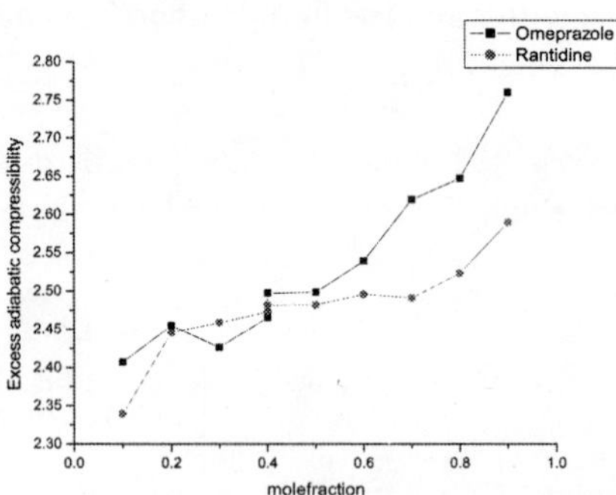

Fig 4. Variation of excess adiabatic with molefraction of HCl

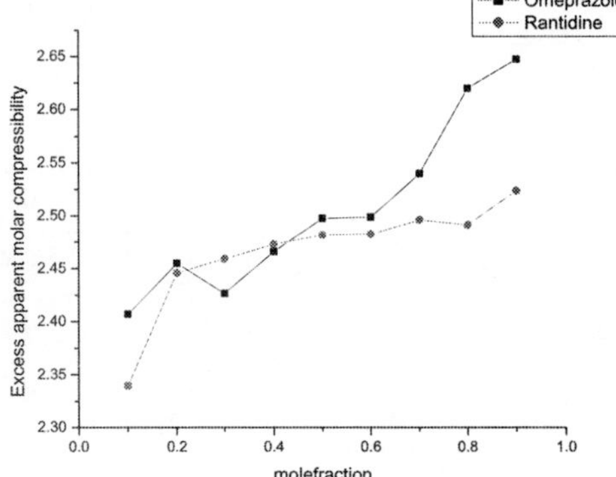

Fig. 5. Variation of excess apparent molar compressibilty with mole fraction of HCl

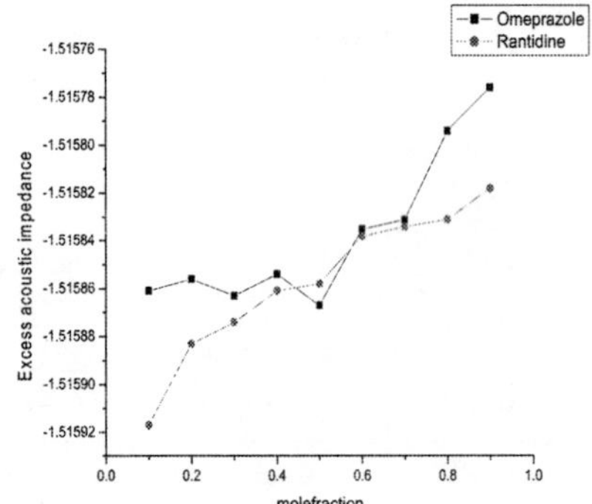

Fig 6. Variation of excess acoustic impedance with mole fraction of HCl

4.   Conclusion

The ultrasonic and excess parameters have been analysed on the basis of dipole-dipole interaction, hydrogen bonding etc. On analysing the above observations it is concluded that omeprazole interact with HCl at the low molefraction but the interaction get weakened at higher mole fractions as compared to rantidine. The use of omeprazole is more effective to decrease the percentage of HCl in the medium that lowers the pH of the system.

5.   References

1.   Dworken, Harvey J Human digestive system: gastric secretion. Encyclopædia Britannica Inc(2016). .

2.   Guyton, Arthur C.; John E. Hall Textbook of Medical Physiology (11 ed.). Philadelphia: Elsevier Saunders. p. 797. ISBN 0-7216-0240-1(2006). .

3.   Comparative effectiveness of proton pump inhibitors". 28 June 2016. Retrieved 14 July 2016.

4.   Laura (1 October 2010). Comparing Proton Pump Inhibitors. PubMed Health. National Center for Biotechnology Information (US). Retrieved (2016).

5.   Prakash, S.,. Thermodynamic and transport properties of binary liquid systems. Ind. J. Chem. 58, 942(1980)

6.   Kondaiah, M., Sreekanth, K., Sravana Kumar, D., Krishna Rao, D: Volumetric and viscometric properties of propanoic acid in equimolar mixtures of N, N-dimethyl formamide + alkanols at T/K = 303.15, 313.15, and 323.15. J. Sol. Chem. 42, 494(2013).

7.   Zorebski, E., Kostka, B.L., 2008. Thermodynamic and transport properties of (1,2-ethanediol + 1-nonanol) at temperatures (298.15 to 313.15) K. J. Chem. Thermodyn. 41, 197(2008).

8.   B. Chandrakant , A. Kumara, A. Singh, Orient. J. Chem., 30,843 (2014)

9.   U. N. Dash and S. Supakar, Acoustic letters, 16, 135, (1992).

10.   A. B. Wood, A Text Book of sound, (G. Bell, London) p. 51, 577.

11.   O.Redlich, A.T.Kister; Ind. Eng. Chem., 40, 345-348(1948).

12.   Kumar R, Mahesh R, Shanmugapriyan B, Kannappan V. Volumetric, viscometeric, acoustic and refractometric studies of molecular interactions in certain binary systems of o-chlorophenol at 303.15K. Ind J Pure Appl Phys 50: 633-640(2012).

13.   Krishna Rao, D., Sreekanth, K.: Study of molecular interactions in the mixtures of secondary alcohols with equimolar mixture of ethanol + formamide from acoustic and thermodynamic parameters. J. Chem. Pharm. Res. 3 (4), 29–41. Nain, A.K., 2008(2011) .

14.   Fort, R.J., Moore, W.R.:. Adiabatic compressibility of binary liquid mixtures. Trans. Faraday Soc. 61, 2102–2111(1965).

Efficacy and Safety of Nab-paclitaxel in Breast Cancer: A Meta-Analysis

Upendra Yadav, Pradeep Kumar, and Vandana Rai*

*Human Molecular Genetics Laboratory, Department of Biotechnology,
VBS Purvanchal University, Jaunpur (UP)– 222 003, India
raivandana@rediffmail.com

ABSTRACT

Worldwide breast cancer is the leading cause of cancer related death in women. Paclitaxel is an effective drug used for the treatment of breast cancer but it has many side effects. Nab-paclitaxel (nanoparticle albumin-bound paclitaxel) is an FDA approved drug for the treatment of breast cancer. Currently many clinical trials are conducted to deliver nab-paclitaxel into the tumor cells. But the efficacy and safety of this nab-paclitaxel over conventional paclitaxel still remains questionable. So, we performed a meta-analysis to evaluate the efficacy and safety of nab-paclitaxel in breast cancer treatment. Electronic databases were searched for the suitable studies using key terms "nab-paclitaxel", "paclitaxel", and "clinical trial" with the combination of "breast cancer" up to August 11, 2019. Risk ratio (RR) and odds ratio (OR) with corresponding 95% confidence intervals (CIs) were calculated. All statistical analyses were performed by the Open Meta-Analyst program. A total of eight studies which fulfilled our criteria were included in this study. For efficacy we retrieved data of 12 months progression free survival, 24 months progression free survival, and overall survival (up to 3 years) and for the safety we took data of nausea, anemia, leukopenia, neutropenia, fatigue, diarrhea and pain. We did not found any difference in efficacy of nab-paclitaxel over paclitaxel (12 months progression free survival- RR_{FE}= 0.86, 95%CI= 0.77-0.97, p= 0.02, I^2= 25.07%; 24 months progression free survival- RR_{FE}= 0.86, 95% CI= 0.64-1.16, p= 0.34, I^2= 0%; and 3 years survival- RR_{FE}= 1.20, 95%CI= 0.92-1.56, p= 0.16, I^2= 37.55%). The meta-analysis of studies used nab-paclitaxel showed reduced adverse effect of anemia (OR_{FE}= 1.66, 95% CI= 1.26-2.19; p= <0.001; I^2= 0%) and leukopenia (OR_{FE}= 1.37; 95%CI= 1.06-1.75; p= 0.01; I^2= 48.63%). However, in case of other adverse effects no significant association was found with nab-paclitaxel (nausea- OR_{FE}=1.15, 95%CI= 0.94-1.41, p= 0.15, I^2= 50.12%; neutropenia- OR_{RE}= 0.75, 95%CI= 0.30-1.87, p= 0.54, I^2= 94.45%; fatigue- OR_{RE}= 1.11, 95%CI= 0.77-1.62, p= 0.55, I^2= 56.02; diarrhea- OR_{FE}= 1.11, 95%CI= 0.77-1.62, p= 0.55; I^2= 34.26; pain- OR_{RE}= 1.15, 95%CI= 0.78-1.69, p= 0.45, I^2= 52.96%). In conclusion the use of nab-paclitaxel has reduces the side effects of anemia and leukopenia in breast cancer treatment in comparison to paclitaxel but nab-paclitaxel has no effect on the overall survival of the patients.

Keywords: Breast cancer; nanomedicine; paclitaxel, clinical trial; meta-analysis.

1.   Introduction

Worldwide breast cancer is the leading cause of cancer related death in women with 2,088,849 new cases and 626,679 deaths recorded in 2018 [1]. Paclitaxel is an effective antitumor taxane agent that is used against a number of cancers along with breast cancer [2]. The taxane binds to the β-subunit of the dimeric protein α,β-tubulin in microtubules in a 1:1 molar ratio, which decreases the dynamic nature of microtubules leads to mitotic arrest and finally results in programmed cell death [3]. The paclitaxel has poor aqueous solubility, hence its commercial formulation consists of the cremophor EL (CrEL) solvent system along with ethanol. Cremophor can aggravate serious toxicities like- nephrotoxicity, neurotoxicity, hypersensitivity and even irreversible sensory neuropathy [4, 5]. To overcome the risk of hypersensitivity reaction caused by cremophor, the CrEL requires a long infusion period along with premedication with steroids and antihistamines [6]. Even after precautions, sometime severe fatal hypersensitivity reactions still occur [7].

In 2005, Food and Drug Administration, USA approved nanoparticle albumin-bound paclitaxel (nab-paclitaxel) for breast cancer treatment. Nab-paclitaxel is cremophor-free drug. This has short infusion and has no CrEL related side effects and allergic reactions.

Various clinical trials were conducted to test effect of nab-paclitaxel in breast cancer. But the efficacy and safety of this nab-paclitaxel over conventional paclitaxel still remains questionable. So, we performed a meta-analysis to evaluate the efficacy and safety of nab-paclitaxel in breast cancer treatment.

2. Materials and Methods

Electronic databases (PubMed, Google Scholar, SpringerLink, ScienceDirect) were searched for the suitable studies using key terms "nab-paclitaxel", "paclitaxel", and "clinical trial" with the combination of "breast cancer" up to August 11, 2019.

3. Inclusion and Exclusion Criteria

Eligible studies had to meet the following criteria: (i) the study should be a clinical trial, and (ii) the articles must report the sample size, number of samples of paclitaxel and nab-paclitaxel. The following exclusion criteria were used: (i) case-control studies; (ii) studies that contained duplicate data; (iii) no usable data reported; (iv) studies conducted on the animal model system; and (v) book chapters or reviews articles etc.

4. Data Extraction

The following information were extracted from all the selected articles: (i) the name of the first author; (ii) year of publication; (iii) country of study; (iv) ethnicity; and (v) distribution of number of samples in paclitaxel and nab-paclitaxel groups. For efficacy we retrieved data of 12 months progression free survival, 24 months progression free survival, and overall survival (up to 3 years) and for the safety we took data of nausea, anemia, leukopenia, neutropenia, fatigue, diarrhea and pain.

5. Statistical Analysis

Meta-analysis was done according to the method given in Rai et al. [8]. Pooled odds ratio (OR) and risk ratio (RR) with its corresponding 95% confidence interval (CI) was calculated to investigate the association between safety and efficacy of nab-paclitaxel and breast cancer risk. Heterogeneity, publication bias and subgroup analysis were done as per the method given in Rai et al. [8]. All p values are two tailed with a significance level at 0.05 and all statistical analyses were undertaken using the freely available program Open Meta-Analyst [9].

6. Results

A total of eight studies [10-17] which fulfilled our criteria were included in this study. We did not found any difference in efficacy of nab-paclitaxel over paclitaxel (12 months progression free survival- RR_{FE}= 0.86, 95%CI= 0.77-0.97, p= 0.02, I^2= 25.07%; 24 months progression free survival- RR_{FE}= 0.86, 95% CI= 0.64-1.16, p= 0.34, I^2= 0%; and 3 years survival- RR_{FE}= 1.20, 95%CI= 0.92-1.56, p= 0.16, I^2= 37.55%) (Figure 1).

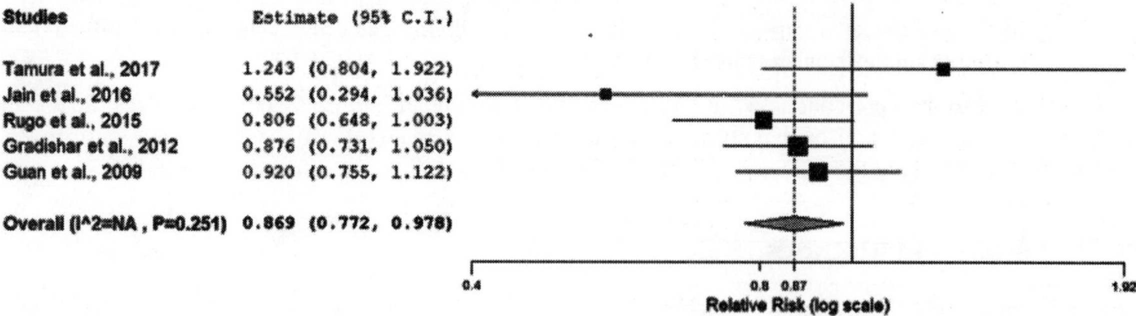

Figure 1 Fixed effect Forest plot of 12 months progression free survival

The meta-analysis of studies used nab-paclitaxel showed reduced adverse effect of anemia (OR_{FE}= 1.66, 95% CI= 1.26-2.19; p= <0.001; I^2= 0%) and leukopenia (OR_{FE}= 1.37; 95%CI= 1.06-1.75; p= 0.01; I^2= 48.63%) (Figure 2). However, in case of other adverse effects no significant association was found with nab-paclitaxel (nausea- OR_{FE}=1.15, 95%CI= 0.94-1.41, p = 0.15, I^2= 50.12%; neutropenia- OR_{RE}= 0.75, 95%CI= 0.30-1.87, p= 0.54, I^2= 94.45%; fatigue- OR_{RE}= 1.11, 95%CI = 0.77-1.62, p= 0.55, I^2= 56.02; diarrhea- OR_{FE} = 1.11, 95%CI= 0.77-1.62, p= 0.55; I^2= 34.26; pain- OR_{RE}= 1.15, 95%CI= 0.78-1.69, p= 0.45, I^2= 52.96%) (Table 1).

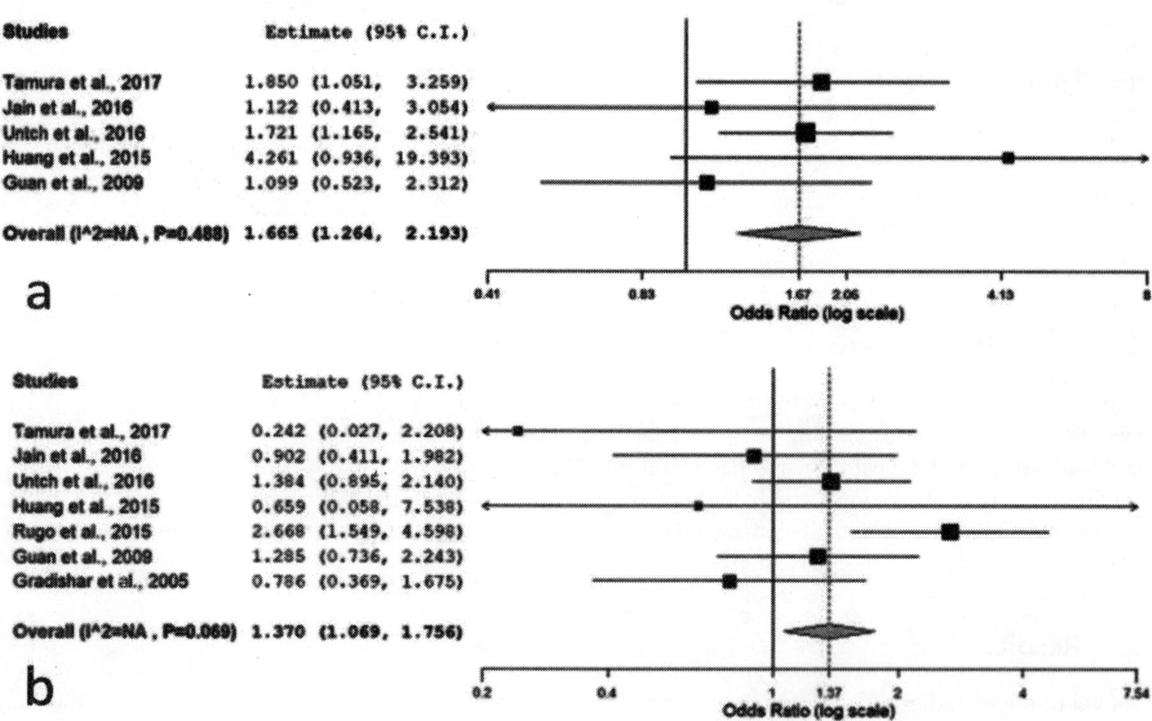

Figure 2. Fixed effect Forest plot of a. Anemia; b. Leukopenia

Table 1. Summary estimates for the odds ratio (OR) of various conditions, the significance level (p-value) of heterogeneity test (Q test) and the I^2 metric.

Condition	Fixed effect	Random effect	I^2 (%)	p (Q)
Nausea	1.15 (0.94-1.41), 0.15	1.29 (0.85-1.97), 0.22	50.12	0.07
Anemia	1.66 (1.26-2.19), <0.001	1.64 (1.24-2.16), <0.001	0	0.49
Leukopenia	1.37 (1.06-1.75), 0.013	1.25 (0.84-1.86), 0.26	48.63	0.06
Neutropenia	1.18 (0.99-1.40), 0.05	0.75 (0.30-1.87), 0.54	94.45	<0.001
Fatigue	1.25 (1.01-1.53), 0.03	1.11 (0.77-1.62), 0.55	56.02	0.05
Diarrhea	1.15 (0.95-1.39), 0.14	1.01 (0.74-1.39), 0.91	34.26	0.19
Pain	1.13 (0.92-1.38), 0.21	1.15 (0.78-1.69), 0.45	52.96	0.07
12 months progression free survival	0.86 (0.77-0.97), 0.02	0.87 (0.76-1.00), 0.05	25.07	0.25
24 months progression free survival	0.86 (0.64-1.16), 0.34	0.87 (0.65-1.16), 0.34	0	0.42
Overall survival (up to 3 years)	1.20 (0.92-1.56), 0.16	1.21 (0.80-1.84), 0.35	37.55	0.20

7.   Discussion

This meta-analysis was designed to compare the effect of nab-paclitaxel and paclitaxel in the treatment of breast cancer. The results showed that the nab-paclitaxel reduces the adverse effects of anemia and leukopenia but failed to demonstrate survival advantages of nab-paclitaxel over paclitaxel. During literature search we found that a meta-analysis was conducted in the year 2017 on the same problem but that study demonstrated that the nab-paclitaxel has no advantage over conventional paclitaxel [18].

Nab-paclitaxel can reach higher tumor accumulation than paclitaxel, due to a receptor-mediated transport process [19-21] and an enhanced permeability and retention (EPR) effect [22]. Also, it exhibits promising tolerability with less side effects than sb-paclitaxel because this formulation is free of cremophor. Therefore, nab-paclitaxel has great advantages in the treatment of cancer and has attracted great attention.

Meta-analysis is a powerful tool for analyzing cumulative data with small and low power studies. During past few years this technique becomes very popular among the geneticists and epidemiologists as it provide concrete evidence for the association of certain disease/disorder with a particular gene or the factor. Several meta-analyses were published which evaluated risk of genetic polymorphism for different diseases and disorders like- prostate cancer [23], schizophrenia [24], Alzheimer's disease [25], digestive tract cancer [26], breast cancer [27], Down syndrome [28], esophageal cancer [29], colorectal cancer [30], prevalence of glucose 6 phosphate dehydrogenase deficiency [31], cleft lip and palate [32] or in the *MTHFR* C677T polymorphism prevalence [33].

The main strengths of our meta-analysis were absence of publication bias, large number of subjects, more studies than the previous meta-analysis. At the same time the present meta-analysis also has some limitations which must be acknowledged like- a) crude odds ratio and risk ratio was used, b) only clinical trials were included, and c) only chemotherapy methods were evaluated other important factors like environmental were not considered.

In conclusion, this meta-analysis demonstrated that nab-paclitaxel has reduces the side effects of anemia and leukopenia in breast cancer treatment in comparison to paclitaxel but at the same time this nab-paclitaxel has no effect on the overall survival of the patients. Finally we recommend that the nab-paclitaxel is an appropriate clinical drug that may achieve greater anticancer efficacy with generally tolerable toxicities than traditional chemotherapy.

8. Acknowledgments

Upendra Yadav is highly grateful to VBS Purvanchal University, Jaunpur for providing financial assistance to him in the form of PDF.

9. References

1. Bray, F., Ferlay, J., Soerjomataram, I., et al.: Global Cancer Statistics 2018: GLOBOCAN Estimates of Incidence and Mortality Worldwide for 36 Cancers in 185 Countries. CA: Cancer J Clin 68, 394-424 (2018).

2. Mollinedo, F., Gajate, C.: Microtubules, microtubule-interfering agents and apoptosis. Apoptosis 8(5), 413-450 (2003).

3. Jordan, M.A.: Mechanism of Action of Antitumor Drugs that Interact with Microtubules and Tubulin. Curr Med Chem Anticancer Agents 2(1), 1-17 (2002).

4. Weiss, R.B., Donehower, R.C., Wiernik, P.H., et al.: Hypersensitivity reactions from taxol. J Clin Oncol 8, 1263-1268 (1990).

5. Ten Tije, A.J., Verweij, J., Loos, W.J. et al.: Pharmacological effects of formulation vehicles: implications for cancer chemotherapy. Clin Pharmacokinet 42, 665-685 (2003).

6. Socinski, M.A.: Single-agent paclitaxel in the treatment of advanced non-small cell lung cancer. Oncologist 4, 408-416 (1999).

7. Tan H, Hu J, Liu S. Efficacy and safety of nanoparticle albumin-bound paclitaxel in non-small cell lung cancer: a systematic review and meta-analysis. Artif Cells Nanomed Biotechnol 47(1), 268-277 (2019).

8. Rai, V., Yadav, U., Kumar, P., et al.: Maternal methylenetetrahydrofolate reductase C677T polymorphism and Down syndrome risk: a meta-analysis from 34 studies. Plos One 9(9), e108552 (2014).

9. Wallace, B.C., Dahabreh, I.J., Trikalinos, T.A., et al.: Closing the gap between methodologists and endusers: R as a computational back-end. J Stat Software 49, 1-15 (2013).

10. Gradishar, W.J., Tjulandin, S., Davidson, N., et al.: Phase III trial of nanoparticle albumin-bound paclitaxel compared with polyethylated castor oil-based paclitaxel in women with breast cancer. J Clin Oncol 23(31), 7794-7803 (2005).

11. Guan, Z.Z., Li, Q.L., Feng, F., et al.: Superior efficacy of a Cremophor-free albumin-bound paclitaxel compared with solvent-based paclitaxel in Chinese patients with metastatic breast cancer. Asia Pac J Clin Oncol 5(3), 165-174 (2009).

12. Gradishar, W.J., Krasnojon, D., Cheporov, S., et al.: Phase II trial of nab-paclitaxel compared with docetaxel as first-line chemotherapy in patients with metastatic breast cancer: final analysis of overall survival. Clin Breast Cancer 12(5), 313-321 (2012).

13. Huang, L., Chen, S., Yao, L., et al.: Phase II trial of weekly nab-paclitaxel and carboplatin treatment with or without trastuzumab as nonanthracycline neoadjuvant chemotherapy for locally advanced breast cancer. Int J Nanomedicine 10, 1969-1975 (2015).

14. Rugo, H.S., Barry, W.T., Moreno-Aspitia, A., et al. Randomized Phase III Trial of Paclitaxel Once Per Week Compared With Nanoparticle Albumin-Bound Nab-Paclitaxel Once Per Week or Ixabepilone With Bevacizumab As First-Line Chemotherapy for Locally Recurrent or Metastatic Breast Cancer: CALGB 40502/NCCTG N063H (Alliance). J Clin Oncol 33(21), 2361-2369 (2015).

15. Jain, M.M., Gupte, S.U., Patil, S.G., et al. Paclitaxel injection concentrate for nanodispersion versus nab-paclitaxel in women with metastatic breast cancer: a multicenter, randomized, comparative phase II/III study. Breast Cancer Res Treat 156(1), 125-134 (2016).

16. Untch, M., Jackisch, C., Schneeweiss, A., et al. Nab-paclitaxel versus solvent-based paclitaxel in neoadjuvant chemotherapy for early breast cancer (GeparSepto-GBG 69): a randomised, phase 3 trial. Lancet Oncol 17(3), 345-356 (2016).

17. Tamura, K., Inoue, K., Masuda, N., et al. Randomized phase II study of nab-paclitaxel as first-line chemotherapy in patients with HER2-negative metastatic breast cancer. Cancer Sci 108(5), 987-994 (2017).

18. Liu, Y., Ye, G., Yan, D., et al.: Role of nab-paclitaxel in metastatic breast cancer: a meta-analysis of randomized clinical trials. Oncotarget 8(42), 72950-72958 (2017).

19. Schnitzer, J.E., Oh, P.: Albondin-mediated capillary permeability to albumin. Differential role of receptors in endothelial transcytosis and endocytosis of native and modified albumins. J Biol Chem 269, 6072-6082 (1994).

20. Desai, N., Trieu, V., Yao, Z., et al.: Increased antitumor activity, intratumor paclitaxel concentrations, and endothelial cell transport of cremophor-free, albumin-bound paclitaxel, ABI-007, compared with cremophor-based paclitaxel. Clin Cancer Res 12, 1317-1324 (2006).

21. Li, H.H., Li, J., Wasserloos, K.J., et al.: Caveolae-dependent and -independent uptake of albumin in cultured rodent pulmonary endothelial cells. PloS One 8, e81903 (2013).

22. Matsumura, Y., Maeda, H.: A new concept for macromolecular therapeutics in cancer chemotherapy: mechanism of tumoritropic accumulation of proteins and the antitumor agent smancs. Cancer Res 46, 6387-6392 (1986).

23. Yadav, U., Kumar, P., Rai, V.: Role of MTHFR A1298C gene polymorphism in the etiology of Prostate cancer: A systematic review and updated meta-analysis. Egypt J Med Hum Genet 17, 141-148 (2016).

24. Rai, V., Yadav, U., Kumar, P., et al.: Methylenetetrahydrofolate Reductase A1298C Genetic Variant and Risk of Schizophrenia: an updated meta-analysis. Indian J Med Res 145, 437-447 (2016).

25. Rai, V.: Methylenetetrahydrofolate Reductase (MTHFR) C677T Polymorphism and Alzheimer Disease Risk: a Meta-Analysis. Mol Neurobio 54, 1173-1186 (2017).

26. Yadav, U., Kumar, P., Rai, V.: NQO1 gene C609T polymorphism (dbSNP: rs1800566) and digestive tract cancer risk: A meta-analysis. Nutr Cancer 70(4), 557-568 (2018).

27. Rai, V., Yadav, U., Kumar, P.: Impact of Catechol-O-Methyltransferase Val 158Met (rs4680) Polymorphism on Breast Cancer Susceptibility in Asian Population. Asian Pac J Cancer Prev 18(5), 1243-1250 (2017).

28. Rai, V., Yadav, U., Kumar, P.: Null association of maternal MTHFR A1298C polymorphism with Down syndrome pregnancy: An updated meta-analysis. Egypt J Med Hum Genet 18(1), 9-18 (2017).

29. Kumar, P., Rai, V.: Methylenetetrahydrofolate reductase C677T polymorphism and risk of esophageal cancer: An updated meta-analysis. Egypt J Med Hum Genet 19(4), 273-284 (2018).

30. Rai, V.: Evaluation of the MTHFR C677T Polymorphism as a Risk Factor for Colorectal Cancer in Asian Populations. Asian Pac J Cancer Prev 16(18), 8093-8100 (2015).

31. Kumar, P., Yadav, U., Rai, V.: Prevalence of Glucose-6-phosphate dehydrogenase deficiency in India: an updated meta-analysis. Egypt J Med Hum Genet 17, 295-302 (2016).

32. Rai, V.: Strong association of C677T polymorphism of methylenetetrahydrofolate reductase gene with nosyndromic cleft lip/palate (nsCL/P). Ind J Clin Biochem 33(1), 5-15 (2018).

33. Yadav, U., Kumar, P., Gupta, S., et al.: Distribution of MTHFR C677T gene polymorphism in healthy North Indian population and an updated meta-analysis. Indian J Clin Biochem 32(4), 399-410 (2016).

Temperature Dependent Nature of Silica Nanoparticles Obtain from Rice Husk

Anil Kumar Singh[1,*] and Annu Kumari[2]

[1]Nano-science Centre, University Department of Physics, V.K.S. University, Ara, Bihar, India.802301
[2]Department of Physics, Veer Kunwar Singh University, Ara, Bihar, India.
*E-mail:anilkrvksu.ara@gmail.com

ABSTRACT

In present study, we first of all, prepared solid nanoparticles of silica from rice husk using acid leaching of rice husk ash (RHA). Silica is the major constituent of Rice Husk Ash (RHA). In rice husk ash the formation of crystalline and amorphous nature of silica nanoparticles depended upon temperature. At lower temperature at 500°C the amorphous nature was observed. When amorphous silica nanoparticles were heated at 700°C (i.e. annealing muffle furnace temperature 700°C for one hours and three hours respectively) the structure of the silica was observed to be shifted towards crystallinity and it appeared to have the Triclinic structure. By heating at higher temperatures, the unburned carbon had been removed from the ashes and this led to the crystallization of the ash from amorphous silica into crystalline form (cristobalite or tridymite).

It was further, observed that at temperature around 700°C crystalline structure was obtained and it contained certain amount of tridymite and cristobalite. The purity of silica obtained was 91% as confirmed from XRD experiments. The purpose of these studies is to develop contrast agent based on solid nanoparticle for ultrasound imaging system.

Keywords: Solid nanoparticles, Crystalline silica nanoparticles, amorphous silica nanoparticles, Rice Husk Ash.

1. Introduction

Rice husk upon burning yields 14–20% ash, which contains 80–95% silica in the crystalline form together with trace amounts of metallic impurities[1]. Silica is the major constituent of Rice Husk Ash (RHA) [1,9]. It exists in many different forms that can be crystalline as well as amorphous. Generally, amorphous silica is formed at lower temperature, but at higher temperature, crystalline silica is obtained [2]. Silica has many applications, such as sources for synthetic adsorption materials[3,5], carriers, medical additives, fillers in composite materials[6,7] etc.

Several investigators have observed that the crystalline and amorphous nature of silica depends on temperature and time of combustion[8,9]. At lower temperature, the amorphous nature of rice husk ash silica was reported[8]. Further, Della, et al., reported that the relative amount of silica was increased after burning out the carbonaceous material at different times and temperatures [9]. By heating at higher temperatures, the unburned carbon can be removed from the ashes [10] but this leads to the crystallization of the ash from amorphous silica into cristobalite or tridymite[11].

2. Materials and Methods

Rice husk (RH) collected from rice mill was washed with purified water and dried up in sunlight then the sample was grinded in a mixer and dried up in open air. Thereafter it was burnt at nearly 100 °C for one hour and cooled to prepare rice husk ash (RHA). Then the sample was subjected to acid leaching process for nearly one hour by 1.0 N Hcl in order to remove impurities and metal oxides, especially K, Ca and Phosphate oxides. After this, the acidic water was removed and water rinsing treatment was carried out until the pH 7 was obtained. It was then dried up using oven. Further, 6.25N NaOH was mixed in it. The solution was heated on hot plate for 2 hours. Its pH was brought down to 7 by washing it with deionized water. The sample, thus obtained was also dried up in hot air oven for 1 hour at 100°C. Now 0.71N H_2SO_4 and ammonia was added drop by drop in it until pH value becomes 8. Once again the sample was placed on hot plate for 90 minutes, after this the solution was filtered and washed with deionized water. The yield of this reaction was silica. The filtrate was oven dried (hot air oven at 100°C) for 5 hours and the sample was left at room temperature for 72 hours.

Thus sample obtain was silica, it was devided into three groups for annealing at different temperatures. The sample one was placed for annealing it for one hour at 500°C another two samples for one hour and three hours respectively at 700°C in a muffle furnace. Finally, silica was obtained (white colour) and the sample was characterized using XRD (D8 Advance Bruker, Germany).

3. Results and Discussion

The X-ray diffraction (XRD) pattern was recorded for different samples. Diffraction peaks at different values of 2θ are indicated in Fig. 1, Fig. 2 and Fig 3.

Fig.1 presents the XRD spectrum of Nano-silica. From the figure we observed that there are diffraction peaks at different values of 2θ corresponding to the different planes (011), (111), (012), (020), (013), (022), (113), (122), (023), (123), (131), (032), (024) and (230). Thus, XRD pattern in Fig.1 shows crystalline form of nano-silica,

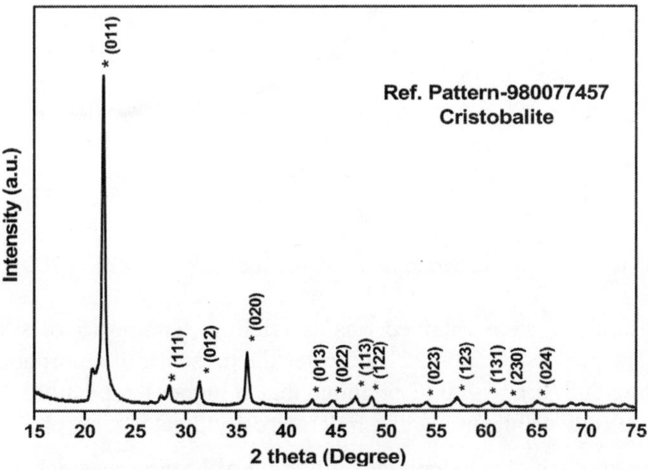

Figure 1   XRD Spectrum of Nano silica (annealing muffle furnace at 700 °C for 3 h).

With the help of Scherrer equation we calculated size of the nano-silica. It turn out to become 20 nm (19.9). Here the crystal structure of the nano-silica obtained as tetragonal The purity of nano-silica obtained was 93% as confirmed from XRD.

Fig 2 indicates X-ray diffraction pattern of the silica sample heated at 500 °C for one hour. In this patter we obtained peak point was at 2θ ≈ 21-22°, this in turn indicates the presence of amorphous silica nanoparticles produced from RHA. Size of the particle in this case was estimated to be 20nm. The purity of silica obtained was found to be 67% as confirmed from XRD. This may indicate that the crystalline nature is affected by impurities.

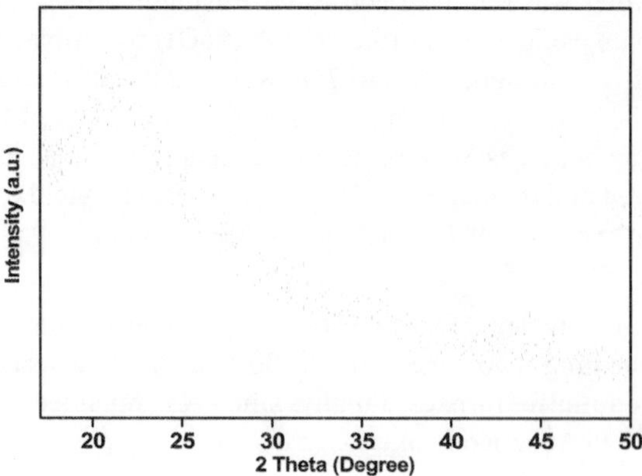

Figure 2 X- ray diffraction pattern of silica (annealing muffle furnace at 500 ⁰C for 1 hour).

In third case, once again we kept temperature same (i.e.700 °C) but duration of heat treatment was reduced (i.e. annealing muffle furnace temperature at 700 °C for 1 hours). Fig. 3.0 indicates X-ray diffraction pattern of silica.

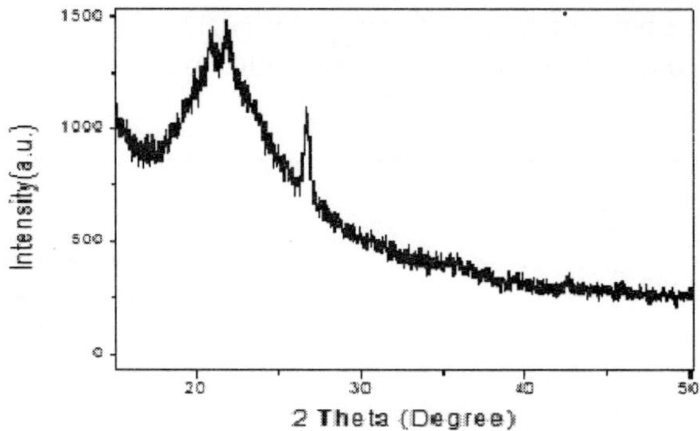

Figure 3 X- ray diffraction pattern of silica (annealing muffle furnace at 700 °C for 1 hour).

In this case the structure of the silica obtained was as Triclinic. The purity of silica obtained was 91% as confirmed from XRD. The peak point $2\theta \approx 22^0$, indicates the presence of amorphous silica. Comparing both XRD peaks at temperature 500 °C and 700 °C be found that at higher temperature the structure of nano silica is shifting towards crystallinity. While at lower temperature it indicated amorphous nature only.

Comparing with the first case we concluded that if duration of heating was enhanced from 1.0 hr to 3.0 hr, amorphous nature was converted into crystalline nature of silica. As already indicated in Fig.1, in which we obtained sharp diffraction peaks at different values of 2θ corresponding to different planes. This is, because, a crystalline material always exhibit sharp diffraction peaks corresponding to diffraction from different planes, while amorphous does not. For amorphous nano-silica the peak point $2\theta \approx 21\text{-}22^0$ as indicated in Fig 2.0. In Fig. 3.0 also no sharp peak could have been observed. At the best we can say that they are shifting towards crystalline nature. In XRD broadening of peak represents amorphous state but sometimes nanoparticles can be caused for the same.

By heating at higher temperatures, the unburned carbon has been removed from the ashes, but this leads to the crystallization of the ash from amorphous silica into cristobalite or tridymite.

4.   References

1.   Chandrasekhar S., Pramada P. and Praveen L.: Effect of organic acid treatment on the properties of rice husk silica, Journal of Materials Science, 40(24), 6535-6544, (2005) .

2.   Omatola KM. and Onojah AD.: Elemental analysis of rice husk ash using X-Ray fluorescence technique, International Journal of Physic Science, 4, 189-93, (2009).

3.   Jang H.T. Park Y., Ko Y.S., Lee J.Y. Margandan B. : Highly siliceous MCM-48 from rice husk ash for CO2 adsorption, Int J Greenhouse Gas Control, 3, 545–549, (2009).

4.   Wongjunda J., Saueprasearsit P.: Biosorption of chromium (VI) in rice husk ask and modified rice husk ash, Environ Res J, 4(3), 244–250 , (2010).

5.   Lakshmi U.R., Vimal Chandra S., Indra Deo M., Lataye D.H.: Rice husk ash as an effective adsorbent: evaluation of adsorptive characteristics for Indigo Carmine dye, J Environ Manage, 90, 710–720 , (2009).

6.   Liu Y. L., Hsu C.Y., Hsu K.Y. : Poly (methylmethacrylate)-silica nanocomposites films from surface-functionalized silica nanoparticles, Polymer, 46, 1851–1856, (2005).

7.   Shin Y., Lee D,, Lee K., Ahn K. H., Kim B. : Surface properties of silica nanoparticles modified with polymers for polymer nanocomposite applications, J Ind Eng Chem, 14, 515–519, (2008).

8.   Adil Elhag Ahmed and Farook Adam: Indium incorporated silica from rice husk and its catalytic activity, Microporous and Mesoporous Materials, 103 (1-3), 284-295, (2007).

9.   Della V. P., Kuhn I. and Hotza D. : Rice husk ash as an alternate source for active silica production, Materials Letters, 57(4), 818- 821 (2002).

10.   Krishnarao R. V., Subrahmanyam J. and Jagadish Kumar T. : Studies on the formation of black particles in rice husk silica ash, Journal of the Europian Ceramic Society, 21(1), 99-104 , (2001).

11.   Real C., Alcala M., Criado J. M. : Preparation of silica from rice Husks, Journal of the American Ceramic Society, 79(8), 2012–2016, (1996).

Nondestructive Inspection (NDI) of Adhesive Joints using Ultrasonic Technology

Sonal Patil, Lingeshvaran Ravi, Raghavendra Haresamudram and Indrajit Malvade

John Deere India Pvt. Ltd., Regional Office, Sangamvadi, Pune-411001, India

ABSTRACT

With the advancement in Manufacturing technologies like adhesive and additive, similar development in quality area is needed. This will help to qualify the parts manufactured using these technologies and provide appropriate feedback to manufacturing process. Current methods in the industry are primarily destructive in nature as the adhesive within the part is invisible. We have explored technologies like Computed Tomography and use of Ultrasonics. In this paper, we are going to discuss about the techniques to inspect adhesively bonded parts, advantages and disadvantages to use these techniques. With the production systems moving with these new technologies, it is imperative to develop a quick and easy feedback mechanism that can be integrated into production lines.

Keywords: Ultrasonic, adhesive, inspection.

1. Introduction

1.1 Adhesive Bonding

Adhesive bonding is used to fasten two surfaces together, usually producing a smooth bond. This joining technique involves glues, epoxies, or various plastic agents that bond by evaporation of a solvent or by curing a bonding agent with heat, pressure, or time.

Whether bonding metal to metal, plastic, glass, rubber, ceramic, or to another substrate material, adhesives distribute stress load evenly over a broad area, reducing stress on the joint. As they are applied inside the joint, adhesives are invisible within the assembly. They resist flex and vibration stresses, and form a seal as well as a bond, which can protect the joint from corrosion, adhesives easily join irregularly shaped surfaces, decrease the weight of an assembly, create virtually no change in part dimensions or geometry, and quickly and easily bond dissimilar substrates and heat sensitive materials.

Adhesives are one-size-fits-all, and assembly can be easily automated. Limitations include the amount of time required for adhesives to fixture and develop full strength, surface preparation requirements, with joint disassembly and the problems associated adhesive layer thickness.

Based on various studies within the industry, it is known fact that the adhesive joint strength depends on adhesive layer thickness. The strength of adhesive joint gets reduced with higher adhesive layer thickness. During assembly of adhesively bonded parts, the adhesive layer thickness may change locally due to part tolerances, fixturing etc. Therefore, it is necessary to measure adhesive layer thickness at a specific location in the assembly.

To accomplish the above objectives, the various attributes that determine the bond strength must be identified. A nondestructive inspection (NDI) method must be developed that can be used in manufacturing environment to gain confidence in use of adhesive joining. Business Impact – The wider use of adhesive joining will result in reduced vehicle weight, increased body stiffness, and improved crashworthiness. Adhesives are also a critical enabler for the joining of dissimilar materials

2.   NDI Methods and Techniques

Over the last 20 years, a large amount of NDI research and development (R&D) has been conducted to determine how to detect and predict the quality of bond in adhesively bonded structure. These methods include primarily,

- Ultrasonic
- Radiography
- Thermography
- Industrial computed tomography

2.1   Industrial computed tomography (CT)

CT scanning is any computer-aided tomographic process, usually X-ray computed tomography, that uses irradiation to produce three-dimensional internal and external representations of a scanned object. Industrial CT scanning has been used in many areas of industry for internal inspection of components. Some of the key uses for industrial CT scanning have been flaw detection, failure analysis, metrology, assembly analysis and reverse engineering applications. Just as in medical imaging, industrial imaging includes both non tomographic radiography (industrial radiography) and computed tomographic radiography (computed tomography). CT uses two types of scanning

2.1.1 Internal Flaw detection using CT

Traditionally, without destructive testing, full metrology has only been performed on the exterior dimensions of components, such as with a coordinate-measuring machine or with a vision system to map exterior surfaces.

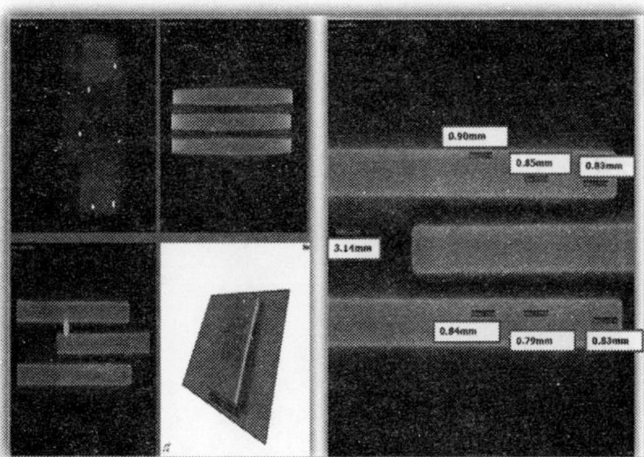

Internal inspection methods would require using a 2D X-ray of the component or the use of destructive testing. Industrial CT scanning allows for full non-destructive metrology.

Image-based finite element method converts the 3D image data from X-ray computed tomography directly into meshes for finite element analysis. Benefits of this method include modelling complex geometries (e.g. composite materials) or accurately modelling "as manufactured" components at the micro-scale.

2.1.2 Experimental Procedure using Computed Tomography

1. Two samples of adhesively bonded joints were used to scan and interpret information (Refer image)
2. Sample with Aluminum as base metal provided better results as compared to Steel

3. Three-dimensional data was available to analyze further on the thickness of adhesive layer and the location of flaws in the joints

4. Though this process provides accurate and reliable results, it has limitation of part size, base material properties and ability to use in the production setup.

2.2　Ultrasonic techniques

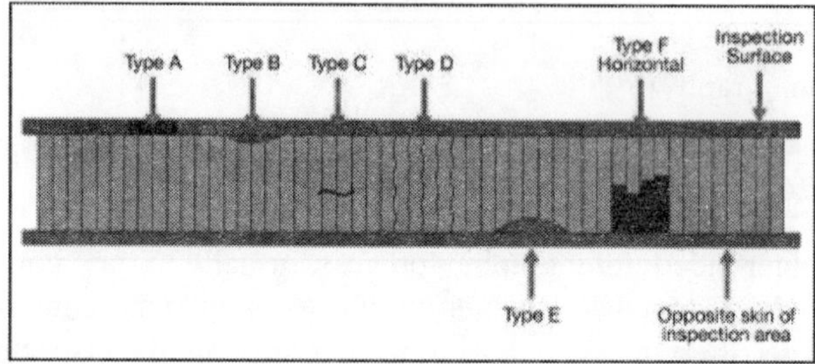

The Ultrasonic Test technique involves an ultrasonic transducer and transmitter. The ultrasonic pulse which is generated is expressed in terms of burst length or cycles, most typically ranging from 2 to 10 MHz. The ultrasound wave propagates through the bond joint and reaches defects and other non-homogeneous characteristics. The transmitted wave undergoes attenuation and sometimes extinction. The ultrasound receiver will detect transmission and reflection of the wave. The intensity of the wave received correlates with defect size and specific adhesion properties. The time of flight (travel time) correlates with the depth of a defect. The surface of the bonded component is scanned with a test head to assess the position of the defects. A coupling agent, such as water, honey, or oil (viscous medium) is employed.

2.2.1 Experimental Procedure using Ultrasonic Thickness measuring instrument

1. 4 samples (known missing areas) of adhesively bonded plates were developed

2. The adhesive bonded area was divided in 8 mm x 8 mm grid

3. The height of back wall reflection was set to 80 % to full screen height in non-bonded area from both sides (A & B). The height of back wall reflection was measured in each grid

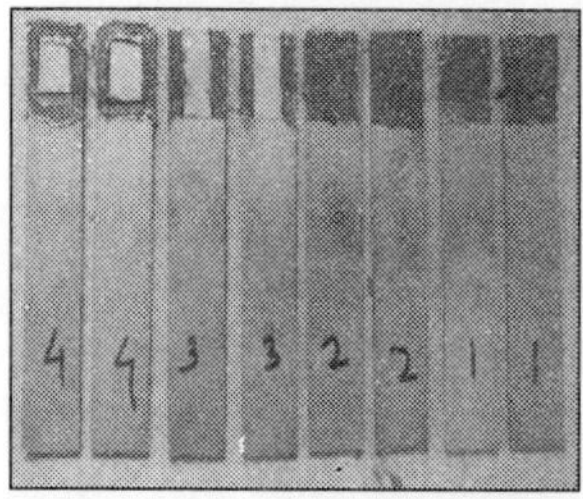
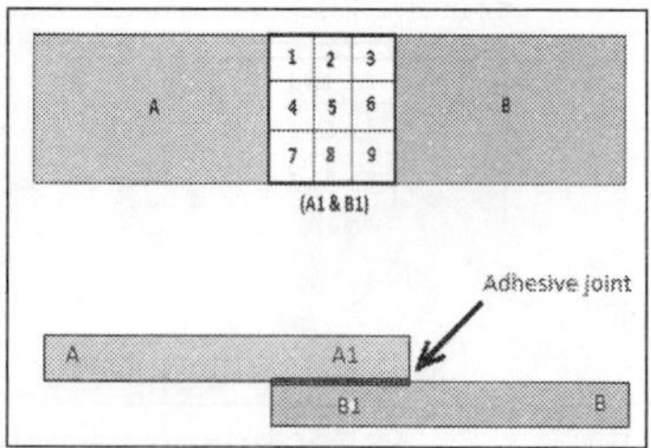

4. The area with no bond showed back wall reflection height equal to or more than 80% of full screen height. The area with good bonds showed the reduction in back wall.

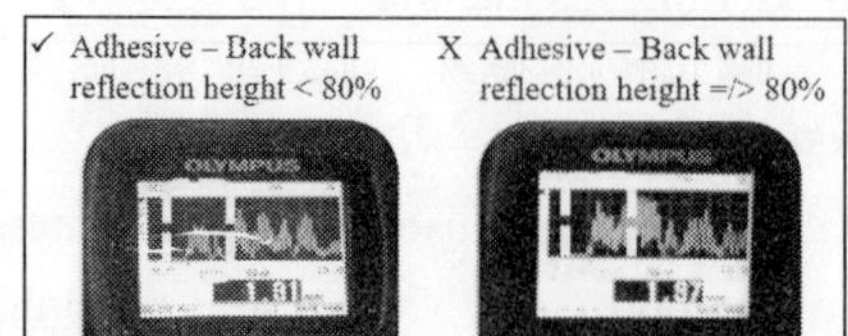

Height of Back wall Reflection on adhesive joint (A1)			
Sr. No.	Plate 1 in %	Plate 2 in %	Plate 3 in %	Plate 4 in %
1	73	71	73	76
2	74	74	71	71
3	76	72	68	72
4	70	71	**80**	78
5	72	75	**80**	**87**
6	72	72	**84**	78
7	70	72	72	74
8	75	78	76	73
9	76	75	71	76

Height of Back wall Reflection on adhesive joint (B1)			
Sr. No.	Plate 1 in %	Plate 2 in %	Plate 3 in %	Plate 4 in %
1	72	73	75	66
2	70	72	78	68
3	71	70	73	70
4	72	74	**81**	73
5	73	74	**84**	**85**
6	74	69	**80**	75
7	70	68	74	68
8	72	70	76	76
9	72	72	75	74

3. References

1. http://www.adhesives.org/adhesives-sealants/fastening-bonding/fastening-overview/adhesive-bonding
2. https://en.wikipedia.org/wiki/Industrial_computed_tomography
3. http://www.dtic.mil/dtic/tr/fulltext/u2/a210051.pdf

Bearing Fault Detection by Support Vector Classifier

Sandip Kumar Singh

Department of Mechanical Engineering, V B S Purvanchal University, Jaunpur-222001
sandipkumarsingh25@gmail.com

ABSTRACT

The bearing is an essential part of all rotating machinery. The early detection of faults in bearing by using vibration signals saves a significant amount of financial loss. Many approaches have been used to overcome this problem in past, but they succeeded to only some extent to identify the faults occurring on outer race, inner race, and rollers/balls. None of them is capable of diagnosing these faults accurately. Machine Learning-based Data-driven methods have shown better results as compared to signal processing-based techniques. In this paper we are presenting a Support Vector Classifier (SVC) which is capable of detecting faults with an accuracy of 99.47%. The results are shown in terms of Area Under Curve (AUC) of the precision-recall curve. A comparison with Multinomial Logistic Regression (MLR) is also shown.

Keywords: Support Vector Classifier (SVC), Multinomial Logistic Regression (MLR), Area Under Curve (AUC)

1. Introduction

Bearing fault detection, using vibration data has gained the focus of mechanical engineers. Samanta and Al-Balushi [1] and Samanta *et al.* [1] analyzed the third and fourth central moments, i.e., skewness and kurtosis. The authors employed ANN and SVM for the diagnosis of bearing faults and summarized that both the even and odd moments are equally capable of representing bearing health effectively. Abbasion *et al.* [2] classified the single level fault severities in rolling element bearings. The authors' employed wavelet transform (WT) for the denoising of vibration signals. The classification has been performed using SVM and faults in various components have been classified. Liu *et al.* [5] and Bordoloi and Tiwari [3] employed SVM for the fault classification in rolling contact elements. Various statistical features viz. kurtosis, standard deviation, range, mean value are also utilized for the diagnosis of rolling element bearings by Kankar *et al.* [7]; Gangsar *et al.* [4] and Yaqub *et al.* [6]. These investigations utilized SVM and ANN (Artificial Neural Networks) and proposed that the selected features are sensitive to provide considerable fault identification accuracy. Here, we propose a new method based on augmented data processing before the SVC. The sequential augmentation of data improves the performance of SVC significantly.

2. The Proposed Method

Classifying data is a prime task of machine learning. Support vector machines (SVM) are used as binary classifiers. They are used both as supervised learning methods and unsupervised learning methods. When the data is labelled, classification by SVM is called SVC that is support vector classifier. In case of unsupervised learning where data is unlabelled, it is clustered in two distinct groups with the help of SVM.

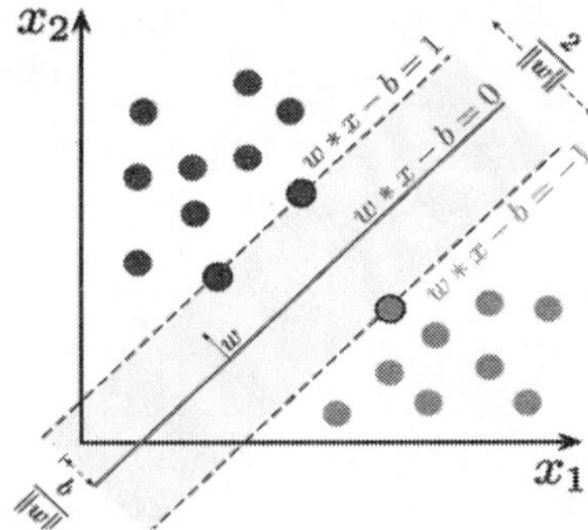

Figure-1 The SVC Classification

A hyperplane separates two different kinds of data in linear SVC. The distance of the nearest data is maximized in from hyperplane. Such SVC is also called maximum margin classifier. In linear SVC a p-dimensional data set is separated from (p-1)-dimensional hyperplane. If the training data set is separable linearly, two parallel hyperplanes are drawn which show a hard margin between the classified data. For clear classification, no data point falls inside the margin. Larger is the distance between the two hyperplanes better is the quality of classification.

Vapnik proposed this hard margin classification algorithm for the linear classifier. Recently sub- gradient descent and coordinate descent algorithms have been used for SVC. We are using a data augmented pre-processing before applying SVC in our proposed method.

3.   Results and Analysis

The Table-1 shows the precision-recall parameters along with training and testing accuracy of the proposed method. We observe that all performance parameters improve significantly with augmented data SVC. The Figure-2 shows the precision-recall curve for SVC with 100%,200% and 400% data augmentation. We get maximum AUC (area under curve), and testing accuracy (99.47%) for 400% augmented data SVC. The Multinomial Logistic Regression (MLR) shows the accuracy of 95.5%. Thus, SVC based method provides better classification performance. The Table-2, showing the confusion matrix for test data also validates the capability of bearing fault classification.

Table 1 Performance of SVC and MLR

SVC 100% data Training Accuracy: 0.955					SVC 200% data Training Accuracy: 0.982				
Class	precision	recall	f1-score	support	Class	precision	recall	f1-score	support
0	0.96	1	0.98	55	0	1	1	1	148
1	0.97	0.97	0.97	147	1	0.98	0.99	0.99	298
2	0.92	0.92	0.92	200	2	0.99	0.96	0.98	419
3	0.95	0.95	0.95	310	3	0.98	0.99	0.99	559
avg / total	0.95	0.95	0.95	712	avg / total	0.98	0.98	0.98	1424

SVC 400% data Training Accuracy: 0.994					MLR (Multinomial Logistic Regression) Training Accuracy: 0.958				
Class	precision	recall	f1-score	support	Class	precision	recall	f1-score	support
0	1	1	1	276	0	0.96	1	0.98	55
1	1	1	1	582	1	0.97	0.96	0.97	147
2	0.98	1	0.99	868	2	0.94	0.94	0.94	200
3	1	0.99	0.99	1122	3	0.96	0.96	0.96	310
avg / total	0.99	0.99	0.99	2848	avg/ total	0.96	0.96	0.96	712

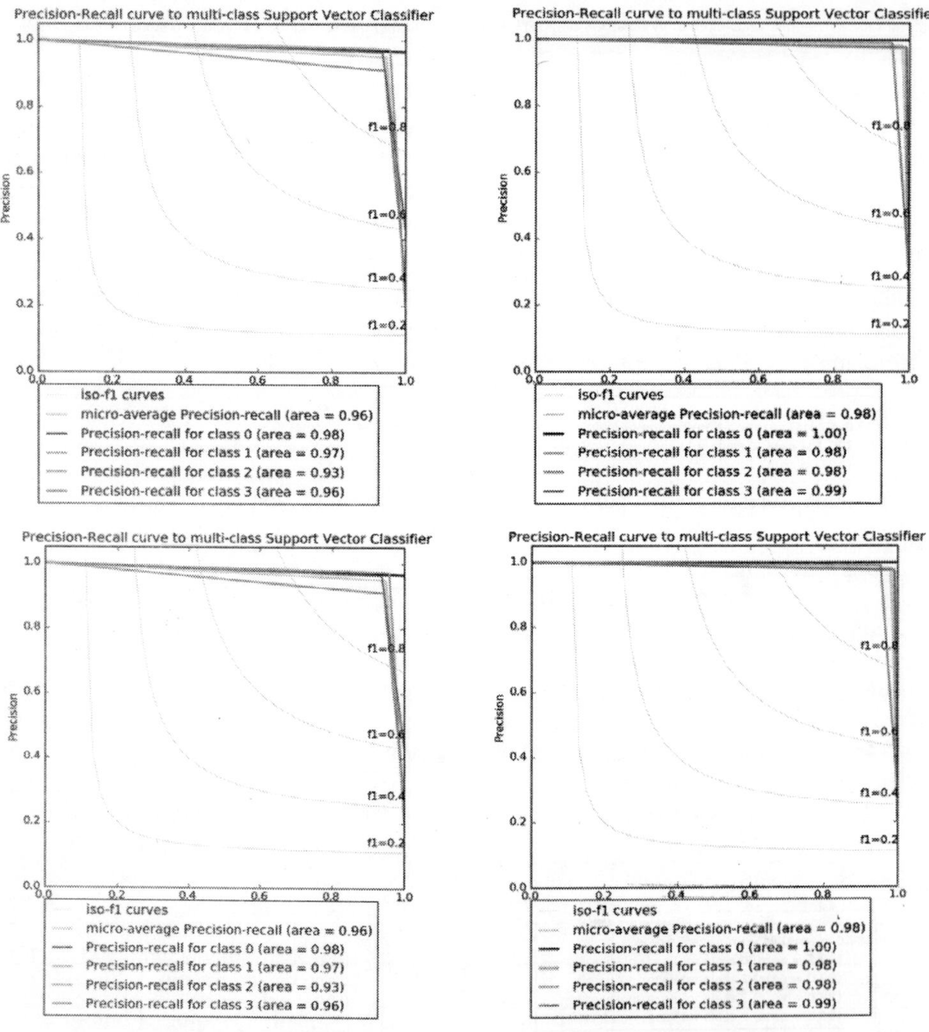

Figure 2. Precision -recall curves for bearing with SVC and MLR

The above results have been validated by applying on open source data of Case Western University data repository. Class 0 is for normal bearing, 1 is for outer race fault, 2 is for inner race fault and 3 is for roller fault.

Table 2 Confusion matrix for SVC and MLR for bearing fault

<table>
<tr><td colspan="10" align="center">CONFUSION MATRIX</td></tr>
<tr><td colspan="5" align="center">SVC 100% data</td><td></td><td colspan="5" align="center">SVC 200% Data</td></tr>
<tr><td>Class</td><td>0</td><td>1</td><td>2</td><td>3</td><td></td><td>Class</td><td>0</td><td>1</td><td>2</td><td>3</td></tr>
<tr><td>0</td><td>55</td><td>0</td><td>0</td><td>0</td><td></td><td>0</td><td>148</td><td>0</td><td>0</td><td>0</td></tr>
<tr><td>1</td><td>0</td><td>142</td><td>2</td><td>3</td><td></td><td>1</td><td>0</td><td>296</td><td>0</td><td>2</td></tr>
<tr><td>2</td><td>0</td><td>5</td><td>184</td><td>11</td><td></td><td>2</td><td>0</td><td>7</td><td>403</td><td>9</td></tr>
<tr><td>3</td><td>2</td><td>0</td><td>13</td><td>295</td><td></td><td>3</td><td>0</td><td>0</td><td>4</td><td>555</td></tr>
<tr><td colspan="5" align="center">Testing accuracy = 94.9438202247191</td><td></td><td colspan="5" align="center">Testing accuracy = 98.455056179775283</td></tr>
<tr><td colspan="5" align="center">SVC 400% Data</td><td></td><td colspan="5" align="center">MLR</td></tr>
<tr><td>Class</td><td>0</td><td>1</td><td>2</td><td>3</td><td></td><td>Class</td><td>0</td><td>1</td><td>2</td><td>3</td></tr>
<tr><td>0</td><td>276</td><td>0</td><td>0</td><td>0</td><td></td><td>0</td><td>55</td><td>0</td><td>0</td><td>0</td></tr>
<tr><td>1</td><td>0</td><td>582</td><td>0</td><td>0</td><td></td><td>1</td><td>0</td><td>141</td><td>3</td><td>3</td></tr>
<tr><td>2</td><td>0</td><td>0</td><td>867</td><td>1</td><td></td><td>2</td><td>0</td><td>3</td><td>187</td><td>10</td></tr>
<tr><td>3</td><td>0</td><td>0</td><td>14</td><td>1108</td><td></td><td>3</td><td>2</td><td>1</td><td>10</td><td>297</td></tr>
<tr><td colspan="5" align="center">Testing accuracy = 99.4733146067415</td><td></td><td colspan="5" align="center">testing accuracy = 95.50561797752809</td></tr>
</table>

4.   Conclusion

From the above tables and figures, it is observed that the proposed method is a versatile approach for bearing fault identification at early stages. It is equally capable of detecting faults on the outer and inner race along with roller faults. The machine learning performance metrics show high precision and recall simultaneously. It validates the predictive capability of the SVC based proposed approach. The method is simple and less time-consuming. The pre-processing technique used is also novel and can be used for smaller size of available data. For future work the proposed method can be tested for compound faults of bearings.

5.   References

1.   Samanta, B., Al-Balushi, K.R. and Al-Araimi, S.A., Artificial Neural Networks and Support Vector Machines with Genetic Algorithm for Bearing Fault Detection, Engineering Applications of Artificial Intelligence, Vol. 16(7-8), 2003, 657-665.

2.   Abbasion, S., Rafsanjani, A., Farshidianfar, A. and Irani, N., Rolling Element Bearings Multi-Fault Classification Based on the Wavelet Denoising and Support Vector Machine, Mechanical Systems, and Signal Processing, Vol. 21(7), 2007, 2933-2945.

3.   Bordoloi, D.J., and Tiwari, R., Optimum Multi-Fault Classification of Gears with Integration of Evolutionary and SVM Algorithms, Mechanism and Machine Theory, Vol. 73, 2014 (a), 49-60.

4.   Gangsar, P. and Tiwari, R., Multiclass Fault Taxonomy in Rolling Bearings at Interpolated and Extrapolated Speeds Based on Time Domain Vibration Data by SVM Algorithms, Journal of Failure Analysis and Prevention, Vol. 14(6), 2014, 826837.

5.   Liu, Z., Cao, H., Chen, X., He, Z. and Shen, Z., Multi-Fault classification based on Wavelet SVM with PSO Algorithm to Analyze Vibration Signals from Rolling Element Bearings, Neurocomputing, Vol. 99(1), 2013, 399-410.

6.   Yaqub, M.F., Gondal, I. and Kamruzzaman, J., Machine Fault Severity Estimation based on Adaptive Wavelet Nodes Selection and SVM, in Proceedings of the IEEE International Conference on Mechatronics and Automation, Beijing, China, 2011, 1951-1956.

7.   Kankar, P.K., Sharma, S.C. and Harsha, S.P., Fault Diagnosis of Ball Bearings using Machine Learning Methods, Expert Systems with Applications, Vol. 38(3), 2011(b), 1876-1886.

Simultaneous Multielemental Analysis of the Pointed Gourd (parwal) by Direct Current arc Optical Emission Spectroscopy

Akhilesh Singh, Chhavi Baran, Aradhana Tripathi, Sweta Sharma, S. Kumar and K. N. Uttam[*]

Saha's Spectroscopy Laboratory, Department of Physics, University of Allahabad, Allahabad
**E-mail: kailash.uttam@rediffmail.com*

ABSTRACT

The present account describes methodological work that exploits the utility of supremacy of the direct current arc optical emission spectroscopy technique for the investigation of the elemental profile of pointed gourd (parwal). The emission spectrum of powder sample of parwal has been recorded in the spectral region 300-700 nm by exciting direct current under optimized experimental condition and analyzed. The recorded spectrum shows persistence lines of calcium, sodium, potassium, iron, manganese, magnesium, chromium and titanium with varying intensities thus confirming the presence of these elements with different concentration in the parwal. Curve fitting analysis has been used for the relative quantitative estimation of the elements present in parwal. The presence of significant amount of chromium and magnesium in the parwal might be responsible for its antihyperglycemic properties. In addition, the presence of copper and iron makes it useful for other enzymatic and metabolic activities in humans.

Keywords: Pointed gourd (Parwal), direct current arc optical emission spectroscopy, elemental analysis, curve fitting, nutrients and trace elements

1. Introduction

Vegetables are the important parts of the human diet. The green vegetables are the rich source of biochemicals and minerals (nutrients, trace elements etc.) that are consumed to reduce chronic, viral, epideomic and cardiovascular diseases. Pointed gourd (parwal) fruits are widely consumed as vegetable by humans and are used in traditional medicines to treat various types of human ailments. It contains a number of bioactive phytochemicals including peptides, triterpenes, sterols, saponin, tannins, flavonoids due to which it posses antihyperglycemic, antihyperlipidemic, antitumor, cytotoxic, arsenic poisoning ameliorative, anti-inflammatory and antidiarrheal properties.

The therapeutic and medicinal importance/applications of the vegetables are attributed due to their elemental and biochemical constituents present in the vegetable. Vegetables contain large amount of the organic elements while the level of inorganic elements are quite small. This poses challenges in the investigation of the elemental constituents of the biosamples like vegetables. An extensive work has been done on the investigation of biochemical constitution of this plant but little is known about its elemental profile. Since the elemental constituents of the fruits are very important in determining their pharmaceutical applicability therefore it is very important to investigate the elemental profile of the fruits. For investigating the elemental profile of the plant tissues, the choice of the techniques is a key factor which depends upon the accuracy and repeatability, time duration of analysis and procedure involved in sample pre-processing. There are a number of challenges in the elemental investigation of the biomaterials such as presence of large amount of water, low volatile organic compounds, heterogeneous distribution of the biochemical, and trace amount of the inorganic elements compared with the organic elements, large difference among the melting and boiling point of the different constituents. Therefore there is a need of new probes that can address all the difficulties simultaneously together with the cost effectiveness, user friendly, free from sample preparation, multielemental, faster data generation, reproducibility, accuracy, sensitive, eco-friendly. One such technique is direct current arc optical emission spectroscopy.

Recently direct current arc optical emission spectroscopy has drawn the attention of analysts due to its supremacies such as digestion free, rapid simultaneous multi-component detection of elements with high sensitivity and accuracy. In direct current arc emission spectroscopy, a sample is excited by direct current and emitted radiations are recorded with the help of optical spectrometer. The analysis of the procured spectrum provides the information of the elemental constituents and their concentration without any sample pre-treatment. The positions, line shapes and intensities of the peaks present in the spectrum gives abundant useful information for the investigation of the properties of biomaterials. In comparison to the other methods, the direct current arc optical emission spectroscopy can give more information without the additional treatment and with much less time and cost.

The present account deals with the assessment of nutrient profile of the pointed gourd by recording the emission spectrum in the spectral region 300-700 nm using direct current arc optical emission spectroscopy and reports the health benefits of the detected nutrients and trace elements.

2.   Materials and Method

The experimental arrangement used for the assessment of the constituents of the pointed gourd (parwal) is described elsewhere [1, 2]. For this, the fresh samples of pointed gourds were purchased from the local vegetable market, Katra, Prayagraj. The collected samples were washed with tap water followed by distilled water to remove the surface impurity and dried at room temperature. Then the samples were cut into small pieces and kept in a hot air oven at a temperature of about 80^0C to evaporate water and other low volatile organic elements. Then the samples were homogenized by pastel and motor arrangement in powder form. The obtained powder was used for the experimental purpose. This process increased the concentration of inorganic elements in the sample used for the investigation and reduced matrix effect.

A small amount of the powder sample was kept inside the cavity of the carbon electrode of the arc arrangement. The electrodes were connected with the direct current supply together with the controlling resistance (ballast). As the voltage was built up across the electrodes, radiations were emitted. These emitted radiations were recorded with the help of Photon Control Fibre Optic Multichannel Spectrometer equipped with two grating in the spectral region 300-700 nm at a resolution of 0.3 nm. The obtained data were processed for the base line correction, smoothing and peak fitting with the help of Origin 8.0 software package.

3.   Results and Discussion

Figure 1 presents recorded emission spectrum of the powder of the pointed gourd (parwal) in the spectral region 300-700 nm. The simultaneous presence of strong and weak spectral signatures (atomic lines) depicts rich presence of the elements in the pointed gourd. The position and peak intensity of the observed spectral signatures provide information about the identity of the elements and their concentration present in the sample. The spectral signatures have been identified with the help of NIST spectral database. The identified elements are displayed in marked spectrogram (Figure 1). The scrutiny of the spectrum reveals the presence of persistent lines of calcium (393.1, 396.6, 422.4, 442.4, 443.3, 445.3, 610.2, 616.1, 643.5, 645.8, 671.5 nm) sodium (9589.5 nm), potassium (404.4 nm), iron (385.8, 438.1 nm), magnesium (383.1, 517.1, 518.3 nm), manganese (403.1 nm) and chromium (357.8, 359.3, 360.5, 425.2, 427.2, 428.7 nm) which confirm the presence of these elements in the pointed gourd sample. The peak intensity of the spectral profile has been used for the determination of the relative fraction of the presence of these elements in the pointed gourd sample. The concentration of elements is found in the same order as reported by other methods. A small deviation is due to the local metrological and geographical factors such as temperature, humidity, soil, and water quality used for growth and development of pointed gourd. It is important to discuss the role of detected elements for maintenance the human health.

The presence of strong and several lines of calcium in the d c arc spectrum of parwal indicates that it is a rich source of calcium. Calcium is important for healthy bones and teeth. It helps in relaxation and contraction of the muscles, nerve functioning, strengthening immune system, blood clotting, and blood pressure regulation. Potassium is needed for proper fluid balance, nerve transmission, muscle contraction, suitable maintenance of blood pressure and water elimination. Sodium is needed for the maintenance of electrolyte balance and fluid balance, heat function and specified metabolic activities, muscle contraction and nerve transition. Chromium is important for the metabolism of fats and carbohydrates, brain functioning and other body processes, stimulated fatty acid and cholesterol synthesis; works closely with insulin to regulate blood sugar (glucose) levels. Iron is needed for the formation of haemoglobin in red blood cells which carries oxygen from the lungs to the body cells needed for energy metabolism, a transport medium for electrons within cells; an integrated part of important enzyme systems in various tissues. Manganese is a part of many enzymes; important for the normal functioning of the brain and nervous system throughout the body; vital for proper and normal growth of human bone structure; useful for post-menopausal women and preventing osteoporosis. Magnesium is found in bones; needed for the formation of protein, muscle contraction, immune system health and nerve transmission.

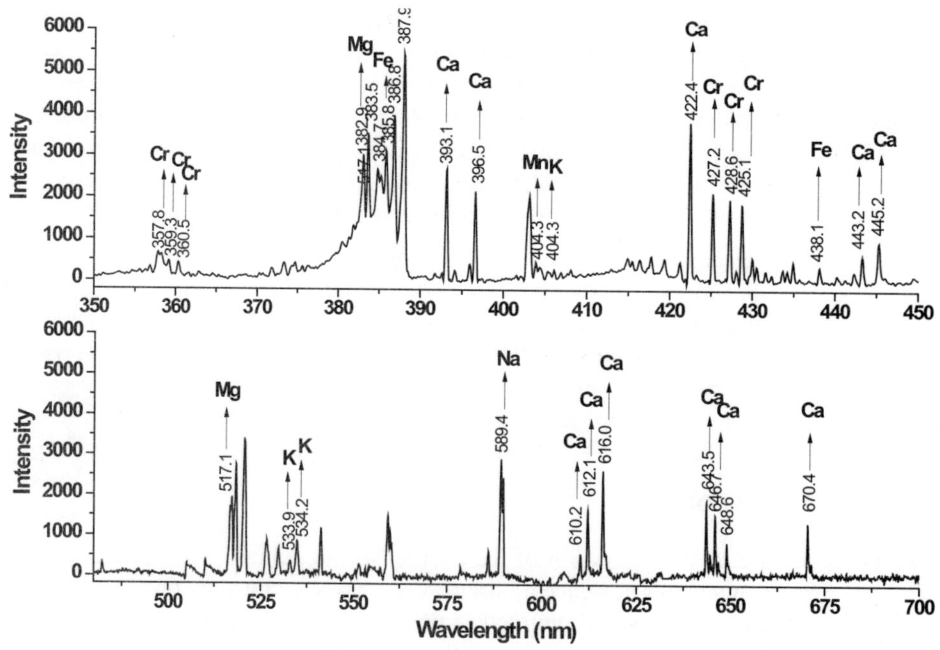

Figure 1: Recorded optical emission spectrum of the pointed gourd by d c arc optical emission spectroscopy

4.   References

1.   Sweta Sharma, Nidhi Shukla, Abhi Sarika Bharti and K. N. Uttam, Simultaneous multielemental analysis of the leaf of moringa oleifera by direct current arc optical emission spectroscopy, Natl. Acad. Sci. Lett. 41, 65–68 (2018).

2.   Shuchi Srivastava, Pavitra Tandon, Renu Singh, H C Gupta and K N Uttam, Elemental composition of gallstone by d c arc optical emission spectroscopy, National Academy Science Letter, 36, 397-402 (2013).

3.   Shuchi Srivastava, Pavitra Tandon, Renu Singh, S Kumar and K N Uttam, Elemental composition of radish by dc-arc optical emission spectroscopy, Science and Technology Journal, 1, 41-44 (2013).

4.   Abhi Sarika Bharti, Sweta Sharma, Nidhi Shukla, M. K. Tiwari and K. N. Uttam, Elemental investigation of the leaf and seed of coriander plant by synchrotron radiation X-ray fluorescence spectroscopy, Natl. Acad. Sci. Lett., 40, 373–377 (2017).

5.   Syed Mohammad, Taghi Gharibzahedi and Seid Mahdi Jafari, The importance of minerals in human nutrition: bioavailability, food fortification, processing effects and nanoencapsulation, Trends in Food Technology 62, 119-132 (2017).

Therapeutic siRNA Delivery for Cancer Therapy Using Nanoparticles

Pradeep Kumar*, Vandana Rai

Human Molecular Genetics Laboratory, Department of Biotechnology,
VBS Purvanchal University, Jaunpur-222003 (UP), India.
*E-mail: pradipk14@yahoo.co.in

ABSTRACT

According to World Health Organization diseases Cancer, among non-communicable diseases, is one of the leading causes of global death in many countries. Mortality due to cancer increases due to delayed diagnosis and treatment. Early and accurate detection and successful treatment of cancer can save millions of lives. Last two decades has witnessed improved treatment of cancer due technological advancement and a better understanding of molecular biology of the cancer. Treatment of cancer involves surgery, radiotherapy, anticancer drug chemotherapy and targeted therapy. siRNA via the phenomenon of RNA interference can inhibit specific cancer promoting gene (i. e post transcriptional silencing) and has proved to be successful as a result many siRNA based anticancer drugs are in clinical trials and many are under preclinical research. Despite many advantages over chemotherapeutic drugs for cancer treatment like safety, high efficacy, and high specificity, siRNA therapeutics for cancer treatment faces many limitations especially their poor delivery. Clinical translation of naked siRNA for cancer treatment is affected by several barriers like intravascular enzymatic degradation, recognition by immune system renal filtration and short half life reduced uptake by cells unstable under physiological conditions. In addition large size, hydrophilic nature and negative charge on naked siRNA molecules prevent them to diffuse across biological membranes. A chemical modification of the siRNA molecule or a delivery vehicle or carrier is required for efficient uptake of siRNA by target cells. Nanomaterials can be used as drug delivery vehicles targeting cancer. Currently nanocarriers like liposomes dendrimers polymeric nanoparticles polymeric micelles inorganic nanoparticles containing anticancer agents such as drug or siRNA molecule have proven to have many advantages compared to other drug delivery system. Many lipid nanoparticles RNAi drugs and cyclodextrin polymer based nanoparticle delivery systems for siRNA are under clinical trials. In recent times scientists have attempted microbubble and ultrasound mediated delivery of miRNA and siRNA for cancer therapy. Ultrasound mediated nanoparticle delivery will be a promising option for targeted delivery of therapeutics like si RNA into target cells with reduced toxicity and systemic dose.

Key words: siRNA, nanoparticles, cancer, therapy

1.   Introduction

Cancer is generic term used for a group of diseases caused by abnormal proliferation of cells. Cancer cells are different from normal (finite) cells as they grow and divide in an uncontrolled and unregulated manner and invade normal tissues and organs and destroy normal body tissue (1,2). Major risk factors that may increase the chances of cancer include age, tobacco use, alcohol use, radiation, infectious agents (like HPV), exposure to chemicals(cacinogens), hormones, unhealthy diet, lack of physical activity and high body mass index(3).

Common types of cancer are lung cancer, breast cancer, colorectal cancer, prostate cancer, skin stomach etc.(1) Cancer survival rate is increasing for many types of cancer, due technological advancement and improvement in the understanding and screening of the disease and its treatment. Different types of treatment available for cancer include surgery, chemotherapy, radiation therapy, targeted and hormonal therapy, and stem cell transplants (4, 5). siRNA drugs for cancer treatment can offer many advantages over chemotherapeutic anticancer drugs, like high degree of safety, high efficacy and can be designed to target and silence any disease causing gene and also the non-druggable targets. A major drawback with the traditional drugs, protein, antibody and small-molecule drugs for cancer therapy is their production whereas synthetic siRNAs are easy to produce by large-scale chemical synthesis (11).

Andrew Fire and Craig Mello was awarded noble prize in physiology or medicine in 2006 for their discovery of RNA interference-double stranded RNA (dsRNA) mediated gene silencing. Since then siRNA has become a powerful tool to study gene function and for gene silencing in protozoans, invertebrates, vertebrates, plants fungi and algae (6,7). The siRNA molecule is 21-25 nucleotides long and is comprised of two strands bonded to each other by hydrogen bonds (Watson–Crick base pairing)(8). Gene silencing by double stranded RNA via RNA interference is a two step process. In the first step double stranded RNA (dsRNA) is cleaved into short 21-25 nucleotides long small interfering RNA(siRNA) by a protein complex DICER(ribonuclease of RNase III family). In the second step these double standed siRNA (21-25 nucleotides long) are unwound and one strand is preferentially incorporated into RNA-induced silencing complex(RISC). This strand binds with complimentary sequence of the target mRNA and is degraded by an RNase present in the RISC. Out of the two strands of siRNA the guide (antisense) strand and the passenger (sense)strand, the guide strand is incorporated into RISC and induces selective silencing of the gene, whereas the passenger strand is cleaved by argonaute proteins(9,10).

In the past, studies in animal models have proved disease genes silencing by local and systemic administration of siRNA(11). Currently scientists are investigating the therapeutic application of siRNA in cancer, infectious and hereditary diseases but delivery of siRNA poses many challenges. There are multiple biological barriers for effective and enhanced delivery of siRNA to the site of action. (i) Naked siRNA molecules are too large (molecular weight is around ~13 kDa; size <10 nm) hydrophilic and at normal pH SiRNA are polyanionic (negatively charged) so they cannot pass through the cellular membranes. (ii) siRNA molecules are susceptible to RNases both ex and in vivo. They are easily degraded by the endogenous RNases, which cleave the phosphodiester linkage of the siRNA molecule in the body fluids. Experimentally it has been proved that without affecting the gene silencing ability of the molecule chemical modification of SIRNA at the 2' –position of the ribose and or phosphate group on the phosphodiester backbone enhances its stability in biological fluids and increases resistance to nucleases. (iii) siRNA molecules are recognized as foreign by innate immune system which leads to activation of the system and generation of an immune response. This can be overcome by designing a modified sequence of siRNA molecule and using smart carrier molecules for delivery of these molecules. (iv) Si RNA molecules are rapidly cleared by the kidney because of small particle size(<10nm) and hydrophilic nature.

Nanoparticles as delivery vehicles for siRNA

Different types of nanoparticle systems are extensively used to enhance the delivery efficiency of siRNA both in vitro and in vivo. Currently most common nanoparticle systems used are lipid based nanoparticle delivery systems (12). Liposomes are widely used as drug delivery systems because of their lipid bilayer structure which allows the entrapment and encapsulation of biological materials and drugs. Cationic lipids can interact with anionic lipids and can destabilize biological membranes facilitating the intracellular delivery of siRNA. Different types of nanoparticle delivery systems have been evaluated for delivering siRNA drugs to silence targets in vivo including polythyleneimine complexes(14,15), PEG–siRNA conjugate(16), Self-assembled nanoparticles(17), chitosan/quantum dot nanoparticles(18), Bionanocapsule/ liposome complexes (19), Solid lipid nanoparticles (SLNs) and Stable nucleic acid lipid particles (SNALPs) (20), Lipid/protamine nanoparticles (21), Chitosan nanoparticles (22). Among all the nanoparticle system, lipid nanoparticles(LNP) have shown promising results in effectively delivering Si RNA drugs to target cells of liver, silencing the gene in rodents and non-human primates(23, 24, 25, 26, 27).

RNAi -based therapeutics in clinical trials

Many siRNA therapeutics with nanoparticle delivery system are in different phases of clinical trials and (Table 1).

Table 1. RNAi therapeutics (drugs) in clinical trial (28, 29, 30, 31)

Therapeutic Si RNA name	Disease/Condition(s)	Delivery/ Carrier system	Targeted Gene	Sponsor/ Pharmaceutical Company	Phase	Status	ClinicalTrials.gov identifiers NCT ID
siG12D-LODER	Pancreatic ductal adenocarcinoma, pancreatic cancer	Polymeric matrix	KRAS G12D	Silenseed ltd	II	Recruiting	NCT01676259
TKM-080301	Hepatocellular carcinoma, hepatoma, liver cancer, liver cell carcinoma, neuroendocrine tumors, cancers with hepatic metastases	lipid noparticle (LNP)	PLK1	Arbutus biopharma corporation	I/II	Completed	NCT02191878, NCT01262235, NCT01437007
ALN-VSP02	Solid tumors,	LNP (Dlin-DMA)	VEGF, KSP	Alnylam Pharmaceuticals	I	Completed, Program hold	NCT00882180, NCT01158079
Atu027	Carcinoma, pancreatic ductal	Cationic lipoplex	PKN3	Silence therapeutics	I/II	Completed	NCT01808638
SPC2996	Chronic lymphocytic leukemia	Naked siRNA	*Bcl-2*	Santaris Pharma A/S	II	Completed	NCT00285103
siRNA–EphA2–DOPC	Advanced cancers	Lipid nanoparticle (LNP)	*EphA2*	M.D. Anderson Cancer Center	I	Recruiting	NCT01591356
SV40 vectors carrying siRNA	Chronic myeloid leukemia	Pseudoviral (SV40) particles	Bcr-Abl	Hadassah medical organization	Not specified	Completed	NCT00257647
Proteasome siRNA	Metastatic melanoma, absence of CNS metastases	DC cells, in vitro transfection	LMP2, LMP7, and MECL1	Scott Pruitt, Duke University	I	Complete	NCT00672542
PSCT19 (MiHA-loaded PD-L-silenced DC vaccination)	Hematological malignancies	Ex vivo transfection	PD-L1/L2	Radboud University	I/II	Recruiting	NCT02528682
Patisiran (ALN–TTR02)	Transthyretin-mediated amyloidosis	LNP	*TTR*	Alnylam Pharmaceuticals	III	Completed	NCT01960348

2.   Conclusion and Future Perspectives

ONPATTRO (Patisiran; lipid complex injection), is a medicine, used in adults only, for the treatment of polyneuropathy caused by hereditary transthyretin-mediated (hATTR amyloidosis). It is the first RNA interference (RNAi) therapeutic of Alnylam Pharmaceuticals' approved by United States Food and Drug Administration (FDA), European Commission (EC), Health Canada, Canada and Japanese Ministry of

Health, Labour and Welfare, Japan. The medicine was approved in August 2018 in USA. Patisiran has proved the potential of RNAi technology in treating diseases (32, 33, 34, 35). Ultrasound mediated nanoparticle delivery will be a promising option for targeted delivery of therapeutics like siRNA into target cells with reduced toxicity. Several scientists have investigated the delivey of siRNA by ulatrasound(36, 37, 38, 39). The success of the therapeutic siRNA depends upon the safe and efficient delivery of the siRNA into the cytoplasm of the cancer cell. A smart nanocarrier engineered in such a way that can efficiently deliver siRNA drug with minimum toxicity is required. The success story of Patisiran has brought a ray of hope for the pharmaceutical companies to develop siRNA based therapeutics in future.

3. References

1. https://www.who.int/health-topics/cancer#tab=tab_1.

2. Cooper, G.M.: The Cell: A Molecular Approach, Fourth Edition pp.719 (2007).

3. https://www.cancer.gov/about-cancer/causes-prevention/risk

4. https://breast-cancer.ca/metsurv-stat/

5. https://www.cancer.gov/about-cancer/treatment/types

6. https://www.nobelprize.org/prizes/medicine/2006/summary/

7. Agrawal, N., Dasaradhi, P.V., Mohmmed, A., Malhotra, P., Bhatnagar, R.K., Mukherjee, S.K.: RNA interference: biology, mechanism, and applications. Microbiol Mol Biol Rev67: 657–685 (2003).

8. Gallas, A., Alexander, C., Davies, M. C., Puri, S., Allen, S.: Chemistry and formulations for siRNA therapeutics. Chemical Society reviews 42, 7983–7997, 10.1039/c3cs35520a (2013).

9. Matranga, C., Tomari, Y., Shin, C., Bartel, D.P., Zamore, P. D.: Passenger strand cleavage facilitates assembly of siRNA into Ago2-containing RNAi enzyme complexes. Cell 123, 607–620(2005).

10. Siomi, H., Siomi, M. C.: On the road to reading the RNA-interference code. Nature 457, 396 –404(2009).

11. Bumcrot, D., Manoharan, M., Koteliansky, V. & Sah, D. W. Y. RNAi therapeutics: a potential new class of pharmaceutical drugs. Nature Chem. Biol. 2, 711–719 (2006).

12. Li, J., Xue, S., Mao, Z.W.: Nanoparticle delivery systems for siRNA-based therapeutics. J. Mater. Chem. B. 4,6620–6639(2016).

13. Dohmen, C., Frohlich, T., Lachelt, U., Rohl, I., Vornlocher, H.-P., Hadwiger, P., Wagner, E.: Defined folate-PEG-siRNA conjugates for receptor-specific gene silencing. Mol. Ther. Nucleic Acids 1 (2012) e7.

14. Lee, H., Lytton-Jean, A.K.R., Chen, Y., Love, K.T., Park, A.I., Karagiannis, E.D., Sehgal, A., Querbes, W., Zurenko, C.S., Jayaraman, M., Peng, C.G., Charisse, K., Borodovsky, A., Manoharan, M., Donahoe, J.S., Truelove, J., Nahrendorf, M., Langer, R., Anderson, D.G.: Molecularly self-assembled nucleic acid nanoparticles for targeted in vivo siRNA delivery, Nat. Nanotechnol. 7, 389–393 (2012).

15. Kim, J.S., Oh, M.H., Park, J.Y., Park, T.G., Nam, Y.S.: Protein-resistant, reductively dissociable polyplexes for in vivo systemic delivery and tumor-targeting of siRNA. Biomaterials 34, 2370–2379 (2013).

16. Li, J.M., Wang, Y.Y., Zhang, W., Su, H., Ji, L.N., Mao, Z.W.: Low-weight polyethylenimine cross-linked 2-hydroxypopyl-beta-cyclodextrin and folic acid as an efficient and nontoxic siRNA carrier for gene silencing and tumor inhibition by VEGF siRNA, Int. J. Nanomedicine 8, 2101–2117 (2013).

17. Willibald, J., Harder, J., Sparrer, K., Conzelmann, K.-K., Carell, T.: Click-modified anandamide siRNA enables delivery and gene silencing in neuronal and immune cells. J. Am. Chem. Soc. 134, 12330–12333 (2012).

18. Tan, W.B., Jiang, S. Zhang., Y.: Quantum-dot based nanoparticles for targeted silencing of HER2/neu gene via RNA interference, Biomaterials 28, 1565–1571 (2007).

19. Yoon, H.Y., Kim, H.R., Saravanakumar, G., Heo, R., Chae, S.Y., Um, W., Kim, K., Kwon, I.C., Lee, J.Y., Lee, D.S., Park, J.C., Park, J.H.: Bioreducible hyaluronic acid conjugates as siRNA carrier for tumor targeting, J. Control. Release 172, 653–661 (2013).

20. Kanasty, R., Dorkin, J.R., Vegas, A., Anderson, D.: Delivery materials for siRNA therapeutics, Nat. Mater. 12, 967e977(2013).

21. Li, S.-D., Chen, Y.-C., Hackett, M.J., Huang, L. Tumor-targeted delivery of siRNA by self-assembled nanoparticles, Mol. Ther. 16, 163–169 (2007).

22. Nascimento, A.V., Singh, A., Bousbaa, H., Ferreira, D., Sarmento, B., Amiji, M.M.: Mad2 checkpoint gene silencing using epidermal growth factor receptor-targeted chitosan nanoparticles in non-small cell lung cancer model, Mol. Pharm.11(10), 3515-27(2014).

23. Tabernero, J., Shapiro, G.I., LoRusso, P.M., Cervantes, A., Schwartz, G.K., Weiss, G.J., Paz-Ares, L., Cho, D.C., et al.: First-in-humans trial of an RNA interference therapeutic targeting VEGF and KSP in cancer patients with liver involvement. Cancer Discov. 3, 406–417 (2013).

24. Wolfrum, C., Shi, S., Jayaprakash, K.N., Jayaraman, M., Wang, G., Pandey, R.K., et al.: Mechanisms and optimization of in vivo delivery of lipophilic siRNAs . Nat Biotechnol 25, 1149 – 57(2007) .

25. Akinc, A., Querbes, W., De S., Qin, J., Frank-Kamenetsky, M., Jayaprakash, K.N, et al.: Targeted delivery of RNAi therapeutics with endogenous and exogenous ligand-based mechanisms . Mol Ther18(13),64 (2010).

26. Zimmermann, T.S. , Lee, A.C., Akinc, A., Bramlage, B., Bumcrot, D., Fedoruk, M.N., et al.: RNAi-mediated gene silencing in non-human primates. Nature 441,111–4 (2006).

27. Li, J., Xue, S., Mao, Z.W.: Nanoparticle delivery systems for siRNA-based therapeutics. J. Mater. Chem. B 4, 6620–6639 (2016).

28. Aghamiri, S., Mehrjardi, K.F., Shabani, S., Keshavarz-Fathi, M., Kargar, S., Rezaei, N.: Nanoparticle-siRNA: a potential strategy for ovarian cancer therapy? Nanomedicine (Lond). 15,2083-2100(2019).

29. Yu, A., Jian, C., Yu, A.H., Tu, M.: RNA Therapy: are we using the right molecules? Pharmacol Ther. 196, 91-104(2019).

30. Weng, Y., Xiao, H., Zhang, J., Liang, X.J., Huang, Y.: RNAi therapeutic and its innovative biotechnological evolution. Biotechnol. Adv. 37, 801–825(2019).

31. Xu, C., Wang, J.: Delivery systems for siRNA drug development in cancer therapy. Asian Journal of Pharmaceutical Sciences;10(1),1-12(2015).

32. http://investors.alnylam.com/news-releases/news-release-details/alnylam-announces-first-ever-fda-approval-rnai-therapeutic

33. http://investors.alnylam.com/news-releases/news-release-details/alnylam-pharmaceuticals-announces-initiation-apollo-b-phase-3

34. Crooke, S.T., Witztum, J.L., Bennett, C.F., Baker, B.F.: RNA□targeted therapeutics. Cell Metab. 2018;27:714□739.

35. Ledford, H.: Gene□silencing technology gets first drug approval after 20□year wait. Nature 560,291□292(2018).

36. Bai, M., Shen, M., Teng, Y., Sun, Y., Li, F., Zhang, X., et al.: Enhanced therapeutic effect of Adriamycin on multidrug resistant breast cancer by the ABCG2-siRNA loaded polymeric nanoparticles assisted with ultrasound. Oncotarget 6, 43779-43790(2015).

37. Carson, A.R., McTiernan, C.F., Lavery, L., Grata, M., Leng, X., Wang, J., Chen, X., Villanueva, F.S.: Ultrasound-targeted microbubble destruction to deliver siRNA cancer therapy. Cancer Res. 72, 6191–6199(2012).

38. Negishi, Y., Endo, Y., Fukuyama, T., Suzuki, R., Takizawa, T. Omata, D., Maruyama, K., Aramaki, Y.: Delivery of siRNA into the cytoplasm by liposomal bubbles and ultrasound. J. Control. Release 132, 124–130 (2008).

39. Endo-Takahashi, Y., Negishi, Y., Kato, Y., Suzuki, R., Maruyama, K., Aramaki, Y., Efficient siRNA delivery using novel siRNA-loaded bubble liposomes and ultrasound, Int. J. Pharm. 422, 504–509 (2012).

Elemental Assessment of the Sattu by Direct Current arc Optical Emission Spectroscopy

Shashwat Seth[1], Shivam Mishra[1], Abhi Sarika Bharti[1], Sweta Sharma[1], Renu Singh[1], S. Kumar[2] and K. N. Uttam[1,*]

[1]Saha's Spectroscopy Laboratory, Department of Physics, University of Allahabad, Allahabad
[2] Department of Physics, IET, VBS Purvanchal University, Jaunpur
*E-mail: kailash.uttam@rediffmail.com

ABSTRACT

In the current study, the phytoelements present in the sattu have been investigated with the help of direct current arc optical emission spectroscopy and their concentration determined qualitatively. For this, the sattu powders were procured from the local market of Katra, Prayagraj. A small quantity of the powdered sattu was kept inside the cavity of the carbon electrode of the arc. The optical emission spectrum of the sattu was recorded in the spectral region 200-700 nm at a resolution of 0.3 nm by exciting sample with the help of direct current. The recorded spectrum shows spectral signature of the elements potassium, magnesium, manganese, sodium, calcium, iron, and chromium thus confirming the occurrence of these elements in the sattu sample. The role of detected elements has been discussed in maintaining the human health.

1. Introduction

Sattu is a traditional Indian local food which is made up of roasted and ground gram. It is considered as poor man's protein and due to its nutritional qualities it is now being considered as global super food. The process of sattu manufacturing keeps the nutritional value of its constituents intact that can be stored for longer periods. Sattu is a rich source of protein and complex carbohydrates and is gluten free. It is widely consumed during summer as it prevents the body from overheating and brings down the body temperature significantly. The high amount of insoluble fibre in Sattu is great for the intestine. It helps in cleaning the colon, detoxifying greasy food, rejings digestion and mixing flatulence, constipation and acidity. Sattu is a low-glycaemic index food and is a great option for diabetics as it helps maintaining sugar level and blood pressure. Sattu helps in preventing osteoporosis. It also helps in building muscle mass and muscle strength rapidly. The various digestive curative and therapeutic applications of Sattu are attributed due to the presence of phytochemicals and phytoelements.

Nowadays various optical spectroscopic techniques are used for the elemental investigation of cereals and foodstuff in search of novel minimal or noninvasive probes. Recently direct current arc optical emission spectroscopy has drawn the attention of analysts due to its supremacies such as digestion free, rapid simultaneous multi-component detection of elements with high sensitivity and accuracy. In direct current arc emission spectroscopy, a sample is excited by direct current and emitted radiations are recorded with the help of optical spectrometer. The analysis of the procured spectrum provides the information of the inorganic constituents and their concentration without any sample pre-treatment. The positions, line shapes and intensities of the peaks present in the spectrum give useful information for the investigation of the properties of biomaterials. In comparison to the other methods, the direct current arc optical emission spectroscopy can give more information without the additional treatment and with much less time and cost [1-3].

In the present paper, the phytonutrients present in the Sattu have been investigated with the help of direct current arc optical emission spectroscopy and determined their concentration quantitatively.

2.   Experimental

The direct current arc optical emission spectroscopy technique has been utilised to access the level of element present in the Sattu. The experimental arrangement for recording the emission spectra of the Sattu is shown in Fig.1 and describes elsewhere [2]. For this, Sattu in form of powders were procured from the local market of Katra, Praygraj. To avoid any kind of degradation and mixing of the pesticide or preservatives commonly used for preservation of edible materials long duration, Sattu powders were purchased from the locally made supply so that the typical aroma could be sensed by the human sense organ "nose". A little amount of the Sattu powder was kept inside the cavity of carbon electrode. The electrodes were connected with the d c arc power supply. As soon as the power was built up, the characteristic radiation of the Sattu samples were emitted. The emitted radiations were recorded with the help of fibre optic coupled Photon Multi Channel spectrometer in the spectral region 200-700 nm at a resolution of the 0.3 nm. The obtained spectral data were processed with the origin 8.0 software package for the base line correction, smoothing, peak spectral analysis and identified with the help of standard reference spectra or NIST spectral database.

3.   Results and Discussion

The emission spectrum of the Sattu powder sample was recorded by exciting direct current in carbon arc in the spectral region 300-700 nm and is reproduced in Fig.2. The recorded spectra depict the presence of number of lines with varying intensities showing the presence of number of elements in the Sattu sample. The obtained lines have been identified with the help of NIST spectral database. The position of the line gives element while intensity depicts level of concentration. The lines of elements having strong intensity are more abundant while those having weak intensity are smaller in quantity. The scrutiny of the spectra show the presence of persistent atomic lines of the potassium (403.0 nm), calcium (393.1, 396.7, 422.4, 443.4, 445.2, 610.2, 612.2, 616.3, 643.5, 645.8 and 670.7 nm), magnesium (383.6 nm), manganese (404.3 nm), sodium (589.3 nm), chromium (357.8 and 360.8 nm) and iron (385.8 and 438.1 nm). The presence of persistent lines confirms the presence of these elements in the Sattu sample.

Calcium is a key nutrient abundantly stored in bones and teeth of human body. It is also involved in vascular contraction, blood clot formation, muscle functions, conduction of nerve impulses, vasodilation, intracellular signalling, and hormonal secretion. It plays major role in the cation-anion balance and acts as an activator of the several enzymes systems in the protein synthesis and carbohydrates transfer. Potassium is one of the most important and abundant macronutrient in the human body after calcium and phosphorus. It assists in maintaining blood pressure, body fluid and electrolyte balance, normal gastrointestinal motility, nerve impulse conduction and muscle contraction. Potassium is also important component of cardiac muscle fiber. Manganese is an important constituent of many enzymes and antioxidants which are involved in controlling nervous system functions, blood sugar and cholesterol level. Iron is involved in oxygen transport, DNA synthesis and electron transport. It is an essential component of hemoglobin and other proteins such as transferrin, ferretin. Enzymes involved in the production of new cells, amino acids, hormones and neurotransmitters are also dependent upon the availability of iron. Sodium is needed for the maintenance of electrolyte balance and fluid balance, heat function and specified metabolic activities, muscle contraction and nerve transition. Chromium is important for the metabolism of fats and carbohydrates, brain functioning and other body processes, stimulated fatty acid and cholesterol synthesis; works closely with insulin to regulate blood sugar (glucose) levels. Magnesium is found in bones; needed for the formation of protein, muscle contraction, immune system health and nerve transmission [3-5].

The results of the present study demonstrate the applicability of d c arc optical spectroscopy as a rapid data generation, sensitive and multielement detection technique for the simultaneous detection of minerals, trace metals and heavy metals in the food samples like sattu in any physical state. The results also give important insight about the elemental profile of sattu and it is observed that sattu is an abundant source of calcium, manganese, iron, potassium. It also contains trace amounts of chromium and magnesium.

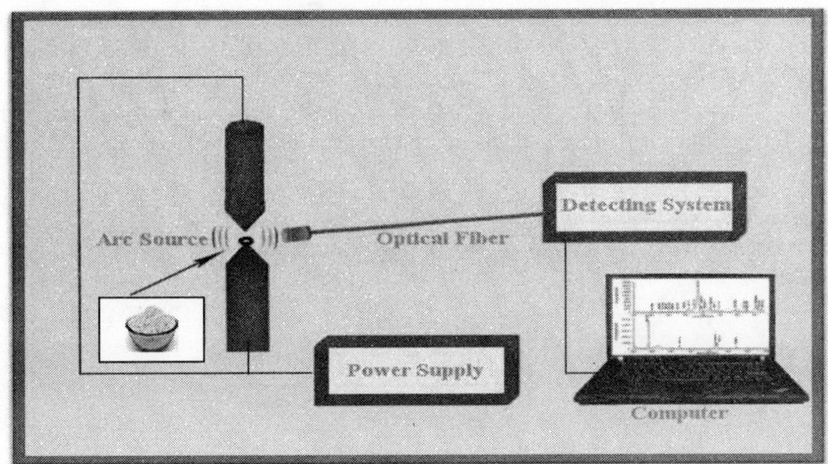

Figure 1 Schematic arrangement of the d c arc optical emission spectroscopy

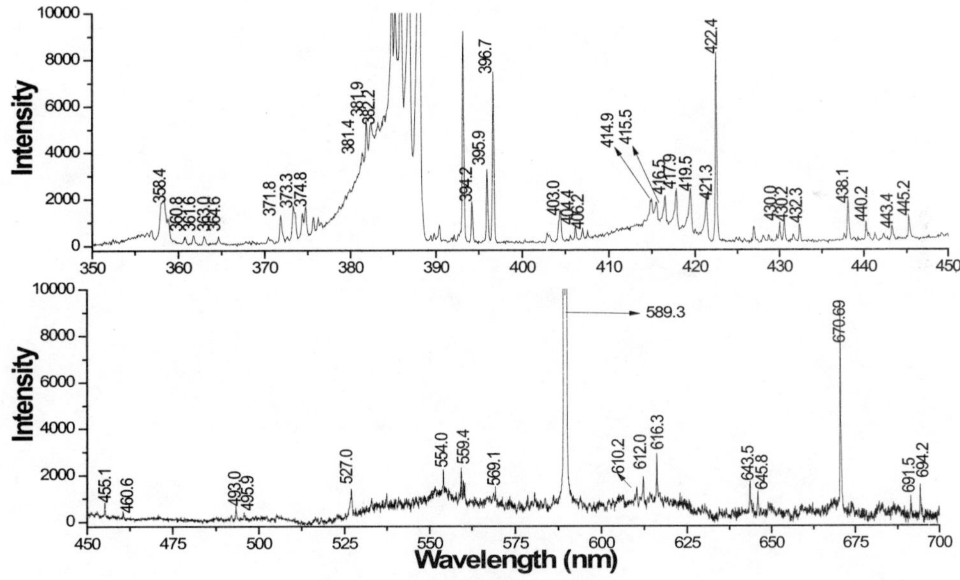

Figure 2: Recorded optical emission spectra of the sattu using d c arc optical emission spectroscopy

4.   References

1.   Sweta Sharma, Nidhi Shukla, Abhi Sarika Bharti and K. N. Uttam, Simultaneous multielemental analysis of the leaf of moringa oleifera by direct current arc optical emission spectroscopy, Natl. Acad. Sci. Lett. 41, 65–68 (2018).

2.   Shuchi Srivastava, Pavitra Tandon, Renu Singh, H C Gupta and K N Uttam, Elemental composition of gallstone by d c arc optical emission spectroscopy, National Academy Science Letter, 36, 397-402 (2013).

3.   Shuchi Srivastava, Pavitra Tandon, Renu Singh, S Kumar and K N Uttam, Elemental composition of radish by dc-arc optical emission spectroscopy, Science and Technology Journal, 1, 41-44 (2013).

4.   Abhi Sarika Bharti, Sweta Sharma, Nidhi Shukla, M. K. Tiwari and K. N. Uttam, Elemental investigation of the leaf and seed of coriander plant by synchrotron radiation X-ray fluorescence spectroscopy, Natl. Acad. Sci. Lett., 40, 373–377 (2017).

5.   Syed Mohammad, Taghi Gharibzahedi and Seid Mahdi Jafari, The importance of minerals in human nutrition: bioavailability, food fortification, processing effects and nanoencapsulation, Trends in Food Technology 62, 119-132 (2017).

Ultrasonication Assisted Synthesis of Silver Nanoparticles Functionalized by Bovine Silver Nanoparticles for the Colorimetric Sensing of Fe^{2+} Ions in Aqueous Media

Aarti Jaiswal[1,*], Sweta Sharma[2], Abhishek Bhardwaj[3], Renu Singh and K N Uttam[2,**]

[1]Centre of Material Science, IIDS, University of Allahabad, Allahabad
[2]Saha's Spectroscopy Laboratory, Department of Physics, University of Allahabad, Allahabad
[2]Department of Environmental Science, VBS Purvanchal University, Jaunpur
E-mail: *aartijaiswal276@gmail.com; **kailash.uttam@rediffmail.com

ABSTRACT

Silver nanoparticles functionalized by bovine serum albumin have been synthesized by ultrasonic assisted method. For this, silver nitrate solution was mixed with dilute solution of bovine serum albumin and ultrasonicated. The change in colour of the solution from milky white to black was observed which indicated the reduction of silver from the silver nitrate solution. The ultraviolet- visible spectrum of the synthesised colloidal solution depict broad absorption in the spectral region 400-600 nm with peak maxima at 408 nm due to the surface plasmon resonance band of metallic nanoparticles that confirms the nano character of the synthesized material. The synthesized nanoparticles were further subjected to characterization by ultraviolet visible spectroscopy. The synthesized silver nanoparticles have been used for detecting calorimetrically the presence of metal ions like Fe^{2+} in aqueous solution.

*Keywords: **Ultrasonic assisted synthesis of nanoparticle, colorimetric sensor, functionised nanoparticles, ultraviolet-visible spectroscopy.***

1. Introduction

The pollution of metal ions in aqeous environment is increasing day by day due to the anthropogenic perturbances such as agricultural runoff, vehicular exhaust, discharge of industrial and domestic effluents and mining and smelting activities, acid mine drainage [1-3]. Iron is the second most abundant element in the earth's crust. It is basically found as Fe^{2+} and Fe^{3+} ions and readily combines with oxygen and sulphur to form oxides, hydroxides, carbonates and sulphides. It is naturally present in the water bodies but sometimes its concentration is elevated due to anthropogenic sources. Major sources of iron in water includes construction material, inter alia for drinking water pipes, pigments in paints and plastics, compounds used in food colouring, supplements for curing iron deficiency and coagulants used in the treatment of water. The presence of excess Fe^{2+} ion may cause serious damage including poisoning. *Fe^{2+} overload can be particularly damaging* to the heart, liver, effects on human plasma cholinesterase and generates reactive oxygen species in a biological system and causes reproductive, neurological, cardiac and mental disorders. Therefore it is very essential to detect the presence of Fe^{2+} ions in the environment in rapid, sensitive and cost effective manner.

Nowadays nanoparticles displaying surface Plasmon resonance properties like silver and gold are highly desired for chemosensing applications particularly toxic metal ions in different environments. Silver nanoparticles have gained significant attention in recent years due to their unique features and wide range of applications in the different fields like catalysis, biosensing, imaging, surface enhancement and antibacterial activity. In addition the conjugation of nanoparticles with biomolecules like proteins, amino acids, carbohydrates and phenolic compounds that can change the optical and binding properties of the nanoparticles is an emerging research problem. The conjugation of proteins like bovine serum albumin acts as good surface binder and significantly alters the properties of silver nanoparticles which can be effectively used in sensing applications in order to reduce their harmful effect/impact on the environment and human health [4-5].

To meet this objective, there is an urgent need to develop a low cost, user friendly free from costlier instruments and protocols for the synthesis of the nanoparticles and sensing systems. Silver nanoparticles have been synthesized by many approaches such as physical and chemical methods like sol-gel, hydrothermal, microwave assisted and laser ablation [6]. Although these methods are effective, they are limited by tedious labour and time intensive protocols and requirements of toxic chemicals. In view of these limitations, ultrasonic assisted synthesis has been recently recognized as a potential approach for the pure nanomaterial synthesis in a rapid, simple, and cost effective manner.

Here we report a sensing system based on silver nanoparticles functionalized by bovine serum albumin for the detection of Fe^{2+}. The silver nanoparticles have been synthesized by ultrasonic assisted method using silver nitrate as precursor and sodium borohydride as a reducing agent. The synthesized silver nanoparticles have been functionlized by bovine serum albumin and have been used for colorimetric sensing of Fe^{2+} ions in aqueous media.

2.   Materials and Method

All the chemicals were purchased from the Merck Ltd, Mumbai, India of the analytical grade. They were used without any further treatment of purity. The 10 mM silver nitrate and bovine serum albumin solutions were mixed together in a 20 ml beaker and was sonicated for 10 minutes. After 10 minutes, 10 mM sodium borohydride solution was mixed in it followed by sonication for the duration of 30 minutes. Then after 30 minutes, the colour of the solution turns black indicating the formation of silver colloidal solution functionalized by bovine serum albumin. This synthesized silver colloidal solution was used for the colorimetric detection of the Fe^{2+} metal ions. For this, 2.5 ml solution of iron sulphate ($FeSO_4$) containing Fe^{2+} ions of different concentration (2, 10, 20, 40, 60, 80 and 100 µM) was prepared in distilled water. To this solution, the synthesized silver colloidal solution functionalized by bovine serum albumin (BSA) was added and the change in the colour of the mixed solution was noticed by naked eye. The colour of the solution of turned yellow immediately after the addition of colloidal silver solution. Further it was observed that the yellow colour of the solution intensified as the concentration of Fe^{2+} ions increased in the solution.

The ultraviolet-visible spectrum of the synthesized silver colloidal solution and different concentration of the metal ions mixed silver colloidal solution was recorded in absorbance mode with the help of fiber optic spectrometer (Avasoft 3646, Avantee, Netherland) in the spectral region 200-800 nm at a spectral resolution 2.3 nm. The obtained spectra have been pre-processed by smoothing and baseline correction using Origin 8.0 software package.

3.   Results and Discussion

The recorded ultraviolet-visible spectrum of the synthesised silver colloidal solution functionalized by BSA is displayed in Figure 1. The spectrum shows the presence of a sharp band at 408 nm which arises due to the characteristic surface Plasmon band of silver nanoparticles. Metal nanoparticles exhibit strong absorption bands in the ultraviolet and visible region due to the surface Plasmon resonance or interband transitions and they are the characteristic properties of the nanoparticles [7]. The occurrence of single symmetrical shape of the surface Plasmon band depicts that the synthesised silver nanoparticles are in spherical, similar shape, size and monodisperse in nature.

For the detection of Fe^{2+} ions in the aqueous solution, the synthesized silver colloidal solution functionalized by bovine serum albumin (BSA) was added. It was noticed that colour of the Fe^{2+} ion solution turned yellowish after the addition of silver colloidal solution. The intensity of the colour enhanced as the concentration of Fe^{2+} ions increased in the solution (Shown in Figure 2). The change and enhancement in the colour of the Fe^{2+} ion solution was observable by the naked eye. This change in colour is due to the aggregation of the silver nanoparticles in the medium by the Fe^{2+} ions. The amine and hydroxyl functional groups present in the BSA helps in binding Fe^{2+} ions onto the surface of silver ions and helps in aggregation processes. The aggregation leads to the change in the optical properties of the silver colloidal solution which is observable in the form of yellow colour. No such colour changes were observed for the Zn^{2+}, Cu^{2+}, Co^{2+} and Pb^{2+} ions indicating its specificity for the colorimetric detection of Fe^{2+} ions.

To investigate the optical properties of the formed aggregates, the ultraviolet-visible spectra of the resultant Fe^{2+}- silver colloidal solution have been recorded (Figure 3). The recorded optical spectra depicts that the addition of Fe^{2+} ion at 2-100 µM concentration does not shift the peak of silver colloidal solution at 408 nm while an increase in the absorbance of the band is observed with distortion in the band shape indicating the formation of aggregates. The increase in the absorbance value is directly proportional to concentration of Fe^{2+} ions in the medium upto 60 µM concentrations. Beyond 60 µM concentration, the absorbance value decreases but it is still greater than the control silver colloidal solution. This could also be accounted by the Beer Lambert's law.

The observations of the present study shows that ultrasonic assisted method of synthesising silver nanoparticles is a highly efficient, user friendly, cost effective, reproducible and ecofriendly approach for the synthesis of metallic nanoparticles like silver. In addition, the silver nanoparticles functionalized by proteins like bovine serum albumin can be a promising cost effective rapid colorimetric sensing system for the detection of trace levels of Fe^{2+} ions in the aqueous solution with high sensitivity which can be observed even by the naked eye.

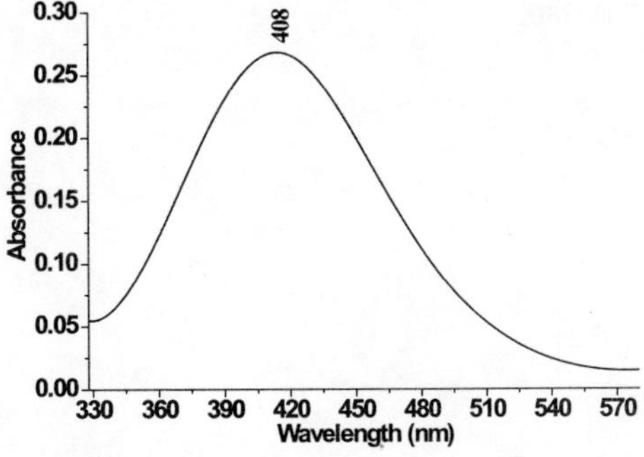

Figure 1. Recorded ultraviolet-visible spectrum of the synthesised silver nanoparticles functionalized by BSA

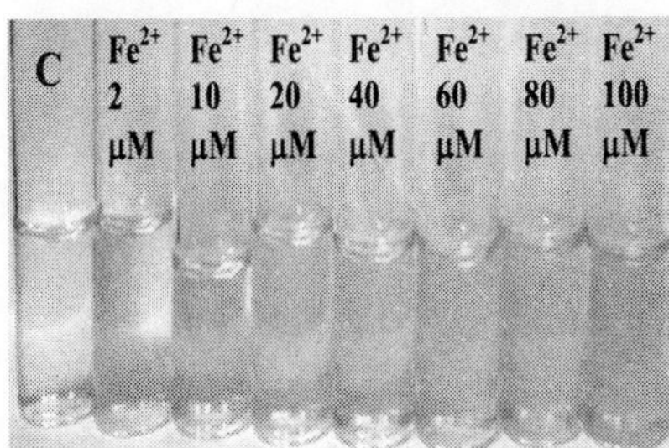

Figure 2. Silver colloidal solution containing different concentrations (2-100 µM) Fe^{2+} ions.

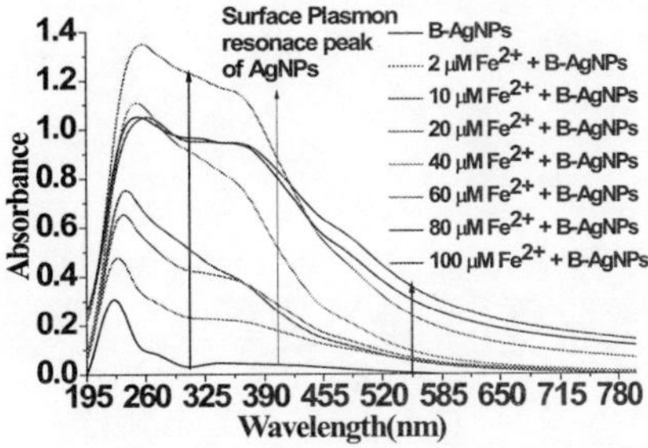

Figure 3. Recorded ultraviolet-visible spectra of the silver colloidal solution mixed with different concentration of Fe^{2+} ions in the spectral region 200-800 nm.

4.   References

1.   A. K. Bhardwaj, A. Shukla, K. N. Uttam, and R. Gopal, Biosynthesis and characterization of silver nanoparticles by surface enhanced Raman spectroscopy, Proceedings of National Laser Symposium (NLS-26), BARC, Mumbai, 20-23 Dec, 2017, CP-10.18

2.   Abhishek Shukla, Abhishek K. Bhardwaj, Sweta Sharma, K. N. Uttam and R. Gopal, Synthesis, structural and optical properties of Manganese Oxide nanoparticles, Proceedings of National Laser Symposium (NLS-26), BARC, Mumbai, 20-23 Dec, 2017, CP-06.01

3.   Abhishek Shukla, Abhishek K. Bhardwaj, S.C Singh, K. N. Uttam, Nisha Gautam, A. K. Himanshu, Jyoti Shah, R. K. Kotnala and R. Gopal, Microwave assisted scalable synthesis of titanium ferrite nanomaterials, Journal of Applied Physics, 123, 161411 (2018)

4.   Abhishek Kumar Bhardwaj, Abhishek Shukla, Shweta Maurya, Subhash Chandra Singh, Kailash N Uttam, Shanthy Sundaram, Mohan P Singh, Ram Gopal, Direct sunlight enabled photo-biochemical synthesis of silver nanoparticles and their Bactericidal Efficacy: Photon energy as key for size and distribution control, Journal of Photochemistry and Photobiology B: Biology, 188, 42-49 (2018)

5.   S Maurya, A K Bhardwaj, K K Gupta, S Agarwal, A Kushwaha, V Chaturvedi, R K Pathak, R Gopal, K N Uttam, A K Singh, V Verma and M P Singh, Green synthesis of silver nanoparticles using Pluerotus and its Bactericidal Activity, Cellular and Molecular Biology, Cell Mol Biol 62, 3, (2016)

6.   Abhishek Shukla, Abhishek K. Bhardwaj, S.C. Singh, K.N. Uttam and R. Gopal, PVA-assisted pulsed laser ablation synthesized manganese ferrite nanomaterials, Proceedings of National Laser Symposium (NLS-5) KIIT, Bhubneshwar, 20-23 Dec 2016, CP-6.16

7.   Abhishek K. Bhardwaj, Abhishek Shukla, Rohit K. Mishra, S. C. Singh, Vani Mishra, K. N. Uttam, Mohan P. Singh, Shivesh Sharma and R. Gopal, Power and time dependent microwave assisted fabrication of silver nanoparticles decorated cotton (SNDC) fibers for bacterial decontamination, Frontiers in Microbiology 8: 330, 2017, doi: 10.3389/fmicb.2017.00330.

Theoretical Perspective of Modified Nucleic Bases Stability While Interacting with Boron Nitride Graphene

Asheesh Kumar* and Devesh Kumar

Department of Physics, Babasaheb Bhimrao Ambedkar University (A Central University), Lucknow (U.P.) 226025, INDIA
*E-mail: akdap235@gmail.com

ABSTRACT

Graphene, a two dimensional material has been a word of mouth among the researchers due to its wide range of applications like high electron mobility and its inherent ability to interact with other molecules. Graphene has been used as a promising candidate for biosensors. Modified nucleic bases (MNBs) like Uric acid (UA), Caffeine (CAF), Hypoxanthine (HX), and Xanthine (X) were subjected to interact with boron nitride graphene. In this study, we report the interaction of the modified nucleic bases with Boron Nitride graphene (BNG) using the density functional theory (DFT) calculations. Highly benchmarked basis sets have been used to calculate the single point energy calculation and to explore the interaction between the boron nitride graphene and modified nucleic bases.

Keywords: Boron Nitride Graphene (BNG) and Modified Nucleic Bases (MNBs).

1.   Introduction

Graphene, a mono-atomic thick material owing sp_2 bonded carbon atoms seems to be in a honeycomb fashion. Graphene of nanometer size exhibits some remarkable chemical and electronic properties [1,2]. It also shows some noteworthy thermal and mechanical strength[3,4]. Graphene has been used for various applications like biosensors [5,6], chemical sensors[7], transparent conductors[8] and finds a range of biological applications. It is well known that the graphene of nanometer size owes a low hydrophobicity, its edges however are quite polar and faces are significantly more hydrophobic in nature [9-12] and it also can pass through the biological systems.

Noncovalent interactions have the significant role for the molecular self assembly and molecular recognition. The various components are responsible for the noncovalent interactions like electrostatic, hydrogen bonding, van der Walls and stacking interactions. Among these components, the dispersion interaction which is the main part of the van der Waals interaction among the non polar molecules plays the key role. It is well established that the dispersion interaction that pervades between the amino acid and DNA, RNA bases in stacked position can sometimes be higher or approximately equal to the strength of H-bonding. Various DNA sensors have been proposed that uses the pi-pi interaction [13,14].

Gowtham et al. [15] utilized the DFT formalism incorporating the pseudo potential for the plane wave taking into account of the periodic lattice of the graphene-nucleobases complexes. Varghese et al. [16] optimized the geometries of graphene nucleobases complexes by employing the H-F method. Sastry et al. [17] established that the interaction energy depends upon the curvature. They studied the CNTS of different diameters and different graphene models by employing the ONIOM methodology as implement in Gaussian 09 software package[18]. Singh et al. [19] showcased the interaction of graphene with the green house gases using the density functional theory. Kumar et al.[20] utilized the density functional theory to study the interaction of nucleic bases with carbon nanotube.

2.   Computational Methods

In the present work, boron nitride graphene model consisting of 21 Nitrogen and 21 Boron atoms have been considered in this study to explore the interaction with the modified nucleic bases. The full geometry optimizations have been performed using the Gaussian 09 software package. Initially all the geometries were subjected to the optimization followed by the single point energy calculations. All the geometries were optimized at M06-2X/6-31+G**. The single point energy were calculated at three different basis sets M06-2X/6-311+G**, WB97XD/6-311+G** and B3LYP-D/6-311+G** to have a greater insights on the interaction.

The interaction energies (I.E.) were calculated by using the formula

$$I.E. = \left[E_{AB} - (E_A + E_B) \right] \tag{4.1}$$

where E_{AB} is energy of the complex formed between MNBs and boron nitride graphene, E_A is the energy of the boron nitride graphene and E_B is the energy of the MNBs.

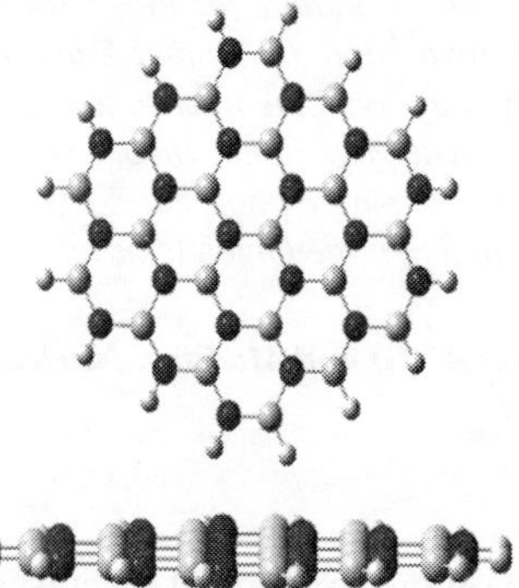

Figure 1. Optimized geometry of the Boron Nitride Graphene (BNG) (Top and Lateral View).

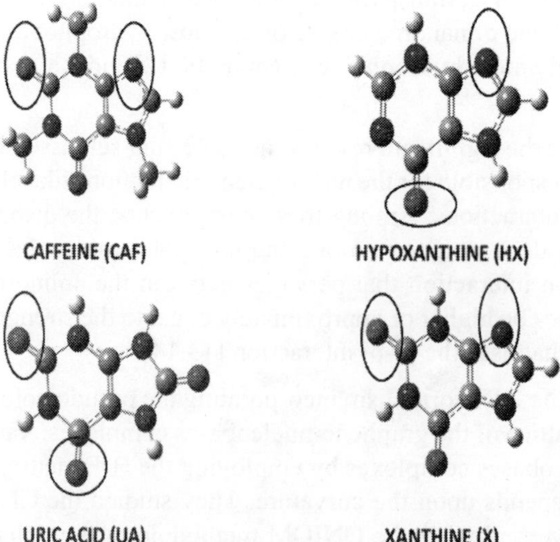

Figure 2. Optimized geometries of the Modified nucleic bases with active sites (encircled).

DNA and RNA are comprised of purine bases i.e. Adenine and guanine. Hypoxanthine, uric acid and xanthine are oxidation products that may be found in the purine metabolism of the humans. On drinking the coffee and tea, caffeine is introduced into our body. Serious health diseases like pneumonia, gout, hyperuricaemia, xanthinuria etc., the levels of these modified nucleobases like uric acid, caffeine, hypoxanthine, and caffeine from the samples of bold and urine proved to be strong indicators to detect such states. Hence the clinical prediction of these indicator levels with accuracy is essential.

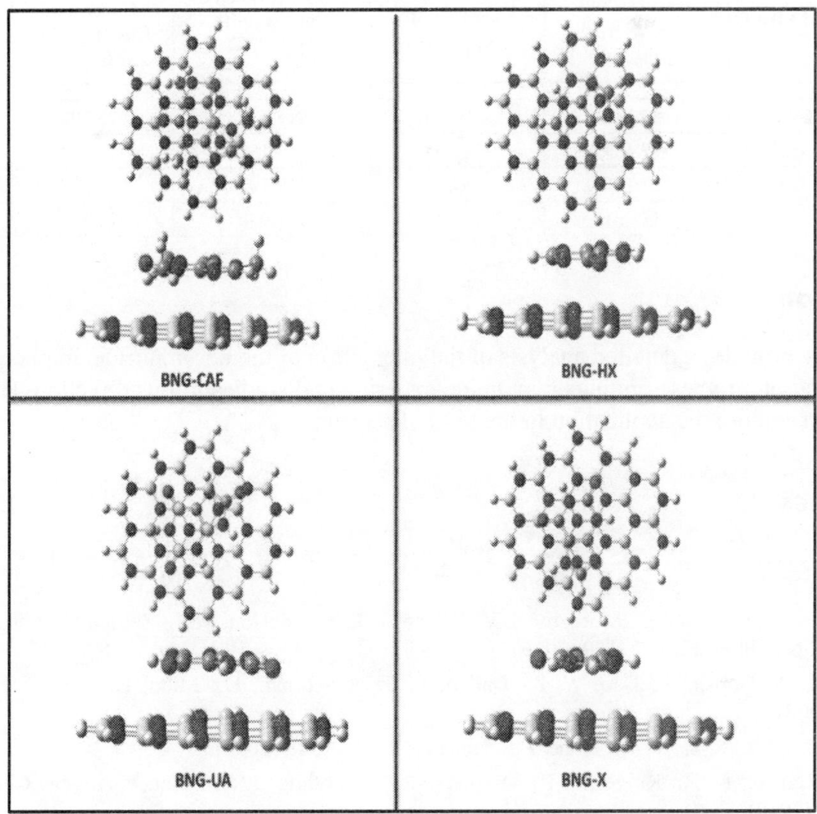

Figure 3. Interaction of modified nucleic bases with boron nitride graphene (Top and side views).

3.   Results and Discussion

The active centers of the MNBs were placed parallel to the graphene surface at a certain distance around 3Å. The set of geometries obtained in this way were optimized at M06-2X/6-31+G** level. It is quite noteworthy that all the MNBs interacted with the different graphene models via the π-π (stacking) interaction. The interaction energies calculated are shown in Table 1. The interaction energies were corrected for the basis set superposition error (BSSE). The interaction energy of all the complex systems were calculated and thereafter were corrected for the basis set superposition error (BSSE). The preferential order of binding of the modified nucleic bases is different for the three basis sets considered in this study. The order is CAF>UA>X>HX for the basis set B3LYPD, CAF>UA>HX>X for basis set WB97XD, while for M062X it is CAF>UA>X>HX. The HOMO LUMO gap is the gap between the highest occupied molecular orbital and the lowest unoccupied molecular orbital. It ranges from 6.70 to 7.30 eV.

Table 1. Calculated interaction energy (kcal/mol) of MNBs with Boron Nitride Graphene (BNG) at M06-2X/6-311++G**(BS1) and WB97XD/6-31++G** (BS2) and B3LYPD/6-31++G**(BS3) with and without basis set superposition error (BSSE).

Model	MNBs	BSSE Uncorrected Energy with M06-2X	BSSE corrected Energy with M06-2X	BSSE corrected Energy with WB97XD	BSSE Corrected Energy with B3LYPD	HOMO LUMO Gap in eV
BNG	CAF	-22.195	-18.220	-25.076	-25.302	6.967
	HX	-17.489	-13.903	-18.158	-18.134	7.309
	UA	-18.770	-15.055	-19.102	-19.328	6.701
	X	-17.491	-13.984	-17.970	-18.136	7.305

4. Conclusion

The present study provides a detailed analysis of the interaction of the boron nitride graphene with modified nucleic bases. Therefore, these findings may guide experimental studies in this direction. Hence, this study may be helpful to explore the application in the field of sensors.

5. References

1.   Hernández Rosas, J. J.; Ramírez Gutiérrez, R. E.; Escobedo- Morales, A.; Chigo Anota, E. J. Mol. Model., 17, 1133−1139 (2011).

2.   Novoselov, K. S.; McCann, E.; Morozov, S. V.; Fal'ko, V. I.; Katsnelson, M. I.; Zeitler, U.; Jiang, D.; Schedin, F.; Geim, A. K. Nat. Phys., 2, 177−180 (2016).

3.   Balandin, A. A; Ghosh, S.; Bao, W. Z.; Calizo, I.; Teweldebrhan, D.; Miao, F.; Lau, C. N. Nano Lett., 8, 902−907(2008).

4.   Lee, C.; Wei, X. D.; Kysar, J. W.; Hone, J. Science , 321, 385−388 (2008).

5.   Yang, W.; Ratinac, K. R.; Ringer, S. P.; Thordarson, P.; Gooding, J. J.; Braet, F. Angew. Chem., Int. Ed., 49, 2114−2138 (2010).

6.   Shao, Y.; Wang, J.; Wu, H.; Liu, J.; Aksay, I. A.; Lin, Y. Electroanalysis, 22, 1027−1036 (2010).

7.   Fowler, J. D.; Allen, M. J.; Tung, V. C.; Yang, Y.; Kaner, R. B.; Weiller, B. H. ACS Nano, 3, 301−306 (2009).

8.   Wassei, J. K.; Kaner, R. B. Mater. Today, 13, 52−59 (2010).

9.   Yang, H.; Fung, S. Y.; Pritzker, M.; Chen, P. PLoS One, 2, e1325 (2007).

10.   Panigrahi, S.; Bhattacharya, A.; Bandyopadhyay, D.; Grabowski, S. J.; Bhattacharyya, D.; Banerjee, S. J. Phys. Chem. C., 115, 14819−14826 (2011).

11.   Banerjee, S.; Sardar, M.; Gayathri, N.; Tyagi, A. K.; Raj, B. Phys. Rev. B, 72, 075418 (2005).

12.   Banerjee, S.; Bhattacharyya, D. Comput. Mater. Sci., 44, 41−45 (2008).

13.   Brett, A. M. O.; Chiorcea, A. M. Langmuir, 19, 3830− 3839 (2003).

14.   Akca, S.; Foroughi, A.; Frochtzwajg, D.; Postma, H. W. C. PLoS ONE, 6, e18442 (2011).

15.   Gowtham, S.; Scheicher, R. H.; Ahuja, R.; Pandey, R.; Karna, S. P. Phys. Rev. B, 76, 033401 (2007).

16.   Varghese, N.; Mogera, U.; Govindaraj, A.; Das, A.; Maiti, P. K.; Sood, A. K.; Rao, C. N. Chemphyschem., 1, 206−210 (2009).

17.   Umadevi, D.; Sastry, G. N. J. Phys. Chem. Lett., 2, 1572−1576 (2011).

18.   Gaussian 09, Revision A.02, M. J. Frisch, G. W. Trucks, H. B. Schlegel, G. E. Scuseria, M. A. Robb, J. R. Cheeseman, G. Scalmani, V. Barone, B. Mennucci, G. A. Petersson, H. Nakatsuji, M. Caricato, X. Li, H. P. Hratchian, A. F. Izmaylov, J. Bloino, G. Zheng, J. L. Sonnenberg, M. Hada, M. Ehara, K. Toyota, R. Fukuda, J.

Hasegawa, M. Ishida, T. Nakajima, Y. Honda, O. Kitao, H. Nakai, T. Vreven, J. A. Montgomery, Jr., J. E. Peralta, F. Ogliaro, M. Bearpark, J. J. Heyd, E. Brothers, K. N. Kudin, V. N. Staroverov, R. Kobayashi, J. Normand, K. Raghavachari, A. Rendell, J. C. Burant, S. S. Iyengar, J. Tomasi, M. Cossi, N. Rega, J. M. Millam, M. Klene, J. E. Knox, J. B. Cross, V. Bakken, C. Adamo, J. Jaramillo, R. Gomperts, R. E. Stratmann, O. Yazyev, A. J. Austin, R. Cammi, C. Pomelli, J. W. Ochterski, R. L. Martin, K. Morokuma, V. G. Zakrzewski, G. A. Voth, P. Salvador, J. J. Dannenberg, S. Dapprich, A. D. Daniels, O. Farkas, J. B. Foresman, J. V. Ortiz, J. Cioslowski, D. J. Fox, Gaussian, Inc., Wallingford CT, (2009).

19. D. Singh, A. Kumar, D. Kumar, Bull. Mater. Sci., 40, 1263 (2017).

20. A. Kumar, D. Singh, D. Kumar, D. Kumar, Adv. Sci. Lett., 24, 802 (2018).

Challenges of Nanotechnology; Nanomedicine: Nanorobots

Alok Kumar Dash*, Jhansee Mishra

Department of Pharmacy, V.B.S. Purvanchal University, U.P., India
*E-mail: alokkudash@yahoo.co.in

ABSTRACT

Nanotechnology is a fascinating science for many scientists as it offers them many challenges. One such challenge is Nanorobots, which once thought to be a fantasy has come into reality now. The proposed application of nanorobots can range from common cold to dreadful disease like cancer. Some such examples can be Respirocyte, Microbivores, Chromallocyte and many more. The study of nanorobots has lead to the field of Nanomedicine. Nanomedicine offers the prospect of powerful new tools for the treatment of human diseases and the improvement of human biological systems. Thepresent era of Nanotechnology has reached to a stage where scientists are able to develop programmable and externally controllable complex machines that are built at molecular level which can work inside the patient's body. By the help of nanotechonology engineers prepare nano robot which navigate the human body, transport important molecules, manipulate microscopic objects and communicate with physicians by way of miniature sensors, motors, manipulators, power generators and molecular-scale computers. Nanorobots have remarkable applications in health care and environmental monitoring. In future, nanorobots will be useful or applicable in treating various diseases like cancer, diabetes, tumour or respiration related diseases.

1.   Introduction

1.1   What Are Nanorobots

Nanorobots are nanoelectromechanical systems designed to perform a specific task with precision at nanoscale dimensions. Its advantage over conventional medicine lies on its size. Particle size has effect on serum lifetime and pattern of deposition. This allows drugs of nanosize to be used in lower concentration and has an earlier onset of therapeutic action. It also provides materials for controlled drug delivery by directing carriers to a specific location. The typical medical nanodevice will probably be a micronscale robot assembled from nanoscale parts (WiseGEEK, n.d.). Nanorobots will be used for maintaining and protecting the human body against pathogens. They will have a diameter of about 0.5 to 3 microns and will be constructed out of parts with dimensions in the range of 1 to 100 nanometres. The main element used will be carbon in the form of *diamond*-because of the strength and chemical inertness of these forms (Bhargava, n.d.) (Figure 1).

1.2   Types of Nanorobots

Various forms of nanorobots are used in different field, but in medical field we use only three main types of nanorobots are (Freitas, 1998):

1.   Respirocyte - An Artificial Oxygen Carrier Nanorobot

2.   Microbivores Nanorobots Artificial Phagocytes

3.   Chromallocyte Mobile Cell-Repair Nanorobot

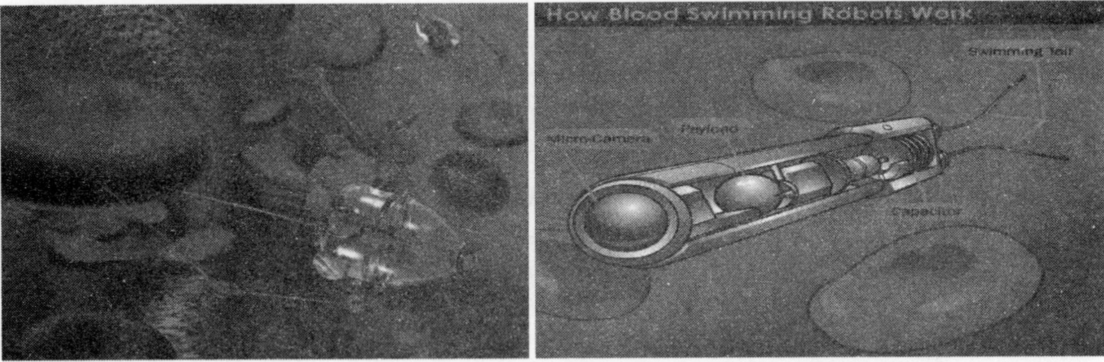

Figure 1 Nanorobots with Red Blood Cells (Google, n.d.a) **Figure 2.** Nanorobots in Blood Stream (Google, n.d.a)

1.3   Components of Nanorobots

The various components in the nanorobot design may include onboard sensors, motors, manipulators, power supplies, and molecular computers (Figure 2). Here are afew of the items you might find inside a nanorobot:

1.3.1. Medicine Cavity

A hollow section inside the nanorobot might hold small doses of medicine or chemicals. The robot could release medication directly to the site of injury or infection.

1.3.2. Probes, Knives and Chisels

To remove blockages and plaque, a nanorobot will need something to grab and break down material. They might also need a device to crush clots into very small pieces.

1.3.3. Microwave Emitters and Ultrasonic SignalGenerators

To destroy cancerous cells, doctors need methods that can kill a cell without rupturing it. A ruptured cancer cell might release chemicals that could cause the cancer tospread further.

1.3.4. Electrodes

Two electrodes protruding from the nanorobot could kill cancer cells by generating an electric current, heating the cell up until it dies (Strickland, n.d.a).

1.3.5. Lasers

Tiny, powerful lasers could burn away harmful material like arterial plaque, cancerous cells or blood clots. The lasers would literally vaporise the tissue. The two biggest challenges and concerns scientists have regarding these small tools are: How to making them effective and safe. For instance, creating a small laser powerful enough to vaporise cancerous cells is a big challenge, but designing it so that the nanorobot doesn't harm surrounding healthy tissue makes the task even more difficult. While many scientific teams have developed nanorobots small enough to enter the bloodstream but that is only the first step to making nanorobots (Strickland,).

1.4   Approaches for the Construction of Nanorobots

There are two main approaches to building at the nanometer scale: Positional assembly

•   Self-Assembly

1.5　Mechanism of Action

Different molecule types are distinguished by a series of chemotactic sensors whose binding sites have a different affinity for each kind of molecule. The control system must ensure a suitable performance. The target has surface chemicals allowing the nanorobots to detect and recognize it (Wasielewski et al, 1997; Hazana et al, 2000 and Curtis et al, 2006). Manufacturing better sensors and actuators with nanoscale sizes makes them find the source of release of the chemical. A Software called Nanorobot Control Design (NCD) simulator was developed for nanorobots in an environments with fluids dominated by Brownian motion and viscous rather than inertial forces

1.6　Uses

Currently nanorobots are used in:

- Cancer Detection and Treatment,· Diagnosis and Treatment of Diabetes
- Controlling Glucose Level,To cure skin diseases, a cream containing nanorobots may be used

In future nanorobots may be used:

- To seek and break kidney stones
- To locate atherosclerotic lesions in blood vessels'(Leary et al, 2006)
- In surgeries
- Nanorobots equipped, with Nanosensors, could be developed to deliver anti-HIV drugs (Menezes et al, 2001)
- In cell targeted delivery
- In treatments for hypoxemia and respiratory illness, dentistry (Requicha, 2003), bacterial infections, physical trauma, gene therapy via chromosome replacement therapy etc.

1.7　Scope of the Nanorobots (Bhargava, n.d.)

Nanorobotics is concerned with:

- Manipulation of nanoscale objects by using micro or macro devices
- Construction and programming of robots with overall dimensions at the nanoscale (or with microscopic dimensions but nanoscopic components) Its advantage over conventional medicine lies on its size. Particle size has effect on serum lifetime and pattern of deposition. This allows drugs of nanosize to be used in lower concentration and has an earlier onset of therapeutic action. It also provides materials for controlled drug delivery by directing carriers to a specific location (WiseGEEK, n.d.). The typical medical nanodevice will probably be a micron-scale robot assembled from nanoscale parts. These nanorobots can work together in response to environment stimuli and programmed principles to produce macro scale results (Freitas, 1998)

2.2　Design of Nanorobots

The various components in the nanorobot design may include onboard sensors, motors, manipulators, power supplies, and molecular computers (Figure 3). Many light elements such as hydrogen, sulphur, oxygen, nitrogen, fluorine, silicon, etc. will be used for special purposes in nanoscale gears and other components (Freitas, 1998).Drexler (1981) evidently was the first to point out, that complex devices resemble biological models in theirstructural components. The manipulator arm can also be driven by a detailed sequence of control signals, just as the ribosome needs mRNA to guide its actions. These control signals are provided by external acoustic, electrical or chemical signals that are received by the robot arm via an onboard sensor using a simple "Broadcast Architecture" (Drexler, 1992; Bryson et al, 1995 and Freitas, 1996a), a technique which can also be used to import power. Biological cell may be regarded as an example of a broadcast architecture in which the nucleus of the cell send signals in the form of mRNA to ribosomes in order to manufacture cellular proteins. Assemblers are molecular achine systems that could be described as systems capable of performing molecular manufacturing at the atomic scale whichrequires control signals provided by an onboard nanocomputer. This programmable nanocomputer must be able to accept stored instructions, which are sequentially executed to direct the manipulator arm to place the correct moiety or nanopart in the desired position and orientation, thus giving precise control over the timing and locations of chemical reactions or assembly operations (Bryson et al, 1995).

2.3   Powering of Nanorobots (Strickland, n.d.b)

Just like the navigation systems, these are used as power sources both internal & external. Nanorobots could get power directly from the bloodstream. A nanorobot could use the patient's body heat to create power but there would need to be a gradient of temperatures to manage it. Power generation would be a result of the Seebeck effect like the joining of two different conductors at different temperatures.

2.4   Nanorobots' Pharmacological Action Mechanism

The target has surface chemicals allowing the nanorobots to detect and recognize it. manufacturing better sensors and actuators with nanoscale sizes makes them find the source of release of the chemical. NCD simulator was developed, which is software for nanorobots in environments with fluids dominated by Brownian motion and viscous rather than inertial forces. First, as a point of comparison, the scientists used the nanorobots' small Brownian motions to find the target by random search. In a second method, the nanorobots monitor for chemical concentration significantly above the background level. After detecting the signal, a nanorobot estimates the concentration gradient and moves toward higher concentrations until it reaches the target. In the third approach, nanorobots at the target release another chemical, which others use as an additional guiding signal to the target. With these signal concentrations, only nanorobots passing within a few microns of the target are likely to detect the signal (Hazana et al, 2000 and Leary et al, 2006).

2.5   Strategies Employed by Nanorobots for Evading the

Immune System

Every medical nanorobot placed inside the human body will encounter phagocyticcells many times during its mission. Thus all Nanorobots, which are of a size capable of ingestion by phagocytic cells, must incorporate physical mechanisms and operational protocols for avoiding and escaping from phagocytes. The initial strategy for medical nanorobots is first to avoid phagocytic contact or recognition. The most direct approach for a fully functional medical nanorobot is to employ its motility mechanisms to locomote out of, or away from, the phagocytic cell that is attempting to engulf it. This may involve reverse cytopenetration, which must be done cautiously (e.g., the rapid exit of nonenveloped viruses from cells can be cytotoxic). Medical nanorobots, therefore, may also need to employ simple but active defensive strategies to forestall granuloma formation. In a clinical environment, another option would be externally supplied acoustic energy. When the task of the nanorobots is completed, they can be retrieved by allowing them to exfuse themselves via the usual human excretory channels or can also be removed by active scavenger systems (Freitas, 2005 and Drexler, 1986).

2.6 Different Forms of Nanorobots

2.6.1. Respirocytes (Drexler, 1992)

The artificial mechanical red cell, "Respirocyte" (Figure 4) is an imaginary nanorobot, floats along in the blood stream. These atoms are mostly carbon atoms arranged as diamond in a porous lattice structure inside the sphDrexleral shell. The Respirocyte is essentially a tiny pressure tank that can be pumped full of oxygen (O_2) and carbon dioxide (CO_2) molecules. Later on, these gases can be released from the tiny tank in a controlled manner. The gases are stored onboard at pressures up to about 1000 atmospheres. There are also gas concentration sensors on the outside of each device. When the nanorobot passes through the lung capillaries, O_2 partial pressure will be high and CO_2 partial pressure as low, so the onboard computer tells the sorting rotors to load the tanks with oxygen and to dump the CO_2. Therefore, the injection of a 5 cm3 dose of 50% Respirocyte aqueous suspension into the bloodstream can exactly replace the entire O_2 and CO_2 carrying capacity of the patient's entire 5,400 cm3 (5.4Litres) of blood. Respirocyte will have pressure sensors to receive acoustic signals from the doctor, who will use an ultrasound-like transmitter device to give the Respirocyte commands to modify their behaviour while they are still inside the patient's body (Freitas, 2005)

2.6.1.1. Mechanism of Respirocytes

These devices have sensors on the surface, which can detect changes in the environment and the onboard minicomputer will regulate the intake and output of the oxygen and carbon dioxide molecules. Reciprocates exchange gasses via molecular sorting rotors. The rotors have specially shaped tips to catch particular types of molecules. Gas molecules are stored tightly in tanks. Each respirocyte has three types of rotors. One gathers oxygen at the lungs or in production before introduction to the body and releases it while travelling through the body. Another captures carbon dioxide while in the bloodstream and releases it at the lungs. The third takes in glucose from the bloodstream, which is burned in a reaction similar tocellular respiration in order to power the respirocyte (Freitas, 1996b).

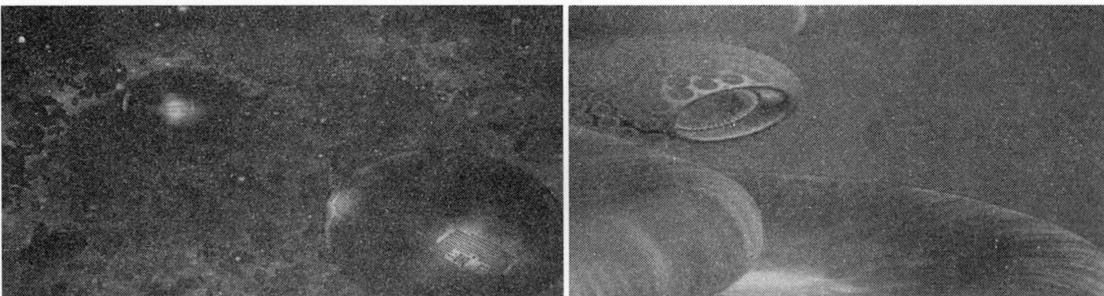

Fig. 4 Respirocytes with Red Blood Stream in Blood Stream **Fig. 5** Microbivores with Red Blood Stream in Blood Stream

2.6.2. Microbivores (Artificial Phagocytes)

A microbivore (Figure 5) has been described, whose primary function is to destroy microbiological pathogens found in the human bloodstream, using the "digest and discharge" protocol. Nanorobotic artificial hypothetical phagocytes called "Microbivores" could patrol the bloodstream, seeking out and digesting unwanted pathogens including bacteria, viruses, or fungi. Microbivores when given intravenously (I.V) would achieve complete clearance of even the most severe septicemic infections in hours or less. (Drexler, 1992). This "digest and discharge" protocol is conceptually similar to the internalization and digestion process practiced by natural phagocytes, except that the artificial process should be much faster and cleaner. For example, it is well known that macrophages release biologically active compounds during bacteriophagy, whereas well-designed microbivores need only release biologically inactive effluent (Drexler, 1986).

2.6.3. Chromallocyte (Mobile Cell Repair Nanorobots)(Freitas, 2007)

Another nanorobot, the Chromallocyte (Figure 6) would replace entire chromosomes in individual cells thus reversing the effects of genetic disease and other accumulated damage to our genes, preventing aging. Chromallocyte is a hypothetical mobile cell-repair nanorobot, capable of limited vascular surface travel into the capillary bed of the targeted tissue or organ, followed by extravasation, histonatation, cytopenetration, and complete chromatin replacement in the nucleus of one target cell, and ending with a return to the bloodstream and subsequent extraction of the device from the body, completing the cell repair mission. Inside a cell, repair machine will first size up the situation by examining the cell's contents and activity, and then take action by working along molecule-by-molecule and structure-by structure; repair machines will be able to repair the whole cell. By working along cell-by-cell and tissue-by-tissue, they (aided by larger devices, where need be) will be able to repair whole organs. By working through a person, organ by organ, they will restore health. Because molecular machines will be able to build molecules and cells from scratch, they will be able to repair even cells damaged to the point of complete inactivity (Robert et al, 2007).

2.6.3.1. Mechanism of the Chromallocyte

The 3 hours chromosome replacement process to be performed by each chromallocyte during Phase IV includes a 26-step sequence of distinct semi-autonomous sensor-driven activities, described below (Scribd, n.d.):

2.6.3.1.1. Injection

The nanorobots are introduced through a flexible telescoping nanocannula(similar to transdermal microcannula but including biochemical and chemotactic nanosensors and nanomotorized guidance) into a small blood vessel located near the target organ.

2.6.3.1.2. Extravasation

The nanorobots employ controlled diapedesis to penetrate the local endothelium of the capillary bed nearest to or within the target organ to gain entry into the tissues.

2.6.3.1.3. ECM immigration

The nanorobots proceed through the Extra Cellular Matrix (ECM), if transit through a cellular tissue is required,moving toward the target cell.

2.6.3.1.4. Cytopenetration

Upon reaching its target cell, the chromallocyte fully enters the cell by cytopenetrating through the plasma membrane and minimal leakage.

2.6.3.1.5. Block Mechanotransduction

Mechanical deformation of the plasma membrane or nuclear envelope can transmit signals either into the nucleus, altering gene expression or into the cytoskeleton, eliciting reaction from cell signalling pathways in the cytosolic compartment.

2.6.3.1.6. Nuclear Localization

Once inside the cell, the chromallocyte exposes, at the anterior end of the device, a set of semaphores, which will bind to outer nuclear membrane (ONM) surface but to no other surface inside the cell.

2.6.3.1.7. Nucleopenetration

The Inner Nuclear Membrane (INM) is lined and stabilized by the nuclear lamina layer, which constitutes a filamentous protein meshwork of 20-80 nm deep.

2.6.3.1.8. Block Apoptosis

Chromallocyte activities that surgically remove DNA from cells resemble mechanical or chemical injuries to chromosomes and appurtenant protein structures that can trigger cell apoptosis.

2.6.3.1.9. Block DNA Repairs

Chromallocyte activities in the nucleus could be misinterpreted by natural biological systems as causing "damage".

2.6.3.1.10. Block Inflammation Signals

Necrotic or damaged cells release signal molecules such as the chromatin-associated High Mobility Group Box 1

(HMGB1) protein that binds with high affinity to RAGE (the Receptor for Advanced Glycation End-products). RAGE exists on the extracellular surface of endothelial cells, smooth muscle cells, mesangial cells, mononuclear phagocytes and certain neurons and thus is a potent mediator of inflammation outside the cell that must be blocked.

2.6.3.1.11. Deactivate Transcription

DNA transcription activities in the nucleus (producing mRNA for export to cytoplasm) must be halted, although ribosomal translation of extant mRNA into protein will continue in the extra nuclear compartment. Chromatin organization does not require ongoing transcription.

2.6.3.1.12. Detach Chromatin

The nanorobot can use molecular sorting rotors to assimilate all free molecules of the synthetic caspase-6- specific inhibitor released earlier. Lamina-Associated Polypeptide (LAP2), a DNA binding protein too, proteolysis might be required for the complete detachment of chromatin from the nuclear envelope.

2.7   Applications of Nanorobots

Some possible applications using nanorobots (respirocytes) are as follows (Drexler, 1981):

2.7.1. Transfusions & Perfusions

Respirocytes may be used as the active oxygen-carrying component of a universally transfusable blood substitute that is free of disease vectors such as hepatitis, venereal disease, malarial parasites or AIDS, storable indefinitely and readily available with no need for cross-matching.

2.7.2. Treatment of Anemia (Drexler, 1981)

Oxygenating respirocytes offer complete or partial symptomatic treatment for virtually all forms of anemia.

2.7.3. Fetal and Child-Related Disorders

Respirocytes may be useful in perinatal medicine, as for example infusions of device suspension to treat fetal anemia (erythroblastosis fetalis), neonatal hemolytic disease.

2.7.4. Respiratory Diseases

The devices could provide an effective long-term drug-free symptomatic treatment for asthma, and could assist in the treatment of hemotoxic (pit viper) and neurotoxic (coral) snake bites; hypoxia, stress polycythemia and lung disorders. Respirocytes could also be used to treat conditions of low oxygen availability to nerve tissue, as occurs in advanced atherosclerotic narrowing of arteries, strokes, diseased or injured reticular formation in the medulla oblongata (controlling autonomic respiration).

2.7.5. Cardiovascular and Neurovascular Applications(Drexler, 1981)

Respirocyte perfusion could be useful in maintaining tissue oxygenation during anesthesia, coronary angioplasty, organ transplantation, siamese-twin separation, other aggressive heart and brain surgical procedures, in postsurgical cardiac function recovery, and in cardiopulmonary bypass solutions.

2.7.6. Tumour Therapy and Diagnostics (Freitas, 1996b)

Cancer patients are usually anemic. X-rays and many chemotherapeutic agents require oxygen to be maximally cytoxic, so boosting systemic oxygenation levels into the normal range using respirocytes might improve prognosis and treatment outcome. The technique can also be used to eliminate the tumours. The specified goal will be able to destroy timorous tissue in such a way as to minimize the risk of causing or allowing a recurrence of the growth in the body. The technique is intended to be able to treat tumours that cannot be accessed via conventional surgery, such as deep brain tumours (Requicha, 2003).

2.8. Other Applications

Nanorobots are also applicable in many other diseases like: The development of nanorobots may provide remarkable advances for diagnosis and treatment of cancer. Glucose carried through the blood stream is important to maintain the human metabolism working healthfully, and its correct level is a key issue in the diagnosis and treatment of diabetes.

- A mouthwash full of smart nanomachines could identify and destroy pathogenic bacteria while allowing the harmless flora of the mouth to flourish in a healthy ecosystem (Requicha, 2003). · Medical nanodevices could augment the immune system by finding and disabling unwanted bacteria and viruses (Requicha, 2003). · Devices working in the bloodstream could nibble away at arteriosclerotic deposits, widening the affected blood vessels. This would prevent most heart attacks.

2.   Conclusion

Nanotechnology as a diagnostic and treatment tool for patients with cancer and diabetes showed that how actual developments in new manufacturing technologies are enabling innovative works, which may help in constructing and employing nanorobots most effectively for biomedical problems. Nanorobots applied to medicine hold a wealth of promise from eradicating disease to reversing the aging process (wrinkles, loss of bone mass and age related conditions are all treatable at the cellular level); nanorobots are also candidates for industrial applications. Manipulating matter at molecular scale and influencing their behaviour (dynamics and properties) is the biggest challenges for the nanorobotic systems. This field is still in very early stages of development and still a lot has to be figured out before any substantial outcome is produced. The future of bio nanorobots (molecular robots) is bright. We are at the dawn of a new era in which many disciplines will merge including robotics, mechanical, chemical and biomedical engineering, chemistry, biology, physics and mathematics so that fully functional systems could be developed. However, challenges towards such a goal abound. Developing a complete database of different biomolecular machine components and the ability to interface or assemble different machine components are some of the challenges to be faced in thenear future.

3. References

1. Bhargava, A. (n.d.) Nanorobots: Medicine of the Future [Internet]. Available from: <http://ewh.ieee.org/r10/bombay/news3/page4.html> [Accessed 30 December 2009].

2. Bryson, J.W., Betz, S.F., Lu, H.S., Suich, D.J., Zhou, H.X.,O'Neil, K.T., and DeGrado, W.F. (1995) Protein Design:A Hierarchic Approach, Science, 270, pp. 935-941.

3. Curtis, A.S.G., Dalby, M., and Gadegaard, N. (2006) Cell signaling arising from nanotopography: implications fornanomedical devices. Nanomedicine Journal, Future Medicine, 1(1), pp. 67-72.

4. Drexler, K.E. (1981) Molecular Engineering: An Approach to the Development of General Capabilities for MolecularManipulation. Proc. National Academy of Sciences, USA, 78(9), pp. 5275-5278.

5. Drexler, K.E. (1986) Engines of Creation: The Coming Era of Nanotechnology. New York, Anchor ress/Doubleday.

6. Drexler, K.E. (1992) Nanosystems: Molecular Machinery, Manufacturing, and Computation. New York, John Wiley & Sons.

7. Freitas, Jr. R.A. (1996a) Respirocytes; A Mechanical Artificial Red Cell: Exploratory Design in Medical Nanotechnology [Internet], Palo Alto, Foresight. Available from: <http://www.foresight.org/Nanomedicine/Respirocytes1.html> [Accessed 2 January 2010].

8. Freitas, Jr. R.A. (1996b) Respirocytes; A Mechanical Artificial Red Cell: Exploratory Design in MedicalNanotechnology [Internet], Palo Alto, Foresight. Available from: <http://www.foresight.org/Nanomedicine/Respirocytes4.html> [Accessed 8 January 2010].

9. Freitas, Jr. R.A. (1998) Nanomedicine [Internet], Palo Alto, Foresight. Available from: <http://www.foresight.org/Nanomedicine> [Accessed 27 December 2009].

10. Freitas, Jr. R.A. (1999) Nanomedicine, Volume I: Basic Capabilities [Internet], Georgetown, Landes Bioscience. Available from: <http://www.nanomedicine.com/NMI.htm > [Accessed 9 January 2010].

11. Freitas, Jr. R.A. (2005) Microbivores: artificial mechanical phagocytes using digest and discharge protocol. J. Evol.Technol., 14, pp. 55-106

12. Freitas, Jr. R.A. (2007) The Ideal Gene Delivery Vector: Chromallocytes, Cell Repair Nanorobots for ChromosomeReplacement Therapy. Journal of Evolution and Technology, 16, pp. 1-97.

Plasmonic Enhancement of the Photocatalytic Degradation of Methylene Blue Dye by using NiO/Ag Composite

Suresh Kumar Pandey*, Manish Kumar Tripathi, Dhanesh Tiwary

Department of Chemistry, IIT (BHU), Varanasi-221005, India
*E-mail: sureshkrpandey.rs.chy17@itbhu.ac.in

ABSTRACT

In this work, we synthesized NiO based nanocomposite (NA) with silver nanoparticle via the solvothermal method and characterized by using XRD, UV-visible, TEM, UV-DRS, as well as SEM instrumental techniques. The prepared nanocomposite was utilized for the photocatalytic degradation of methylene blue dye. The crystallite size of the composite was 31 nm obtained from XRD by Scherrer equation, and the particle size are calculated 20±5 nm from TEM analysis. The rate constant of nanocomposite (NA) correspond to methylene blue is 1.67×10^{-2} minute^{-1}. The nanocomposite NA shows an excellent efficiency for the degradation of organic dyes with visible-light and also provide stability for degradation of methylene blue in an aqueous medium.

Keywords: Photocatalysis, semiconductor, methylene blue (MB).

1.   Introduction

Synthetic organic dyes are broadly used in different kinds of industries like Textile, paint, cosmetics, drugs, food industries, etc. The effluents from these industries are directly discarded into the river or ocean, which affects the properties of water [1]. The high photochemical stability and non-biodegradable nature of these effluents are cause severe problems to the humans and also make imbalance in the aquatic ecosystem [2, 3]. Many nitrogen-containing dyes (like methylene blue, congo red, rhodamine B, and malachite green, etc.) are able to resist photolysis and generate many carcinogenic products in between the degradation process [4]. In recent time, resolving the water contamination problem is the main current issue because the whole world is facing water cries problem at a very high level. For removal of these dyes, many conventional methods (like precipitation, adsorption, chemical oxidation, coagulation-flocculation, filtration, etc.) and some biological methods were used. However, these methods suffer from some severe drawback and required further treatment [5]. So in place of the above methods, some advanced processes such as photo Fenton, semiconductor-based catalysis, Fenton, ozonolysis and photolysis through H_2O_2 are used to remove dye from water. Among all the methods, Photocatalytic processes are remarkably and more suitable techniques for the degradation of organic effluents. These processes generally utilize some oxidizing species (i.e., hydroxyl radical) in the presence of light and degrade the dyes substrate. [5]. In literature, numerous metals and their oxide (like TiO_2, Fe_2O_3, and Co_3O_4, etc.) nanoparticles were used as photocatalyst or adsorbent substrate. But they suffer from some limitations like very less transmittance of light and aggregation of nanoparticles. Resulting, dispersibility of nanoparticles is decreased along with surface area which is responsible for the weak catalytic activity of nanomaterials. The photocatalytic property mainly depends on size, the functionality of surface, defects, shape, and crystallinity of the nanoparticles [6]. A smaller nanoparticle contains a large surface area resulting to provide more active sites for photochemical reactions; thus, the efficiency of photo-catalysts is exceeded [7]. According to El- Kemary et al., NiO nanoparticles are a very active catalyst and adsorbent substrate because of their super durability, strong photosensitivity as well as its high absorptivity affinity [8].

In this work, we synthesized NiO based nanocomposite (NA) with silver nanoparticle via the solvothermal method with enhanced photocatalytic efficiency towards methylene blue degradation. The kinetic study of the degradation of methylene blue explains the photocatalytic efficiency of nickel oxide nanocomposite with respect to NiO nanoparticle.

2. Experimental

2.1 Reagents

Nickel nitrate hexahydrate $Ni(NO_3)_2 \cdot 6H_2O$, Citric acid, sodium hydroxide [NaOH] and methylene blue were purchased from Merck, India. Silver nitrate [$AgNO_3$] and $NaBH_4$ were obtained from Sigma Aldrich, India. All solutions were prepared in deionized water. The pH of solutions was maintained with the help of 0.1 M HCl and 0.1 M NaOH.

2.2 Synthesis of NiO and Ag/NiO nanoparticles

1.74 g $Ni(NO_3)_2 \cdot 6H_2O$ [0.2M] was dissolved in 30mL double distilled water. 20 mL of 0.2 M citric acid was added dropwise with adjustment of pH into it. The resulting homogeneous and transparent solution was subject to stirring via slow evaporation at 70-80 °C until a highly viscous gel was obtained. After that it was dried at 105°C for 8 hours, the collected material was ground in a pestle mortar and calcined in a muffle furnace at 400°C for 4 hours. Further, the synthesis of Ag/NiO nanocomposite was done by dispersing 0.5g NiO in 50 mL water with ultrasonication for 1h and then 10 mm of $AgNO_3$ Solution was added under stirring. After 20 min of vigorous stirring 25 mL of 20 mg $NaBH_4$ was added and kept stirring for 30 minutes. Composite was obtained by the centrifugation which was washed 3-4 times with water and ethanol. the nanocomposite was dried overnight at 70° C. Photocatalytic degradation of Methylene Blue (MB) dye was carried out in a standard quartz cuvette of 1cm path length. In this 3 ml of 2×10^{-5} M MB solution was taken. The cuvette containing the dye solution was maintained at 308 K. Then 0.33 mg of the prepared Ag/NiO was added to it and kept in cool Philips white LED photocatalytic chamber (approximately 94 mW/cm^2). The absorption spectrum of the reaction mixture was recorded after every ten-minute time interval in the range of 200-800 nm.

3. Characterization

Thermo Scientific Evolution 201 UV-Vis spectrophotometer was utilized to record the UV-Vis absorbance spectra of Ag/NiO NPs dispersed in water, and degradation measurement. X-ray diffraction pattern was obtained by Rigaku Mini-X 600 Japan. from 2θ esteem $30° - 90°$, at the output pace of 1° for every minutes and the progression size was 0.02. Transmission electron microscopy imaging of synthesized Ag/NiO NPs was done with TECNAI 20 G2-electron magnifying lens working at a voltage of 200 kV. The emission spectra were recorded from 420 nm to 800 nm at an excitation wavelength of 440 nm. The cuts widths were the same (0.4 nm) for shower excitation and discharge. The solid-state UV−visible estimations were performed by utilizing Shimadzu Pharmaspec UV-1700 model, working in 200−800 nm spectral range.

4. Results and Discussion

XRD Analysis. Fig. 1 (a) gives the X-ray diffraction pattern of the powder sample of Ag-NiO nanocomposite and NiO to identify the phase(s) formed. The crystallite size of the composite was 31 nm obtained by applying the Scherrer equation. Diffraction peaks correspond to NiO was at the 2Θ values 37.34°, 43.32°, 62.93°, and

75.48° and after addition of Ag, the most intense peak was appeared at 2Θ angle 38.13°, which confirmed the Ag phase introduced into the NiO phase (JCPDS Card No. 89-7390 and 96-110-0137 respectively). FTIR spectra [Fig. 1(b)] confirms the bonding of oxygen with Ni [9] through the appearance of a peak at 400 cm^{-1} and 850 cm^{-1} [10].

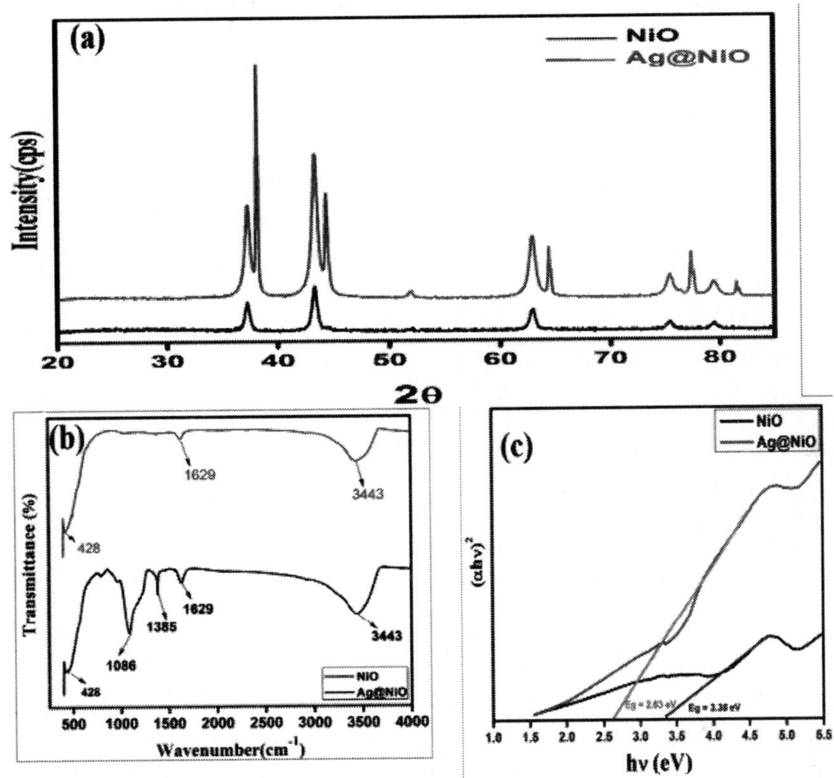

Figure 1 (a) Normalized XRD pattern of NiO & Ag/NiO; (b) FTIR spectra of Ag/ NiO NPs; (c) Band gap energy of Ag/NiO nanocomposite.

The detailed information about the grains microstructure and morphology of the synthesized nanocomposite, TEM observation was carried out. Figure 2 shows the HR-TEM images of the synthesized nanocomposite. A TEM image of this sample shows a high yield of Ag/NiO heterostructure nanocrystals consisting of metallic Ag nanoparticles and NiO nanoparticle, as presented in Fig. 2(a). The NiO nanoparticles assembled with Ag nanoparticles on the surface. Moreover, Ag aggregation are also not found in our TEM observations, indicating that all metallic Ag nanoparticles are entirely dispersed in NiO NPs. Fig. 2(b) shows the metallic Ag nanoparticle size distribution of the sample. It was evident that the diameters of nanocomposites (NA) are in the range of 12-25 nm and the average diameter of was about 18.5 nm (Fig. 2(c)). A typical magnified TEM image of an individual Ag/NiO heterostructure reveals that the metallic Ag nanoparticle is embedded in the NiO NPs (i.e., the formation of a dimer-type heterostructure). The high-resolution TEM (HRTEM) image (Fig. 2(a)) from Fig. 2b shows a distinguished interface and the continuity of lattice fringes between the NiO NPs and metallic Ag nanoparticles, confirming the formation of chemical bonds between them. It also shows the uniform lattice structure and single-crystalline nature of the NiO NPs. The spacing between adjacent lattice fringes is 0.208 nm, which is close to the d spacing of the [002] plane. On the other hand, as to the nanoparticle of the heterodimer (Fig. 2b), lattice fringes with an interplanar spacing of 0.236 nm corresponding to the [111] planes of fcc Ag are observed.

Bandgap energy of the synthesized nanocomposite was 2.63 eV calculated from Tauc plot. It indicates that this was in a visible region. The bandgap of the NiO NPs was lying in UV region (3.35 eV) which shows very less activity towards organic pollutants.

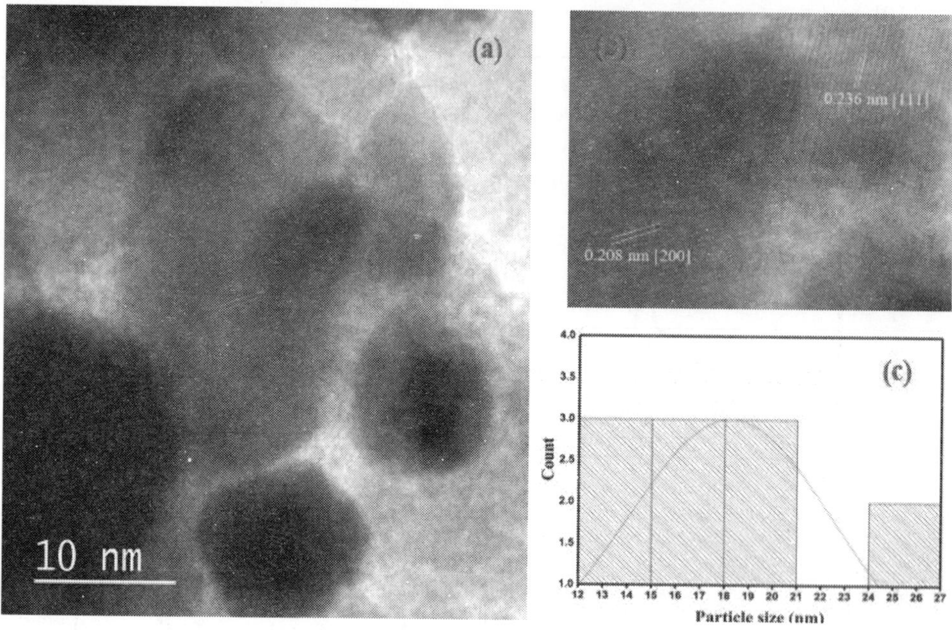

Figure 2 (a) HRTEM image of Ag/NiO NPs; (b) d spacing of the Ag/NiO heterostructure nanocrystal fringes; (c) Particle size of Ag nanoparticle in Ag/NiO heterostructure

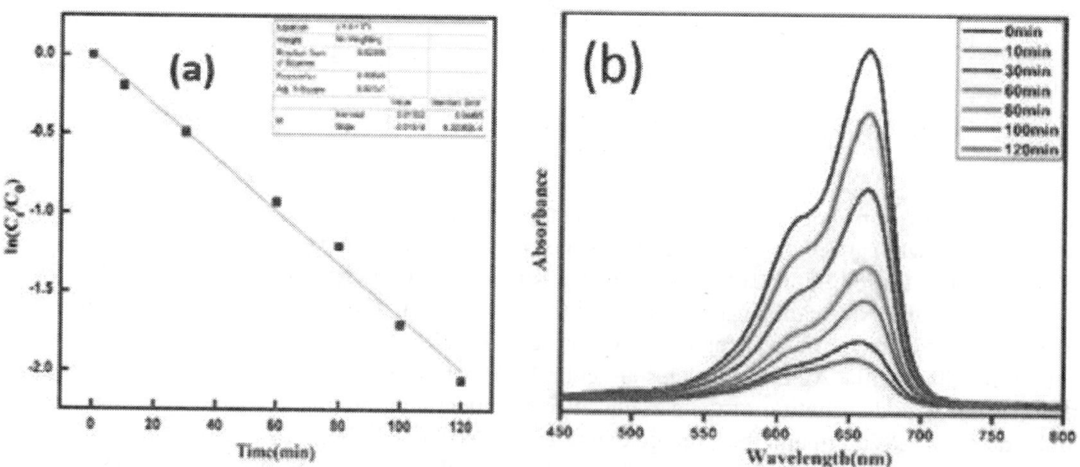

Figure 3 (a) Kinetics plot for MB degradation with Ag-NiO. (b) UV-visible absorption spectra for MB degradation with Ag-NiO nanocomposites

From Fig. 3(b) we say that, the degradation of MB with Ag/NiO heterostructure nanocatalysts exhibit higher photocatalytic activity compared to pure NiO; for example, 87.22 % decolorization of MB with Ag/NiO as photocatalysts was found in 120 min, while 59.64 % Degradation was found with pure NiO nanocrystals. The synthesized Ag/NiO nanoparticles shows excellent activity which is easily viualised form Fig. 4.

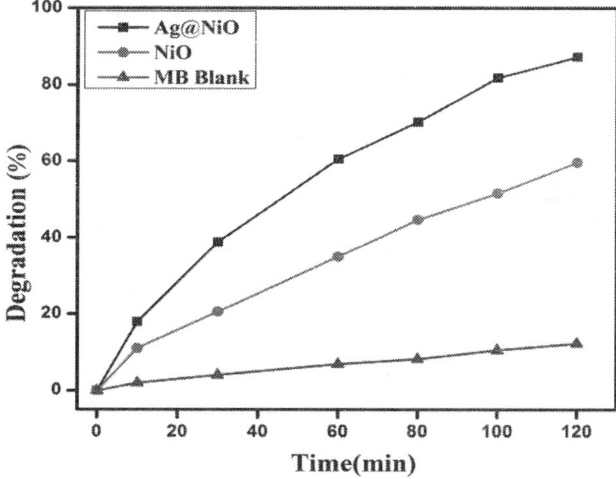

Figure 4. Relative percentage degradation percentage of MB with Ag/NiO, NiO and without catalyst.

When the Ag/NiO heterostructure nanocatalysts are dispersed in the solution with an organic pollutant, the surface electrons on Ag nanoparticles should eventually transfer to the dye in the dark. However, when these catalysts are radiated by cooled white light with photon energy higher or equal to the bandgap of NiO nanocrystals, electrons (e-) in the valence band (VB) can be excited to the CB with simultaneous generation of the same amount of holes (h^+) in the VB. The energy level of the bottom of the CB is higher than the new Fermi energy level of the Ag/NiO heterostructure, so the photoexcited electrons could transfer from NiO NPs to Ag nanoparticles due to the irradiation energy. The electronic acceptors like adsorbed O_2 can easily trap the photoelectrons to produce a superoxide radical ($\cdot O_2^-$) [11] Goto et al. have concentrated on analyzing molecular oxygen reduction to $\cdot O_2^-$, which determined the overall photocatalytic reaction [12]. The photoinduced holes can be easily trapped by OH^- to further produce a hydroxyl radical ($\cdot OH$), which is a powerful oxidant component for the partial or complete mineralization of organic chemicals [13].

5.   Conclusion

Heterostructured nanocomposite Ag/NiO particles of the average diameter of 18.5 nm have been prepared in an aqueous medium by utilizing the solvothermal method. The synthesized nanoparticle demonstrates efficient visible-light driven photocatalytic activity and also provides stability for degradation of methyl blue in an aqueous medium. In contrast to the majority of reports in the literature, MB degradation in the presence of this photocatalyst follows the first-order kinetics. The photocatalytic rate constant shows superlinear (with Ag/NiO NPs of 0.0167 minute^{-1}) with light intensity. This is because of the localized surface plasmon resonance phenomenon (LSPR) of the Ag component is able to explore the radiation on the rest of the heterostructured nanocomposite for higher exciton generation rates with the intensity of incident light.

6.   References

1.   K.M. Dooley, S.Y. Chen, J.R. Ross, J. Catalys., 1994, 145, 402–408.

2.   H.X. Yang, Q.F. Dong, X.H. Hu, J. Power Sources, 1999, 79, 256–261.

3.   E.L. Miller, R.E. Rocheleau, J. Electrochem. Soc., 1997, 144, 3072–3077.

4.   G. Wang, X. Lu, T. Zhai, Y. Ling, H. Wang, Y. Tong, Y. Li, Nanoscale, 2012, 4, 3123–3127.

5.   M. El-Kemary, N. Nagy, I. El-Mehasseb, Mate. Sci. Semicondu. Process., 2013, 16, 1747–1752.

6.   D. Wang, C. Song, Z. Hu, X. Fu, J. Phys. Chem. B, 2005, 109, 1125–1129.

7.   R.J. Russell, M.V. Pishko, C.C. Gefrides, M.J. McShane, G.L. Cote, Analyt. Chem., 1999, 71, 3126– 3132.

8.   M. Ramesh et al., J. Mater. Res., 2018, 33, 601-610.

9.   S. Adhikari et al. J. Photochem. Photobiol. A 2018, 357, 118-131.

10.   Z. Sabouri, A Kbari, et al. J. mol. Structure. 2018, 1173, 931-936

11.   Ryu, J.; Choi, W. EnViron. Sci. Technol. 2004, 38, 2928.

12.   Goto, H.; Hanada, Y.; Ohno, T.; Matsumura, M. J. Catal. 2004, 225, 223.

13.   Yatmaz, H. C.; Akyol, A.; Bayramoglu, M. Ind. Eng. Chem. Res. 2004, 43, 6035.

Role of Science Communication in Application of Earthworm on Agricultural Soil Restoration

Manoj Mishra[1]* and Sudhir K. Upadhyay[2]

[1]Department of Mass Communication, V.B.S. Purvanchal University, Jaunpur-222003, India
[2]Department of Environmental Science, VBS Purvanchal University, Jaunpur-222003, India
*Email: manjulmanoj1@gmail.com

ABSTRACT

Earthworm is essential living ingredients for agricultural soil system; it has eco-friendly capability to enhance the soil health. In the present study, OC, N, P and yield of vegetable crops were observed at five different sites of district Jaunpur in year 2016, and all the formers were applied uncontrolled pesticides dose. In vitro experiments of different concentration of soil and varied population of earthworms reveled that OC, N, P of the soil increased while concentration of pesticides were reduced after 20DAS followed by 10DAS as compared with control. Keeping the views of indiscriminate uses of pesticides; we initiated a campaign to educate the formers to utilize only vermicompost and interesting results were observed in the year 2017 and 2018. Organic carbon, total nitrogen, total phosphorous of the treated soil and yield of vegetables crop were increase 26, 25, 13, and 30% respectively, in the year of 2018 followed by 2017.

Keywords: Earthworm, soil health, nutrient, communication and pesticide.

1. Introduction

About 3500 species of earthworms are reported worldwide with diverse habitat, earthworms are the member of order haplotaxida and phylum is annelid (Paoletti, 1999). Toe role of earthworms are increasing aeration and draining in soil, they utilize energy, nutrients and habitat from soil (Lavelle, 1988; Pechnik, 2010). Most of the organic matters from soil are ingested by earthworms; they also feed living organisms like nematodes, microfloraetc (Curry and Schmidt, 2007). Earthworms prefer to ingest plant tissues/ residues but selective for most of the organic compounds/matter (Bonkowski *et al.,* 2000). Earthworms able to mix soil horizons, digest organic matter, dig burrows they deposit cast etc. these activities increase soil porosity, structural stability of soil and nutrition (Lavelle, 1988). Due to the worms selecting the nutrients that they consume, it results in their casts having higher soil organic matter, nutrient contents (Lavelle *et al.,* 1998) and even protecting the soil from erosion (Bernier, 1998). They also have an influence on the processes of aggregation, residue decomposition, nutrient mineralization, aeration, and water infiltration (Fonte *et al.,* 2009).The presence of earthworms may alter the structure of plant communities as well. Since earthworms manage the distribution of organic matter, plant root foraging is affected (Scheu, 2003). However, because earthworms release casts that have nutrients, plants grown better when earthworms are present (Scheu, 2003). Due to the heavy machinery in use today, there have been controls on earthworm growth and survival. These new techniques such as tillage and fertilization have been impacting the earthworm population in a negative way (Fonte *et al.,* 2009).Earthworms play a large role in soil structure and diversity. They have been called ecosystem engineers because they are an integral part of the soil ecosystem. This makes them a very important species that will continue to dominate soil ecosystems. Modern agricultural is based on proper irrigation, seed quality, synthetic fertilizers along with augmentation of pesticides and insecticides, massive use of pesticides uses are started since 1960 through green revolution. Most of the developing countries including India, peoples engaged in agricultural practices and maximum number of formers have less cultivated land area and they dependent on agriculture for their social and economical development

(Pimentel, 2005). The excessive and indiscriminate use of pesticides/insecticides and synthetic fertilizers led to severe environmental contaminations and affected water, funa, flora, soil, disease etc (Mahmood *et al.,* 2016). They are chemically active compounds which kill to the target organisms, and enter in trophic level as the bioaccumulation /biomagnifications mechanism (Palis *et al.,* 2006). Keeping this view the present objectives are (i) Observation of selected formers and their agriculture practices, (ii) evaluation of pesticides supplemented soil with earthworm in pot experiment (iii) communicate and educate among formers to apply the earthworm treated soil (vermicompost) in agricultural field (v) evaluate the soil health and yield with treated soil in agricultural field.

2.   Materials and Methods

Study sites, use of pesticides/insecticides and synthetic fertilizers

Five different sites namely S1=Baksha block, S2=Karanja Kala block, S3=Sikrara block and S4=Badalapur block and S5=Khuthan block of Jaunpur district [25.7490° N, 82.6987° E] U.P were selected as sites for evaluation of pesticides/insecticides uses and synthetic fertilizer application.

Soil analysis

Soil pH, ECe were observed as earlier described mehod of APAH, (2012). Organic carbon was examined by spectrophotometer at 660 nm Datta *et al.*, (1962). The available nitrogen of soil samples were estimated by the method described by Subbiah and Asija, (1956). Available phosphorus in agricultural soil was estimated with earlier described method (Olsen, 1954). Potassium content was measured flame photometer. Demibras, (1998) has earlier described method for spectrophotometric analysis of carbaryl in soil; Carbaryl on hydrolysis gave 1-naphthol which reacted with diazotized sulphanilic acid to form a product showing absorption at λmax475 nm.

Experimental design and communication of earthworm's uses

Earthworms were taken from K.V.K. Baksha block, Jaunpur and different treatments were prepared in pot inoculated with varied population of earthworms. Treatment T1 was 100gm of agricultural soil+5 nos of earthworms, T2 was 500gm of agricultural soil+5 nos of earthworms, T3 was 1000gm of agricultural soil+5 nos of earthwarms, T4 was 100gm of agricultural soil+10 nos of earthworms, T5 was 500gm of agricultural soil+10 nos of earthworms, and T6 was 1000gm of agricultural soil+10 nos of earthworms. All the treated pot sublimated with 100 and 200pmm of carbaryl pesticides respectively. Control was without pesticides and earthworm.

3.   Results and Discussion

In the present study, organic carbon, total nitrogen, total phosphorous of the soil and yield of vegetables crop were observed at five different sites of district Jaunpur in year 2016 (Table 1). A descriptive and cross sectional observation was observed on questionnaire based survey revealed that maximum farmers of chosen sites were applied pesticides in vegetables grown field for production (table 1). This is an alarming situation for environment due to contamination of pesticides to aquifer as well as it enters in trophic level and reach upto human beings and induces several disorders. FAO (2008) /WHO (2009) have defined the class of hazardous pesticides/insecticides which their specific characteristic which responsible for several problems, few convention like Stockholm (2001), Rotterdam (2004) drawn the attention of the organic pollutants and pesticides globally. It has been reported earlier about the exposure of highly hazardous pesticides / insecticides among the agriculture and peoples who involved in their practiced (handling, dilution, mixing etc) are suffering from kidney, liver, bronchial disorder etc. Exposures to pesticides /insecticides and their root of exposures both are induces high health risk in human being (Safi, 2002; Palis *et al.*, 2006; Rastogi *et al.*, 2010) like dermal disorders through sprays, mouth and teeth through contaminated food etc (WHO, 2006). Keeping this views we planned to examine the role of earthworm in quality of pesticide used soil. Different treatment reveled that organic carbon, total nitrogen, total phosphorous of the soil increase due to inoculation of earthworms after 20DAS followed by 10DAS (Figure 2) and concentration of pesticides were reduced at 20DAS followed by 10DAS (Figure 3). These significant results become a base for communication among the formers of chosen site to use earthworm treated soil (vermicompost) shown in figure 1. Vermicompost is the end product of a process called vermicomposting, which uses earthworms to increase the speed of the composting process and ensure higher-quality compost. In addition to vermicompost there is vermicast, which is slightly different. Vermicast, also known as worm castings, is the excrement from the worms, minus the rest of the compost. After 2016 we initiated a campaign to educate the formers to utilize only vermicompost and interesting results were observed in the year 2017 and 2018. Organic carbon, total nitrogen, total phosphorous of the treated soil and yield of vegetables crop were increase 26, 25, 13, 12, and 30% respectively in year of 2018 followed by 2017 (Figure 4a and 4b). Lavelle *et al.*, (1998) earlier reported that casts of earthworms have rich soil organic matter and nutrient they also help to maintain soil health, increase aggregation, reduce decomposition and protection of soil erosion (Bernier, 1998; Fonte *et al.*, 2009).

Table 1 Evaluation of soil status, of organic carbon (OC), Total Nitrogen (N), Phosphorous (P), Potassium content (K), pesticides use and yield among formers. (Y=formers satisfied their yield); S1=Baksha block, S2=Karanja Kala block, S3=Sikrara block and S4=Badalapur block and S5=Khuthan block of Jaunpur district.

Without application of Earthworm treated soil, year: 2016						
Study Sites	**OC**	**N**	**P**	**K**	**PU (%)**	**Yield**
S1	3.5	1.6	1.3	1.1	>89	Y
S2	2.9	2.1	1.5	0.6	>85	Y
S3	3.8	2.3	1.1	1.1	>90	Y
S4	3.5	2.1	1.6	1	>82	Y
S5	2.2	1.3	1.2	1	>88	Y

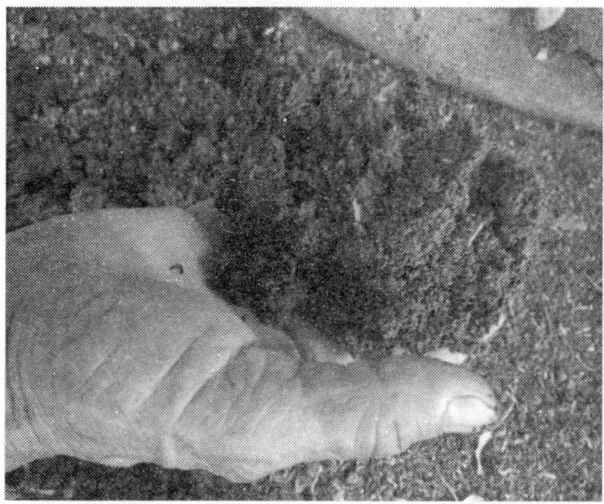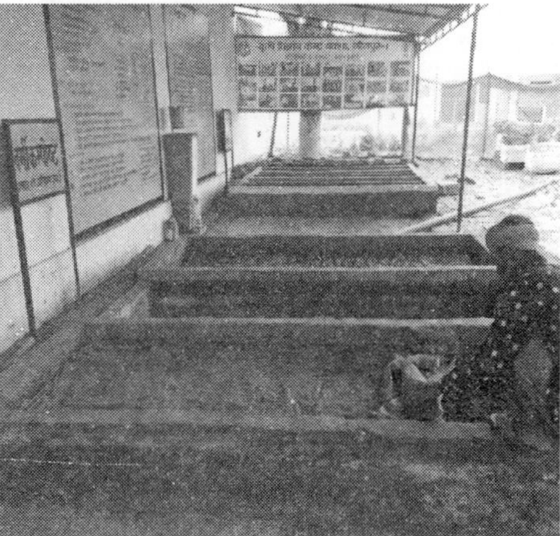

Figure 1 Preparation of Earthworm treated soil (vermi compost) at Bakha Block, jaunpur.

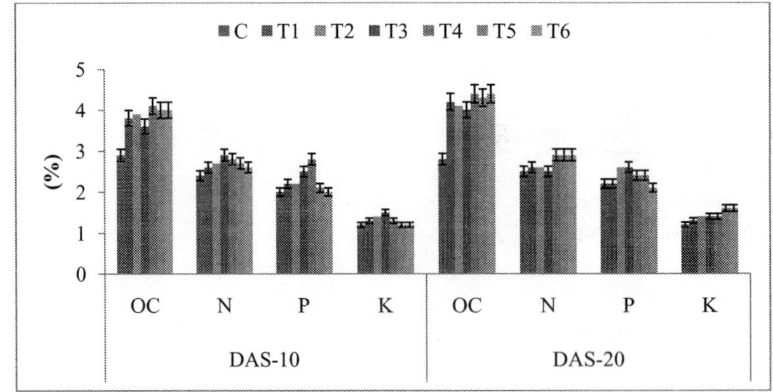

Figure 2 Organic carbon (OC), total nitrogen (N), phosphorous (P) and potassium content in soil under different treatment with earth warm after 10and 20 days respectively. C=control; 100gm soil without earthworm, T1=100gm soil with 5 nos of earthworm, T2= 500gm of soil with 5 nos of earthworm, T3=1000gm soil with 5 nos of earthworm, T4=100gm soil with 10 nos of earthworm, T5=500gm soil with 10 nos of earthworm, T6=1000gm soil with 10nos of earthworm, DAS=days after inoculation of earthworm.

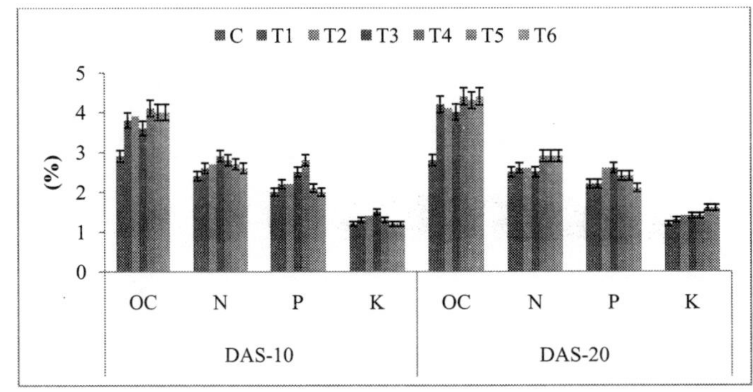

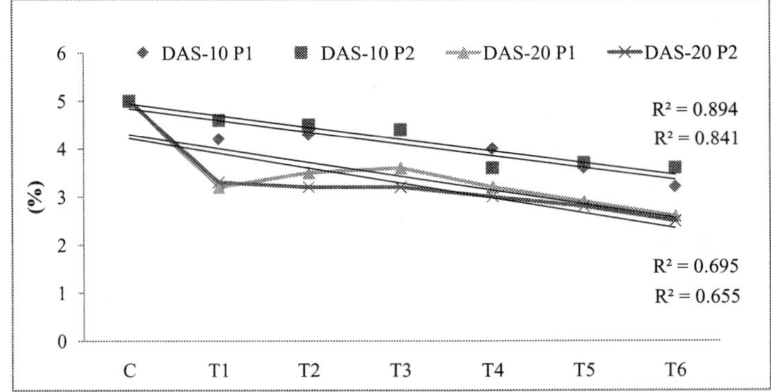

Figure 3 Evaluation of pesticides load in soil after treatment of earthworm. C=control; 100gm soil without earth warm, T1=100gm soil with 5 nos of earthworm, T2= 500gm of soil with 5 nos of earthworm, T3=1000gm soil with 5 nos of earthworm, T4=100gm soil with 10 nos of earthworm, T5=500gm soil with 10 nos of earthworm, T6=1000gm soil with 10nos of earthworm, DAS=days after inoculation of earthworm. P1 and P2 =concentration of pesticides [P1=100ppm and P2=200ppm].

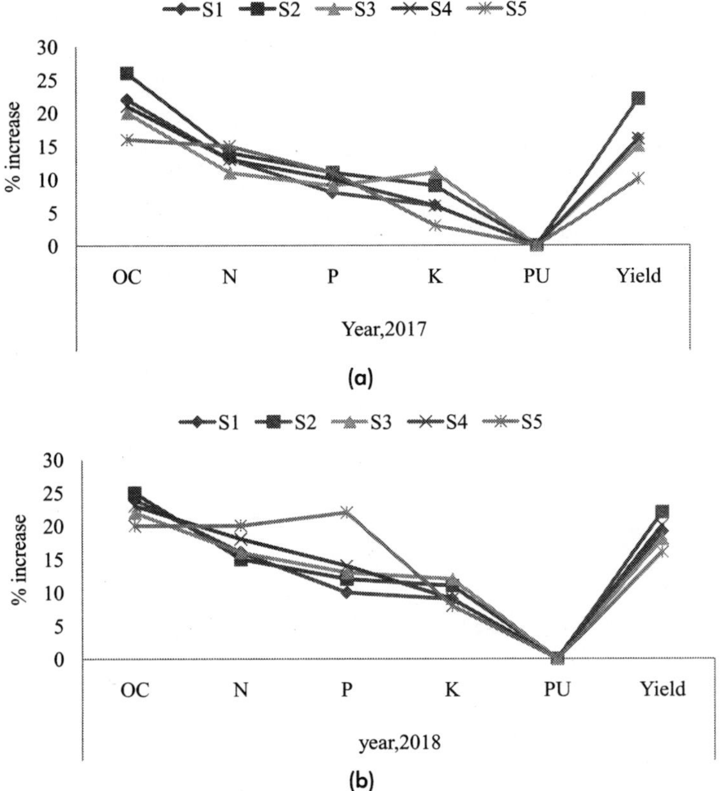

Figure 4 Evaluation of soil status and yield of vegetable crop under application of earthworm treated soil; Percent increase of organic carbon (OC), Total Nitrogen (N), Phosphorous (P) and Potassium content , PU (pesticide uses) and crop yield. Figure a represent of year 2017 and figure b represent of year 2018.

4.   Conclusion

Indiscriminate use of pesticides and fertilizers are badly affects the agriculturally soil health, earthworms are natural ingredients which able to increase the soil health. Earthworms have also capable to reduce pesticides concentration in soil and enhances organic carbon, total nitrogen, total phosphorous, earthworm treated soil are significantly increase yield of vegetables corps. Continuous communication among the formers to educate them for apply earthworm treated soil could be effective tool to minimize the pesticide load in agricultural field.

5.   References

1.   Bernier N (1998) Earthworm feeding activity and development of the humus profile. Biology and Fertility of Soils .26, 215-223.

2.   Bonkowski M, Griffiths BS, and Ritz K (2000) Food preferences of earthworms for soil fungi.Pedobiologia. 44, 666-676.

3.   Curry JP, Schmidt O (2007) The feeding ecology of earthworms – A review. Pedobiologia. 50, 463-477.

4.   Datta NP, Khera MS, Saini TR (1962) A rapid calorimetric procedure for the determination of the organic carbon in soils. J Indian Soc Soil Sci. 10,67–74.

5. Demirbaş A, Sci. Total Environ. 220 (1998) 235.

6. Demirbas A (1998) Spectrophotometric determination of carbaryl pesticide and its hydrolysis product in soil and strawberry samples. Sci Total Environ. 220,235–241.

7. FAO/WHO (2008) Second session of the FAO/WHO meeting on pesticide management and 4th session of the FAO panel of experts on pesticide management. Recommendations. Rome, Food and Agriculture Organization of the United Nations; Geneva, World Health Organization.

8. FAO/WHO (2009) JMPR: Joint FAO/WHO Meeting on Pesticide Residues. Rome, Food and Agriculture Organization of the United Nations; Geneva, World Health Organization.

9. Fonte SJ, Winsome T, Six J (2009) Earthworm populations in relation to soil organic matter dynamics and management in California tomato cropping systems. Applied Soil Ecology .41, 206-214.

10. Lavelle P (1988) Earthworm activities in the soil system. Biology and Fertility of Soils. 3, 237-251.

11. Lavelle P, Pashanasi B, Charpentier F, Gilot C, Rossi JP, Derourard L, Andre L, Ponge JF, Bernier N (1998) Large-scale effects of earthworms on soil organic matter and nutrient dynamics. Earthworm Ecology . 103-122.

12. Mahmood I, Imadi SR, Shazadi K, Gul A, Hakeem KR (2016) Effects of Pesticides on Environment. Plant, Soil and Microbes . 253-269.

13. Olsen SR, Cole CV, Wantanable FS and Dean LA (1954) Estimation of available phosphorus in soil by extraction with Sodium bicarbonate. United State Dept. of Agric. CIRC., Washinton, D.C., 939.

14. Palis F G, R J Flor, H Warburthon and M Hossain (2006) Our farmers at risk: behavior and belief system in pesticide safety. Journal of Public Health . 28(1), 43–48.

15. Paoletti MG (1999) The role of earthworms for assessment of sustainability and as bioindicators. Agriculture, Ecosystems & Environment . 74,137-155.

16. Pechenik J A (2010) Biology of Invertebrates.Sixth Edition.McGraw Hill Higher Education. 357-358.

17. Pimentel D (2005) Environmental and economic costs of the application of pesticides primarily in the United States'. Environment, Development and Sustainability. 7, 229–52.

18. Rastogi S K, S Tripathi, and D Ravishanker (2010) A study of neurologic symptoms on exposure to organophosphate pesticides in the children of agricultural workers. Indian Journal of Occupational and Environmental Medicine .14(2), 54.

19. Rotterdam Convention on the Prior Informed Consent Procedure for Certain Hazardous Pesticides and Industrial Chemicals in International Trade. Geneva and Rome, Secretariat of the Rotterdam Convention 2004.

20. Safi J M (2002) Association between chronic exposure to pesticides and recorded cases of human malignancy in Gaza Governorates (1990–1999). Science of the total environment .284(1), 75□84.

21. Scheu S (2003) Effects of earthworms on plant growth: patterns and perspectives: The 7th international symposium on earthworm ecology· Cardiff· Wales· 2002. Pedobiologia .47, 846-856.

22. Stockholm Convention on Persistent Organic Pollutants (POPS). Geneva, Secretariat of the Stockholm Convention 2001.

23. Subbaiah BV and Asija GL, (1956) A rapid procedure for the estimation of available nitrogen in soil. Curr. Sci. 25, 259.

24. WHO/UNEP (2006) Sound management of pesticides and diagnosis and treatment of pesticide poisoning. A resource tool. Geneva, World Health Organization and United Nations.

Investigation of Zirconium Nanowires by Elastic, Thermal and Ultrasonic Analysis

Mohit Gupta[1,*], Sudhanshu Tripathi[2], Devraj Singh[3] and R.R.Yadav[1]

[1]Department of Physics, University of Allahabad, Prayagraj-211002, India
[2]Department of ICE, Amity School of Engineering and Technology, Noida-201313, India
[3]Department of Physics, AIAS, Amity University Uttar Pradesh, Noida-201313, India
*E-mail: mohitauphy89@gmail.com

ABSTRACT

The zirconium nanowire (Zr-NWs) has been investigated by elastic, thermal and ultrasonic analysis at room temperature along unique direction. The second and third order elastic constants of Zr-NWs have been figured out using the Lennard-Jones Potential model. The second order elastic constants were used to find out the Young's modulus, bulk modulus, shear modulus, tetragonal modulus, Poisson's ratio, Pugh's indicator, ultrasonic velocities, Breazeale's non-linearity parameters. Further these associated parameters of Zr-NWs have utilized to find out the Grüneisen parameters, thermal conductivity, thermal relaxation time, acoustic coupling constants and ultrasonic attenuation. On the basis of analyzed properties of Zr-NWs, the chosen material is ductile in nature and having metallic characteristics.

Keywords: Zirconium nanowires, elastic constants, thermal conductivity, ultrasonic attenuation

1. Introduction

In recent years nanoscience has become one of the most exciting fore-fronts fields in physics, chemistry, engineering, and biology. Quite understudy research in this area begins with developing an understanding of materials with novel characteristics at the nanoscale. Attempts have been made to achieve control over conductivity, capacity, strength, ductility, reactivity etc. in different combination of matters. This has led to radical changes and departures in the fundamental understanding of matter. Single crystalline NWs are the important class of the nanostructure materials due to unique properties. The magnetic NWs attract attention of scientists and engineers in last years. The most demanded NWs applications are high density magnetic storage media, GMR sensors [1,2], biomagnetic [3,4] and medical devices [5]. The ultrasonic techniques have been the most widely used non-destructive methods for characterization of the bulk materials in general. A complete understanding of the behavior of ultrasonics in a material is prerequisite for any material characterization scheme. The structural inhomogeneities, non-linear elastic properties, dislocations, grains, phase transformations, electrical properties, thermal properties, size of particles in nanostructured materials, vacancies in the lattice sites in intermetallics are well related to ultrasonic attenuation and velocity and other related parameters at different physical conditions like temperature, orientation, magnetization etc. [6-8]. The ultrasonic studies at nanoscale are rarely found in the literature. Only few studies have been reportedin literature [9,10].Hu et al. [11] constructed EAM-type many-body potentials for ten hexagonal close packed metals. These potentials reproduce for each metal considered the experimentally observed equilibrium density, c/a ratio, cohesive energy, five independent second-order elastic constants and, approximately, the vacancy formation energy. A modification term has been also introduced for describing metals with negative Cauchy pressure. Finnis-Sinclair (F-S) type many-body potentials have been constructed for eight hexagonal metals: Co, Zr, Ti, Ru, Hf, Zn, Mg and Be by Igarashi et al. [12]. They found that each of the constructed potentials has been represented by a stable hexagonal close-packed lattice with a particular non-ideal c/a ratio. As per authors information, no one has studied the zirconium-nanowires (Zr-NWs) for its mechanical, thermal and acoustical properties and this is motivation to study these additional properties of the Zr-NWs.

In present investigation, first of all, we computed the second and third- order elastic constants (SOECs and TOECs) for Zr-NW with Lennard-Jones potential model. The obtained values of SOECs have been applied to find out the Young's modulus, bulk modulus, shear modulus, Poisson's ratio, Breazeale's non-linearity parameter, ultrasonic velocities and thermal conductivity. Further, these evaluated parameters have been used to find out thermal relaxation time, acoustic coupling constants and ultrasonic attenuation due to phonon-phonon (p-p) interaction and thermal relaxation mechanisms. Obtained results have been presented and discussed with available findings on Zr-NWs at room temperature and along unique axis.

2. Theory

The chosen material Zr-NWs is wurtzite hexagonal close packed (hcp) with lattice parameter a=3.23 Å and c=5.14 Å.6 SOECs and 10 TOECs have been computed with Lennard-Jones interaction potential as detailed in our previous paper [13]. These SOECs are used to find out the Young's modulus (Y), bulk modulus (B), shear modulus (G), Poisson's ratio (υ), Zener anisotropic factor (Z_A), angle dependent longitudinal, shear and quasi shear ultrasonic velocities and thermal conductivity using the expressions of our previous paper [13]. The SOECs and TOECs have been used to find the ultrasonic Grüneisen parameters (UGPs). The expressions to find the UGPs are given in literature [14]. The specific heat per unit volume (Cv) and energy density (E_0) were calculated using the tables for the ratio of Debye temperature and room temperature in AIP handbook [15]. Further these parameters have been applied to calculate the ultrasonic attenuation due to phonon-phonon interaction and thermoelastic relaxation mechanisms in Zr-NWs using the modified Mason's approach [16].

3. Results and Discussion

The SOECs and TOECs have been obtained using Lennard-Jones interaction potential with Lennard-Jones interaction constant (b_0) 1.7764×10⁻⁶⁵ erg cm⁷and constants (m, n) 6, 7 respectively. SOECs are presented in Table 1.

Table 1. SOECs (in GPa) of Zr nanowire at 300K

Temp. (K)	C_{11}	C_{12}	C_{13}	C_{33}	C_{44}	C_{66}
300	190.45	74.44	61.30	175.24	46.20	77.84
[1]						
[2]	144	74	67	166	33.4	-

From the Table 1, it is noticeable that the second order elastic constants of Zr-NWs have been found nearly same with previous value given by Hu et al. [11]. This confirms the validation the approach to compute the SOECs. The SOECs have been utilized to compute the mechanical parameters Y, B, G, υ and Z_A of Zr-NWs. These values of the mechanical parameters with TOECs are given in Table 2. Further the value of Pugh's indicator i.e., B/G (1.80) is greater than 1.75, which approves the ductile nature of Zr-NWs. The Zener anisotropic ratio (Z_A) deviates from the unity, which settles the anisotropic behavior of Zr-NWs.

Table 2. TOECs, Y, B, G and v at 300K of Zr-NWs

Temp.	C_{111}(GPa)	C_{112}(GPa)	C_{113}(GPa)	C_{123}(GPa)	C_{133}(GPa)	C_{344}(GPa)	C_{144}(GPa)	C_{155}(GPa)
300 K	-3105.6	-49.23	-98.81	-125.58	-592.96	-555.89	-146.32	-97.527
	C_{222}(GPa)	C_{333}(GPa)	Y(GPa)	B(GPa)	G(GPa)	υ	Z_A	
	-2457.3	-2111.5	142.75	105.14	58.33	0.26	0.76	

The ultrasonic velocities (V_L, V_{S1} and V_{S2}: here L stands for longitudinal wave, S1 for shear wave and S2 for quasi shear wave) have been computed with the help of the SOECs and the density of Zr-NWs for the ultrasonic wave propagation at different orientation from the unique axis of Zr-NWs. The values of the ultrasonic velocities are shown in Fig. 1.

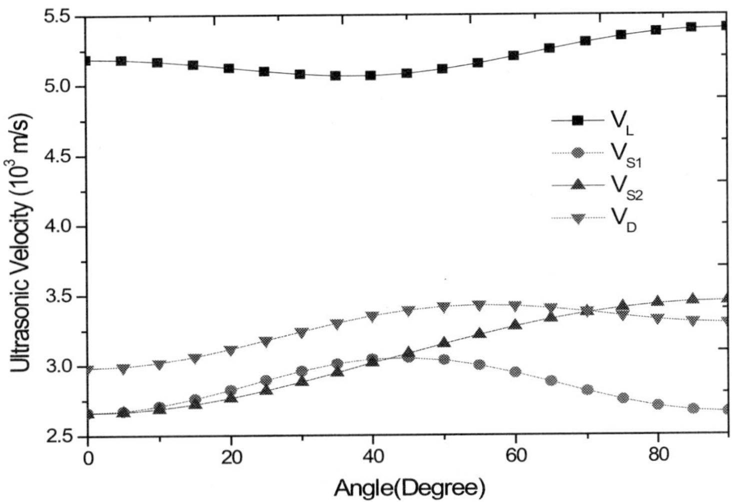

Figure 1. Angle dependent ultrasonic velocities

It is depicted from Fig. 1 that the minimum longitudinal and maximum quasi shear velocities values have been found at 40° and the maximum value of Debye average velocity is at an angle 50°. As we know that Debye average velocity has been obtained by combined values of V_L, V_{S1} and V_{S2}. Although, no direct data is available to compare the velocities of Co-NWs, but the trend of the graph (Fig. 1) has been found similar to other wurtzite hcp materials ZnO and BeO [13, 17].The values of E_0, C_V have been computed from the AIP Handbook [15]. The values of E_0, C_V, acoustic coupling constants (D_L and D_S) with ultrasonic velocities values are given in Table 3.

Table 3. Specific heat per unit volume(10^5 Jm^{-3}), energy density (10^6 Jm^{-3}K^{-1}), acoustic coupling constants and ultrasonic velocities (10^3 ms^{-1}) of Zr NWs at 300K.

C_V	E_0	D_L	D_S	V_L	VS1=V_{S2}	V_D
15.28	249.01	174.87	54.80	5.18	2.66	2.98

The thermal conductivity (κ) has been evaluated using the Morelli and Slack approach [18]. These all associated parameters now have been put to find out the thermal relaxation time (τ) and ultrasonic attenuation due to phonon-phonon interaction and thermoelastic relaxation mechanisms. These parameters have been presented in Table 4.

Table4. Temperature dependent thermal Conductivity (Wm^{-1}K^{-1}), thermal relaxation time (ps) and ultrasonic attenuation (10^{-16} Nps^2 m^{-1}) of Zr-NWs

T(K)						
	τ	κ	$(\alpha/f^2)_L$	$(\alpha/f^2)_s$	$(\alpha/f^2)_{th}$	$(\alpha/f^2)_{Total}$
300	5.08	24.6	32.13	37.17	0.073	69.38

Here it is observable that the values of ultrasonic attenuation due to thermoelastic relaxation mechanism $[(\alpha/f^2)_{th}]$ is negligible in comparison to ultrasonic attenuation due to phonon-phonon interaction $[(\alpha/f^2)_L$ and $(\alpha/f^2)_S]$. The total attenuation is found less in comparison to other studied wurtzitehcp materials ZnO [13] and BeO [17].

4. Conclusion

Based on the theoretical calculation of this reveals thefollowing inferences;

- The moderate growth in the ultrasonic velocity (V_{S2}) with the incremented levels of angle has been revealed than the loftier progress with the longitudinal wave ultrasonic velocity.

- The theoretical approach also validates the application of studied zirconium nanowires under the varying conditions of elastic, thermal and ultrasonic analysis.

- The ultrasonic attenuation is predominant over the thermoelastic loss in Zr-NWs.

- This can also be declared that on the basis Pugh's indicator (B/G) analysis thatZr-NWs is stable.

- The predicted value of Zener anisotropic ratio (Z_A) is less than one(unity), which confirms the anisotropic behaviour of Zr -NWs.

The obtained results of elastic constants, ultrasonic velocities, thermal relaxation time and ultrasonic attenuation will be used to get further investigation of various transport properties of Zr -NWs.

5. References

1. M. Albrecht, A. Moser, C.T. Rettner, S. Anders, T. Thomson, B.D. Terris, 2002, Appl. Phys.Lett., 80, 3409-3413.
2. F. Nasirpouri, P. Southern, M. Ghorbani, A Irajizad, W. Schwarzacher, 2007,J..Magn.Magn.Mat., 308, 35–39.
3. A. Hultgren, M. Tanase, C.S. Chen, G.J. Meyer, D.H. Reich 2003, J. Appl. Phys., 93, 7554- 7556.
4. D.H. Reich, M. Tanase, A. Hultgren, L.A. Bauer, C.S. Chen, G.J. Meyer, 2003, J. Appl. Phys., 93, 7275-7280.
5. P.D. McGary, L. Tan, J.Zou, B. Stadler, P.R. Downey, A.B. Flatau, 2006. J. Appl. Phys., 99, 08B310.
6. D. Singh, D.K. Pandey, D.K. Singh, R.R.Yadav, 2011, Applied Acoutics, 72, 737-741.
7. D.K. Singh, D.K. Pandey, D. Singh, R.R. Yadav, 2012,J..Magn.Magn.Mat.,,324, 3662–3667.
8. S.K. Verma, D.K. Pandey, R.R. Yadav, 2012, Physica B: Physics of Condensed Matter, 407, 3731-3735.
9. G. Mishra, D. Singh, P.K. Yadawa, S.K. Verma, R.R. Yadav, 2013, Platinum Metals Rev., 57, 186-191.
10. V. Pandey, G. Mishra, S.K. Verma, M. Wan, R.R. Yadav, Open Acoustic J.2012, 3, 664-668.
11. W. Hu, B. Zhang, B. Huang, F. Gao and D. J Bacon, J. Phys.: Condens. Matter 13 (2001) 1193–1213.
12 M. Igarashi, M. Khantha and V. Vitek, Philos. Mag. B 63 (1991) 603-627.
13. S. Tripathi, R. Agarwal and D.Singh, Johnson Matthey Tech. Rev. 63 (2019) 166-176.
14. M. Nandanpawar and S. Rajagopalan, J. Acoust. Soc. Am. 71, 1469-1472 (1982).
15. D.E. Gray, American Institute of Physics Hanbook, IIIrd Edition, McGraw-Hill Book Company Inc. (1957).
16. C. P. Yadav, D.K. Pandey and D. Singh, Indian J. Phys. 93 (2019) 1147-1153.
17. S. Tripathi, R. Agarwal and D.Singh, J. Pure Appl. Ultrason. 41 (2019) 44-50.
18. D. T. Morelli and G.A. Slack, High Lattice Thermal Conductivity Solids (in: High Thermal Conductivity Materials) (Ed. S.L. Shinde and J.S. Goela), Springer, New York, Ch.2, p.37 (2006).

Dependence of Negative Index Materials on Electric Permittivity and Magnetic Permeability by Effective Medium Theory

Girijesh N. Pandey[1]*, Khem B. Thapa[2], Anil Kumar Shukla[3] and Suresh K Sharma[4]

[1]*Department of Physics, AIAS, Amity University Uttar Pradesh, Noida-201313, India
[2]Department of Physics, Babasaheb Bhimrao Ambedkar University (A central University), Lucknow-226025, India
[3]Department of Electronics and Telecommunication, ASET, Amity University Uttar Pradesh, Noida-201313, India
[4]Department of Physics, Harcourt Butler Technical University, Kanpur
*E-mail: gnpandey2009@gmail.com

ABSTRACT

We have theoretically studied and calculated the impedance and effective refractive index of the split ring resonator (SRR) in host materials medium by applying effective medium theory. Such calculations have made very easy to fabricate artificial structure of the negative index materials containing SRR. By changing the length of the host as well as the thickness of the SRR material, we simulate the effective parameters of metamaterials like effective permittivity, effective permeability. With these parameters, we also concluded that the effective parameters ε and μ are responsible for to change the value of negative index materials. On calculations, we have found that the effective medium theory of periodic structure is more powerful tool to calculate the μ_{eff} and ε_{eff} by calculating the reflectance and transmittance.

OCIS codes: Photonics; metamaterial, split ring resonator

1.   Introduction

The refractive index is described as the interaction between the light and materials. The electron and atom in any material interact with the electromagnetic wave of light and due to this, an index of refraction for specific is arises in the material. As we know that refractive index is frequency dependent and have value greater than 1 for all naturally occurring materials. Is negative index of refraction is possible? [1]. First time Veselago, in 1968 [2] predicted the concept of left-handed material (LHM) which was composed with simultaneously negative electrical permittivity (ε) and magnetic permeability (μ) for the certain frequency range. Smith and Pendry et al. [3, 4] who are developed and designed the structures which are magnetically active, are known as split-ring resonator (SRR) structure. The SRR is made up of metallic rings with gaps which have been widely used for creating negative μ.

Pandey et al. [5-9] have mathematically simulated and studied the reflectance properties, band structures, group velocities and optical properties of one dimensional photonic crystal (1-D PC) containing metamaterials using translational matrix method (TMM). They theoretically observed the abnormal behaviors of the group velocity of such structure which has larger value than the speed of light in certain range of normalized frequency of the 1-D PC containing negative index materials. C. M. Soukoulis et al. [10, 11] studied numerically with an improved version of TMM method. The absorption, reflection, transmission and phase of reflection are simulated and compared with experimental value for both single SRR with negative permeability and negative index materials. Wiltshire et al, artificially constructed the negative index materials which has become of interest, because these materials can exhibit electromagnetic characteristics12]. Lopez and Barrera have established the general condition under which negative refraction occurs and studied some properties of refraction, refraction and their potential applications [13]. In 2007, Liu et al. [14] examined the field-averaging approach to the homogenization of meta-materials.

In this present approach, we have theoretically studied the effect of effective permittivity and permeability of the medium using effective medium theory. The frequency dependence of the effective electromagnetic parameters of left-handed and related meta-materials are studied [15, 16] of the split ring resonator and wire type. By varying the width of inserted material as well as the host material, we have calculated the effective parameters like effective permittivity and effective permeability. Using these parameters we have also calculate the refractive index and impedance of the medium.

2. Theory and Methodology

The effective permittivity ε_{eff} having an effective plasma frequency can be written in Drude's form:

$$\varepsilon_{eff}(\omega) = 1 - \frac{\omega_p^2}{\omega(\omega + i\Gamma)} \tag{1}$$

where ω_p represent the effective plasma frequency and Γ is the effective damping constant of the wire medium.

The effects of spatial dispersion are obtained due to the variation of phase of the applied electromagnetic field along the direction of perpendicular to the planes. In these conditions, the effective refractive index and the impedance both has exhibit spatial dispersion.

The geometry of the model of the considered structure is shown in Fig.1.

The one dimensional (1-D) transfer for considered structure can be defined as

$$F' = TF \tag{2}$$

where

$$F = \begin{pmatrix} E \\ H_{red} \end{pmatrix} \tag{3}$$

where E and H_{red} are the complex electric and magnetic field amplitudes

The transfer matrix for a homogeneous 1-D slab can be expressed as

$$T = \begin{pmatrix} \cos(nkd) & -\dfrac{z}{k}\sin(nkd) \\ \dfrac{k}{z}\sin(nkd) & \cos(nkd) \end{pmatrix} \tag{4}$$

Where the refractive index in n and z is the wave impedance of the slab. We know the n and z are related to the local relative permittivity and permeability

$$n = \sqrt{\varepsilon\mu}, z = \sqrt{\mu/\varepsilon} \tag{5}$$

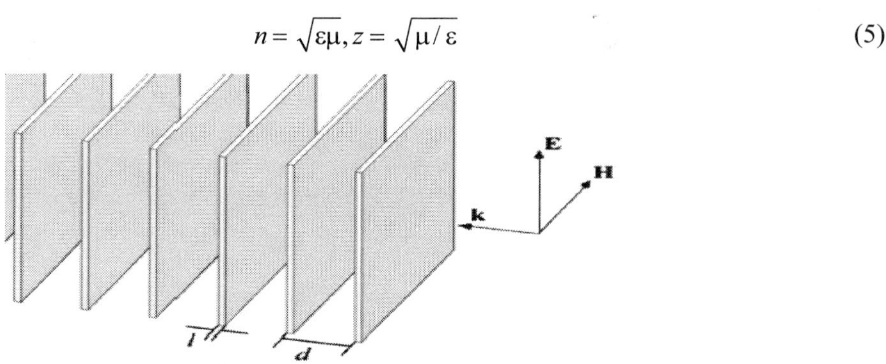

Fiure.1 The schismatic periodic structure of electrically or magnetically polarized sheets and the electromagnetic wave is to propagate along the direction normal to the sheets.

Similarly we can write transfer matrices in each region as

$$T_{tot} = T_{vacuum} T_{material} T_{vacuum} \tag{6}$$

where

$$T_{vacuum} = \begin{pmatrix} \cos\left(\dfrac{kd}{2}\right) & -\dfrac{1}{k}\sin\left(\dfrac{kd}{2}\right) \\ k\sin\left(\dfrac{kd}{2}\right) & \cos\left(\dfrac{kd}{2}\right) \end{pmatrix} \tag{7}$$

and

$$T_{material} = \begin{pmatrix} \cos(nkl) & -\dfrac{z}{k}\sin(nkl) \\ \dfrac{k}{z}\sin(nkl) & \cos(nkl) \end{pmatrix} \tag{8}$$

Bloch impedance and the propagation factor is obtained when the transfer-matrix formalism is considered,

$$2\cos(\alpha d) = T_{11} + T_{22} \tag{9}$$

and

$$Z_{B,red}^2 = \frac{T_{12}}{T_{21}} \tag{10}$$

We can find in wave-representation for T_0 for a single slice of vacuum and T_{slab} for a single slice of homogeneous material of the thickness d,

$$T_0(d) = \begin{pmatrix} e^{ikd} & 0 \\ 0 & e^{-ikd} \end{pmatrix}, \quad T_{slab}(d) = \begin{pmatrix} \alpha(d) & \beta(-d) \\ \beta(d) & \alpha(-d) \end{pmatrix}$$

where

$$\alpha(d) = \cos(qd) + \frac{i}{2}\left(z + \frac{1}{z}\right)\sin(qd) \tag{11}$$

By using the interrelation between the transfer matrix and the scattering matrix, we can define the refection $r_{\mp}$ and transmission $t_{\pm}$ amplitudes,

$$\beta(d) = \frac{i}{2}\left(z - \frac{1}{z}\right)\sin(qd) \tag{12}$$

$$S = \begin{pmatrix} t_+ & r_+ \\ r_- & t_- \end{pmatrix}, \quad T = \begin{pmatrix} t_+ - r_+ t_-^{-1} r_- & r_+ t_-^{-1} \\ -t_-^{-1} r_- & t_-^{-1} \end{pmatrix} \tag{13}$$

The reflection and transmission amplitudes for a considered structure can be calculated which is composed of a left vacuum slice of length 'a' of N homogeneous unit cells of length L in propagation direction and terminated by a right vacuum slice of length 'b',

$$t_- = \frac{e^{-ikNL}}{\alpha(-d)e^{-ik(a+b)}} \tag{14}$$

$$r_+ = e^{-ikNL}\beta(-d)e^{-ik(a-b)}t_- \tag{15}$$

The scattering amplitudes R and T after N unit cells can be written as,

$$T = t\_e^{ikNL} = \alpha^{-1}(-d)e^{ik(a+b)} \tag{16}$$

$$R = \beta(-d)e^{-ik(a-b)}T \tag{17}$$

We assume a = b = 0 in the continuum the scattering amplitudes of the homogeneous slab which are typically defined from the considered structure.

We obtained the scattering formulae with given amplitudes R and T obtained from the parameters impedance z(ω) and index of refraction n(ω). Then we have

$$z_{eff}(\omega) = \pm\sqrt{\frac{(1+R)^2 - T^2}{(1-R)^2 - T^2}} \tag{18}$$

$$n_{eff}(\omega) = \pm\frac{1}{kL}\arccos\left(\frac{1-R^2+T^2}{2T}\right) + \frac{2\pi}{kL}m \tag{19}$$

For known $n_{eff}(\omega)$ and $z_{eff}(\omega)$ the effective permeability μ and permittivity ε can be defined as

$$\mu_{eff}(\omega) = n_{eff}(\omega)z_{eff}(\omega) \tag{20}$$

$$\mu_{eff}(\omega) = n_{eff}(\omega)z_{eff}(\omega) \tag{21}$$

3.   Results and Discussion

By applying effective medium theory, we have studied and calculated the effective refractive index and impedance of the split ring resonator (SRR) in host materials medium. In the present study, we have verified the electric permittivity and magnetic permeability of the SRR periodic structure. This SRR structure is inserted in the host medium and calculates the effective permittivity and effective permeability of the SRR in the presence of the host medium as well as the SRR artificial structure itself.

The negative refractive index due to the artificial structure of SRR at microwave frequency is [17],

$$\varepsilon_H(\omega) = 1 - \frac{\omega_{ep}^2 - \omega_e^2}{\omega^2 - \omega_e^2 + i\gamma\omega} \tag{22}$$

$$\mu_H(\omega) = 1 - \frac{\omega_{mp}^2 - \omega_e^2}{\omega^2 - \omega_m^2 + i\gamma\omega} \tag{23}$$

The variation of the electric permittivity (ε), magnetic permeability (μ) and refractive index of the SRR materials versus angular frequency (ω) are shown in Fig. 2. This figure has three parts, in first part the permittivity versus frequency is depicted that the permittivity is positive for the frequency range from 0 Hz to 117 Hz and it becomes to zero at 120Hz. Above 130Hz frequency, the permittivity starts to have negative value. The second part of this figure is shows the magnetic permeability versus angular frequency. This figure has also same characteristics with different frequency range. The permeability is positive for frequency range from 0 Hz to 165 Hz. Then again it comes to zero. The permittivity starts increasing negative value from above to 170Hz. The third part of the figure represent that the refractive index of the SRR for frequency ranges 20-200Hz. The refractive index versus angular frequency (ω) is found three regions: (i) positive refractive index for range 0 Hz to 118 Hz, (ii) zero refractive index for 118 Hz to 165 Hz and (iii) negative refractive index for 165 Hz to 200Hz. So overall in figure 2, all the ε, m, and n are negative beyond the range of 165 Hz. The unusual behavior of the SRR is the frequency range 118-165Hz where the refractive index is zero. The study of the SRR as a NIM material has contained positive, zero refractive and negative refractive index for certain frequency ranges.

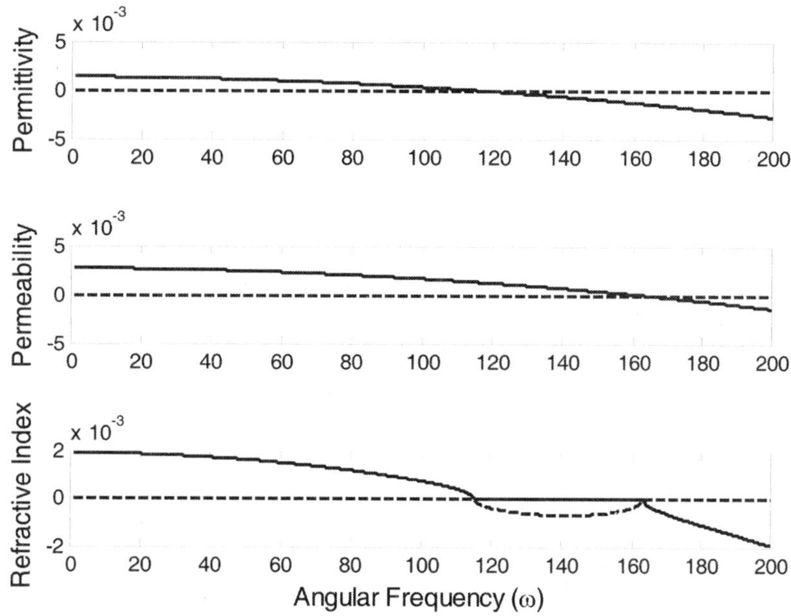

Figure 2. Electric permittivity, magnetic permeability and refractive index of SRR versus angular frequency

Now we have consider split ring resonator (SRR) which are arranged periodically in host material of length L and width of SRR is d as shown in Fig. 3 [18]. Now we study the frequency response of these parameters (ε,μ, n and Z) by varying the thickness of the host material and the inserted material by using effective medium approximation. We observe that when we fix the width of inserted material and increase the thickness of host material, the negativity of ε, μ and n keeps on increasing whereas impedance remains zero.

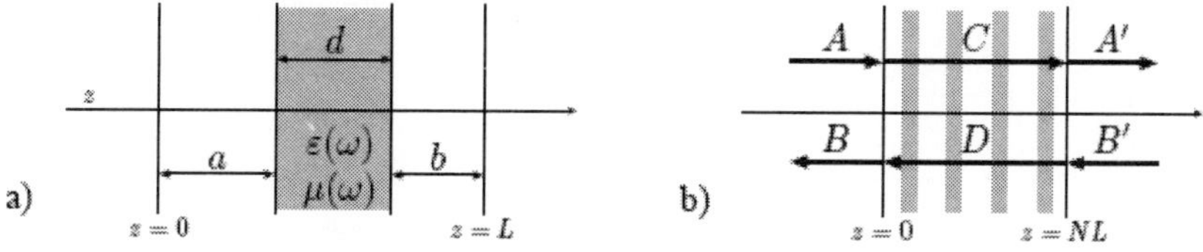

Figure 3. The layouts of the single unit cell

The layouts of the single unit cell (a) and (b) of a finite slab of the periodic structure are shown Fig. 3. The shaded regions indicate The homogeneous core of the width d which is characterized by functions $\mu(\omega)$ and $\varepsilon(\omega)$ shown in shaded part which is sandwiched by two vacuum slabs. L is the length of a single unit cell, N the number of unit cells in the slab. According to the effective medium theory the effective permittivity and permeability of the considered structure is given by;

$$\varepsilon(\omega) = 1 + \frac{L}{d}\left[\varepsilon_H(\omega) - 1\right] \tag{24}$$

$$\mu(\omega) = 1 + \frac{L}{d}\left[\mu_H(\omega) - 1\right] \tag{25}$$

Equations (24) and (25) are calculated by considering the reflectance and transmittance of the composite structure.

The permittivity and permeability for left-handed material are as follows;

$$\varepsilon_H(\omega) = 1 - \frac{\omega_p^2}{\omega^2 + i\gamma\omega} \frac{\omega_{ep}^2 - \omega_e^2}{\omega^2 - \omega_e^2 + i\gamma\omega} \tag{26}$$

$$\mu_H(\omega) = 1 - \frac{\omega_m^2}{\omega^2 + i\gamma\omega} \frac{\omega_{mp}^2 - \omega_m^2}{\omega^2 - \omega_m^2 + i\gamma\omega} \tag{27}$$

The effective refractive index and impedance has been calculated by effective medium theory when the effective permittivity and permeability of the considered structure is calculated from Eqs. (24) and (25).

$$n_{eff}(\omega) = \sqrt{\varepsilon(\omega)\mu(\omega)} \tag{28}$$

$$Z_{eff}(\omega) = \sqrt{\frac{\mu(\omega)}{\varepsilon(\omega)}} \tag{29}$$

Now we calculate the electric permittivity and magnetic permeability of the SRR using Eqs. (24) and (25). We have also calculated the effective refractive index and impedance of the materials using Eqs. (28) and (29).

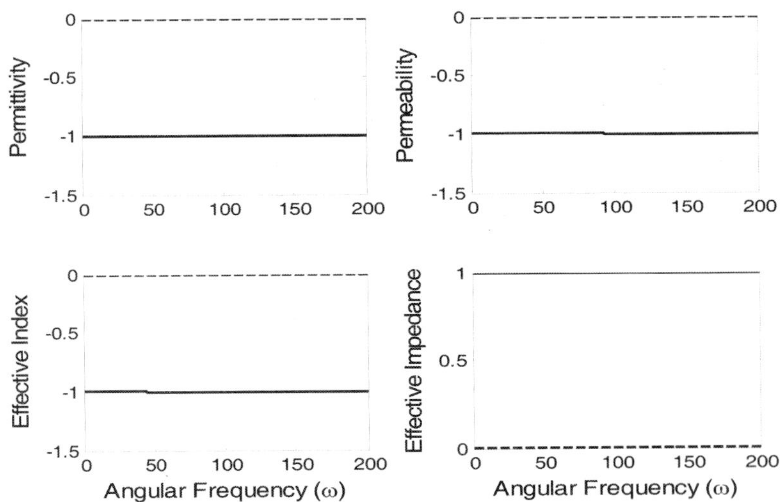

Figure.4 Electric permittivity, magnetic permeability and refractive index of composite material versus angular frequency when L=10mm; d=05mm

By varying the width of the host material, we have several interesting results of SRR by applying effective medium theory. When we kept width of host material L=10mm and width of inserted material d = 5mm, we find a few graphs as shown in Fig. 4. Figure 4 contain four parts, the first part of the figure shows the electric permittivity (ε) versus angular frequency (ω) response of SRR. The electric permittivity (ε) attains a negative value and it is equal to -1. Similar results are obtained for the case of magnetic permeability (μ) in above given conditions. The magnetic permeability is also attains a negative value of -1.

The remaining two parts of the Fig. 4 shows the response of effective refractive index n_{eff} and effective impedance Z_{eff} versus angular frequency (ω). From the third part of figure 4, it is clear that effective index is also -1. The last part of Fig. 4 shows the behavior of effective impedance with respect to the angular frequency. Now we increased the width of host material (L) and keeping the thickness of inserted material d same as in earlier case. In this particular case when we have fixed L=20mm and d=5mm, we obtained several results which are shown in Fig. 5.

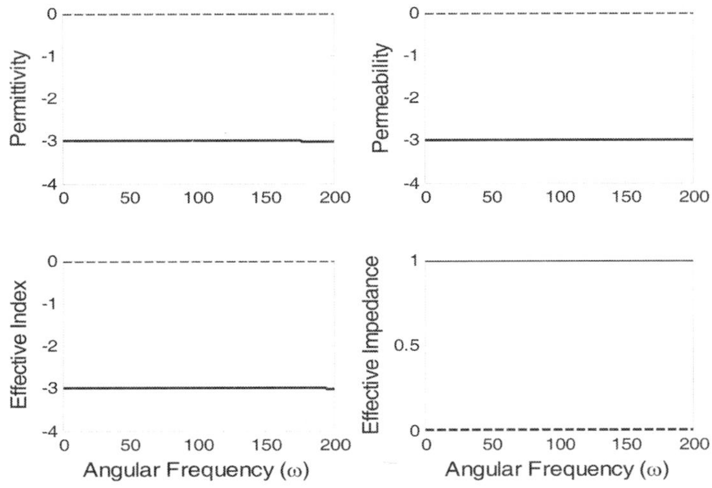

Figure 5. Electric permittivity, magnetic permeability and refractive index of composite material versus angular frequency on taking L=20mm; d=05mm

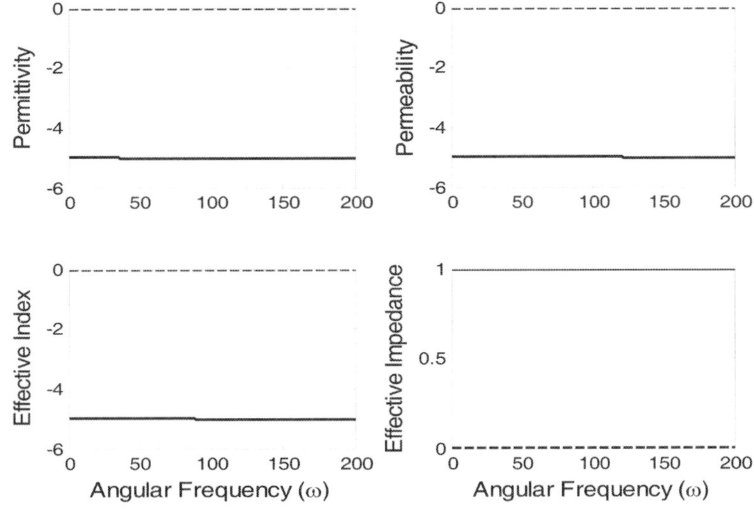

Figure 6 Electric permittivity, magnetic permeability and refractive index of composite material versus angular frequency for L=30mm; d=05mm

In first two parts of Fig. 5, the response of electric permittivity and magnetic permeability with respect to angular frequency are shown. We observe that the electric permittivity attains a value of -3 and magnetic permeability also becomes equal to -3. The remaining two parts of Fig. 5 show how the effective refractive index and impedances are varying with angular frequency. The values of electric permittivity and magnetic permeability thus obtained from the above equation which gives the effective refractive index n_{eff} = -3 and effective impedance Z_{eff}=1.

Again we consider new value of L and keeping the width of inserted material same, i.e. d=5mm. With L=30mm.We obtained one more result having four parts showing the variations of electric permittivity (ε), magnetic permeability (μ), effective refractive index (n_{eff}), and effective impedance (Z_{eff}) with respect to angular frequency (ω). The values of electric permittivity (ε) and magnetic permeability (μ) obtained from above equation which gives the n_{eff} and Z_{eff} same as it is shown in last figure 6.

4. Conclusion

The SRR has the negative refractive index due to the negative permittivity and negative permeability at certain frequency. The negative value of the SRR can be changed by changing the length of the host as well as the thickness of the SRR material. Such study is very useful to fabricate the structure of the SRR with different thickness and host materials as the experimentalist wants. We have calculated the all the parameters of the NIMs using the effective medium theory which is very useful for the future. We concluded that the effective parameters ε and μ are responsible for to change the value of negative index materials. On calculations, we have found that the effective medium theory of periodic structure is more powerful tool to calculate the μ_{eff} and ε_{eff} by calculating the reflectance and transmittance.

5. References

1. A. Schuster, An Introduction to the Theory of Optics (Arnold, London, 1904)
2. V. G. Veselago, Sov Phys., Usp 10:509–514, 1968.
3. D. R. Smith, W. J. Padilla, D. C. Vier, S. C. Nemat-Nasser, S. Schultz , Phys. Rev. Lett., 84:4184–4187, 2000.
4. J. B. Pendry, Phys. Rev. Lett., 85, 3966, 2000.
5. G.N. Pandey, Khem B. Thapa, Sanjeev K Srivastava and S.P. Ojha, Pro. Electroma. Rese. M, 2, 15–36, 2008
6. S. K. Srivastava, G. N. Pandey and S. P. Ojha, Optik119, 117-121 (2008).
7. G. N. Pandey and S. P. Ojha, Optik - International Journal for Light and Electron Optics, Volume 124, Issue 18, Sept. 2013, Pages 3514-3519.
8. G N Pandey, Thesis: Thesis on the topic «Some Optoelectronic Devices Based on Photonic Band Gap Materials» submitted to Lucknow University, India, 2007.
9. G N Pandey, Int. J. Adv.Electron. Electron. Eng., 3, 965-970, 2013
10. P. Marks and C M Soukoulis, Phys. Rev. B, 65, 033401, 2001.
11. N.H. Shen, T. Koschny, M.Kafesaki and Phys. Rev. B, 85, 075120, 2012.
12. D.R.Smith, J.B.Pandry and M.C.K. Wiltshira, Science, 305, 788, 2004.
13. C.P.Lopez and R.G.Barrera, Phys. Status Solidi B, 249, N0.6, 1110-1118, 2012.
14. R. Liu, T. J. Cui, D. Huang, B. Zhao, and D. R. Smith, Phys. Rev. E, 76, 026606, 2007.
15. S. A. Ramakrishna, Physics of negative refractive index materials, Rep. Prog. Phys. 68, 449–521, 2005.
16. T. Koschny, P. Markoš, E. N. Economou, D. R. Smith, D. C. Vier, and C. M. Soukoulis, arXiv:cond-mat/0411590v1, 2004.
17. R. Aylo, Thesis on the topic «Wave propagation in negative index materials» submitted to University of Dayton, Ohio, 2010
18. D. R. Smith,Phy. Rev. E, 81, 036605, 2010

Synthesis and Optical Properties of SnS Nanoparticles

B. K. Pandey[1, 2, *], Ram Gopal[1]

[1]Department of Physics, University of Allahabad, Prayagraj-211002, India
[2]Department of Physics, Dr. Shyama Prasad Mukherjee Govt. Degree College, Prayagraj-211013, India
*E-mail: bishnu.pandey750@gmail.com

ABSTRACT

We have successfully synthesized undoped and manganese (Mn) doped tin sulphide (SnS) nanoparticles (NPs) using chemical precipitation method. Herein, we have studied optical properties of SnS NPs using UV-Visible absorption and photoluminescence (PL) spectroscopy. We have studied effect of Mn doping on optical bandgap of SnS NPs. Optical band gap of SnS NPs get widen at different percentage (0.5, 2.0 and 5.0 %) of Mn doping. PL spectra at 665 nm suggest band to band transition which supports UV-visible absorption findings.

Keywords: SnS NPs, bandgap, optical properties, PL spectra,

1.   Introduction

Since last decades, photovoltaic phenomena showed promising potential to fulfill energy need of the future generations. SnS is one of the important materials for the fabrication of near infra red (NIR) photodetector due to narrow-band gap energy [1]. SnS nanomaterials belong to narrow-band gap and large optical absorption coefficient (10^4 cm^{-1}) and high photoelectric current efficiency (25 %) [2-4]. Owing to these properties, it is very promising material for the application in solar absorber for fabrication of solar cell application [5-6]. SnS nanomaterials is none toxic to avoid adverse effect on environment, it may be one of the basis for this materials to use in narrowband semiconductor in photovoltaic and solar absorber. Optical property of SnS nanocrystals depends very much on synthesis rout, for example, optical band gap of SnS nanomaterials range from 1.0 eV to 1.80 eV depending on tin and sulfur ratio. SnS is a p type semiconductor with layered orthorhombic structure. In layered SnS tin and sulfur atom are tightly bounded with Vander walls forces [7]. Sulfur and tin ratio decides density of states of conduction and valence band further density of state is responsible to maintain the gap between conduction and valence band.

2.   Material, Method

All the chemicals were analytical grade and used as such without further purification and all the experiments were performed in open air atmosphere. Doubled distilled water is used as a solvent while Manganese chloride ($MnCl_2$) were used as a Mn dopant precursor. Mn doped SnS nanoparticles were prepared by using simple precipitation method. In the typical procedure, different molar concentrations of aqueous solution of $MnCl_2$ with respect to $SnCl_2.2H_2O$ were prepared. This prepared solution was mixed into the aqueous solution of $SnCl_2.2H_2O$ with stirring around an hour to get homogeneous mixing of Mn ions in solution. The resulting solution was added drop wise into another containing Na_2S (Qualigens 50% assay) with constant magnetic stirring. To study the effect Mn doing into SnS, three samples S2, S3 and S4 are prepared of mol concentration of 1 mM, 2 mM and 5 mM $MnCl_2$ solutions respectively and one sample S1 is prepared without $MnCl_2$ solutions to compared with doped samples. The precipitate was centrifuged and washed several times, with double distilled water and ethanol, to remove unreacted reactants and impurities. The precipitate collected from centrifuged are dried at 55° C for few hours to obtain dried powders, which are used to record XRD pattern and PL spectra. These powders are uniformly dispersed in ethanol by ultrasonification for recording UV–vis spectra and TEM image.

3.   Results and Discussion

3.1   X-ray diffraction

Figure 1 shows the X-ray diffraction pattern of as synthesized samples S and S3 after baseline correction. Diffraction pattern reveals no extra XRD peak position after doping of 5% Mn in sample S3, because Mn atoms have found positions at SnS lattice site and Mn atoms are not participation any reaction and forming any complexes.

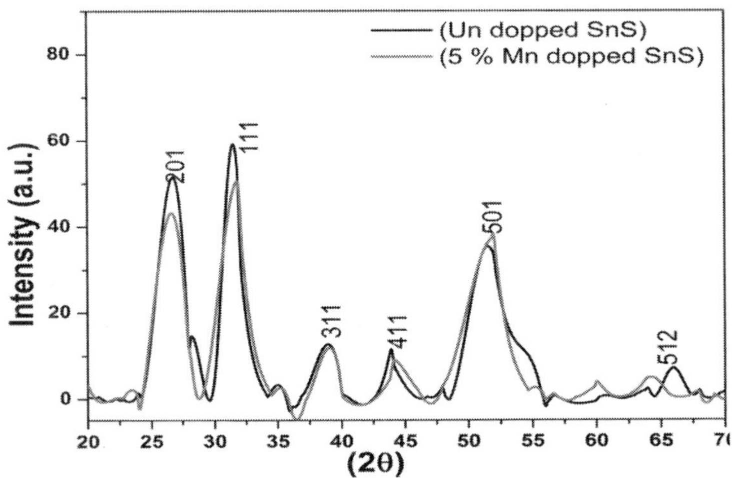

Figure 1 X-Ray diffraction of S and S3 samples

We have estimated crystallite size of SnS NPs using Scherrer's formula given in equation (1).

$$D = K\lambda / \beta\cos\theta \tag{1}$$

Where the constant K is taken to be 0.94, $\lambda = 1.5406$ Å is the wavelength of X-ray used, and β the full width at half maximum of the diffraction peak corresponding to 2θ. Using Eq. (1), the average crystalline size found to be in the range of 3-17 nm. Table 1(a and b) shows the comparative study of peak position, plane spacing, FWHM and particle size of sample S and S3. Plane spacing (d values) of both samples S and S3 of respective different peak positions are similar but a few values are quite different which indicates that Mn doping can alter lattice parameters. The FWHM values of sample S are smaller than sample S3 due to larger particle size formation.

3.2   UV-visible absorption

The UV-visible absorption spectra of as synthesized samples S, S1, S2, and S3 in the range of 200-800 nm are shown in the Fig.2. SnS powder was dispersed in double distilled water before UV-Visible absorption measurements. The absorption band edge of all samples starts from 700 nm and increases upto 265 nm. Similar UV-Visible absorption spectra and optical band gap have been reported by zou at al [9-10].

The optical band gap (*Eg*) of the SnS nanoparticles can be determined by the Touch equation:

$$\alpha h n = (h\nu - E_g)^n \tag{2}$$

where $h\nu$ is the photon energy, α is the absorption coefficient and n is either 1/2 for a direct transition or 2 for an indirect transition. The $(\alpha h\nu)^2$ versus $h\nu$ curve for the sample is shown in Fig. 3, the best linear relationship is obtained by plotting $(\alpha h\nu)^2$ against $h\nu$ indicating that the optical band gap of these nanoparticles is due to a direct allowed transition. The value of the band gap has been determined from the intercept of the straight line at $\alpha = 0$. The optical band gap of as synthesized samples S, S1, S2, and S3 is determined 1.48, 1.52, 1.54, and 1.78 eV respectively.

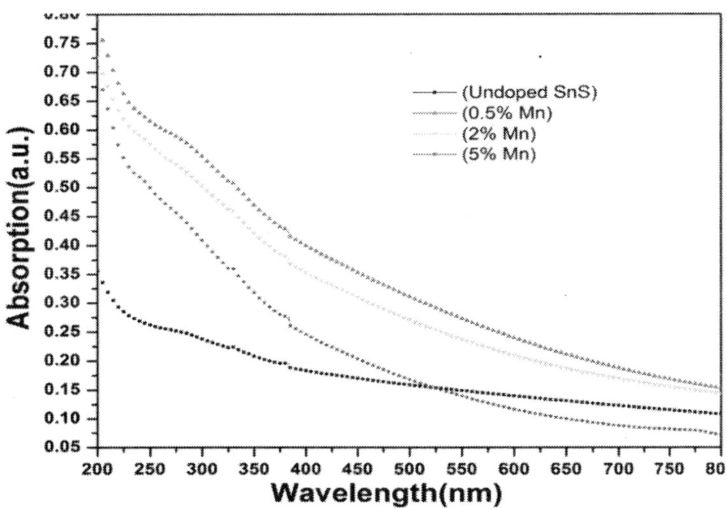

Figure 2 UV-Visible absorption spectrum of S, S1, S2, S3 samples

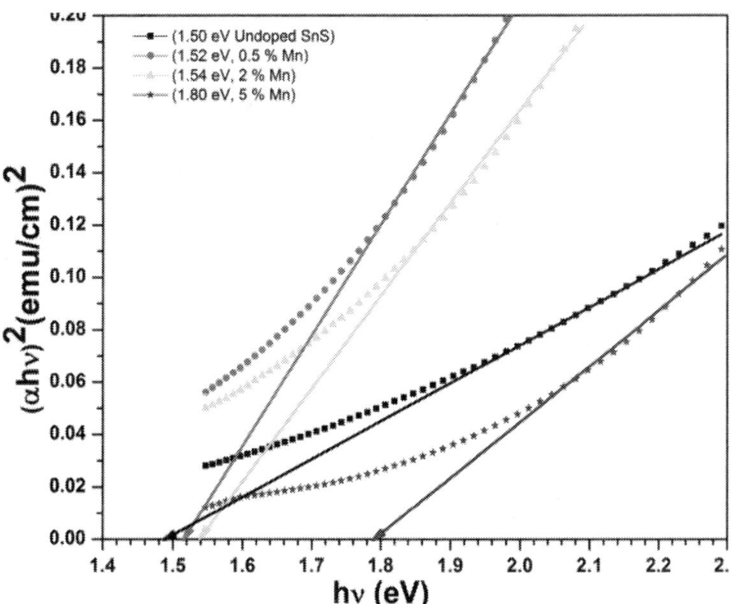

Figure 3 Optical band gap calculated by tauc's relation of S, S1, S2, and S3 samples.

4.   References

1.   W. Albers, C. Haas, F. van der Maesen, Phys. Chem. Solid.15, 306 (1960).

2.   M.M. El-Nahass, H.M. Zeyada, M.S. Aziz, N.A. El-Ghamaz, , Opt. Mater. 20, 159 (2002).

3.   A. Tanusevski, Semicond. Sci. Technol., 18, 501 (2003).

4.   A. Tanusevski, D. Poelman, Sol. Energy Mater. Sol. Cells 80,297 (2003).

5.   T, Rauch, M. Bo"berl, S. F. Tedde, J. Fu"rst, M. V. Kovalenko, G. Hesser, U. Lemmer, W. Heiss, O. Hayden, ,Nat. Photon. 3, (2009), 332.

6.   A. H. Souici, N. Keghouche, J. A.Delaire, H. Remita, A. Etcheberry, M. Mostafavi, , J. Phys. Chem. C 113,(2009), 8050.

Attenuation of Ultrasound in B1 and B2 Structures of CdO

Jyoti Bala[1], Vyoma Bhalla[2,*], Devraj Singh[2,3], C. P. Yadav[4], and D.K. Pandey[4]

[1]University School of Information and Communication Technology, Guru Gobind Singh Indraprastha University, New Delhi-110078, India
[2]Amity School of Engineering and Technology Delhi, A.U.U.Premises, Noida-201313, India
[3]Department of Physics, AIAS, Amity University Uttar Pradesh, Noida-201313, India
[4]Department of Physics, P.P.N. (P.G.) College, Kanpur-208001, India
*E-mail: bhallavyoma@gmail.com

ABSTRACT

The attenuation of ultrasonic waves has been estimated in rocksalt type (B1) and CsCl type (B2) structures of CdO at room temperature along <100>, <110> and <111> directions. First of all, the higher order elastic constants have been computed using Born model with Mori and Hiki approach. Then, the second order elastic constants (SOECs) were applied to compute the mechanical constants such as shear modulus, Young's modulus, bulk modulus, tetragonal modulus, Poisson's ratio, Pugh's indicator for finding performance of CdO. Numerous physical quantities, such as ultrasonic velocity, Debye temperature, thermal conductivity, ultrasonic Gruneisen parameter and acoustic coupling constants have been determined for the chosen material. Finally, the attenuation of ultrasonic waves has been compared in B1 and B2 phases of CdO and discussed in correlation with available findings.

Keywords: Cadmium oxide, elastic constants, thermal properties, ultrasonic properties.

1. Introduction

Over the past few years metal oxides semiconductors have received enormous attention due to their interesting electrical and optical properties in several technologically challenging areas. One of the important semiconductor material is Cadmium Oxide (CdO). It is the transparent conductive oxides (TCOS) and are of high interest from industrial applications such as liquid crystal display (LCD), photoelectric devices, gas sensors, IR detectors, etc. It normally crystallizes into rock-salt structure (NaCl) under pressure [1-4]. Sahoo et al. [5] carried out Ab initio calculations on structural, elastic and dynamic stability of CdO at high pressures and concluded the transformation of CdO from B1 to B2 phase under hydrostatic pressure of ~87 GPa. Bhardwaj [6] studied the structural and thermophysical properties of cadmium oxide using the Three-Body Potential (TBP) model. Jentys et. al. [7] studied the structural properties of CdO and CdS clusters in zeolite Y. The structural properties of CdO in the rock-salt (sodium chloride), cesium chloride etc was studied using first-principles total energy calculations by Moreno et. al. [8]. Dou et. al. [9] performed the experimental and theoretical investigation of the electronic structure of CdO using periodic Hartree-Fock and density functional methods. Piper et. al. [10] studied the electronic structure of single-crystal rocksalt CdO by soft x-ray spectroscopies and ab initio calculations.

In the present study, a computational approach has been followed for the investigation of ultrasonic attenuation in order to study the inherent properties of CdO. The Coulomb and Born- Mayer potentials model have been used to determine the elastic, mechanical and thermo-physical properties at room temperature. The van der Waals' forces of interaction have been neglected. To the best of our knowledge, no calculation has been done on the temperature dependent study of CdO using this model.

2. Theory

The temperature dependent elastic, mechanical and ultrasonic properties at room temperature have been studied using simple Coulomb and Born-Mayer interionic potential models [11-12].

The evaluation of second- and third-order elastic constants (SOECs and TOECs) have beeb done using Mori and Hikki approach [13].

The elastic constants computed helps in the evaluation of mechanical properties such as Bulk Modulus (B), Young's modulus (Y), shear modulus (S), Poisson's ratio (σ), anisotropy (A) etc. using the approach followed in our previous work [11,12].

The relation used for finding the ultrasonic velocities for waves propagating along <100> direction for B1- and B2- type structured CdO is given in our previous work [12, 14].

The ultrasonic attenuation due to phonon–phonon interaction (Akhieser loss) for longitudinal and shear modes is given by Mason [11].

3. Results and Discussion

The SOECs and TOECs for B1 and B2 structures of CdO are computed at room temperature using the nearest neighbour distance (r_0) as 1.927Å and hardness parameter (b) as 0.123Å. The results obtained have been listed in Table 1.

Table 1 Second and third elastic constants [in x10^{11} N/m²] for CdO at room temperature.

CdO→ SOEC/TOEC↓	B1	B2
C_{11}	10.64	13.66
C_{12}	2.87	2.40
C_{44}	3.299	4.17
C_{111}	-160.22	-97.42
C_{112}	-11.87	-51.87
C_{123}	3.185	-59.83
C_{144}	5.459	-20.98
C_{166}	-13.44	-20.74
C_{456}	5.355	-49.67

From Table 1, the elastic constant C_{11} represents elasticity in length and is found more in B2-CdO. A longitudinal strain at room temperature produces a change in C_{11}. The elastic constants C_{12} and C_{44} are related to the elasticity in shape, which is a shear constant. A transverse strain with temperature causes a change in shape without a change in volume. Therefore, from the values of C_{12} and C_{44} in B1 and B2-CdO these are less sensitive to temperature as compared to C_{11}.

Elastic modulus B, Y, G, σ , λ , μ , B/G and Anisotropy (A) are also calculated at room temperature using evaluated SOECs and are presented in Table 2. From Table 1 the value of C_{44} >0 thus, the CdO is stable at room temperature according to Born stability criterion [11]. The elastic constants helps in determining the response of the crystal to external forces. They play major role in determining the strength of the material. The single crystal shear moduli for the {100} plane along the [010] direction and for the {110} plane along the [110] direction are simply given by $G_{\{100\}} = C_{44}$ and $G_{\{110\}} = (C_{11} - C_{12})/2$, respectively. It is found that the shear moduli G{100} are always lower than G{110}. The obtained ν values are less than the lower limit value of 0.25 which indicate that the interatomic forces in the B1 and B2-CdO are non-central forces. B/G for the chosen materials must be between 1.56 and 1.59 to be brittle in nature and thus, B1-CdO is more brittle from Table 2.

Table 2 Mechanical properties of CdO at 300K.

CdO	B (GPa)	Y (GPa)	G (GPa)	λ (GPa)	H (GPa)	C_p (GPa)	B/G	s	A	P (gm/cm³)	$G_{\{100\}}$	$G_{\{110\}}$
B1	54.6	86.9	35.2	31.17	6.23	-4.23	1.55	0.235	0.849	8.48	3.299	3.88
B2	61.5	112.4	47.0	30.1	9.55	-17.7	1.31	0.195	0.741	3.724	4.17	5.63

From Table 3, it is observed that the Debye average velocity (V_D) and Debye temperature (T_D) is highest for B2-CdO. The specific heat per unit volume (C_V) and crystal energy density (E_0) have been computed from θ_D/T tables of AIP Handbook[11]. The values for C_V in $10^7 Jm^{-3}K^{-1}$ is equal to 1.58 and 0.67 for B1 and B2 CdO respectively. The value of E_0 is 3.43×10^9 Jm^{-3} for B1-CdO and 1.34×10^9 Jm^{-3} for B2-CdO. The acoustic coupling constants D_L and D_S (for longitudinal and shear waves) which assess the ability of thermal phonons to absorb energy from sound wave have been measured along <100> directions and is listed in Table 3. The total ultrasonic attenuation is higher for B1-CdO and the thermoelastic losses are more as compared to the values of B2-CdO in Table 3.

Table 3 Ultrasonic velocities, thermal conductivity and D_L, D_S, α/f^2 (in $10^{-16} Nps^2m^{-1}$) along <100> direction of CdO compounds at 300K.

CdO→ Parameters↓	B1	B2
V_L (10^3 m s⁻¹)	3.54	6.06
V_S (10^3 m s⁻¹)	1.97	3.34
V_D (10^3 m s⁻¹)	2.196	3.728
T_D (K)	281	363
K (Wm⁻¹K⁻¹)	0.917	0.549
D_L	13.99	8.95
D_S	1.054	19.63
$(\alpha/f^2)_L$	6.01	0.336
$(\alpha/f^2)_S$	1.313	2.184
$(\alpha/f^2)_{th}$	0.021	0.002
$(\alpha/f^2)_{Total}$	7.345	2.522
τ_s (X10⁻¹⁴s)	3.59	1.75

4.   Conclusion

On the basis of above discussion following point can be drawn:

- B1-CdO is more brittle in nature as compared to B2-CdO.

- Anisotropic factor, A is found to be smaller than unity for B1 and B2 CdO. So these are completely anisotropic materials.

- Thermal conductivity and thermal relaxation time plays an important role for total attenuation in these materials and is higher for B1-CdO.

- The elastic, mechanical, thermal and ultrasonic properties of CdO may be used for further investigation and in the manufacturing industries.

5. References

1. Quiñones-Galván J. G., Lozada-Morales R., Jiménez-Sandoval S., Camps E., Castrejón-Sánchez V. H., Campos-González E., Zapata-Torres M., Pérez-Centeno A., Santana-Aranda M. A.: Physical properties of a non-transparent cadmium oxide thick film deposited at low fluence by pulsed laser deposition. Mater. Res. Bull. 76, 376-383, 2016

2. Sagadevan S., Veeralakshmi A.: Synthesis, structural, anddielectric characterization of cadmium oxide nanoparticles. Int. J. Chem. Mol. Eng. 8, 1492-1495, 2014.

3. Yang, Y., Jin, S., Medvedeva, J. E., Ireland, J. R., Metz, A.W., Ni, J., Hersam, M. C., Freeman, A. J. and Marks, T. J.: CdO as the archetypical transparent conducting oxide. Systematics of dopant ionic radius and electronic structure effects on charge transport and band structure. J. Am. Chem. Soc. 127, 8796-8804, 2005.

4. Sarma, H. and Sarma, K. C.: Structural characterization of cadmium oxide nanoparticles by means of X-ray line profile analysis. J. Basic A Eng. Res. 2, 1773-1780, 2015.

5. Sahoo B. D., Joshi K. D., Gupta S. C.: Ab initio calculations on structural, elastic and dynamic stability of CdO at high pressures. J. Appl. Phys. 112, 093523, 2012.

6. Bhardwaj P: Structural and thermophysical properties of cadmium oxide. ISRN Thermodynamics. 2012, 1-4, 2012.

7. Jentys A., Grimes R.W., Gale J. D., Catlow C. R. A.: Structural Properties of CdO and CIS Clusters in Zeolite Y. J. Phys. Chem. 97, 13535-13538, 1993.

8. Moreno R. J. G., Takeuchi N.: First principles calculations of the ground-state properties and structural phase transformation in CdO. Phys. Rev. B 66, 205205, 2002.

9. Dou Y., Egdell R. G., Law D. S. L., Harrison N. M., Searle B. G.: An experimental and theoretical investigation of the electronic structure of CdO. J. Phys. Condens. Matter. 38, 8447, 1998.

10. Piper L. F. J., DeMasi A., Smith K. E., Schleife A., Fuchs F., Bechstedt F., Zuniga-Pérez J. and Munoz-Sanjosé V.: Electronic structure of single-crystal rocksalt CdO studied by soft x-ray spectroscopies and ab initio calculations. Phys. Rev. B 77, p.125204, 2008.

11. Bhalla V., Kumar R., Tripathy C. and Singh D.: Mechanical and thermal properties of praseodymium monopnictides: an ultrasonic study. Int. J. Mod. Phys. B 27, p.1350116, 2013.

12. Bhalla V., Singh D., Jain S. K.:Mechanical and thermophysical properties of cerium monopnictides. Int. J. Thermophys. 37, p.33, 2016.

13. Mori S., Hiki Y.: Calculation of the third-and fourth-order elastic constants of alkali halide crystals. J. Phys. Soc. Jpn. 45, 1449-1456, 1975.

14. Singh D., Pandey D. K.: Ultrasonic investigations in intermetallics. Pramana-J.Phys. 72, 389-398, 2009.

Ultrasonic Attenuation in Lanthanum Monopnictides

Chinmayee Tripathy[1, 2,*], Devraj Singh[3] and Rita Paikaray[1]

[1]Department of Physics, Ravenshaw University, Cuttuck-753003, India
[2]Department of Applied Physics, HMR Institute of Technology & Management, Hamidpur, Delhi-110036, India
[3]Department of Physics, AIAS, Amity University Uttar Pradesh, Noida-201313, India
*E-mail: chinmayeetripathy2011@gmail.com

ABSTRACT

Ultrasonic attenuation study is used to characterize the lanthanum monopnictides materials. The causes of attenuation in these solids at higher temperature are due to phonon-phonon interaction known as Akhieser loss, and due to thermoelastic relaxation. The ultrasonic attenuation for lanthanum monopnictides had been calculated along different <100>, <110>, <111> crystallographic directions.

Keywords: *Ultrasonic attenuation, lanthanum monopnictides, thermoelastic relaxation.*

1. Introduction

The ultrasonic attenuation technique is one of the versatile tool in studying the microstructural and mechanical properties of solids. The lattice imperfections, ferromagnetic, ferroelectric, NMR, thermal relaxation, thermoelastic loss, are the several causes of attenuation at different temperatures in different types of solids. The most important causes of ultrasonic attenuation in solids are due to electron-phonon, phonon-phonon, interaction and that due to thermoelastic relaxation. At high temperature the ultrasonic attenuation is caused due to phonon-phonon interaction known as Akhieser loss and also due to thermoelastic relaxation.

Rare earth compounds have unusual optical, magnetic, phonon and anomalous phase transition properties. The presence of partially filled f-electron orbital is the cause of this unusual behaviour. The f-electron orbitals are highly delocalised under pressure. Rare earth compounds undergo structural phase transition under pressure. There had been a large no of studies of Lanthanum monopnictides found in literature[1-6].

G. Vaitheeswaran et.al. [1] had analysed the electronic structure and structural properties of LaSb and LaBi by the self-consistent tight binding linear muffin tin orbital method. G. Pagare et. al. [2] had studied the theoretically the pressure induced structural phase transition of lanthanum mono pnictides LaP, LaAs, LaSb from their initial NaCl (B1) phase to body centered tetragonal (BCT) phase at high pressure .Second order elastic constants for all the three compounds had also been calculated in this study. The structural, elastic, electronic, thermodynamical and vibrational properties of LaAs and LaP in the rock-salt (B1) structure were investigated by E Deligöz et.al. [3]. They also calculated second order elastic constants, electronic band structure, bulk modulus, Young's modulus, Poisson's ratio, anisotropy factor, sound velocities, and Debye temperature performing ab initio calculations. G. Vaitheeswaran,et.al. [4] theoretically calculated the electronic structure and the relative stabilities of LaP and LaAs at high pressures in the rocksalt, primitive tetragonal and CsCl structures. The first principles calculation results of the second order elastic constants and lattice dynamics of two lanthanum monopnictides, LaN and LaBi, which crystallize in rock-salt structure (B1 phase) are presented by Gökhan Gökoglua, Aytaç Erkisi [5] . Theoretical calculations were based on plane wave basis sets and pseudopotential methods in the framework of Density Functional Theory (DFT) with generalized gradient approximation. D. Varshney[6], investigated the pressure induced structural phase transition from NaCl-type (B1) to CsCl-type (B2) structure and elastic properties of lanthanum pnictides LaN, LaP, LaAs, LaSb, LaBi.

In the present work the ultrasonic attenuation due to phonon- phonon interaction over frequency $(\alpha/f^2)_{Akh}$ and ultrasonic attenuation due to thermoelastic relaxation $(\alpha/f^2)_{Th}$, over frequency of lanthanum monopnictides LaX (LaN, LaP, LaAs, LaSb, LaBi) in NaCl structure had been investigated along <100>, <110>, <111> directions at room temperature . For the evaluation of the ultrasonic coefficients the second and third order elastic constants (SOECs and TOECs) are also calculated using Coulomb and Born Mayer [7] potentials.

2.   Theory

The second and third order elastic constants (SOECs and TOECs) are calculated using Coulomb and Born Mayer [7] potentials.

$$\phi(R) = \phi(C) + \phi(B) \tag{1}$$

Where $\phi(C)$ is the Coulomb potential and $\phi(B)$ is the Born- Mayer potential, given by

$$\phi(C) = \pm \frac{e^2}{r} \text{ and } \phi(B) = A \exp\left(-\frac{r}{b}\right) \tag{2}$$

Where e is the electronic charge, r is the nearest neighbour distance, b is the hardness parameter, and A is the strength parameter[10].

 Following Brugger's definition of elastic constants at absolute zero the SOECs and TOECs are obtained. We get higher order elastic constants at particular temperature[8,9] by adding vibrational energy contribution to the static elastic constants i.e

$$C_{ij} = C_{ij}^0 + C_{ij}^{vib} \text{ and } C_{ijk} = C_{ijk}^0 + C_{ijk}^{vib} \tag{3}$$

Here 0 and vib represents the static and vibrational contribution of elastic constants. The detail expression for C_{ijk} and C_{ij} are given in our previous paper[10].

The Debye temperature Θ_D defines the limits of lattice stability and is used to characterize the lattice thermal phonons. From Debye average velocity Debye temperature Θ_D is calculated. The expression for Debye temperature is

$$\theta_D = \frac{h}{K_B} \left(\frac{3pN\rho}{4\pi M}\right)^{\frac{1}{3}} V_D \tag{10}$$

Where p = no of atoms per molecule, N= Avogadro's number, ρ= Density of the material,

M = mass of molecule.

From Debye temperature many thermal properties like thermal conductivity, specific heat, thermal energy density, relaxation time and attenuation are calculated.

When ultrasonic wave is propagating in solid medium there is attenuation of waves because of lattice imperfections, phonon-phonon interaction, electron- phonon interaction and thermoelastic mechanism. Generally at higher temperature (>100K) there is no electron phonon interaction as there is no coupling between electron and phonon mean free path. The phonon-phonon interaction and thermoelastic phenomenon are the main cause of ultrasonic attenuation at higher temperature. The total attenuation is sum of attenuation due to phonon-phonon interaction (Akhieser loss) and thermoelastic loss.

Ultrasonic attenuation due to phonon-phonon interaction (Akhieser loss) is

$$\left(\frac{\alpha}{f^2}\right)_{long} = \frac{4\pi^2 \tau_l E_0 D_L}{6\rho V_l^3} \tag{11}$$

$$\left(\frac{\alpha}{f^2}\right)_{Shear} = \frac{4\pi^2 \tau_s E_0 D_S}{6\rho V_S^3} \tag{12}$$

Ultrasonic attenuation due to thermoelastic mechanism is given by

$$\left(\frac{\alpha}{f^2}\right)_{th} = \frac{4\pi^2 <\gamma_i^j>^2 KT}{2\rho V_L^5} \tag{13}$$

Where K is thermal conductivity, ρ is density, V_L and V_S are the ultrasonic velocity for longitudinal and shear waves respectively, E_0 is the thermal energy density, τ_1, $\tau_S = \tau_{th}$ the thermal relaxation time for longitudinal and shear waves respectively. τ_{th} is the thermal relaxation time for the exchange of acoustic and thermal energy [11] by considering the condition wt<<1. The expression for thermal relaxation time is

$$\tau_{th} = \frac{3K}{C_V V_D^2} \tag{14}$$

$$\frac{1}{2}\tau_L = \tau_S \tag{15}$$

The acoustic coupling constant D, which is a measure of acoustic energy conversion into thermal energy

$$D = 9<\gamma_i^j>^2 - \frac{3<\gamma_i^j>^2 C_V^T}{E_0} \tag{16}$$

Where Cv is the specific heat per unit volume, E_0 is the thermal energy density which can be obtained using Θ_D /T Table of AIP handbook[12].

3.   Results and Discussion

The SOECs and TOECs for lanthanum monopnictides LaX (LaN, LaP, LaAs, LaSb, LaBi) at room temperature from Burgger's definition of elastic constants and presented in our previous paper [13]. From SOECs the other mechanical parameters and ultrasonic velocities along different crystallographic directions are presented in our previous paper[13]. The calculated values of Debye average velocity from ultrasonic velocities are presented in Table-2. Debye temperature is one of the important parameter and is used to characterize the thermal phonons and describes various lattice phenomena. Debye temperature had been calculated by the formula given by Eq. (7) from Debye average velocity and Grüneisen parameter and presented in our previous paper [13]. The variation of Debye average velocity with direction is shown in Fig 1. Fig 1 shows that LaN has the highest value of Debye temperature . It shows that the value of Debye temperature is decreasing with the molecular weight of the compounds. From Mason's Grüneisen parameter [14]tables the ultrasonic Grüneisen parameters were calculated using SOECs and TOECs. The acoustic coupling constants are evaluated using the average Grüneisen parameter $<\gamma>$ and the square average Grüneisen parameter $<(\gamma)^2>$ along different crystallographic directions for longitudinal and shear waves. The relaxation time for all the compounds had been calculated using the formula given by Eqs. (14)-(15) for longitudinal and shear waves and presented in Table-2. Table-2 shows that the relaxation time for shear waves is equal to the thermal relaxation time, while longitudinal waves have relaxation time about twice that of for shear waves for all the compounds . The thermal relaxation time for all lanthanum monopnictides is in the range of 10^{-12}sec which shows the semimetalic nature of the chosen compounds. This type of behaviour was observed in other rare earth compounds like, cerium monopnictides [15], neptunium monopnictides [16], berkelium monopnictides[11].

Table 1. Debye average velocity(in 10^3 m/s), Debye temperature(in K), thermal relaxation time (10^{-12}s) of lanthanum monopnictides(LaX) along different crystallographic directions at room temperature.

Materials	Directions	V_D	Θ_D	$\tau_s = \tau_{th}$	τ_L
LaN	<100>	1.9	269.19	2.6	5.2
	<110>	2.14	303.11	2.1	4.2
	<111>	1.91	271.27	2.6	5.2
LaP	<100>	1.67	209.26	3.0	6.0
	<110>	1.91	244.82	2.2	4.4
	<111>	1.94	242.95	2.2	4.4
LaAs	<100>	1.01	124.24	2.8	5.6
	<110>	1.22	149.93	1.9	3.8
	<111>	1.44	176.63	1.4	2.8
LaSb	<100>	1.29	149.81	3.8	7.6
	<110>	1.53	177.79	2.7	5.7
	<111>	1.62	163.93	2.4	4.8
LaBi	<100>	1.11	126.47	4.4	8.8
	<110>	1.32	150.47	3.1	6.2
	<111>	1.41	161.44	2.7	5.4

The ultrasonic attenuation due to thermo elastic mechanism and due to phonon-phonon interaction , which is also known as Akhieser loss for longitudinal and shear waves had been evaluated at room temperature and presented in Table 2. Table 2 shows that the ultrasonic attenuation due to thermo elastic mechanism is much less than ultrasonic attenuation due to phonon-phonon interaction. This shows that phonon-phonon interaction is the dominant cause of attenuation in these compounds. The variation of total attenuation with direction is shown in Fig. 2 for all the monopnictides. Figure 2 shows that the attenuation is minimum along <110> direction for all the compounds. Hence <110>direction is the suitable direction for ultrasonic wave propagation.

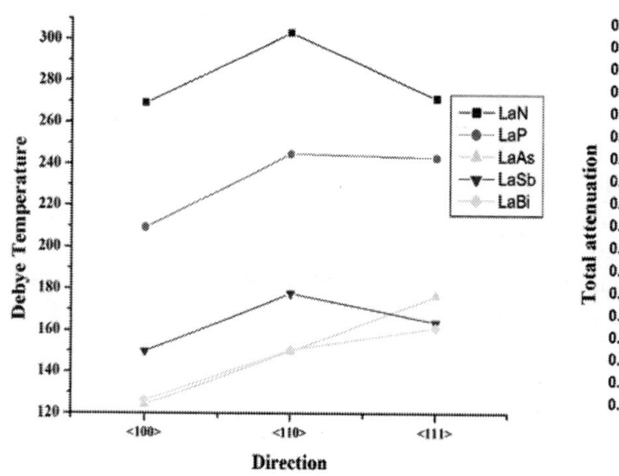

Fig1. Variation of Debye Temperature with direction.

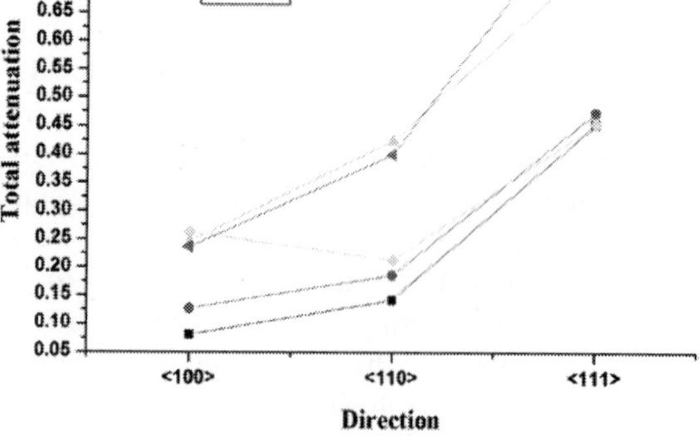

Fig 2. Variation of Total attenuation with direction.

Table 2. Acoustic coupling constant, thermoelastic attenuation$(\alpha/f^2)_{th}$, ultrasonic attenuation due to p-p interaction $(\alpha/f^2)_{Akh(l)}$, $(\alpha/f^2)_{Akh(S1)}$, $(\alpha/f^2)_{Akh(S2)}$ and Total attenuation in $10^{-16}Nps^2\,m^{-1}$, along <100>, <110>, <111> direction at room temperature

Materials	Directions	D_L	D_{S1}	D_{S2}	$(\alpha/f^2)_L$	$(\alpha/f^2)_{S1}$	$(\alpha/f^2)_{S2}$	$(\alpha/f^2)_{Th}$	Total(α/f^2)
LaN	<100>	13.41	1.04	1.04	0.05	0.0025	0.0025	0.00024	0.05524
	<110>	15.99	1.07	22.13	0.06	0.01011	0.0711	0.0007	0.1422
	<111>	15.07	16.60	16.60	0.07	0.190	0.190	0.0005	0.45356
LaP	<100>	15.67	1.04	1.04	0.08	0.003	0.003	0.00016	0.08499
	<110>	18.55	0.87	27.52	9.007	1.378	7.460	7.017	0.17915
	<111>	16.39	20.04	20.04	0.088	0.192	0.192	0.0007	0.47302
LaAs	<100>	20.94	1.13	1.13	0.17	0.076	0.076	0.00017	0.24505
	<110>	25.69	0.74	39.52	2.666	3.8714	1.4925	1.1467	0.09863
	<111>	20.03	27.59	27.59	0.002	0.003	0.003	0.00196	0.01012
LaSb	<100>	35.41	1.07	1.07	0.26	0.0055	0.0055	0.00019	0.26247
	<110>	20.78	0.80	31.38	15.28	2.268	10.729	0.0979	0.21256
	<111>	17.62	22.53	22.53	0.135	0.263	0.263	0.001196	0.45366
LaBi	<100>	17.84	1.07	1.07	0.17	0.061	0.061	0.00025	0.23598
	<110>	21.3819	0.7925	32.31	21.5	3.1788	14.643	0.1279	0.39998
	<111>	17.97	23.09	23.09	0.183	0.3448	0.34479	0.00161	0.8739

4. Conclusion

In this present study the ultrasonic attenuation of LaN, LaP, LaAs, LaSb, LaBi were calculated at room temperatures by a simple method. The ultrasonic attenuation is minimum along <110> direction for all the monopnictides. The phonon-phonon interaction is the dominant cause of ultrasonic attenuation. The thermoelastic attenuation is almost negligible as compared to attenuation due to phonon-phonon interaction. The order of thermal relaxation time is of the order of pico seconds, which proves the semimetallic nature of these compounds. The calculated value of Debye temperature is found to be highest for LaN for all directions. The higher values of Debye temperature corresponds to the lowest value of attenuation. Hence LaN is having lowest attenuation along all the directions. The knowledge of these properties are useful for many practical applications like thermo-elastic stress, load deflection, internal strain, fracture toughness, material characterization etc.

5. References

1. G. Vaitheeswaran, V. Kanchana, M. Rajagopalan, Physica B 315 (2002) 64–73

2. Gitanjali Pagare, Sankar P. Sanyal , P.K. Jha. J. Alloys Comp. 398 (2005)16–20

3. E Deligoz, K. Colakog˜lu, Y O¨ C, iftc,i and H O¨ zıs,ık, J. Phys.: Condens. Matter 19 (2007) 436204 (11pp)

4. G. Vaitheeswaran, V. Kanchana, M. Rajagopalan, J. Alloys Comp. 336 (2002) 46–55

5. Gökhan Gökoglu, Aytaç Erkisi Solid State Communications 147 (2008) 221–225

6.   D. Varshney, S. Shriya, and M. Varshney. Eur. Phys. J. B (2012) 85: 241

7.   K. Brugger, J. Phys. Rev. 133, 6A (1964).

8.   S. Mori and Y. Hiki, J. Phys. Soc. Jpn. 45, No.5, 1449 (1975).

9.   P.B. Ghate. Phys. Rev. 139, A1666(1965).

10.   D. Singh, D.K. Pandey Pramana.72 (2009) 389-398.

11.   D.Singh, S.Kaushik, S.Tripathi, V.Bhalla and A.K.Gupta. Arab.J.Sci. Eng.39 (2014) 485-494.

12.   Gray, D. E. 1981. American Institute of Physics Handbook (McGraw-Hill Book Company, Inc., New York)

13.   C.Tripathy, D.Singh, R.Paikray, J.Pure. Appl.Ultrason. 38(2016).

14.   W. P. Mason, Physical Acoustics, Vol. 3B, Academic Press, New York,1965, p.237.

15.   Bhalla V., Singh D. and Jain S.K. Int.J. Thermophys., 37 (2016) 33.

16.   D. Singh, G. Mishra, R. Kumar and R. R. Yadav,VNU. J. Sci.Maths. Phys. 32, (2016)43-53.

Ultrasonic and Thermal Properties of Cobalt Nanowires

Mohit Gupta[1,*], Sudhanshu Tripathi[2], Devraj Singh[3] and R.R.Yadav[4]

[1]Department of Physics, University of Allahabad, Prayagraj-211002, India
[2]Department of ICE, Amity School of Engineering & Technology, Noida-201313, India
|[3]Department of Physics, AIAS, Amity University Uttar Pradesh,, Noida-201313, India
*E-mail: mohitauphy89@gmail.com

ABSTRACT

We have computed elastic, mechanical, thermal and ultrasonic properties of hexagonal close packed (hcp) cobalt nanowires (Co-NWs) in high temperature regime. The second and third order elastic constants were calculated using the Lennard-Jones potential model at 300K. These elastic constants are used to find out mechanical properties, ultrasonic velocities, ultrasonic Grüneisen parameters and thermal conductivity for the stability and bonding properties of Co-NWs. Further the relaxation time, non-linearity parameter and ultrasonic attenuation have been computed using the associated parameters. The achieved results of the present investigation have been analyzed with other NWs systems.

Keywords:Co-NWs, elastic properties, thermal properties, ultrasonic properties

1.   Introduction

In current years, cobalt nanowires, as a ferromagnetic material, have fascinated significant care because of their unresolved magnetic properties and brilliant performance in applications [1] in high-density magnetic storage media [2,3], in immune magnetic separation [4], in gene delivery [5] and as targeted drug carrier [6]. The uniform linear cobalt nanowires with a mean diameter of about 100 nm were obtained with chemical reduction in aqueous solution with an external magnetic field by Li et al. [1]. Yang et al. [7] fabtricated ordered arrays of cobalt nanowires by electrodepositing the corresponding materials into the pores of anodic aluminum oxide (AAO) membranes. Lavín et al. [8] prepared the arrays of Co nanowires with different lengths and diameters have been prepared by electrodeposition into nanopores of alumina and polycarbonate membranes. Heidelberg et al. [9] introduced a model which precisely accounts for the mechanical properties of Co nanowires in a clamped-clamped beam configuration over the entire elastic range and provides a complete procedure for the examination of a broad range of nanowire systems. Hu et al. [10] constructed EAM-type many-body potentials for ten hexagonal close packed metals. These potentials reproduce for each metal considered the experimentally observed equilibrium density, c/a ratio, cohesive energy, five independent second-order elastic constants and, approximately, the vacancy formation energy. A modification term has been also introduced for describing metals with negative Cauchy pressure. Finnis-Sinclair (F-S) type many-body potentials have been constructed for eight hexagonal metals: Co, Zr, Ti, Ru, Hf, Zn, Mg and Be by Igarashi et al. [11]. They found that each of the constructed potentials has been represented by a stable hexagonal close-packed lattice with a particular non-ideal c/a ratio. As per authors information, no one has studied the cobalt-nanowires (Co-NWs) for its mechanical, thermal and acoustical properties and this is motivation to study these additional properties of the Co-NWs.

In present investigation, firstly, we computed the second- and third- order elastic constants (SOECs and TOECs) with Lennard-Jones potential. The obtained values of SOECs have been applied to find out the Young's modulus, bulk modulus, shear modulus, Poisson's ratio, Breazeale's non-linearity parameter, ultrasonic velocities and thermal conductivity. Futher these evaluated parameters have been used to find out thermal relaxation time, acoustic coupling constants and ultrasonic attenuation due to phonon-phonon (p-p) interaction and thermal relaxation mechanisms. Obtained results have been presented and discussed with available findings on Co-NWs at room temperature and along unique axis.

2.   Theory

The chosen material Co-NWs is wurtzite hexagonal close packed (hcp) with lattice parameter a,c are 2.506 and 4.072 respectively. 6 SOECs and 10 TOECs have been computed with Lennard-Jones interaction potential as detailed in our previous paper [12]. These SOECs are used to find out the Young's modulus (Y), bulk modulus (B), shear modulus (G), Poisson's ratio (υ), Zener anisotropic factor (ZA), angle dependent longitudinal, shear and quasi shear ultrasonic velocities and thermal conductivity using the expressions of our previous paper [12]. The SOECs and TOECs have been used to find the ultrasonic Grüneisen parameters (UGPs). The expressions to find the UGPs are given in literature [13]. The specific heat per unit volume (Cv) and energy density (E_0) were calculated using the tables for the ratio of Debye temperature and room temperature in AIP handbook [14]. Further these parameters are applied to calculate the ultrasonic attenuation due to phonon-phonon interaction and thermoelastic relaxation mechanisms in Co-NWs using the modified Mason's approach [15].

3.   Results and Discussion

The SOECs and TOECs have been obtained using Lennard-Jones interaction potential with Lennard-Jones interaction constant (b_0) 2.8347×10^{-65} erg cm^{7}and constants (m, n) 6,7 respectively.The SOECs,are presented in Table 1. It is depicted from Table 1 that the values of present investigation is varied 10- 20% of the previous values [10, 11]. These are comparable with previous values.

Table 1. Second order elastic constants (GPa) of Co nanowire at 300K

Temp. (K)	C_{11}	C_{12}	C_{13}	C_{33}	C_{44}	C_{66}
300	376.6	150.27	129.03	377.3	95.27	83.94
[10]	319.53	166.11	102.10	373.64	82.41	76.77
[11]	295	159	111	335	71	-

The SOECs have been utilized to compute the mechanical parameters Y, B, G, υ and Z_A of Co-NWs. These values of the mechanical parameters with TOECs are given in Table 2. From the Table 2, it is noticeable that although the value of shear modulus (G) is quite different but the bulk modulus value of Co-NWs is exactly same with previous value given by Hu et al. [10]. This confirms the validation the approach to compute the SOECs and bulk modulus (B). Further the value of Pugh's indicator i.e., B/G (1.53) is less than 1.75, which confirms the brittle nature of Co-NWs. The Zener anisotropic ratio (Z_A) deviates from the unity, which confirms the anisotropic behavior of Co-NWs. The TOECs were also compared with wurtzite hcp zinc oxide nanowires [12]. The Born stability criteria were satisfied by Co-NWs too. This confirm the mechanical stability of the Co-NWs.

The ultrasonic velocities (V_L, V_{S1} and V_{S2}: here L stands for longitudinal wave, S1 for shear wave and S2 for quasi shear wave) have been computed with the help of the SOECs and the density of Co-NWs for the ultrasonic wave propagation at different orientation from the unique axis of Co-NWs. The values of the ultrasonic velocities are shown in Fig. 1.

Table 2. Third order elastic constants, Young Modulus (Y), bulk Modulus (B), shear Modulus (G) and Poisson's ratio at 300K of Co-NWs

Temp. (K)	C_{111}(GPa)	C_{112}(GPa)	C_{113}(GPa)	C_{123}(GPa)	C_{133}(GPa)	C_{344}(GPa)	C_{144}(GPa)	C_{155}(GPa)
300	-6141.4	-973.70	-203.73	-258.93	-1274.7	-1195	-301.69	-201.08
	C_{222}(GPa)	C_{333}(GPa)	Y(GPa)	B(GPa)	G(GPa)	v	Z_A	
	-4859.2	-4732.7	300.16	181.45	118.29	0.26	0.76	
[10]				181.42	74.82	0.31		

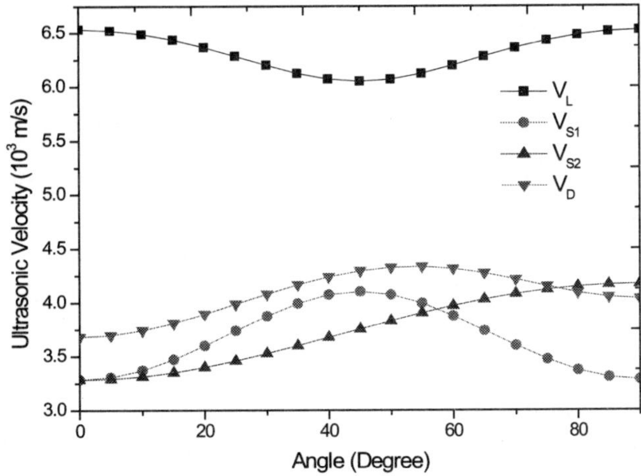

Figure 1. Ultrasonic velocities and Debye velocity vs. angle from the unique axis of Co-NWs.

It is obvious from Fig.1 that the longitudinal velocity (V_L) has been found minimum at 45°, while the quasi shear velocity (V_{S2}) maximum at 45° and Debye average velocity (V_D) has been received maximum at 50°. As we know that Debye average velocity has been obtained by combined values of V_L, V_{S1} and V_{S2}. Although, no direct data is available to compare the velocities of Co-NWs, but the trend of the graph (Fig. 1) has been found similar to other wurtzitehcp materials ZnO and BeO [12, 16]. The values of E0, C_V have been computed from the AIP Handbook [14]. The values of E0, C_V, acoustic coupling constants (DL and DS) with ultrasonic velocities values are given in Table 3.

Table 3. Specific heat per unit volume C_V (10^5 Jm^{-3}), energy density E_0 (10^6 Jm^{-3}K^{-1}), acoustic coupling constants (D_L and D_S) and ultrasonic velocities (10^3ms^{-1}) of Co NWs at 300K.

C_V	E_0	D_L	D_S	V_L	$V_{S1}=V_{S2}$	V_D
25.50	333.29	57.73	1.48	6.53	3.28	3.68

The thermal conductivity (κ) has been evaluated using the Morelli and Slack approach [17]. These all associated parameters now have been put to find out the thermal relaxation time (τ) and ultrasonic attenuation due to phonon-phonon interaction and thermoelastic relaxation mechanisms. These parameters have been given in Table 4.

Table 4. The temperature dependent thermal conductivity (Wm^{-1}K^{-1}), thermal relaxation time (ps) and ultrasonic attenuation of Co-NWs

T(K)						
	τ	κ	$(\alpha/f^2)_L$	$(\alpha/f^2)_S$	$(\alpha/f^2)_{th}$	$(\alpha/f^2)_{Total}$
300	21.36	246.31	21.93	2.21	.0964	24.25

Here it is observable that the values of ultrasonic attenuation due to thermoelastic relaxation mechanism $[(\alpha/f^2)_{th}]$ is negligible in comparison to ultrasonic attenuation due to phonon-phonon interaction $[(\alpha/f^2)_L$ and $(\alpha/f^2)_S]$. The total attenuation is found less in comparison to other studied wurtzitehcp materials ZnO [12] and BeO [16].

4. Conclusion

The conclusions of this work are drawn into the followingpoints as:

- The evaluated SOECs and TOECs validates the approach of computation using the Lennard-Jones potential for Co-NWs.

- On the basis mechanical constants of Co-NWs, it is confirmed that Co-NWs is stable and anisotropic and brittle in nature.

- The restoring time will be minimum for wave propagation along 50° for Co-NWs.

- The comparison for ultrasonic attenuation shows that the Co-NWs is better than the other wurtzitehcp materials ZnO and BeO.

The obtained results of elastic constants, ultrasonic velocities, thermal relaxation time and ultrasonic attenuation will be used to get further investigation of various transport properties of Co-NWs.

5. References

1. X. Li, L. Sun, H. Wang, K. Xie, Q. Long, X. Lai and L. Liao, Beilstein J. Nanotechnol. 7 (2016) 990–994

2. D. Saini, D., R. P. Chauhan and S.J. Kumar, Mater. Sci.: Mater. Electron. 25 (2013) 124–127.

3. N. Liakakos et al., Nano Lett. 14 (2014) 3481–3486.

4. A. Hultgren, M. Tanase, C.S. Chen and D.H. Reich, IEEE Trans. Magn. 40 (2004) 2988–2990.

5. M. P. Raphael et al., Nanotechnology 21 (2010) 285101.

6. W. Gao and J. Wang, J. Nanoscale 6 (2014) 10486–10494.

7. S. G. Yang, H. Zhu, G. Ni, D. L. Yu, S. L. Tang and Y. W. Du, J. Phys. D: Appl. Phys. 33 (2000) 2388–2390.

8. R. Lavín et al., Mol. Cryst. Liq. Cryst. 521 (2010) 293–300.

9. A. Heidelberg et al., Nano Lett. 6 (2006) 1101-1106.

10. W. Hu, B. Zhang, B. Huang, F. Gao and D. J Bacon, J. Phys.: Condens. Matter 13 (2001) 1193–1213.

11. M. Igarashi, M. Khantha and V. Vitek, Philos. Mag. B 63 (1991) 603-627.

12. S. Tripathi, R. Agarwal and D.Singh, Johnson Matthey Tech. Rev. 63 (2019) 166-176.

13. M. Nandanpawar and S. Rajagopalan, J. Acoust. Soc. Am. 71, 1469-1472 (1982).

14. D.E. Gray, American Institute of Physics Hanbook, IIIrd Edition, McGraw-Hill Book Company Inc. (1957).

15. C. P. Yadav, D.K. Pandey and D. Singh, Indian J. Phys. 93 (2019) 1147-1153.

16. S. Tripathi, R. Agarwal and D.Singh, J. Pure Appl. Ultrason. 41 (2019) 44-50.

17. D. T. Morelli and G.A. Slack, High Lattice Thermal Conductivity Solids (in: High Thermal Conductivity Materials) (Ed. S.L. Shinde and J.s. Goela), Springer, New York, Ch.2, p.37 (2006).

Non-linear Elastic, Mechanical and Ultrasonic Properties of Hexagonal Silicon Carbide

Sudhanshu Tripathi[1, 2, *], Rekha Agarwal[3], Devraj Singh[4]

[1]University School of Information Communication and Technology, Guru Gobind Singh Indraprastha University, Dwarka, Delhi-110078, India, [2]Department of Instrumentation and Control Engineering, Amity School of Engineering and Technology, Sector-125, Noida-201313, India, [3]Department of Electronics and Communication Engineering, Amity School of Engineering and Technology, Sector-125, Noida-201313, India, [4]Deaprtment of Physics, AIAS, Amity University Uttar Pradesh, Noida-201313, India
*E-mail:tripathisudhanshu@gmail.com

ABSTRACT

In the present study, the ultrasonic attenuation due to phonon-phonon interaction, thermoelastic relaxation and dislocation damping mechanisms has been investigated in hexagonal 2H-SiC for longitudinal and shear waves. The nonlinear elastic properties (second and third order elastic constants) of single crystalline SiC have been computed using Lennard-Jones Potentials in the high temperature regime. The computed values of the second order elastic constants have been applied to compute the mechanical properties such as bulk modulus (B), shear modulus(G), Young's modulus (Y), Poisson's ratio (ϑ) and anisotropy factor (A) and ultrasonic velocities at room temperature. Further second and third order elastic constants have applied to compute Grüneisen parameter, acoustic coupling constants and ultrasonic attenuation. The Born-Criterion for mechanical stability is satisfied by 2H-SiC. Value of fracture to toughness ratio is 1.54, so 2H-SiC is brittle in nature. Achieved results are discussed in correlation with available theoretical/experimental results.

Keywords: Silicon carbide, elastic constants, mechanical properties, ultrasonic properties

1.   Introduction

SiC is a IV-IV group compound, whish shows polytypism and finds its application in high power[1], hard radiation [2],high temperature [3], and high frequency[4] areas. Due to lattice mismatch the strain developed in SiC governs electrical and optical properties in semiconductor heterostructures [5]. The information about second order elastic constants (SOECs) and their pressure derivatives, as well as third order elastic constants (TOECs) enables to analyze the impact of stress due to crystal growth process and device processing mechanism of semiconductor devices[6]. The impurities also affect the thermal conductivity of SiC. As the differences in the atomic mass between the impurities and substituted atom increases the thermal conductivity decreases[7]. Zhou et al. [8] have reported the stability and electronic structure of single crystalline 2H-SiC at nano scale and their dependency on size, surface effects has been investigated. Termentzidiz el al. [9] have discussed the thermal conductivity of the diameter modulated and polytype modulated SiC nanowires. Temperature dependent mechanical and thermodynamic properties of single crystal SiC polytypes has been presented by Xu et al.[10] using first principle. Jones et al. [11] had studied the pressure dependent nonlinear elastic nature of 2H-SiC. Only few literatures have reported about the nonlinear properties of 2H-SiC.Hence in order to elaborate the nonlinear elastic and thermophysical properties of 2H-SiC further investigations are customary.

In the present investigation, firstly, we computed the second- and third- order elastic constants (SOECs and TOECs) with Lennard-Jones potential. The obtained values of SOECs have been applied to find out the Young's modulus, bulk modulus, shear modulus, Poisson's ratio, Zener anisotropy, ultrasonic velocities and thermal conductivity. Further these evaluated parameters have been used to find out thermal relaxation time, acoustic coupling constants and ultrasonic attenuation due to phonon-phonon (p-p) interaction and thermal relaxation mechanisms. Obtained results have been presented and discussed with available findings on 2H-SiC at room temperature.

2.   Theory

The chosen material SiC is wurtzite hexagonal close packed (hcp) with lattice parameter a ,c are 3.079 and 5.053 respectively. SOECs and TOECs have been computed with Lennard-Jones interaction potential as detailed in our previous paper [12]. These SOECs are used to find out the Young's modulus (Y), bulk modulus (B), shear modulus (G), Poisson's ratio (υ), Zener anisotropic factor (ZA), angle dependent longitudinal, shear and quasi shear ultrasonic velocities and thermal conductivity using the expressions of our previous paper [12]. The SOECs and TOECs have been used to find the ultrasonic Grüneisen parameters (UGPs). The expressions to find the UGPs are given in literature [13]. The specific heat per unit volume (Cv) and energy density (E0) were calculated using the tables for the ratio of Debye temperature and room temperature in AIP handbook [14]. Further these parameters are applied to calculate the ultrasonic attenuation due to phonon-phonon interaction and thermoelastic relaxation mechanisms in SiC using the modified Mason's approach [15].

3.   Results and Discussion

The SOECs and TOECs have been obtained using Lennard-Jones interaction potential with Lennard-Jones interaction constant (b_0) 3.0882×10-64 erg cm^{7}and constants (m, n) 6, 7 respectively. The SOECs, are presented in Table 1. It is depicted from Table 1 that the values of present investigation are varied 10- 20% of the previous values [11,16]. These are comparable with previous values.

Table 1. Second order elastic constants (GPa) of SiC at 300K

Temp. (K)	C_{11}	C_{12}	C_{13}	C_{33}	C_{44}	C_{66}
300	518.20	208.3	102.95	540.27	133.71	211.82
[11]	493	187	91	547	137	153
[16]	541	117	61	586	162	212

The SOECs have been utilized to compute the mechanical parameters Y, B, G, υ and ZA of SiC. These values of the mechanical parameters with TOECs are given in Table 2.This confirms the validation the approach to compute the SOECs and bulk modulus (B). Further the value of Pugh's indicator i.e., B/G (1.54) is less than 1.75, which confirms the brittle nature of SiC. The Zener anisotropic ratio (ZA) deviates from the unity, which confirms the anisotropic behavior of SiC. The TOECs were also compared with wurtzite hcp zinc oxide nanowires [12]. The Born stability criteria were satisfied by SiC too. This confirm the mechanical stability of the SiC.

The ultrasonic velocities (V_L, V_{S1} and V_{S2}: here L stands for longitudinal wave, S1 for shear wave and S2 for quasi shear wave) have been computed with the help of the SOECs. The values of E_0, C_V have been computed from the AIP Handbook [14]. The values of E_0, C_V , acoustic coupling constants (D_L and D_S) with ultrasonic velocities values are given in Table 3.

Table 2. Third order elastic constants, Young Modulus (Y), bulk Modulus (B), shear Modulus (G) and Poisson's ratio at 300K of SiC

Temp. (K)	C_{111}	C_{112}	C_{113}	C_{123}	C_{133}	C_{344}	C_{144}	C_{155}
300	-2812	-1993	-1040	-1089	-1253	-423	-104	-28.2
[11]	-2676	-1040	-1009	-1199	-1219	-392	-97	-16
	C222	C333	Y	B	G	v	Z_A	
300	-2225	-2303	418.33	282.6	174.72	0.26	0.77	
[11]	-2086	-2107	420.7	252.9	172.1	0.22	---	

Table 3. Specific heat per unit volume C_V (10^5 Jm^{-3}), energy density E_0 (10^6 Jm^{-3}K^{-1}), acoustic coupling constants (D_L and D_S) and ultrasonic velocities (10^3ms^{-1}) of SiC at 300K.

C_V	E_0	D_L	D_S	V_L	$V_{S1}=V_{S2}$	V_D
0.81	80.70	51.60	1.73	12.97	6.45	7.24

The thermal conductivity (κ) has been evaluated using the Morelli and Slack approach [17]. These all associated parameters now have been put to find out the thermal relaxation time (τ) and ultrasonic attenuation due to phonon-phonon interaction and thermoelastic relaxation mechanisms. These parameters have been given in Table 4.

Table 4. The temperature dependent thermal conductivity (Wm^{-1}K^{-1}), thermal relaxation time (ps) and ultrasonic attenuation of SiC

T(K)	τ	κ	$(\alpha/f^2)_L$	$(\alpha/f^2)_S$	$(\alpha/f^2)_{th}$	$(\alpha/f^2)_{Total}$
300	59.03	339.22	4.6116	0.6295	0.0289	5.27

Here it is observable that the values of ultrasonic attenuation due to thermoelastic relaxation mechanism [(α/f2)th] is negligible in comparison to ultrasonic attenuation due to phonon-phonon interaction [(α/f2)L and (α/f2)S].

4.   Conclusion

The conclusions of this work are drawn into the following points as:

- The evaluated SOECs and TOECs validates the approach of computation using the Lennard-Jones potential for SiC.

- The comparison for ultrasonic attenuation shows that the SiC is better than the other wurtzite hcp materials .

- On the basis mechanical constants of SiC, it is confirmed that SiC is stable and anisotropic and brittle in nature.

The obtained results of elastic constants, ultrasonic velocities, thermal relaxation time and ultrasonic attenuation will be used to get further investigation of various transport properties of SiC.

5.   References

1.   Bragg, J.W., Sullivan III, W.W., Mauch, D., Neuber, A.A. and Dickens, J.C.: All solid-state high power microwave source with high repetition frequency. Review of Scientific Instruments, 84(5), 054703 (2013).

2.   Mandal, K.C., Muzykov, P.G., Krishna, R., Hayes, T. and Sudarshan, T.S.: Thermally stimulated current and high temperature resistivity measurements of 4H semi-insulating silicon carbide. Solid State Communications, 151(7), 532-535 (2011).

3.   Pushpakaran, B.N., Hinojosa, M., Bayne, S.B., Veliadis, V., Urciuoli, D., El-Hinnawy, N., Borodulin, P., Gupta, S. and Scozzie, C.: High temperature unclamped inductive switching mode evaluation of SiC JFET. IEEE Electron Device Letters, 34(4),526-528 (2013).

4.   Swamy, M.M., Kume, T. and Takada, N.: An efficient resonant gate-drive scheme for high-frequency applications. IEEE Transactions on Industry Applications, 48(4), 1418-1431,(2012).

5.   Tse, G., Pal, J., Monteverde, U., Garg, R., Haxha, V., Migliorato, M.A. and Tomić, S.: Non-linear piezoelectricity in zinc blende GaAs and InAs semiconductors. Journal of Applied Physics, 114(7), 073515,(2013).

6.   Łepkowski, S.P., Majewski, J.A. and Jurczak, G.: Nonlinear elasticity in III-N compounds: Ab initio calculations. Physical Review B, 72(24), 245201,(2005).

7.   Kawamura, T., Hori, D., Kangawa, Y., Kakimoto, K., Yoshimura, M. and Mori, Y. Thermal conductivity of SiC calculated by molecular dynamics. Japanese journal of applied physics, 47(12R), 8898,(2008).

8.   Zhou, R.L., Zuo, R.Z., Wang, L., Zhang, B.H. and Pan, B.C.: Size-and surface-dependent electronic structures of crystalline SiC nanotubes. Journal of Applied Physics, 109(8), 084318,(2011).

9.   Termentzidis, K., Barreteau, T., Ni, Y., Merabia, S., Zianni, X., Chalopin, Y., Chantrenne, P. and Volz, S.:Modulated SiC nanowires: Molecular dynamics study of their thermal properties. Physical Review B, 87(12), 125410, (2013).

10.   Xu, W.W., Xia, F., Chen, L., Wu, M., Gang, T. and Huang, Y. High-temperature mechanical and thermodynamic properties of silicon carbide polytypes. Journal of Alloys and Compounds, 768, 722-732,(2018).

11.   Jones, S. and Menon, C.S., Non-linear elastic behavior of hexagonal silicon carbide, Physica Status Solidi (b), 251(6), 1186-1191 (2014).

12.   Tripathi, S., Agarwal, R. and Singh, Size dependent elastic and thermophysical properties of Zinc oxide nanowires, Johnson Matthey Technology Review.63 66-176 (2019).

13.   Nandanpawar, M. and Rajagopalan, S. Grüneisen numbers in hexagonal crystals. The Journal of the Acoustical Society of America, 71(6), 1469-1472,(1982).

14.   Gray, D.E.: American Institute of Physics Handbook. McGraw Hill, New York, 1957.

15.   Yadav, C.P., Pandey, D.K. and Singh, D., Ultrasonic study of Laves phase compounds $ScOs_2$ and YOs_2. Indian Journal of Physics, 93, 1147-1153 (2019).

16.   Sarasamak, K., Limpijumnong, S. and Lambrecht, W.R.:Pressure-dependent elastic constants and sound velocities of wurtzite SiC, GaN, InN, ZnO, and CdSe, and their relation to the high-pressure phase transition: A first-principles study. Physical Review B, 82(3), 035201 (2010).

17.   D. T. Morelli and G.A. Slack, High Lattice Thermal Conductivity Solids (in: High Thermal Conductivity Materials) (Ed. S.L. Shinde and J.s. Goela), Springer, New York, Ch.2, p.37 (2006).

Elastic and Ultrasonic Properties of B1 and B2 Phase Boron Monopnictides

Jyoti Bala[1,*], Punit K. Dhawan[2], Giridhar Mishra[2] and Devraj Singh[3,4]

[1] University School of Information, Communication & Technology, Guru Gobind Singh
Indraprastha University, New Delhi–110078
[2]Department of Physics, Prof. Rajendra Singh (Rajju Bhaiya) Institute of Physical Sciences for Study and Research,
Veer Bahadur Singh Purvanchal University, Jaunpur-222003, India
[3] Department of Applied Physics, Amity School of Engineering & Technology Delhi, Noida-201313, India
[4]Department of Physics, AIAS, Amity University Uttar Pradesh, Noida-201313, India
*E-mail: jyoti_pu@yahoo.com

ABSTRACT

We have investigated and evaluated the elastic, ultrasonic and thermo-physical properties of NaCl and CsCl Boron based compounds BX(X=N, P and As) along <100> orientations. In the present study, we evaluate and compared the higher order elastic constants values at room temperature using theoretical approach of Mori and Hiki. The second order elastic constants have been applied to calculate the mechanical properties which confirmed that CsCl is not closely packed structure because of large volume/less density. Also, CsCl based boron compounds are stronger than NaCl based compounds. Further elastic constant have been applied to compute ultrasonic velocities for longitudinal and shear modes, thermal conductivity, Debye velocity and thermal relaxation time at room temperature. Finally ultrasonic attenuation has been estimated using phonon-phonon interaction and thermoelastic relaxation mechanism. We have found that the value of ultrasonic and Debye velocity is highest for CsCl boron based compounds at room temperature. From the result, we conclude that BN is strongest and most fit material for crystallographic study along <100> direction among other boron based compounds in both type of structure. We also found that the chosen materials are semi metallic in nature. The result was obtained and the correlation with available results was discussed on the chosen materials for their future prospects.

Keywords: Elastic property, thermal property, ultrasonic property.

1. Introduction

Boron-based compounds are widely used in electronic field due to the small core size of boron atom and the absence of p electrons. Many theoretical study have been carried out on boron based compounds specially on BP, BAs and BSb which explained their structural and electronic properties in the NaCl phase structure [1-2]. Although very few experimental data on these compounds [3-4] for both phase B1 and B2 are available in literature. Some other properties of these compounds at high pressure were studied by Wentzcovitch et al. [5-7], which also discussed its electronic properties. In the available literature, we did not find temperature dependent theoretical work on these compounds for both structure i.e. B1 and B2 phase. Due to limited theoretical studies on these compounds on both cubic structure (NaCl and CsCl) we got motivated to make new analysis on these materials. In present work we evaluate temperature dependent elastic, ultrasonic and thermal properties of Boron based compounds BX(X=N, P and As) at room temperature for both NaCl and CsCl phase structure. Also, we investigated the mechanical and thermophysical properties of these compounds. Finally the ultrasonic attenuation for boron based compounds was computed at 27°C temperature by using the computed parameters.

2. Computational Approach

In our research, we have followed Mori and Hiki theoretical approach [8-9] to calculate higher order elastic constants outlined by Brugger's potential model. The derive value of SOECs have been used to find out the mechanical constants such as bulk modulus (B), Young's modulus (Y), Poisson's ratio (υ), Lame modulus (λ), Hardness (H) and density at 27^0C temperature using the expression given in literature [10]. Higher order elastic constants are further used to compute ultrasonic properties of boron based compounds in both phase structure (NaCl and CsCl) and expression are explained in our previous paper [11]. C_v is Specific heat per unit volume and E_θ can be obtained from Θ_D/T tables of AIP Handbook [12]. In this paper we evaluate minimum thermal conductivity of material using following expression [13]:

$$\kappa = k_B V_D \times \left(\frac{M}{n\rho N_A} \right)^{-2/3} \tag{1}$$

here k_B = Boltzmann constant, n = number of atomic per unit cell, N_A=Avogadro's number, ρ=density, M=Molecular weight and V_D is Debye velocity.

3. Results and Discussion

The higher order Elastic constants i.e. SOECs and TOECs are analyzed at 27°C temperature using lattice parameter of boron based compounds BX(X=N, P and As) are 3.428 Å, 4.199 Å, 4.475 Å for B1 structure and 3.575 Å, 4.196 Å, 4.510 Å for B2 structure respectively. Table 1 represent that BN has greater elastic moduli than other chosen boron compounds in both phase structure which shows that it's the strongest compounds. The similar type of elastic behavior can be observed in other cubic structure compounds [14-16].

Table 1 SOECs for HFX at 27°C temp (in the unit of 10^{11} Nm^{-2})

Materials	Structure	C_{11}	C_{12}	C_{44}	C_{111}	C_{112}	C_{123}	C_{144}	C_{166}	C_{456}
BN	NaCl	8.86	12.64	13.09	-91.55	-50.25	-17.16	18.37	-51.31	18.13
	CsCl	9.379	5.5670	4.7939	-93.29	-7.619	-3.6178	-2.909	-7.811	-4.269
BP	NaCl	8.52	5.09	5.45	-112.17	-21.02	6.82	8.19	-22.07	8.05
	CsCl	5.653	2.869	2.538	-52.38	-6.564	-4.669	-3.656	-6.178	-5.089
BAs	NaCl	7.89	3.80	4.14	-107.28	-15.79	4.97	6.36	-16.83	6.24
	CsCl	4.490	2.1124	1.987	-40.94	-5.940	-4.597	-3.474	-5.331	-4.917

Using above higher order elastic constants values, we evaluate mechanical properties of boron based compounds presented in Table 2. From the Table 2 we observed that density of boron compounds decreases as we shift from NaCl (FCC) to CsCl (BCC) structure which confirm that BCC lattice is not closely packed structure because of large volume/less density. Also, CsCl boron based compounds are the strongest one compared to NaCl based boron compounds due to the highest value of hardness and bulk modulus factor. We also benchmarked the obtained results with other NaCl and CsCl based compounds and found same mechanical nature of chosen materials[17-18].

Table 2: Mechanical properties of boron based compounds

Materials Parameters	BN		BP		Bas	
	NaCl	CsCl	NaCl	CsCl	NaCl	CsCl
B (10^{11} N/m²)	11.05	6.838	6.23	3.797	5.17	2.905
H (10^{10} N/m²)	0.135	4.604	0.532	2.972	5.22	2.531
ρ (g/cm³)	4.091	1.804	3.748	1.878	6.35	3.103
Poisons ratio(υ)	0.531	0.291	0.267	0.276	0.249	0.265

Table 3. Ultrasonic velocities V_L, V_{s1}, V_{s2} ($10^3 ms^{-1}$), Debye temperature Θ_D (in K), thermal relaxation time τ_l (ps) and acoustic coupling constant (D_L, D_S) at 27°C temperature along <100> direction

Material Parameters	BN		BP		BAs	
	NaCl	CsCl	NaCl	CsCl	NaCl	CsCl
V_l	4.38	7.211	4.77	5.486	3.52	3.804
V_{s1}	5.66	5.155	3.81	3.676	2.55	2.530
V_{s2}	5.66	5.155	3.81	3.676	2.55	2.530
V_D	5.077	5.580	4.05	4.016	2.757	2.767
Θ_D	882.44	738.17	574.26	452.61	367.08	290.13
τ_l	2.37	2.15	2.92	2.93	4.21	4.30
D_L	14.67	5.88	13.27	3.89	12.30	3.43
D_{s1}	9.44	0.88	1.97	0.92	1.34	1.12

From table 3, we found thermal relaxation time is of the order of picosecond which shows the metallic nature of boron based compounds for both phase of structure [19]. We found that the value of ultrasonic velocity is highest for CsCl boron based compounds at room temperature along <100> direction presented in Table 3. Thermal conductivity of chosen compounds is found to decrease with the increase in molecular weight shown in Fig. 1. We also observed that BN has the highest value of thermal conductivity and Debye velocity at 27⁰C temperature for both phase structure. Hence BN material can be used as most thermal-conductive material. Fig 2, helps us to understand further that the value of net attenuation is quite less for BN compound compared to other boron based compounds in the case of NaCl phase structure. We compare our result with other cubic type materials [20-21] and found way more similar to it.

4.   Conclusions

On the basis of above results, analysis and discussion of the obtained results, we can conclude following points

- With respect to other boron based compounds, the elastic properties of BN are predominant
- CsCl based boron compounds are stronger than NaCl based compounds.
- BN is strongest and most fit material for crystallographic study along <100> direction among other boron based
- BN has the highest thermal conductivity which confirms that BN has good thermal performance.
- The thermal relaxation time can be derived in order of picosecond, which further confirms the semi-metallic nature of the chosen materials.

- The thermal conductivity of the materials decreases with increase in the molecular weight of the materials. Also, BN has least value of attenuation in B2 phase.

These results help us to understand the application of these materials for study as well for the industrial uses.

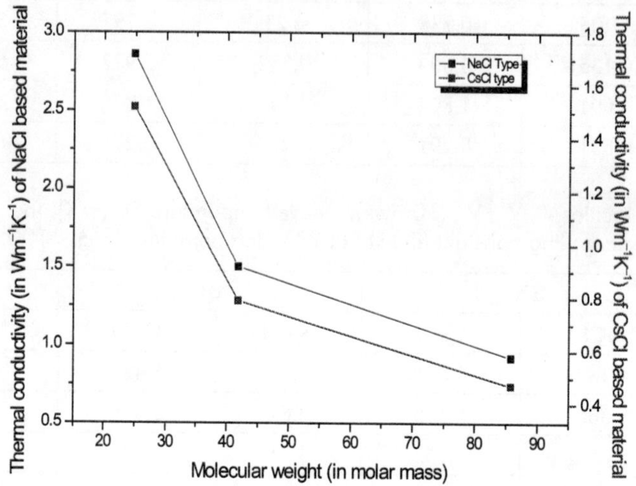

Figure 1　Thermal Conductivity of NaCl and CsCl based materials BMP (MP=N, P, As) with molecular weight at room temperature along <100> direction

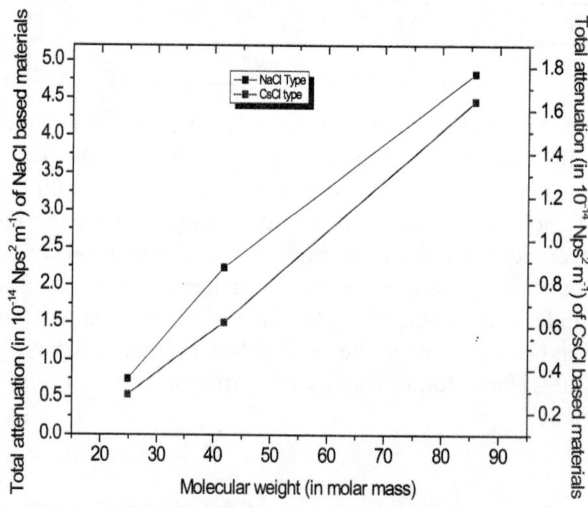

Figure 2　Total Attenuation loss of NaCl and CsCl based materials BMP (MP=N, P, As) with molecular weight at room temperature along <100> direction

5.　References

1.　P. Rodriguez-Hernandez, M. Gonzalez-Diaz, A. Munoz, Phys. Rev. B 51, (1995), 14705.

2.　L. Vel, G. Demazeau, J. Eloumeau, Mater. Sci. Eng. B 10, (1991), 149.

3.　E. Knittle, R.M. Wentzcovitch, R. Jeanloz, M.L. Cohen, Nature (London) 337,(1989), 349.

4.　K. Bencherifa,b, A. Yakoubia and H. Mebtouchea, Acta Phys. Pol. A Acta Phys. Pol. A 131, (2017), 209-212.

5.　R. Wentzcovitch, K.J. Chang, M.L. Cohen, Phys. Rev. B 34, (1986), 1071.

6.   R. Wentzcovitch, M.L. Cohen, J. Phys. C 19, (1986), 6791.

7.   W. Sekkal, B. Bouhafs, H. Aourag, M. Certier, J. Phys.: Condens. Matter 10, (1998), 4975.

8.   K Brugger, Phys. Rev., 133, (1964), A1611–A1612

9.   Bor Max, Mayer J.E, mag. of Phys., 75, (1931), 1-18

10.   R. R. Yadav and D. K. Pandey, Acta Phys. Pol. A 107, (2005), 933.

11.   V Bhalla, D. Singh, Indian J Pure Appl Phys, 54, (2016), 40–45

12.   D. E. Gray, American Institute of Physics Handbook (McGraw Hill: New York) 1981

13.   A Khan, D K Pandey, D. Singh, J. Pure Appl. Phys. 41, (2019), 1-8

14.   D. Singh, V. Bhalla, J. Bala , S. Wadhwa, Z Naturforsch A, 72, (2017), 977-983

15.   D. Singh, A. Kumar, R.K.Thakur, R.Kumar, Proc. Natl. Acad.Sci, India, Sec.A Phys. Sci. (Article in Press, 2019)

16.   C.P. Yadav, D. K. Pandey and D.Singh. Z. Naturforsch. A (2019). doi:10.1515/Zna-2019-0041.

17.   A. Khan, C. P. Yadav, D. K. Pandey, D. Singh and D. Singh, J. Pure Appl. Ultrasonic 41, (2019) 1-8.

18.   D. Singh, D K Pandey, Pramana J. of Physics, 72(2), 2009, 389-398

19.   V. Bhalla, D.Singh, S.K. Jain, R.Kumar, Pramana 86, (2016), 1355-1367.

20.   V Bhalla, D Singh, G Mishra, J Pure Appl Ultrason, 38, (2016), 23–27

21.   C Tripathy, D. Singh, R. Paikaray, Can. J. Phys., 96(5), 2018, 513-518

Analysis of ZnO as Membrane Material for Capacitive Micromachined Ultrasonic Transducer

Sudhanshu Tripathi[1,2*], Rekha Agarwal[2] and Rashmi Vashisth[3]

[1]University School of Information Communication and Technology, Guru Gobind Singh Indraprastha University, Dwarka, Delhi-110078, India
[2]Department of Instrumentation and Control Engineering, Amity School of Engineering and Technology, Sector-125, Noida-201313, India
[3]Department of Electronics and Communication Engineering, Amity School of Engineering and Technology, Sector-125, Noida-201313, India
*E-mail: tripathisudhanshu@gmail.com

ABSTRACT

In this paper, nanostructured w-ZnO has been utilized as the membrane material of the Capacitive Micromachined Ultrasonic Transducer (CMUT) with circular geometry, using the formulated structural and elastic parameters based on ultrasonic theory. The significant factors of ultrasonic transducers like resonant frequency, deflection analysis, capacitance change and pull in voltage have been analyzed using analytical model and FEM simulations. The obtained results has been discussed and correlated with theoretical and experimental results available in literatures.

Keywords: CMUT, Mechanical properties, Ultrasonic properties, Pull in voltage.

1. Introduction

Recently with technological advancement the conventional piezo composite transducers have been replaced by capacitive micromachined ultrasonic transducers (CMUT) [1]. The micromachining techniques enabled to generate high electric fields at micron level, leading to better transduction efficiency, broader bandwidth and higher resolution in correspondence to piezoelectric transducers [2]-[3]. Intensive research on CMUT has been done to improve its performance through device structure, fabrication technology and materials properties [4]-[7]. The CMUTs finds applications in numerous areas like medical imaging, distance finding and non-destructive testing methods [8]. In addition to application in ultrasound detector and generator, CMUT also finds its application in wide areas from consumer electronics to medical imaging systems e.g. blood and intraocular pressure measurement, ultrasonic imaging, thickness of the cornea [9],[10]. The exhaustive potential of CMUT has motivated the researcher towards its modeling under different loading conditions. The electrical and mechanical modeling schemes using the approaches like mathematical modeling, equivalent circuit modeling, modeling using simulations. Now a day's majority of work reported includes modeling and optimization of single devices [11], [12]. J.Wang et al. [13] have developed an analytical model for analysis of membrane deflection profile of CMUT for under water applications. They have also studied the effect of lateral forces on CMUT operating modes and deflection characteristics. Lardiès et al. [14] had proposed two methods for model parameter (e.g. stiffness and damping coefficients, resonance frequency etc.) identification for the membrane of CMUT. The SiC membrane based CMUT has been proposed by Q.Zang et al. [15] and the proper operation of the device fabricated has been demonstrated via electrical and acoustical characterization. The frequency response of the transducer designed has been predicted by simulation and FEM modeling. Thiebert et al. [16] described the manufacturing and mechanical characterization of carbon suspended membrane acting as mobile electrode of CMUT. The thickness of membrane reduced to nanometer range to get significant displacement. In the present work, finite modelling of CMUT is performed with a silicon substrate and w-ZnO (Wurzite Zinc Oxide) as a membrane laid over a small gap filled with air. Frequency domain, time dependent, Eigen frequency and stationary analysis are done in COMSOL. The results obtained are being analyzed with membrane materials existing in literature.

Contrary to piezoelectric transducers, transduction is obtained electrostatically. To the best of author's knowledge, ZnO- based CMUT membrane have not been reported previously. ZnO as a structural material is showing significant interest of researchers due to its mechanical, electronic and thermoelectricity. The large piezoelectricity of ZnO makes it suitable candidate for electro acoustical devices. The mechanical parameters such as Bulk modulus, Young's modulus, Poisson's ratio, elastic constants etc. and their dependency on temperature and size at bulk and Nano level are important parameters for engineering applications. The second order elastic constants of w-ZnO satisfies the Born stability criterion for hcp structured material indicating that w-ZnO is mechanically stable [17]. The Zener anisotropy of w-ZnO founds to be less than 1, indicating the degree of elastic anisotropy. The Poisson's ratio of the w-ZnO material is about 0.31 representing its ionic behavior. The Young's modulus value of w-ZnO lying in the range of 140-200 GPa depending upon its diameter at nano level [18].

The parallel plate structured CMUT is formed with a heavily doped silicon substrate having an insulating layer with inbuilt cavity on it. The cavity can be a vacuum or filled with air for providing damping effect. The insulating layer with cavity is overlaid by a semiconductor or an insulating material of micron thickness forming the membrane. The substrate and the membrane forms a parallel plate capacitor with air as the dielectric. When the DC bias is applied between the two plates of the capacitor, the top electrode is deflected downwards due to the electrostatic forces of the substrate. With the AC bias superimposed on the deflected plate, the plate starts vibrating generating the acoustic waves in the surrounding medium and CMUT works as a transmitter. Conversely, when the deflected plate is subjected to acoustic signals leading to capacitance change, which can be further amplified making CMUT as a receiver [19]. The CMUT membrane can be constructed in various geometries such as circular, square, rectangular, hexagonal etc. and with different materials like silicon, polysilicon, silicon nitride etc. [20].

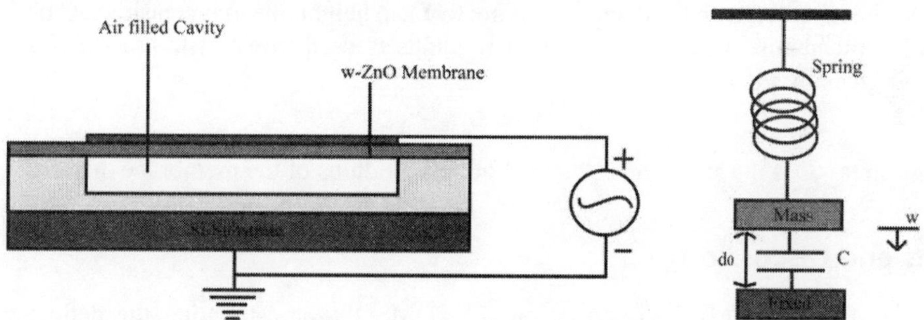

Fig. 1. Single CMUT cell schematic (Left) with Electrical equivalent model (Right)

2.   Theory of Operation

The parallel plate model of CMUT can be modelled as the capacitor, mass and spring as shown in Fig. 1 [21], [22]. Using the force balance, the Mass force is balanced by the sum of capacitive force and the spring force, as shown in Eq. (1)

$$F_{Cap} + F_{Spring} = F_{Mass} \tag{1}$$

The electrostatic force is produced by the DC bias (V) among substrate and the membrane, raises to F_{Cap} and is given by Eq. (2)

$$F_{Cap} = -\frac{d}{dx}\left(\frac{CV^2}{2}\right) = -\frac{\epsilon_0\, AV^2}{2(d_0 - w)^2} \tag{2}$$

Where, V is the applied DC bias among the electrodes, d_0 mentions the original gap between the electrodes, ww is the deflection of membrane along the radius, ϵ_0 is the relative permittivity and A is the area of the electrodes.

Using the Newton's Second Law of motion for mass force, F_{Mass} and Hooke's Law for the spring force, F_{Spring} results in Eq. (3)

$$m\frac{d^2w(t)}{dt^2} = -\frac{\epsilon_0\,AV(t)^2}{2(g_0 - w(t))^2} + kW(t) = 0 \tag{3}$$

The electrostatic forces produced by the bottom electrode are balanced by the inherent mechanical forces of membrane. When the DC bias is increased further, the restoring mechanical forces of membrane are not able to overcome the electrostatic forces of the substrate and the membrane collapse with the substrate and this DC voltage is known as Collapse/Pull in voltage and is calculated as shown in Eq. (4)[21]

$$V_{Pull} - in = \sqrt{\frac{8Kd_0^3}{27E\,\epsilon_0}} \tag{4}$$

When the DC biased membrane is subjected to AC bias the membrane starts vibrating within the cavity and produces acoustic waves. The magnitude of AC bias is much smaller than the DC bias and can be written as Eq. (5)

$$V(t) = V_{DC} + V_{AC}\,Sin(wt) \tag{5}$$

The force due to AC and DC bias on the membrane can be given by Eq. (6)

$$F_{DC+AC} = \frac{\epsilon_0\,AV^2}{2(d_0 - w)^2} = \frac{\epsilon_0\,A(V_{DF} + V_{AC}Sin(wt))^2}{2(d_0 - w)^2} \tag{6}$$

The spring force is increased with the decrease in effective gap height due to increasing DC bias. The w-ZnO is utilized as the membrane material, its young's modulus is used to estimate the stress and strain with Hooke's Law as given by Eq. (7)

$$\sigma = E\epsilon \tag{7}$$

Where, σ is the stress, C is the strain, and E is the Young's modulus of the membrane material.

3.   Results and Discussion

Finite element analysis of CMUT is carried out in COMSOL for estimating the deflection of w-ZnO membrane. The material properties and dimension used for simulation are summarized in Table 1.

Table 1. Dimension and Material Properties used for Analysis

Material	w-ZnO(Wurzite- Zinc Oxide)
Radius, R	45 µm
Thickness, t	1 µm
Young's modulus, E	145.45 GPa
Poisson's Ratio, v	0.31
Density	5680 kg/m³

For finding the maximum frequency with which the membrane vibrates, Eigen frequency study in COMSOL was exploited with Solid mechanics module and it was found the membrane vibrates at 1.39 MHz. Further, using the frequency domain study the maximum deflection of membrane was found to be at 1.39 MHz as shown in Fig. 2. When the electrostatic forces of membrane are not withstand by the mechanical restoring forces of membrane due to increased bias, top plate collapses with the substrate. For finding the collapse voltage of the device with w-ZnO membrane, deflection profile was studied, and analytically it was found the collapse occurs when the deflection of membrane extents the 1/3rd of the initial gap height. A continuous force is subjected on membrane when the DC bias is applied and the magnitude of bias is increased till both the electrodes collapses. With the parametric analysis in coupled fields, on this condition solution fails to converge and the simulations lay off. Before the solution fails, the last voltage signifies to the pull-in voltage. The deflection with increased bias is shown in Fig. 3 with assessed collapse or pull-in voltage. The pull-in voltage solved from deflection graph is 104.94 V.

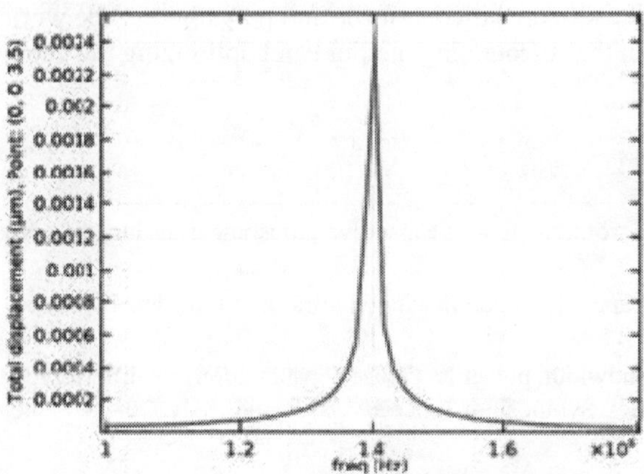

Fig. 2. Frequency Domain plot showing maximum deflection at the resonant frequency (Left)

Fig. 3. Deflection analysis plot for estimating the Pull-in voltage (Right)

With the Eigen frequency results, the time dependent study was performed for the dynamic operation of the membrane, applying both the DC and AC bias (Eq. 5), the membrane deflection obtained is shown in Fig. 4. The alternating waves produced are the acoustic waves transmitted to the surrounding environment.

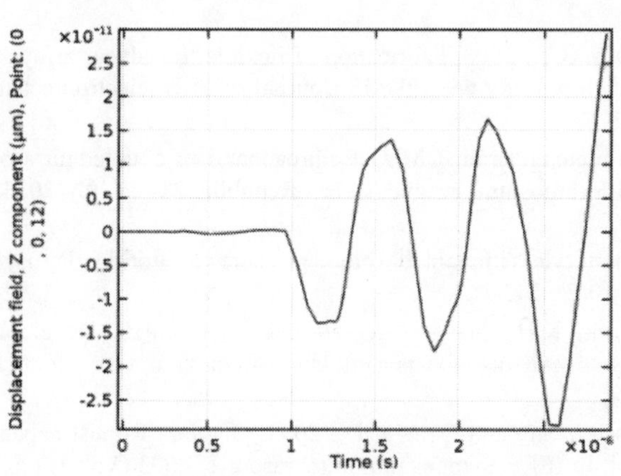

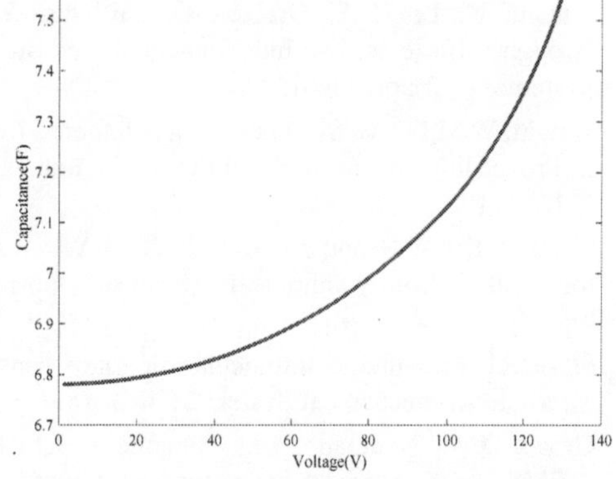

Fig. 5. Acoustic waves generated with application of AC and DC bias (Left)

Fig. 6. Capacitance variation with increasing DC bias (Right)

Fig. 6 displays the capacitance change with increasing DC bias between membrane and substrate. With increasing DC bias the distance between the electrodes is reduced, i.e. w decreases and the capacitance increases. Air filled in cavity acts as the dielectric among the electrodes.

4. Conclusion

FEM analysis of CMUT with w-ZnO membrane was performed, using appropriate boundary conditions. The electrical and structural characteristics as a transmitter were obtained successfully. The mechanical properties of the w-ZnO were found to be suitable to be used as a transducer, which is not reported in literature. Significant characteristics of CMUT with w-ZnO are reported by the authors like pull-in voltage, resonant frequency, capacitance change and acoustic wave generation. It has been found the results obtained are comparable with materials already used for CMUT like silicon, silicon nitride and polysilicon. The work can be extended to analyzing the transduction efficiency in the surrounding medium and optimizing the geometry further.

5. References

1. Jin, X., Ladabaum, I. and Khuri-Yakub, B.T. The microfabrication of capacitive ultrasonic transducers. journal of microelectromechanical systems 7(3), 295-302.

2. Ergun, A.S.; Yaralioglu, G.G.; Khuri-Yakub, B.T. Capacitive micromachined ultrasonic transducers: Theory and technology. J. Aerosp. Eng. 2003, 16, 76–84.

3. Senlik, M.N.; Olcum, S.; Koymen, H.; Atalar, A. Bandwidth, power and noise considerations in airborne CMUTs. In Proceedings of the IEEE International Ultrasonics Symposium Proceedings, Rome, Italy, 20–23 September 2009; pp. 438–441.

4. Eccardt, P.C., Niederer, K., Scheiter, T. and Hierold, C., 1996, November. Surface micromachined ultrasound transducers in CMOS technology. In 1996 IEEE Ultrasonics Symposium. Proceedings (Vol. 2, pp. 959-962). IEEE.

5. Erguri, A.S., Huang, Y., Zhuang, X., Oralkan, O., Yarahoglu, G.G. and Khuri-Yakub, B.T., 2005. Capacitive micromachined ultrasonic transducers: Fabrication technology. IEEE transactions on ultrasonics, ferroelectrics, and frequency control, 52(12), pp.2242-2258.

6. Noble, R.A., Jones, A.D., Robertson, T.J., Hutchins, D.A. and Billson, D.R., 2001. Novel, wide bandwidth, micromachined ultrasonic transducers. IEEE transactions on ultrasonics, ferroelectrics, and frequency control, 48(6), pp.1495-1507.

7. Zhuang, X., Lin, D.S., Oralkan, Ö. and Khuri-Yakub, B.T., 2008. Fabrication of flexible transducer arrays with through-wafer electrical interconnects based on trench refilling with PDMS. Journal of Microelectromechanical Systems, 17(2), pp.446-452.

8. Wright, W.M.D.; McSweeney, S.G. A tethered front-plate electrode CMUT for broadband air-coupled ultrasound. In Proceedings of the Joint UFFC, EFTF and PFM Symposium, Prague, Czech Republic, 21–25 July 2013; pp. 1716–1719.

9. Cong, P., Ko, W.H. and Young, D.J., 2009. Wireless batteryless implantable blood pressure monitoring microsystem for small laboratory animals. IEEE sensors journal, 10(2), 243-254.

10. Shin, K.S., Jang, C.I., Kim, M.J., Yun, K.S., Park, K.H., Kang, J.Y. and Lee, S.H., 2015. Development of novel implantable intraocular pressure sensors to enhance the performance in in vivo tests. Journal of Microelectromechanical Systems, 24(6), 1896-1905.

11. Greve, D.W., Neumann, J.J., Oppenheim, I.J., Pessiki, S.P. and Ozevin, D., 2003, October. Robust capacitive MEMS ultrasonics transducers for liquid immersion. In IEEE Symposium on Ultrasonics, 2003 (Vol. 1, pp. 581-584). IEEE.

12. Lohfink, A., Eccardt, P.C., Benecke, W. and Meixner, H., 2003, October. Derivation of a 1D CMUT model from FEM results for linear and nonlinear equivalent circuit simulation. In IEEE Symposium on Ultrasonics, 2003 (Vol. 1, pp. 465-468). IEEE.

13. Wang, J., Pun, S.H., Mak, P.U., Cheng, C.H., Yu, Y., Mak, P.I. and Vai, M.I., 2016. Improved Analytical Modeling of Membrane Large Deflection With Lateral Force for the Underwater CMUT Based on Von Kármán Equations. IEEE Sensors Journal, 16(17), pp.6633-6640.

14. J. Lardiès, G. Bourbon, P. Le Moal, N. Kacem, V. Walter, T.P. Le, Modal parameter identification of a CMUT membrane using response data only. Mech. Ind. 18(8), (2017) 802

15. Zhang, Q., Cicek, P. V., Allidina, K., Nabki, F., & El-Gamal, M. N. (2013). Surface-micromachined CMUT using low-temperature deposited silicon carbide membranes for above-IC integration. Journal of microelectromechanical systems, 23(2), 482-493.

16. S. Thibert, A. Ghis, M. Delaunay, Mechanical characterization of ultrathin DLC suspended membranes for CMUT applications. Phys. Procedia. 70 (2015) 974-977.

17. Tripathi, S., Agarwal, R., Singh, D. (2019). Size Dependent Elastic and Thermophysical Properties of ZnO Nanowires. Johnson Matthey Technology Review.

18. Fan, S., Bi, S., Li, Q., Guo, Q., Liu, J., Ouyang, Z., Jiang, C. and Song, J., 2018. Size-dependent Young's modulus in ZnO nanowires with strong surface atomic bonds. Nanotechnology, 29(12), 125702.

19. Ergun, A. S., Yaralioglu, G. G., and Khuri-Yakub, B. T., "Capacitive Micromachined Ultrasonic Transducers: Theory and Technology," Journal of Aerospace Engineering, Vol. 16, (2003), 76–84.

20. Rashmi Sharma, Rekha Agarwal, Anil Arora. Evaluation of Ultrasonic Transducer with Divergent Membrane Materials and Geometries. SmartCom, CCIS 2016,628, 779-787.

21. Ladabauni I., Jin X.C., Soh H.T., Atalar A, and Khuri-Yakub B.T.. Surface micromachined capacitive ultrasonic transducers . IEEE Trans. Ultrason, Freq. Control, 1998,45, 678-690.

22. Yaralioglu G. G., Ergun A. S., and Khuri-Yakub B. T., Finite-element analysis of capacitive micromachined ultrasonic transducers. IEEE Trans. Ultrason. Ferroelectr. Freq. Control, 2005, 52(12), 2185–2198.

23. Introduction to COMSOL Multiphysics Users Manual, October, 2012

24. Wong L.L.P., Chen A. I. H., Z Li, Logan A. S. and Yeow J. T. W., A row- column addressed Micromachined ultrasonic transducer array for surface scanning applications. Ultrasonics, 2014, 54(8), 2072-2080.

Synthesis of Silicon Carbide Nanofluids and Study of its Ultrasonic Characterization

N. R. Pawar[1,*], R. D. Chavhan[2], O. P. Chimankar[2] and S. J. Dhoble[2]

[1]Department of Physics, Arts, Commerce and Science College, Maregaon - 445 303, India
[1]Department of Physics, RTM Nagpur University, Nagpur- 440 033, India
* E-mail: pawarsir1@gmail.com

ABSTRACT

Silicon Carbide (SiC) nanofluids were synthesized by two step method. In this method SiC nanopowder was initially prepared and the powder was dispersed in methanol base fluid [1-3]. The nanofluid exhibits much greater properties as compared to base fluid. SiC Nanoparticles exhibits characteristics like high thermal conductivity, high stability, high purity, good wear resistance and a small thermal expansion co-efficient. These traits make it ideal for applications across a wide range of domains, with more being uncovered by the research of academics and engineers.

SiC nanoparticles have been synthesized by sol-gel method [4-5]. The mixture of SiO_2:Mg in the molar ratio1:2 heated in the furnace at 650°C for 6 hours. For an acid etching of the obtained product for 5 hour a mixture of HF 10% wt and HNO_3 4 M were used. Then the mixture is washed with distilled water and dried at room temperature. The final product is SiC in powder form. The prepared sample was characterized by X- ray diffraction (XRD), FTIR and Scanning electron microscopy (SEM). Average particle size has been estimated by using Debye-Scherrer formula [6-8]. It was found to be 50 nm. Nanofluids of SiC in methanol base fluid were prepared and their acoustical studies were made such that different types of interactions could be assessed. Thermo-acoustical parameters of this nanofluids system were computed from ultrasonic velocities, densities and viscosities at temperatures 293K, 298K, 303K, 308K and 313K at fixed frequency 5MHz over the entire range of concentrations. The obtained results of present investigation have been discussed in the light of interactions between the SiC nanoparticles and the molecules of methanol based fluids.

Keywords: Nanofluids, ultrasonic characterization, XRD, FTIR, SEM

1.   Introduction

Silicon Carbide Nanoparticles is known for its stability, refractory properties, wear resistance, thermal conductivity, small thermal expansion co-efficient, and resistance to oxidation at high temperatures. It exhibits characteristics like high thermal conductivity, high stability, high purity, good wear resistance and a small thermal expansion co-efficient. These particles are also resistant to oxidation at high temperatures. SiC nanoparticles have been synthesized by sol-gel method. The prepared sample was characterized by X- ray diffraction (XRD), FTIR and Scanning electron microscopy (SEM). Thermo-acoustical parameters of SiC nanofluid were computed from ultrasonic velocities, densities and viscosities at temperatures 293K, 298K, 303K, 308K and 313K at fixed frequency 5MHz over the entire range of concentrations.

2.   Method of Synthesis of SC Nanofluids

Silicon carbide nanoparticles have been synthesized by sol-gel method [9-10]. The mixture of SiO_2: Mg in the molar ratio 1:2 heated in the furnace at 650°C for 6 hours. For an acid etching of the obtained product for 5 hour a mixture of HF 10% wt and HNO_3 4 M were used. Then the mixture is washed with distilled water and dried at room temperature. The final product is SiC in powder form. SiC nanopowder was initially prepared and the powder was dispersed in methanol base fluid.

3. Spectroscopic Characterization of SiC Nanoparticles

Figure 1 shows the XRD pattern of Silicon carbide (SiC) nanoparticles. It is seen that the materials is well crystalline in nature and well agreed with standard JCPDS file number 029-1129 shown in Fig. 2. The estimate size of SiC nanoparticles using Debye Scherrer formula is found about 50 nm.

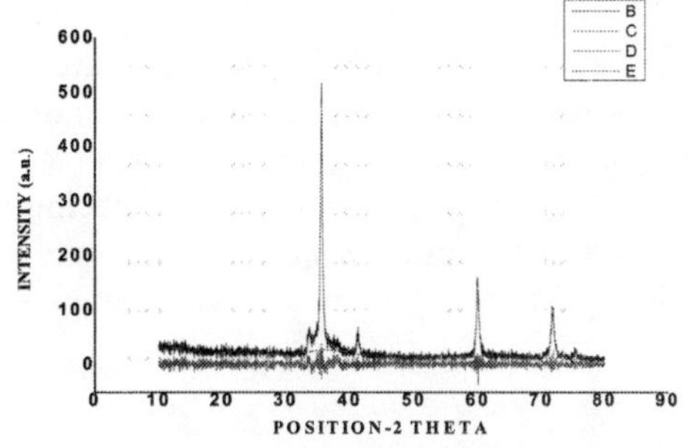

Figure 1 XRD pattern of SiC Nanoparticles

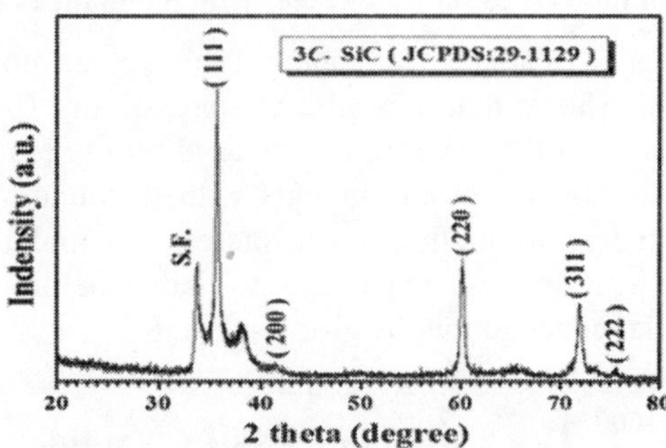

Figure 2 XRD pattern of SiC nanoparticles JCPDS file

FTIR analysis indicated the vibrations of metal oxygen (M–O) groups. FTIR spectroscopy shows the degradation phases and absorption in different regions which indicates structural relationship between them. From Fig. 3 it is seen that the inorganic groups is gradually decomposed at 1078.96 cm^{-1} and 804.12 cm^{-1}. SEM study is carried out to observe the overall surface morphology and crystallite sizes of the prepared nanomaterials shown in Fig. 4.

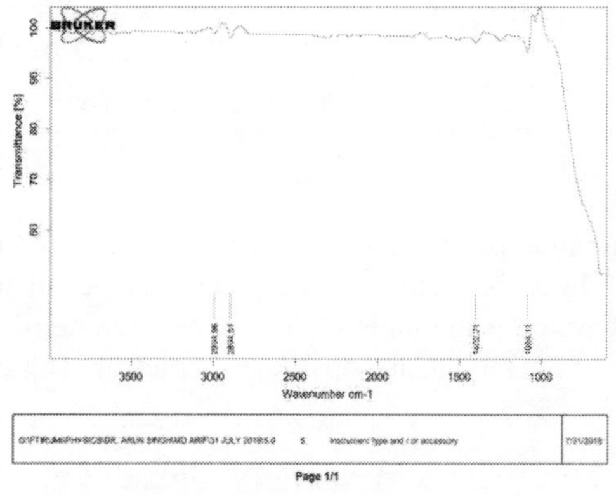

Figure 3. FTIR analysis of SiC nanoparticles

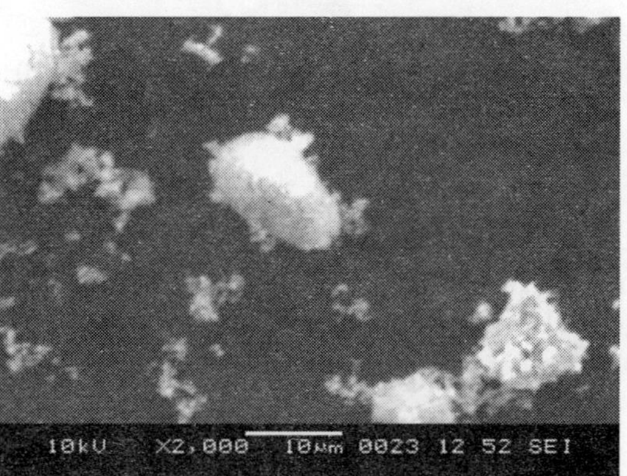

Figure 4. SEM of SiC nanoparticles

4. Results and Discussion

The experimentally measured values of ultrasonic velocity, adiabatic compressibility, density and viscosity are represented graphically in Figs. 5-8.

Ultrasonic velocity gets increases with increasing the molar concentration of the SiC nanoparticles in methanol this shows that the physical parameters of the sample changes by increasing the molar concentration. Nanoparticles suspensions do not settle which provides a long self- life which imparts ultrasonic velocity to them. For SiC nanoparticle the velocity of the nanofluid is higher than methanol and also by increasing the molar concentration of the SiC nanoparticle, peaks obtained at 0.3 and 0.6, the variation is represented in the Fig. 5. Peak at molar concentration 0.3 and 0.6 represents the strong aggregation of SiC nano suspension in methanol based nanofluids. The cause behind this increase of ultrasonic velocity with increase in molar concentration (x) is due to strong interaction between nanosize particle and micro sized fluid molecule and also due to increase in density of nanofluid with increase of molar concentration. Ultrasonic velocity can be interpreted as the nanosize SiC particles have more surfaces to volume ratio and which can absorb more methanol molecules on its surface, which enhances the ultrasonic velocity.

The variation of adiabatic compressibility versus molar concentration of SiC nanoparticles in methanol based nanofluids shows that adiabatic compressibility (β_a) decreases with increase in molar concentration. The surface area of the material is increased by the reduction in particle size. Due to this higher percentage of the SiC Nanoparticles can interact with surrounding fluids. It may due to decrease in interspacing of SiC nanoparticles in nanofluids with increase in molar concentration. It is primarily the compressibility that changes with structure which leads to change in ultrasonic velocity. The variation of adiabatic compressibility with molar concentration is given in Fig. 6.

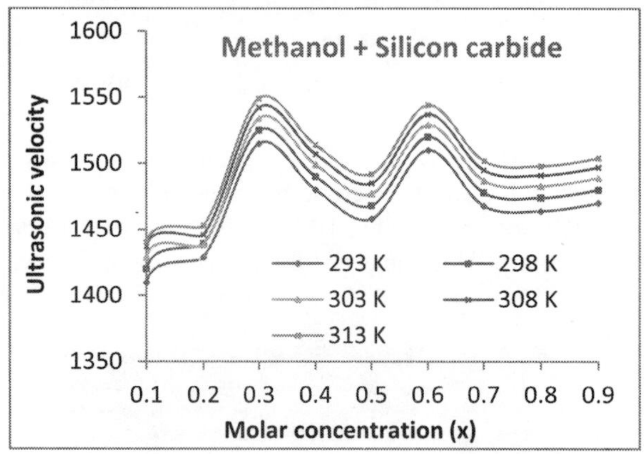

Figure 5 Variation of u versus x

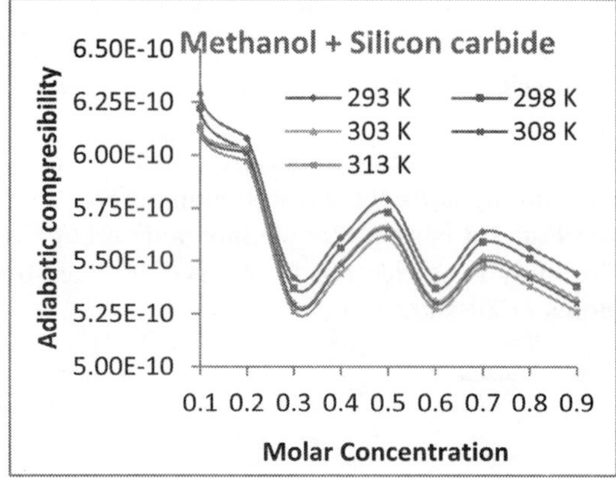

Figure 6 Variation of β_a versus x

Figure 7 shows the variation of density with molar concentration of SiC nanoparticles in methanol. Densities of the nanosuspension are calculated by measuring the weight of the nanofluid using 25 ml of specific gravity bottle and also by using the standard value of density of water. Nanofluids of SiC have more density than methanol. Increase in density indicates the close packing between the SiC nanoparticles in methanol base fluid.

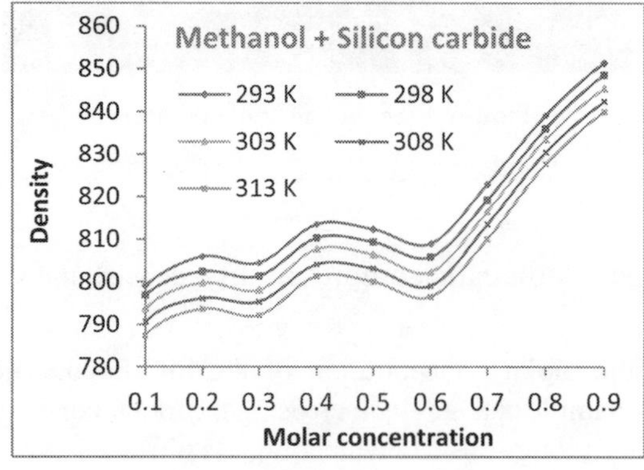

Figure 7 Variation of ρ versus x

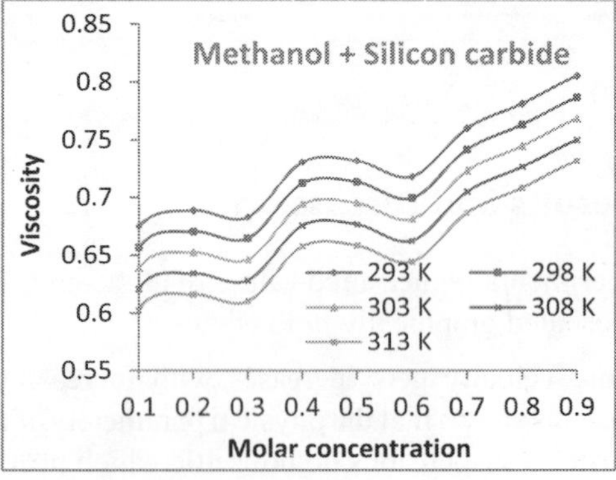

Figure 8 Variation of η versus x

The plot of viscosity (η) versus molar concentrations clearly shows that viscosity slightly increases with increase in molar concentration of SiC nanoparticles in methanol based nanofluids. As the motion of nanoparticles becomes more rapid when the temperature of the medium was raised which lowers the viscosity of the medium as the size of the particles was reduced. Hence viscosity of nanofluids decreases with increase in temperature. The viscosity of SiC nanoparticle strongly depends on structure of SiC nanoparticles and consequently interactions between the SiC nanoparticles and molecules of the fluid.

5.   References

1.   D.H. Kumar, H.E. Patel, V.R.R. Kumar, T. Sundararajan, T. Pradeep and S.K. Das, 2004. Model for heat conduction of nanofluids, Physical Review Letters, 94 (14), 1-3.

2.   S. Rajagopalan, S. J. Sharma and V.Y. Nanotkar. Ultrasonic Characterization of Silver Nanoparticles, Journal of Metastable and Nanocrystalline Materials 2005, 23, 271-274.

3.   C. Peng, J. Zhang, Z. Xiong, B. Zhao, P. Liu, Fabrication of porous hollow γ-Al2O3 nanofibers by facile electro spinning and its application for water remediation, Microporous and Mesoporous Materials, 215, (2015) 133-142.

4.   G. Amaral-Labat, C. Zollfrank, A. Ortona, S. Pusterla, A. Pizzi, V. Fierro, A. Celzard. Structure and oxidation resistance of micro-cellular Si-SiC foams derived from natural resins. Ceramics International. 2013. 39:1941-1851.

5.   W. Guo, H. Xiao, W. Xie, J. Hu, Q. Li, P. Gao. A new design for preparation of high performance recrystallized silicon carbide. Ceramics International. 2012. 38:2475-2481.

6.   R D Chavhan, Abhranil Banerjee, Mrunal Pawar, O P Chimankar and N R Pawar, Synthesis and Ultrasonic Characterization of Boron nitride Nano suspension in organic base fluids, J Pure Appl Ultrason 41 (2019) 80-83.

7.   R D Chavhan, Abhranil Banerjee, Mrunal Pawar, O P Chimankar, S. J. Dhoble and N R Pawar, Synthesis and Ultrasonic Characterization of Silicon carbide Nano suspension in organic base fluids, JETIR, 6, 4 (2019) 309-318.

8.   X. Zhan, M. HonkNEN and E. Leva, 2008. Transition alumina nanoparticles and nanorods from boehmite nanoflakes. J Crystal Growth 310(30), 3674-3679.

9.   G. Amaral-Labat, C. Zollfrank, A. Ortona, S. Pusterla, A. Pizzi, V. Fierro, A. Celzard. Structure and oxidation resistance of micro-cellular Si-SiC foams derived from natural resins. Ceramics International. 2013. 39:1941-1851.

10.   W. Guo, H. Xiao, W. Xie, J. Hu, Q. Li, P. Gao. A new design for preparation of high performance recrystallized silicon carbide. Ceramics International. 2012. 38:2475-2481.

Synthesis, Spectroscopic Characterization and Ultrasonic study of α-Alumina Nanofluids

Mrunal Pawar[1], R. D. Chavhan[2], O. P. Chimankar[2], S. J. Dhoble[2] and N. R. Pawar[3,*]

[1]St.Vincent Pallotti College of Engineering and Technology, Nagpur-441 108, India
[2]Department of Physics, RTM Nagpur University, Nagpur- 440 033, India
[3]Department of Physics, Arts, Commerce and Science College, Maregaon - 445 303, India
*E-mail: pawarsir1@gmail.com

ABSTRACT

Nanofluids are solid-liquid composite materials consisting of solid nanoparticles or nanofibers with sizes typically of 1-100 nm suspended in liquid. Nanofluids have attracted great interest recently because of reports of greatly enhanced thermal properties. When Nanoparticles are mixed with base fluid, some of the particles are remain suspended in the fluid. These suspended particles in the base fluid are considerably changes the transfer characterization and flow of base fluid. The larger surface area of nanoparticles not only increases the thermal transfer but also increases the stability of suspension. Nanoparticles are expected to have a surface to volume ratio given as large surface to volume ratio proportional to the inverse of particle size of nanomaterials changes the role played by the surface atoms in determining their thermodynamic properties [1-3]. α-Al_2O_3 nanoparticles has high dimensional stability, it is widely used in a variety of plastics, rubber, ceramics, refractory products for reinforcement toughening, in particular, significantly to improve the ceramic density, finish, thermal fatigue resistance, fracture toughness, creep resistance and wear resistance. As it is a high performance material of far infrared emission, it is widely used in fibber fabric products and high pressure sodium lamp as far-infrared emission and thermal insulation materials.

Nanoparticles of alpha alumina (α-Al_2O_3) was prepared by sol-gel method [4-7] from Aluminum isopropoxide [Al $(OC_3H_7)_3$] and aluminum nitrate. Starting solution was prepared by adding aluminum isopropoxide [Al $(OC_3H_7)_3$] gradually in 0.2 M aluminum nitrate and solution continuously stirred for 48 hours. Later, Sodium dodecylbenzen sulfonate (SDBS) was added and stirred for one hour. Now this solution were heated up to 60°C and stirred constantly for evaporation process. Now the paste so obtained was heated at 90°C for 8 hours, we get nanoparticles of alpha alumina (α-Al_2O_3) in powder form. The prepared sample was characterized by X- ray diffraction (XRD), FTIR and Scanning electron microscopy (SEM). Average particle size has been estimated by using Debye-Scherrer formula [8-9]. It was found to be 30 nm. Nanofluids of α-Al_2O_3 in methanol base fluid were prepared and their acoustical studies were made such that different types of interactions could be assessed. Thermo-acoustical parameters of this nanofluids system were computed from ultrasonic velocities, densities and viscosities at temperatures 293K, 298K, 303K, 308K and 313K at fixed frequency 5MHz over the entire range of concentrations. The obtained results of present investigation have been discussed in the light of interactions between the α-Al_2O_3 nanoparticles and the molecules of methanol based fluids.

Keywords: Nanofluids, spectroscopic characterization; ultrasonic characterization, XRD, FTIR, SEM

1. Introduction

α-Al_2O_3 nanoparticles has high dimensional stability, it is widely used in a variety of plastics, rubber, ceramics, refractory products for reinforcement toughening, in particular, significantly to improve the ceramic density, finish, thermal fatigue resistance, fracture toughness, creep resistance and wear resistance. As it is a high performance material of far infrared emission, it is widely used in fiber fabric products and high pressure sodium lamp as far-infrared emission and thermal insulation materials. In addition, due to high resistivity and good insulation property, it is widely used as the main components for YGA laser crystal and integrated circuit substrates. The prepared sample was characterized by X- ray diffraction (XRD), FTIR and Scanning electron microscopy (SEM). Thermo-acoustical parameters of α-Al$_2$O$_3$ nanofluid were computed from ultrasonic velocities, densities and viscosities at temperatures 293K, 298K, 303K, 308K and 313K at fixed frequency 5MHz over the entire range of concentrations.

2.   Method of Synthesis of α-Al$_2$O$_3$ Nanofluids

Nanoparticles of alpha alumina (α-Al$_2$O$_3$) was prepared by sol-gel method [10] from Aluminum isopropoxide [Al (OC$_3$H$_7$)$_3$] and aluminum nitrate. Starting solution was prepared by adding aluminum isopropoxide [Al (OC$_3$H$_7$)$_3$] gradually in 0.2 M aluminum nitrate and solution continuously stirred for 48 hours. Later, Sodium dodecylbenzen sulfonate (SDBS) was added and stirred for one hour. Now this solution were heated up to 60°C and stirred constantly for evaporation process. Now the paste so obtained was heated at 90°C for 8 hours, we get nanoparticles of alpha alumina (α-Al$_2$O$_3$) in powder form.

3.   Spectroscopic Characterization of SiC Nanoparticles

Figure 1 shows the XRD pattern of α-Al$_2$O$_3$ nanoparticles. It is seen that the materials is well crystalline in nature and well agreed with standard JCPDS file number shown in figure 2. The estimate size of SiC nanoparticles using Debye Scherrer formula is found to be in the range of 20 nm to 30 nm.

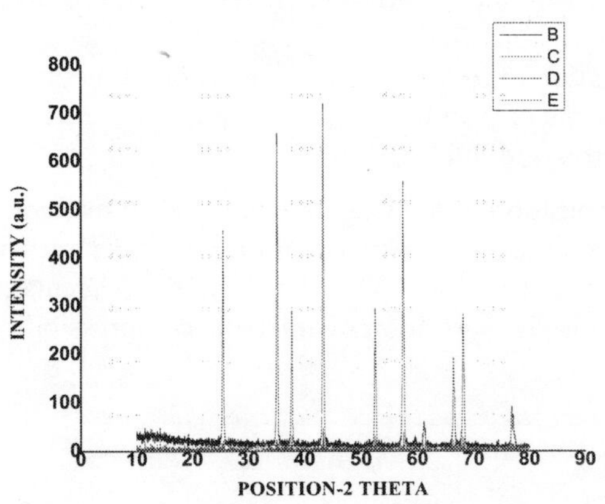

Figure 1 XRD pattern of α-Al$_2$O$_3$ Nanoparticles

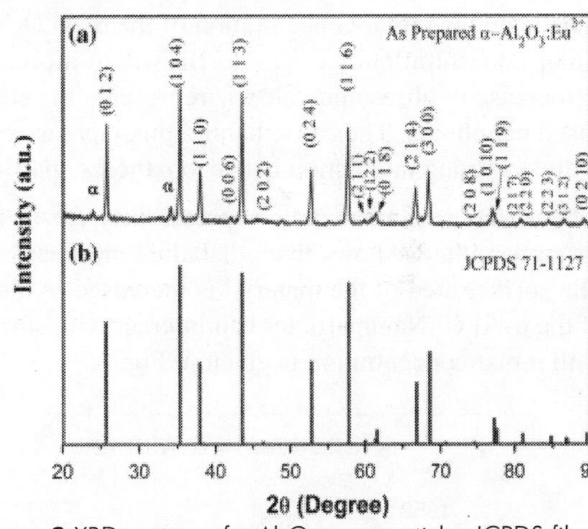

Figure 2 XRD pattern of α-Al$_2$O$_3$ nanoparticles JCPDS file

FTIR analysis indicated the vibrations of metal oxygen (M–O) groups. FTIR spectroscopy shows the degradation phases and absorption in different regions which indicates structural relationship between them. From figure 3 it is seen that the inorganic groups is gradually decomposed at inorganic groups is gradually decomposed at 1084 cm^{-1}. Also the O–H absorption peak observed at 2894.96 cm^{-1}, and a very weak band at about 1402.21 cm^{-1}. SEM study is carried out to observe the overall surface morphology and crystallite sizes of the prepared nanomaterials shown in figure 4.

The experimentally measured values of ultrasonic velocity, adiabatic compressibility, density and viscosity are represented graphically in Figs. 5-8.

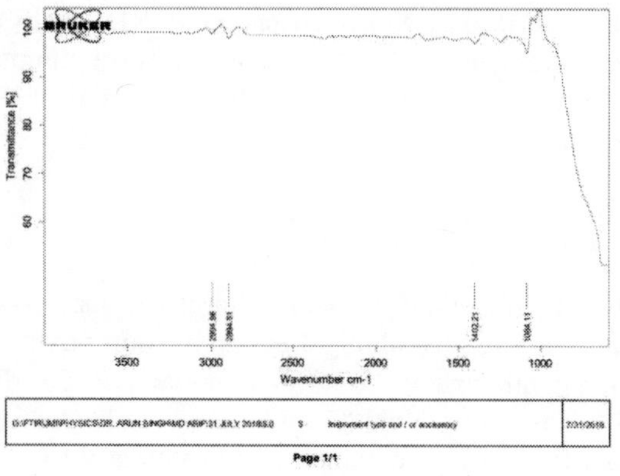

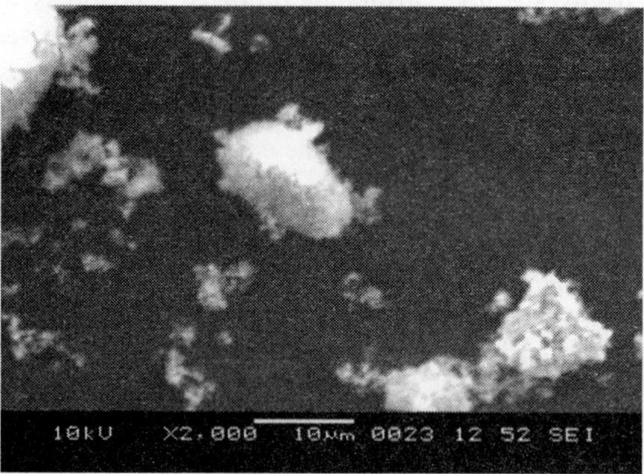

Figure 3. FTIR analysis of α-Al$_2$O$_3$ nanoparticles

Figure 4. SEM image of α-Al$_2$O$_3$ nanoparticles

4.   Results and Discussion

Ultrasonic velocity gets increases with increasing the molar concentration of the α-Al$_2$O$_3$ nanoparticles in methanol. Nanoparticles suspensions do not settle which provides a long self- life which imparts ultrasonic velocity to them. For α-Al$_2$O$_3$ nanoparticle the velocity of the nanofluid is higher than methanol and also by increasing the molar concentration of the α-Al$_2$O$_3$ nanoparticle. Non linear variation ultrasonic velocity with molar concentration may due to Brownian motion of α-Al$_2$O$_3$ nanoparticles; it is represented in the figure 5. Increase in ultrasonic velocity represents the strong aggregation of α-Al$_2$O$_3$ nano suspension in methanol based nanofluids. The cause behind this increase of ultrasonic velocity with increase in molar concentration is due to strong interaction between nanosize particle and micro sized fluid molecule.

The variation of adiabatic compressibility versus molar concentration of α-Al$_2$O$_3$ nanoparticles in methanol based nanofluids shows that adiabatic compressibility (βa) decreases with increase in molar concentration. The surface area of the material is increased by the reduction in particle size. Due to this higher percentage of the α-Al$_2$O$_3$ Nanoparticles can interact with surrounding fluids. The variation of adiabatic compressibility with molar concentration is given in Fig. 6.

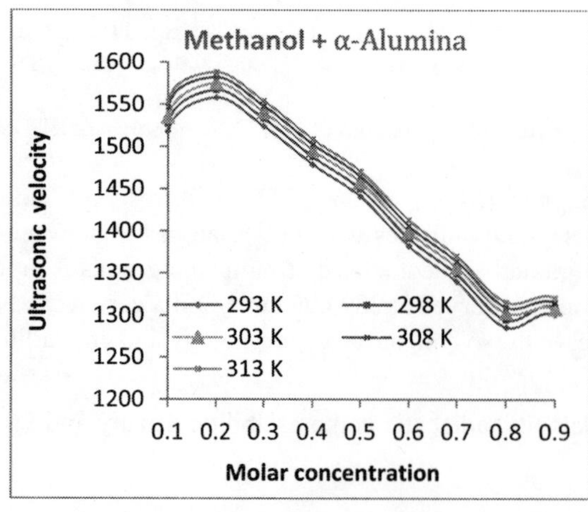

Figure 5 Variation of u versus x

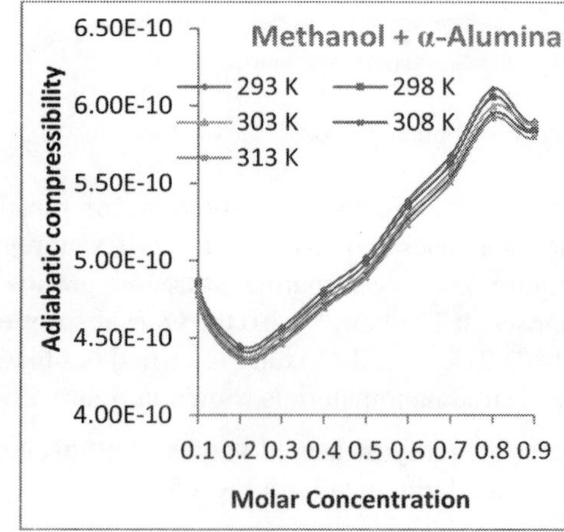

Figure 6 Variation of β$_a$ versus x

Figure 7 shows the variation of density with molar concentration of α-Al$_2$O$_3$ nanoparticles in methanol. Densities of the nanosuspension are calculated by measuring the weight of the nanofluid using 25 ml of specific gravity bottle and also by using the standard value of density of water. Nanofluids of α-Al$_2$O$_3$ have more density than methanol. Increase in density indicates the close packing between the α-Al$_2$O$_3$ nanoparticles in methanol base fluid.

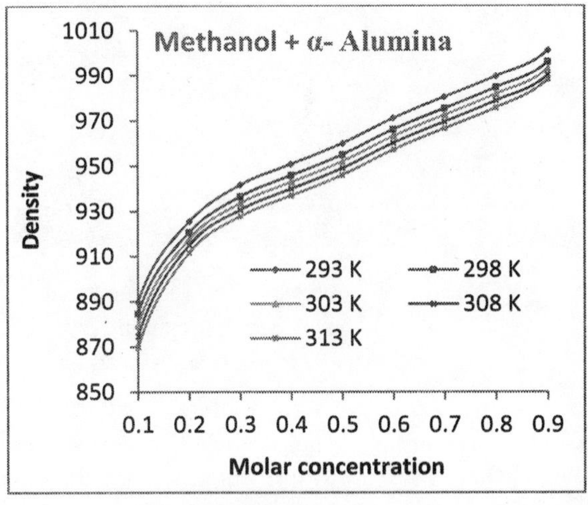

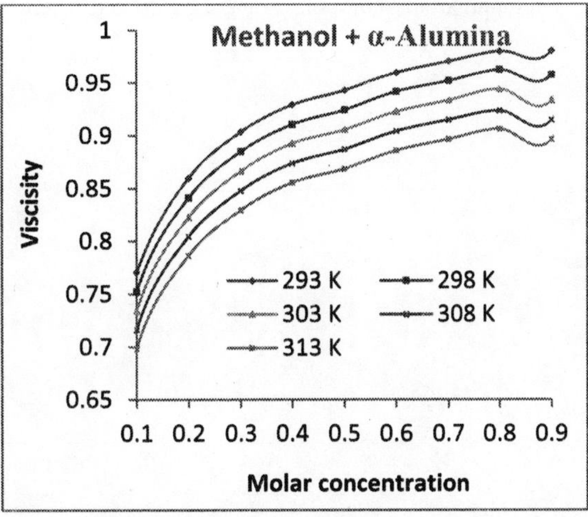

Figure 7 Variation of ρ versus x   **Figure 8** Variation of η versus x

The plot of viscosity (η) versus molar concentrations clearly shows that viscosity slightly increases with increase in molar concentration of α-Al$_2$O$_3$ nanoparticles in methanol based nanofluids. As the motion of nanoparticles becomes more rapid when the temperature of the medium was raised which lowers the viscosity of the medium as the size of the particles was reduced. Hence viscosity of nanofluids decreases with increase in temperature. The viscosity of α-Al$_2$O$_3$ nanoparticle strongly depends on structure of α-Al$_2$O$_3$ nanoparticles and consequently interactions between the α-Al$_2$O$_3$ nanoparticles and molecules of the fluid.

5.   References

1.   B. X. Wang, L. P. Zhou, X.F. Peng, A fractal model for predicting the effective thermal conductivity of liquid with suspension of nanoparticles, Int. J. Heat Mass Transfer, Vol. 46(14), pp. 2665-2672, (2003).

2.   S.U.S. Chooi and Eastman, J. A. Enhancing thermal conductivity of fluids with nanoparticles, International mechanical engineering congress and exhibition, San Francisco, CA, (1995).

3.   S.K. Das, S. U. S. Choi, W.Yu, T. Pradeep, Naofluids, Science and Technology, John Wiley and Sons, Inc,(2008)

4.   Y.K. Park, E.H. Tadd, M. Zubris and R. Tannenbaum, 2005. Size controlled synthesis of alumina nanoparticles from aluminum alkoxides, Materials Reasearch Bulletin, 40 (9), 1512.

5.   D.G. Wang, F. Guo, J.F. Chen, H. Liu and Z. Zhag. Preparation of nano aluminium trihydroxide by high gravity reactive precipitation, Chemical Engineering Journal, 121(2-3), 109-114.

6.   R. Aghababazadeh, A.R. Mirhabibi, J. Pourasad, A. Brown, A. Brydson and N. AmeriMahabad, 2007. Economical synthesis of Nanocrystalline alumina using an environmentally low-cost binder, Journal of Surface Science. 601(13), 2864-2867.

7.   R. Rogojan, E. Andronescu, C. Ghitulica and B. Stefan. Synthesis and characterization of alumina nano-powder by sol-gel method. UPB Sci Bull Ser B. 73 (2, 27), 67-76.

8.   R D Chavhan, Abhranil Banerjee, Mrunal Pawar, O P Chimankar and N R Pawar, Synthesis and Ultrasonic Characterization of Boron nitride Nano suspension in   organic base fluids, J Pure Appl Ultrason 41 (2019) 80-83.

9.   R D Chavhan, Abhranil Banerjee, Mrunal Pawar, O P Chimankar, S. J. Dhoble and N R Pawar, Synthesis and Ultrasonic Characterization of Silicon carbide Nano suspension in

10.   P. Christian and M. Bromfield, 2010. Preparation of small silver, gold and copper nanoparticles which disperse in both polar and non-polar solvents, J. Mater, Chem. 20, 1135-1139.

EPR and Optical Study of Cu^{2+} Doped Potassium Hydrogen Bis Homophathalate

Awadhesh Kumar Yadav[1] and Ram Kripal[2]

[1]Government P.G. College Saidabad, Prayagraj, Uttar Pradesh, 221508
[2]EPR Laboratory, Department of Physics, University of Allahabad, Allahabad, 211002
E-mail: aky.physics@gmail.com; ram_kripal2001@gmail.com

ABSTRACT

EPR study is carried out on Cu^{2+} doped potassium hydrogen bis homophathalate. Only one Cu^{2+} lattice site is observed. The site exhibits one set of four hyperfine lines in all directions. The g factor and hyperfine splitting are calculated from EPR spectra which are: $g_x = 2.0589\pm0.002$, $g_y = 2.0747\pm0.002$, $g_z = 2.1975\pm 0.002$, $A_x = (74 \pm 2)\,'10^{-4}\,cm^{-1}$, $A_y = (78\pm 2)\,'10^{-4}\,cm^{-1}$ and $A_z = (161\pm 2)\,'10^{-4}\,cm^{-1}$. It is found that Cu^{2+} enters the lattice interstitially. The ground state wave function of the Cu^{2+} ion in the lattice is determined from the spin Hamiltonian parameters obtained from EPR study. With the help of the optical absorption study, the nature of bonding in the complex is also discussed.

Keywords: EPR, spin Hamiltonian, absorption, spectra, angular variation, rhombic symmetry.

1. Introduction

EPR gives a detailed description of the ground state of paramagnetic ion and electric field symmetry produced by the ligands around the metal ion [1-5]. Several studies of the cupric ion in octahedral or square planar coordination have been done. However, only few tetrahedrally coordinated cupric complexes have been studied as this ion coordinates mostly in octahedral configuration. A theoretical study of $CuCl_4^{2-}$ [6] indicates that the ground state contains about 8% 4p character and the excited states t_2 contain as large as 18% 4p character. The optical and magnetic investigation of $CuCl_4^{2-}$ ion [7-9] indicates that the t_2 orbitals contain about 12% 4p state admixture. In EPR study of copper (II) a-a' bromo dipyrromethene [10] the 4p admixture was found to be of the order of 20-30%. It is seen that, in these studies, although the g-values are not appreciably different from the typical g-values for distorted octahedral coordination, the copper nuclear hyperfine interaction parameters are markedly different. For a trigonally distorted tetrahedral environment of cupric ion in ZnO, the magnetic parameters are quite different than those in the tetragonally distorted octahedral cases [11-13].

2. Crystal Structure

The crystal structure of potassium hydrogen bis homophthalate, $[K(C_9H_7O_4)_2(H)]$, was reported by Gupta and Dubey [14]. The potassium ion lies on the twofold axis (0, y, ¼) in the monoclinic unit cell with a = 32.66(5), b = 5.51(2), c = 9.97(0) Å, β= 95.9⁰, Z = 4 formula units of $[K(C_9H_7O_4)_2(H)]$; space group C2/c. There is a fourfold coordination around the potassium ion with potassium-oxygen distances ranging from 2.76 to 2.80 Å. The molecules are held together by van der Waals contacts, metal-oxygen ionic linkages and a short hydrogen bond of 2.59 Å between oxygen atoms belonging to carboxyl groups of adjacent homophthalic acid units.

3. Experimental

Single crystals of potassium hydrogen bis homophthalate doped with Cu^{2+} were grown from aqueous solution containing a trace of ethanol by mixing potassium hydroxide with homophthalic acid in stoichiometric amounts and slight admixture of (2%) copper sulphate at room temperature. After a few days, hexagonal thin plate like transparent crystals were formed [14].

The ESR spectra are recorded by using Varian E-1700 EPR spectrometer operating at X-band frequencies with 100 kHz modulation. A Varian flux meter with proton probe having 0.2 cubic centimeters of 0.25 molar solution of $GdCl_3$ in H_2O was used for magnetic field measurement along with a Hewlett-Packard frequency counter. For recording the EPR spectra, the crystal was rotated about a, b and c* axes at an interval of 10^0. c* axis is perpendicular to a and b. The optical absorption spectra were recorded on Unicam-5625 spectrophotometer in the wavelength range 195-1100 nm at room temperature.

4. Results and Discussion

The spectra recorded at room temperature, when the magnetic field is along the **c*** axis, are shown in Fig. 1 (a). The spectra consist of one set of four hyperfine lines, which indicate that there is only one copper complex present in the lattice. Thus an interstitial site of Cu^{2+} ion is expected in the crystal. The lines of the above quartet has triplet structure clearly showing that the triplet is due to the interaction of unpaired Cu^{2+} electron and the two equivalent ^1H (I = 1/2) nuclei. The angular dependence of the superhyperfine constant A^H for rotation of the crystal in all the three planes was investigated. The superhyperfine constant A^H varied from 20.0 to 25.0 G. EPR spectra recorded in ba and bc* planes showed a large anisotropy in A and g values, however, the corresponding variation in c*a plane is very small [15]. The spin Hamiltonian corresponding to rhombic symmetry is of the form

$$H = \beta \left(g_z B_z S_z + g_x B_x S_x + g_y B_y S_y\right) + A_z I_z S_z + A_x I_x S_x + A_y I_y S_y \qquad (1)$$

Computer simulation work has been done using the various parameters obtained from the EPR spectra of copper doped crystal using Schonland procedure [15]. The simulated spectrum using EasySpin [16-17] and spin Hamiltonian parameters $g_x = 2.0589 \pm 0.002$, $g_y = 2.0747 \pm 0.002$, $g_z = 2.1975 \pm 0.002$, $A_x = (74 \pm 2)'10^{-4}$ cm^{-1}, $A_y = (78 \pm 2)'10^{-4}$ cm^{-1} and $A_z = (161 \pm 2)'10^{-4}$ cm^{-1} (Frequency = 9.1 GHz) is given in Fig. 1(b). The simulation was based upon numerical diagonalization of the entire S = 1/2, I = 3/2 energy matrix and the first derivative spectra. Lorentzian first derivative line shapes were used. The simulated spectrum is in good agreement with experimental one. The best-fit spin Hamiltonian parameters are given in Table 1 which are similar to the values in other lattices [7, 18]. The parameter errors may be determined using statistical analysis [19].

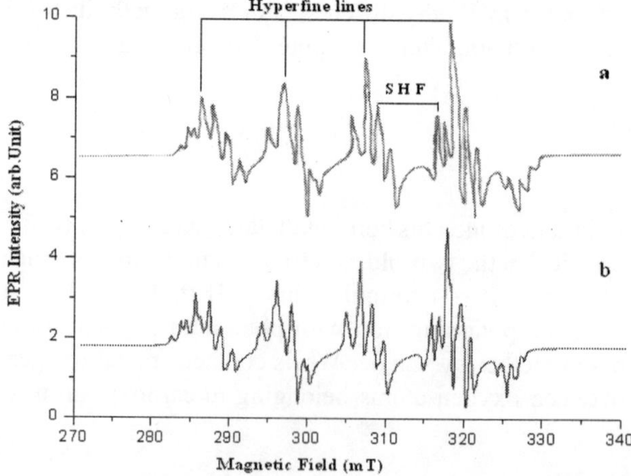

Fig. 1(a) EPR spectra of Cu^{2+} doped potassium hydrogen bis homophthalate for magnetic field along **c***-axis (Frequency = 9.1 GHz). (b) Simulated EPR spectra of Cu^{2+} doped potassium hydrogen bis homophthalate along **c***-axis (Frequency = 9.1 GHz).

Table 1. Spin Hamiltonian parameters for Cu^{2+} ion site I in potassium hydrogen bishomophthalate single crystal

No. Lattice	g_x	g_y	g_z	A_x	A_y $(10^{-4}\ cm^{-1})$	A_z	Ref.
(1) Cs_2ZnCl_4: Cu^{2+}							
	2.058 ±0.004	2.062 ±0.003	2.297 ±0.002	51± 5	46± 5	25± 4	[8]
(2) $C_{12}H_8N_2ZnCl_2$: Cu^{2+}							
	2.058 ±0.002	2.062 ±0.002	2.297 ±0.002	9± 4	9 ± 4	123± 4	[17]
(3) $ZnC_{28}H_{36}N_6O_6$: Cu^{2+}							
	2.0201 ±0.002	2.0900 ± 0.002	2.1634 ± 0.002	30± 2	40 ±2	154± 2	[1]
(4) $[K(C_9H_7O_4)_2(H)]$: Cu^{2+}							
	2.0589 ±0.002	2.0747 ± 0.002	2.1975 ± 0.002	74± 2	78 ±2	161± 2	*

*present study

5. Optical spectrum

The room temperature optical absorption spectrum of Cu^{2+} doped potassium hydrogen bis homophathalate single crystal, in the wavelength range 195-1100 nm is exhibited in **Fig. 2(a), (b)**. There are three bands occurring at n_1 = 9321 cm⁻¹, n_2 = 15567 cm⁻¹, and n_3 = 20582 cm⁻¹, in 325-1100 nm range and four bands in the ultraviolet (UV) range, most of which are weak in intensity, occurring at n_4 = 27463 cm⁻¹, n_5 = 32218 cm⁻¹, n_6 = 37090 cm⁻¹, n_7 = 49904 cm⁻¹.

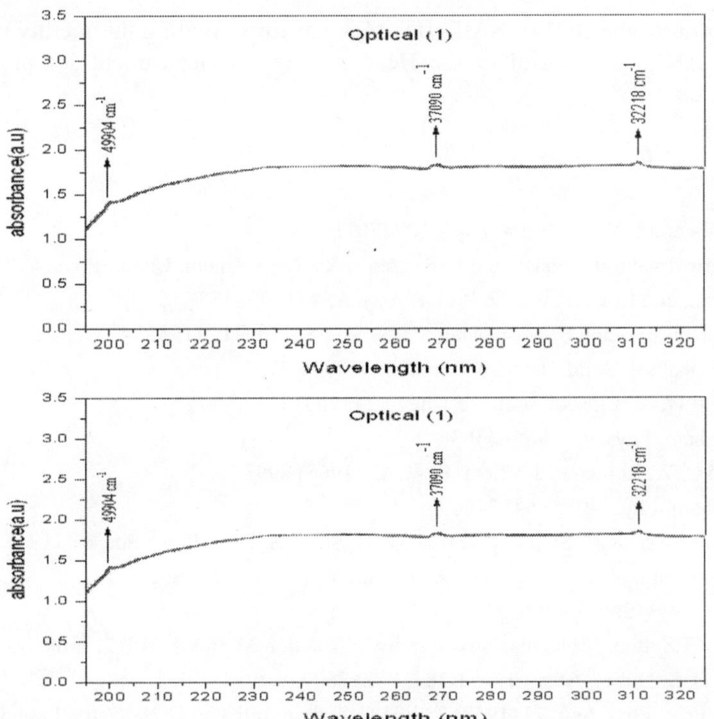

Figure 2 (a) Room temperature absorption spectrum in the wavelength range 195-325 nm. (b) Room temperature absorption spectrum in the wavelength range 325-1100 nm.

From the nature of absorption spectrum, the absorption band at n_1 can be regarded as the d-d transition band between the ground state $|xy\rangle$ and the excited state $|x^2 - y^2\rangle$. The band at v_2 may be regarded as the d-d transition band between the ground state $|xy\rangle$ and the excited state $|xz, yz\rangle$. The other band observed at v_3 is assigned as $|3z^2 - r^2\rangle \leftrightarrow |xy\rangle$ transition band20-22].

The four observed absorption bands in the UV range, occurring at $v_4 = 27463$ cm^{-1}, $v_5 = 32218$ cm^{-1}, $v_6 = 37090$ cm^{-1}, $v_7 = 49904$cm^{-1}, are probably, the charge-transfer transition bands, because they arise from higher-lying energy levels.

6.   Conclusion

EPR together with optical absorption study of potassium hydrogen bis homophathalate single crystal doped with Cu^{2+} has been done .The principal g and A parameters are evaluated from EPR spectra and are fitted to rhombic symmetry spin Hamiltonian. The angular variation plot showed that the Cu^{2+} ion enters the lattice interstitially. The ground state wave function for Cu^{2+} in the lattice is constructed which is found to contain about 34% 4p-state admixture. The optical absorption spectrum has been explained well in terms of a D$_{2d}$ symmetry in the Cu^{2+} complex. The estimated MO coefficients indicate that for the Cu^{2+} complex in potassium hydrogen bis homophathalate lattice, the bonding between the Cu^{2+} ion and the oxygen ligands is strongly covalent while the bonding between the Cu^{2+} ion and its axial ligands is mostly ionic.

7.   Acknowledgement

The authors are thankful to the staff of SAIF, IIT, Mumbai for providing the facility of EPR spectrometer. One of the authors, AKY, is thankful to the Head of Physics Department for providing departmental facilities.

8.   References

1.   R. Kripal, S. Misra and I. Mishra, Mol. Phys. 109 (2011)239.

2.   S. Kiczka, S. K. Hoffmann, J. Goslar, and L. Szczepanska, Phys. Chem. Chem. Phys. 6 (2004) 64.

3.   F. Koksal, I. Kartal, and B. Karabulut, Z. Naturforsch A54 (1999) 177.

4.   M. Korkmaz, O. Korkmaz and S. Kospancali, Phys. Stat. Sol (b) 112 (1982) 423.

5.   H. Kalkan, and F. Koksal, Solid State Commun.103 (1997)137.

6.   L. L. Lohr, Jr., and W. M. Lipscomb, Inorg. Chem. 2 (1963) 911.

7.   M. Sharnoff, J. Chem. Phys. 42(1965) 3383.

8.   M. Sharnoff, and C. W. Reimann, J. Chem. Phys. 43 (1965) 2993.

9.   J. Ferguson, J. Chem. Phys. 40 (1964) 3406.

10.   C. A. Bates, W.S. Moore, K. J. Standley, and K. W. H. Stevens, Proc. Phys. Soc. 79 (1962) 73.

11.   R. E. Deitz, H. Kamiura, M. D. Sturge, and A. Yariu, Phys. Rev. 132 (1962)1559.

12.   C. A. Bates, Proc. Phys. Soc. 79(1962) 69.

13.   G. A. Sim and L. E. Sutton, Molecular Structure by Diffraction Methods, Vol. 2, Roy. Soc. Chem., 1974.

14.   M. P. Gupta and D. S. Dubey, Acta Cryst. B28 (1972) 2677.

15.   D. S. Schonland, Proc. Phys. Soc. 73 (1959) 788; V. Chandramouli, and G. S. Sastry, Indian J. Pure and Appl. Phys. 27 (1989) 101.

16.   J. R. Pilbrow, Mol. Phys. 16 (1969) 307; S. Stoll and A. Schweiger, J. Magn. Reson. 178 (2006)42.

17. S. Stoll, Spectral Simulation in Solid-State EPR, Ph. D. Thesis, ETH, Zurich, 2003.

18. G. K. Kokoszka, C. W. Reimann. and H. C. Allen, Jr., J. Phys. Chem. 71 (1967) 121.

19. S. K. Misra and S. Subramanian, J. Phys. C 15 (1982)7199.

20. J. C. Rivoal, and B. Briat, Mol. Phys. 27 (1974) 1081.

21. A. Abragam and B. Bleaney, Electron Paramagnetic Resonance of Transition Ions, Clarendon Press, Oxford, 1970.

22. S. K. Hoffmann, and J. Goslar, J. Solid State Chem. 44 (1982) 343.

Acoustic Method for the Estimation of Radius, van der Waals Constants and Molecular Dimension of Pure Organic Liquids

Ramakant*, Shekhar Srivastava

Department of Chemistry, University of Allahabad, Prayagraj-211002, India
*Email: ramakantsingh87@gmail.com

ABSTRACT

From the experimental values of density and sound speed of five pure organic liquids (n-hexane, n- heptane, n-dodecane, cyclohexane and toluene), radius (r), van der Waals constants (a), (b) and molecular dimension (d), were computed at five different temperatures ranging from 283.15 K to 333.15 K. The experimental data of density and sound speed were taken from the paper of Romani et al (Phys. Chem. Chem. Phys., 2001, 3, 5230-5236). All the calculated properties were found to vary with temperature.

Keywords: Organic liquids, density, sound speed.

1.   Introduction

Molecular radius is an important parameter of pure organic liquids which reflects their structural features. Molecular radius is not only related to the number of atoms involved but also to the nature of liquids. It is directly or indirectly, an important parameter in the theories of liquids like collision factor theory (CFT) [1,2] and scaled particle theory [3,4]. Molecular radius helps to evaluate important-properties of liquids [5,6].

Acoustic methods are the most powerful tools for the structural and physical – chemical studies of liquids [7]. Ultrasonic velocity and density data are used to calculate molecular radius in pure liquids. The effect of various parameter on molecular radius in pure liquids have been studies earlier [8] using various acoustic methods suggested by Schaaffs' [1,9], van der Waals constant are important parameter in studying molecular dimension as constant 'a' provides a collection for the intermolecular forces constant 'b' adjusts for the volume occurred.

In the present work use have calculated molecular radius by Schaaffs' method and non-acoustical (CF-FCC) method and van der Waals constant with respect to temperature ranging from 283.15 K to 333.15 K of pure organic solvents namely n-hexane, n-pentane, n-dodecane, cyclohexane and toluene.

2.   Theoretical/ Formulation

1.   van der Waals constant [10]

$$a = \frac{\rho u^2 V^2}{\left(\dfrac{B}{A}+1\right)} \tag{1}$$

$$b = V - \frac{RT}{\rho u^2}\left(\frac{B}{A}+1\right) \tag{2}$$

where is density, u is sound velocity and V is molar volume.

2. Dimension [10]

$$d = \left\{ \frac{3}{2N_0\pi} \left[V - \frac{RT}{\rho u^2} \left(\frac{B}{A} + 1 \right) \right] \right\}^{\frac{1}{3}} \tag{3}$$

where N_0 is Avogadro's constant, R is gas constant, T is temperature, is density and u is sound velocity.

3. Radius

a) Schaaffs' relation (Acoustical Methods) [11]

$$r = \sqrt[3]{\frac{M}{\rho N}} \sqrt[3]{\frac{3}{16\pi} \left[1 - \frac{\gamma RT}{Mu^2} \left(\sqrt{1 + \frac{Mu^2}{\gamma RT}} - 1 \right) \right]} \tag{4}$$

b) Non-Acoustical (CP-FCC) methods [12]

$$r = \frac{1}{2} \sqrt[3]{\frac{M\sqrt{2}}{\rho N}} \tag{5}$$

where N is Avogadro's number, ρ is density, u is sound velocity, M is molecular mass and Υ is specific heat ratio.

3. Results and Discussion

The results of radius calculated by acoustical (Schaaffs') and non-acoustical (CP-FCC) method are reported in Table 1.

Table 1. Calculated values of radius by acoustical (Schaaffs') and non-acoustical (CP-FCC) method for different organic liquids at varying temperatures ranging from 283.15K to 333.15K.

T (K)	Acoustical methods (Schaaffs' relation)	Non-acoustical methods (CP-FCC)
	$10^8 \cdot r$	$10^8 \cdot r$
	cm	cm
	n-hexane	
283.15	2.28	3.36
288.15	2.29	3.37
293.15	2.29	3.37
298.15	2.29	3.38
303.15	2.30	3.39
308.15	2.30	3.40
313.15	2.30	3.40
318.15	2.31	3.42
333.15	2.32	3.44
	n-heptane	
283.15	2.38	3.49
293.15	2.38	3.50

298.15	2.39	3.51
303.15	2.39	3.52
308.15	2.40	3.53
313.15	2.40	3.53
318.15	2.42	3.56
333.15	2.42	3.57
n-dodecane		
283.15	2.77	4.04
288.15	2.78	4.05
293.15	2.78	4.06
298.15	2.78	4.06
308.15	2.78	4.07
313.15	2.79	4.08
318.15	2.80	4.10
333.15	2.81	4.11
Cyclohexane		
283.15	2.15	3.15
288.15	2.15	3.16
293.15	2.15	3.17
298.15	2.16	3.17
308.15	2.17	3.19
313.15	2.17	3.19
318.15	2.17	3.20
333.15	2.18	3.22
Toluene		
283.15	2.14	3.14
288.15	2.14	3.14
293.15	2.14	3.15
298.15	2.15	3.15
313.15	2.16	3.17
333.15	2.17	3.19

From Table 1 it is clear than as the temperature increase the value of molecular radius increase slowly showing expansion of liquid to minimum extent. But with increasing chain length n-hexane > n-heptane > n-dodecane > cyclohexane > toluene value increase showing large expansion within the molecule making more voids and volatile in nature.

Table 2 shows the calculated value of van der Waals constant (a & b) and molecular dimension (d) for different organic liquids at varying temperatures ranging from 283.15K to 333.15K.

Table 2. Calculated values of van der Waals constant (a & b) and molecular dimension (d) for different organic liquids at varying temperatures ranging from 283.15K to 333.15K.

T (K)	a	b	10^9 d
	L^2 atm mol^{-2}	L mol^{-2}	cm
n-hexane			
283.15	42.231	0.120	4.560
288.15	42.154	0.121	4.573
293.15	41.550	0.121	4.577
298.15	41.435	0.122	4.585
303.15	40.910	0.122	4.592
308.15	41.185	0.123	4.601
313.15	41.078	0.124	4.610
318.15	42.453	0.125	4.627
333.15	45.121	0.127	4.650
n-heptane			
283.15	53.539	0.135	4.752
293.15	54.871	0.137	4.768
298.15	54.797	0.137	4.775
303.15	55.422	0.138	4.786
308.15	54.598	0.139	4.795
313.15	54.448	0.139	4.798
318.15	55.326	0.142	4.831
333.15	52.893	0.142	4.831
n-dodecane			
283.15	150.267	0.215	5.542
288.15	151.228	0.216	5.552
293.15	150.122	0.216	5.556
298.15	150.268	0.217	5.563
308.15	147.169	0.218	5.570
313.15	148.213	0.220	5.585
318.15	149.625	0.222	5.608
333.15	144.887	0.223	5.615
Cyclohexane			
283.15	39.872	0.100	4.296
288.15	38.904	0.100	4.303
293.15	38.501	0.101	4.307
298.15	37.484	0.101	4.312
308.15	37.831	0.102	4.330
313.15	37.672	0.103	4.332

318.15	37.344	0.103	4.343
333.15	35.839	0.105	4.361
Toluene			
283.15	41.483	0.099	4.279
288.15	41.040	0.099	4.285
293.15	38.913	0.099	4.288
298.15	39.526	0.100	4.294
313.15	41.375	0.101	4.315
333.15	45.202	0.103	4.345

Table 2 shows that with temperature rise the value of a, b and d increases gradually and similar trend is with increasing chain length showing strong intermolecular interaction and compact structure of solvents.

4.   Conclusion

The acoustic methods are helpful in determining the properties on the basis of radius, van der Waals constant the molecular dimension of pure liquids undertaken in our study.

5.   References

1.   Beyer, R.T., Letcher, S.V.: Physical Ultrasonics (Eds Massey, H.S.W. and Bruecner, K.A.) Academic, NY, Chapter 7, 202-230 (1979).

2.   Hartman, B.: Potential energy effects on the sound speed in liquids. J. Acoust. Soc. Am. 65, 1392-1396 (1979).

3.   Sehgal, C.M., Porter, B.B. Greenleaf, J.F.: Ultrasonic nonlinear Parameters of alcohol-water mixtures. J. Acoust. Soc. Am. 79, 566-570 (1986).

4.   Sehgal, C.M., Greenleaf, J.F.: Correlative study of properties of water in biological system using ultrasound and magnetic resonance. Magnetic Resonance in Medicine 3, 976-985 (1986).

5.   Dunn, F., Law, W.K., Frizzell, L.A.: Nonlinear ultrasonic wave propagation in biological materials. IEEE Ultrasonic Symposium, New York, pp. 527-532 (1981).

6.   Yoshiezumi, K., Sato, T., Ichida, N. A.: physiochemical of nonlinear parameters B/A for media predominantly composed of water. J. Acoust. Soc. Am. 82, 302-305 (1987).

7.   Beyer, R.T.: Parameters of nonlinearity in fluids. J. Acoust. Soc. Am. 32, 719-721 (1960).

8.   Coppens, A.B., Beyer, R.T., Ballou, J.: Parameter of nonlinearity in fluids. III. Values of sound velocity in liquid metals. J. Acoust. Soc. Am. 41, 1443-1448 (1966).

9.   Law, W.K., Frizzell, L.A., Dunn, F.: Comparison of thermodynamic and finite amplitude methods of B/A measurement in biological materials. J. Acoust. Soc. Am. 74, 1295-1297 (1983).

10.   Sehgal, C.M.: Non-linear ultrasonics to determine molecular properties of pure liquids. Ultrasonics 33(2), 155-161 (1995).

11.   Schaaffs, W.: Zur bestimmung von moleku"lradien organischer fiussigkeiten aus schallgeschwindigkeit und dichte. Z. Phys. 114, 110-115 (1939).

12.   Mishra, R.L., Pandey, J.D.: Comparision of Factor Theory and Free Length Theory for Binary Liquid Mixture. Ind. J. Pure Appl. Phys. 15, 505-506 (1977).

Thermal and Lattice Dynamical Study of MgO by (VTBFS) Model

U C Srivastava

Department of Physics, Amity Institute of applied Sciences, Amity University, Noida, U.P. -201301, India.
Email: ucsrivastava@amity.edu ,umeshmitul@gmail.com

ABSTRACT

In present manuscript phonon dynamics of alkaline-earth oxides MgO by incorporating the three-body interactions in the framework of 'van der Waals three-body force shell model' (VTBFSM) is based on my thorough theoretical study of the relevant research papers on this topic .The thermal properties, densities of states (DOS) and structurer analysis of magnesium oxide with their results has been theoretically presented .However, a considerable improvement on computational results has been obtained by use of present model and successfully predicted the lattice dynamic of MgO for study of bulk thermo-elastic properties .An excellent agreement has been observed with measured and available experimental data.

Keywords: Phonon, thermal properties, density of state, van der Waals Interaction.

1. Introduction

In recent years, the availability of the phonon dispersion relations for magnesium oxide by means of the inelastic scattering of thermal neutrons has stimulated considerable interest in the study of its lattice dynamics among both theoretical and experimental workers. It is solid of great interest and crystallizes in sodium–chloride structure. The studies of lattice energy and other properties made by Huggins and sakamoto [1] clearly show that it is purely an ionic solid. The pioneer work of Kellerman [2] the lattice dynamics of the alkali halides has provided attentive theoretically as well as experimentally. Lowdin's [3] and Lundqvist's [4] theory of ionic solids leads to many–body force of which the three-body component is the first important term. Lattice dynamic is one of the methods by help of it the complete structural properties can be analyzed. The van der Waals interaction (VWI) potential owes its origin to the correlations of the electron motions in different atoms. Thus, the inclusion of VWI and TBI effects in RSM has utilized in the Hitler, London and the free-electron approximations which is a significant advance over previous lattice models. The interaction systems of the present model thus consist of the long-range screened Coulomb, VWI, TBI and the short-range overlap repulsion operative up to the second-neighbour ions.

2. Theory

The present model is based on the framework of ion polarizable (RSM) proposed by Dick and Over Hauser [5] and Woods et al [6] by two research groups and it successfully applied to study of lattice property, effective up to the second neighbor in short-range interactions. The study of complete dynamical behaviour of MgO has reported by introducing the van der Waals interactions (VWI) effect and expression for the contribution of (TBI) that prove the relevance of use model (VTBFSM),which has been rigorously derived and exactly evaluated in the framework of RSM [7].The relevant expression and general formalism of VTBFSM model given as

$$\Phi = \Phi^C + \Phi^R + \Phi^{TBI} + \Phi^{VWI} \tag{1}$$

Where Φ^C is a long-range Coulomb interaction potential.. Second term Φ^{or} is a short-range overlap repulsion potential. Third term Φ^{TBI} is a three-body interaction potential.This interaction potential is expressed by [8] as

$$\Phi^{TBI} = \alpha_m \frac{Z^2 e^2}{r_0}\left[\frac{2n}{Z} f(r)_0\right] \tag{2}$$

van der Waals interaction potential and owes its origin to the correlations of the electron motions in different atoms closely the method used by Wood et.al[5]..The introduction of VWI and TBI in the framework of RSM leads to the secular determinant:

$$\left|\underline{D}(\bar{q}) - \omega^2 \underline{M} I\right| = 0 \tag{3}$$

Here $\underline{D}$ (q) is the (6 x 6) dynamical matrix for the Rigid Shell model expressed as:

If we consider only the second neighbor dipole-dipole van der Waals interaction energy, then it is expressed as:

$$\Phi_{dd}^{VWI}(r) = -S_v \left|\frac{C_{++} + C_{--}}{6r^6}\right| = \Phi^V(r) \tag{4}$$

Where, S_v is lattice sum and the constants C_{++} and C_{--} are the van der Waals coefficients corresponding to the positive-positive and negative-negative ion pairs, respectively.

2.1   Thermodynamically properties of MgO

Density of state, temperature dependence of free energy, specific heat capacity at constant volume were calculated. Specific heat capacity at constant volume (Cv) was calculated using the following equation [5-6].

$$U = \int_0^{\upsilon_m} \frac{h\upsilon^3}{e^{h\upsilon/kT} - 1} d\upsilon \tag{5}$$

and

$$C_\upsilon = 3 NK_B \frac{\sum_\upsilon \{E(x)\} G(\upsilon) d\upsilon}{\sum_\upsilon G(\upsilon) d\upsilon} \tag{6}$$

Where $E(x)$ is the Einstein function difiend as $E(x) = x^2 \dfrac{e^{(x)}}{\{e^{(x)} - 1\}^2}$ and $\sum_\upsilon G(\upsilon) d\upsilon$ = Total number of frequencies.According to thermodynamics, the equilibrium of a solid at a temperature T is determined by the minimum value of the free energy.

$$F = E - TS \tag{7}$$

2.2   Density of States

To determine the phonon density of states for each polarization is given by VTBFS model.

$$g(\omega) = \frac{dN}{d\omega} = N \int_{BZ} \sum_j \delta\left[\omega - \omega_j(q)\right] dq = \left(\frac{VK^2}{2\pi^2}\right)\cdot\left(\frac{dK}{d\omega}\right) \tag{8}$$

$N = (L/2\pi)^3 (4\pi K^3/3)$, K is wave vector and $L^3 = V$. Where N as a normalization constant such that $\int g(w)dw$ =1 and $g(w)dw$ is the ratio of the number of eigenstates in the frequency interval

3.   Numerical Computations

The input data and the model parameters of MgO reported in table -1taking the values of input constants from [25-26] and calculated the model parameter .The Internal energy, entropy, free energy heat capacity and dispersion relation curve at temperature 500K has shown in Fig .1-3 with the available theoretical and experimental result which has shown parallel to the present calculated results.

Table 1 Input data and model parameters for MgO

Input data (Constants)	Expt. Values[17]	Expt. Values[18]	Model Parameters		
			Parameter	Calculated Values using [17]	Calculated Values using[18]
C_{11} (10^{11} dyn cm^{-2})	30.70[9]	28.917[13]	Z_m	2.00	2.00
C_{12} (10^{11} dyn cm^{-2})	8.50[9]	8.796[13]	$r_o f_o'$	-0.330	-0.152
C_{44} (10^{11} dyn cm^{-2})	15.89[9]	15.461[13]	A	31.319	7.912
r_0 (10^{-8} cm)	4.213[9]	2.106[14]	B	-3.9431	-1.350
a (10^{-24} cm^3)	1.76[11]	0.581	d_1	-0.1371	-0.0962
a_1 (10^{-24} cm^3)	0.094	0.163	d_2	-0.5977	-0.732
a_2 (10^{-24} cm^3)	1.666	1.354	Y_1	1.644	1.350
ϵ_0	9.86[10]	9.86[10]	Y_2	-3.443	-3.334
ϵ_∞	2.956[10]	2.957[15]			
n_L (THz)	21.55[LST]	21.679[16]			
n_T (THz)	11.81[12]	11.870[10]			

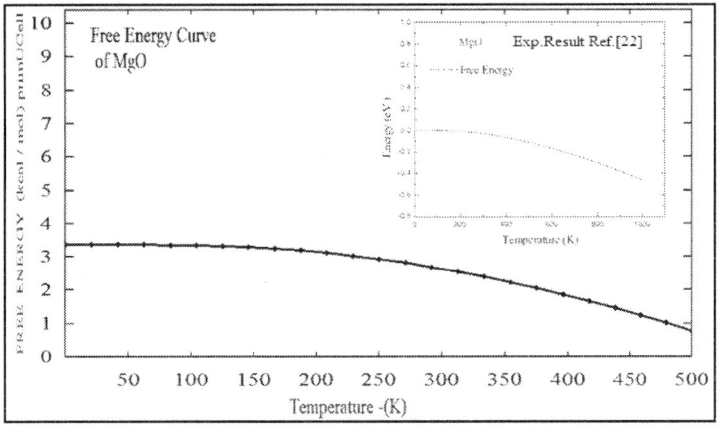

Figure 1 Free Energy curve of MgO

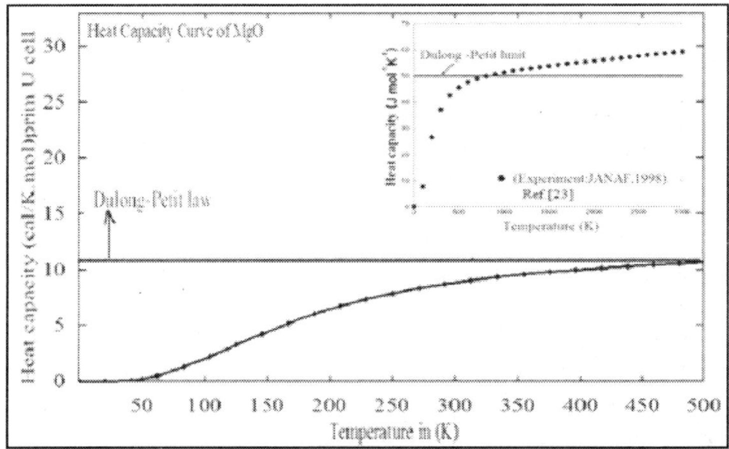

Figure 2 Heat Capacity curve of MgO

On raising the temperature free energy value of MgO is continuously decreasing with increasing temperature. In fig-1. on raising the temperature up to 150K free energy value continuously increasing and then further energy transforms reversibly decreases continuously up to 500K at high temperature energy dissipation more rapidly can be seen.our theoretical reported result is agree well with experimentally reported result by ref. [22]. The heat capacity is raised continuously on increasing in temperature value from 0 to 7 (cal/ k .mole per unit cell) at the temperature range of 50K to 300K.The exponentially increment in specific heat value curve has been observed the value from low-temperatures were smoothly growing on. At 300 K the heat capacity of MgO smoothly increases, but on the other higher value of temperature shown in fig. 2. Heat capacities increases very small and then remain constant for further increases in temperature value up to 500K. As the temperature increases the value of heat capacity increases and approaches a constant at high temperatures that tends to the Dulong-Petit limit [27].In fig .2 the experimental reported result is given by [23] and at lower temperature less number of points available but their nature is similar to theoretical result.

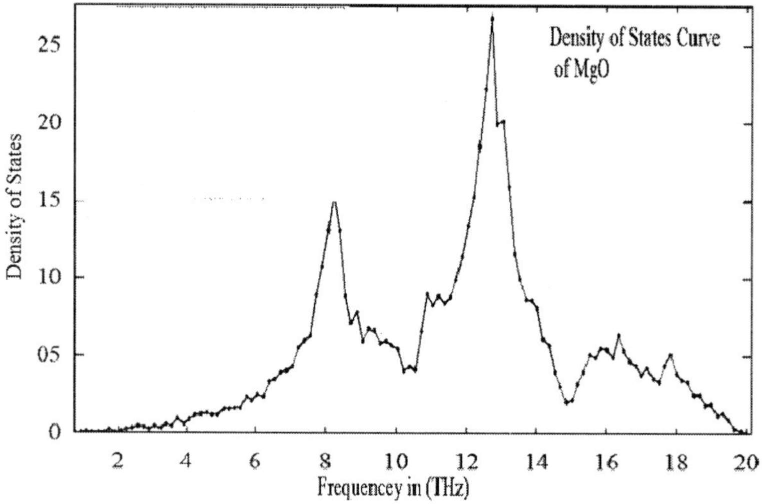

Figure 3 Density of states curve of MgO

The DOS curve with frequency (THz) value is reported in fig .3. At frequency of 13 (Thz) the peak attended the maximum value, there are many states available for occupation and on increasing the frequency value a local density of states (LDS) available, frequency of 8 (Thz) more occupied states are available and less occupied states are above the 14 THz frequency range the gap has been observed after 15 (THz) again distortion in peaks can be seen.The illustrated thermodynamic properties obtained confirmed the characteristics of MgO. If compare to the experimental result the peak at 11 THz are similar to our theoretical result but above this value some sharp electronic peak available from 35 cm-1 to 45 cm-1 so in this range the discrepancy in spectroscopic experimental and lattice dynamical result occurred and rest value the result are approximately similar.

The lattice dynamical calculations for alkaline-earth oxides MgO on the basis of 11 parameters. The uncertainty in the thermal expansion for MgO is seen that using the phonon theory do not converge for $T>2000$ K, whereas those by [28] show convergence up > 3000 K has been observed at high temperature but it does not affect the result.In the present study despite the lower symmetry of MgO and the uncertainty as to the exact nature of the distortion of the lower–temperature structure. Our theoretical study at the lower temperature side shows a better agreement, but at the higher temperature side, slight disagreement may be ascribed to the non-inclusion of the harmonic interactions in using present model, which it may be inferred that the incorporation of van der Waals interactions is essential. The Complete lattice dynamical, thermodynamical property and density of state curve of MgO theoretically reported has agreed with different reported data [13-24]. The present model successfully used by different researcher for theoretically reported the lattice dynamic of alkali halides and semiconductor materials [29-34].

4.   References

1.   Huggins M L , Sakamoto Y J. J Phys Soc Japan. Lattice Energies and Other Properties of Crystals of Alkaline Earth Chalcogenides.;12: 241(1957).

2.   Kellerman E W.Phil Trans Roy Soc (London). Theory of the Vibrations of the Sodium Chloride Lattice.;A238: 513(1940).

3.   Lowdin P O. Ark Mat Astr Fys (Sweden).;35A:30(1947). https://doi.org/10.1021/ac60002a736

4.   Lundqvist S O. Ark Fys (Sweden).;12:263,(1957).

5.   Dick B G, Over Hauser A W.Phys Rev.Theory of the Dielectric Constants of Alkali Halide Crystals.;112: 90. (1958).

6.   Woods A D B,Cochran W,Brockhouse B N. Phys Rev. Lattice Dynamics of Alkali Halide Crystals.;119: 980 (1960).

7.   Verma M P, Singh R K. Phys Stat Sol. The Contribution of Three-Body Overlap Forces to the Dynamical Matrix of Alkali Halides.;33:769(1969).

8.   Kresse G. Journal of Noncrystalline Solids. Ab initio molecular dynamics for liquid metals. 1995;193: 222-229.

9.   Simmons G, Wang H. MIT Press Mass.(1972). https://doi.org/10.7202/700372ar

10.   Sangster M J L, Peckham G, Saunderson D H. J Phys. Lattice dynamics of magnesium oxide. 1970;C 2:1026.

11.   M.P.verma & S.K.Agarwal.Phys.Rev.B84880,(1973).

12.   B.N.N.Achar & G.R.Barsch, Phys. Status Solidi 6, 247,(1971).

13.   R.H.L.Yddane,R.G.Sachs and E.Teller,Phys.Rev.59,673,(1941).

14.   R.E.Stephens and I.H.Malitson,J.Res .Natl.Bur.Std.(U.S),49.249,(1952).

15.   Chung D H. Philosophy Magazine. Elastic moduli of single crystal and polycrystalline MgO;8:833-841(1963).

16.   Stephens R E , Malitson I H. Journal of Research of the National Bureau of standards(U.S). Index of refraction of magnesium oxide .;49:249(1952).

17.   Skinner B J. Am Mineralogist. Science and the Citizen .;232(5):42-45,(1975).

18.   Ghose S, Michael K et.al. Physical Review Letters. Lattice Dynamics of MgO at High Pressure: Theory and Experiment.;96: 035507. (2006).

19.   Oganov A R. Treatise on Geophysics. Theory and Practice – Thermodynamics, Equations of State, Elasticity, and Phase Transitions of Minerals at High Pressures and Temperatures .;2 :121-152,(2007).

20.   Koči L., Ma Y., Oganov A. R., Souvatzis P., Ahuja R. Elasticity of the superconducting metals V, Nb, Ta, Mo, and W at high pressure. Phys. Rev.; B 77: 214101,(2008).

21.   Mirhosseini M M , Reza Khordad. European Physics Journal Plus. Prediction of physical properties of XO (X = Am, Cd, Mg, Zr) compounds using density functional theory .;131: 239,(2016).

22.   Chase M W. Journal of Physical and Chemical refrence data. NIST-JANAF thermochemical tables.;9,(1998).

23.   Tang Xiaoli, Dong Jianjun. Proceedings of the National Academy of Sciences . Lattice thermal conductivity of MgO at conditions of Earth's interior ;107 (10): 4539-4543,(2010).

24.   Coppari F, Smith R F et.al. Nature Geoscience. Experimental evidence for a phase transition in magnesium oxide at exoplanet pressures .;6(11):926-929,(2013).

25.   Albers R C. Nature . An expanding view of plutonium.;410: 759-761 ,(2001).

26.   Agarwal S K.Solid state communication. Crystal dynamics of magnesium oxide.:39(3):513-516,(1981).

27.   Kushwaha M S, Kushwaha S S. Canadian Journal of Physics. Lattice dynamics of ZnTe, CdTe, GaP, and InP;58(3): 35-358,(1980).

28. Karki B B, Wentzcovitch R M, Gironcoli S, Baroni S. Physical Review B. High-pressure lattice dynamics and thermoelasticity of MgO. ;61:8793-8800(2000).

29. Singh R K, Prabhakar N V K. Physics Status Solidi (b). Phase Transition and Anharmonic Properties of Semimagnetic Semiconductors .;146(1): 111-116(1988).

30. Srivastava U C , Upadhyaya K S. Optoelectronics & Advanced Materials (OAM-RC). Van der Waals three-body force shell model (VTSM) for the Lattice dynamical studies of Potassium fluoride;4(9):1336-1341(2010).

31. Wattanasarn H, Seetawan T. Advanced Materials Research. Studies Thermophysical Properties of MgO by First Principle Simulation .; 802:139-143(2013).

32. Srivastava U C. Optoelectronics and Adv. Materials, Rapid Communications . Study of cohesive energy for KX(X=F, Cl, Br & I) crystal structure.;7(9-10):698-701,(2013).

33. Srivastava U C. Int. Journal of Modern Physics B. Dynamical study of Debye temperature and combined density of states of TiO2 .;30:1750020-28,(2016).

34. Srivastava U C. Journal of Science and Arts. Unified study of ND4I by lattice dynamical approach.; 1(42):247-254,(2018).

A Novel Decision Tree-based Method for Phishing Detection

Pravin Kumar Pandey[1*], Sandip Kumar Singh[2]

[1]Department of Computer Science & Engineering, UNSIET, VBS Purvanchal University, Jaunpur-211001, India
[2] Department of Mechanical Engineering, UNSIET, VBS Purvanchal University, Jaunpur-211001, India
*E-mail:pravin108786@gmail.com

ABSTRACT

Phishing is an electronically connected criminal activity in which the attacker steals the user's personal information like username, countersign, internet banking account, credit/debit card number with the expiration date, password, pin, legitimacy, confidential patient record, CVV number, etc. to boon financially. Email-based phishing is the most common and traditional way of phishing scams, in which the phisher will send a suspicious email with an embedded URL and ask the user to click the URL. When the user clicks on the link, the link will be redirected to a spoofed site that looks the same to the original site to steal their credentials and displays some error message. Later the phishing uses those credentials for malicious purposes. To overcome these scams, many anti-phishing tools have developed. Among that the machine learning-based approaches can give a better result. This paper is an extensive study of the various machine learning-based anti-phishing approaches and their results that detect the phishing URL's from the URLs with URLs features. Six most important models of machine learning have been examined for the phishing detection problem. The Decision Tree-based method outperforms other methods.

*Keywords: **Phishing, anti-phishing, machine learning, phishtank, legitimate, suspicious, decision tree.***

1. Introduction

Phishing is a wide term used to describe a group of scam people with their personal information shared such as consumer name, password, credit/debit card number, etc., that manipulate information for disseminating reasons. Earliest contact is sent to a bulky group of people at once, so anyone can be a victim. They will contact their victims with the help of URLs, social media, emails, and phones. The only target through this attack of these people is to send a fake correspondence, which appears to have originated from the actual organization, hoping that a large group will follow the links provided to them from these contacts and disclose their personal information to the phishers. Phishing is an automated detection method used to cheat billions of dollars to outsiders and phishing technology uses human nature as well as the power of the internet to deceive millions of people in the world [1]. The social media platforms are used for deceitful, cultivated and perceptive information from internet users by covering through a legitimate entity. The basic goal of phishing technology is to illegally commit deceitful financial transactions on behalf of internet users [2]. An anti-phishing working group (APWG), which is an NGO community (a non-profitable group) has reported on the 1st quarter of 2019 (January, February, March) that there was 180,768 phishing incident detected [3]. Various methodologies are being adopted at present to identify phishing web sites and emails. Sajid Yousuf Bhat *et al.* proposes an approach for "Spammer classification using ensemble methods over structural social network features" [4]. In [4] finds out whether the URL is spam/legitimate on the social network with community-based features. Mouad Zouina *et al.* proposes an approach for "A novel lightweight URL phishing detection using SVM and similarities index" [5]. In [5] phishing detection from the URL with the help of 6 features. SVM and similarity index is targeted to improve overall recognition of the phishing detection system. Alejandro Correa *et al.* explore "Classifying phishing URLs using recurrent neural networks" [6]. In [6] we explored the use of URLs as input for machine learning models applied for phishing site prediction with the help of 14 features. Suh *et al.* used "Comparing writing style feature-based classification methods for estimating user reputations in social media" it evaluates the performance of classifiers depend on the state-of-art methods 4 writing style features such as lexical, syntactic, structural, content-specific[7]. Gunikhan Sonowal *et al.* using "Masphid: a Model to Assist Screen Reader Users for Detecting Phishing Sites Using Aural and Visual Similarity measures" [8]. In [8] URL is phishing, suspicious or legitimate based on the 10 features. Kshitij Tayal *et al* explore "Particle swarm optimization trained class association rule mining: Application to phishing detection" [9]. In [9] class association rules used to detect the URLs are phished or legitimate.

2.   The proposed method

The following machine learning algorithms have been used for phishing detection problem in recent researches which have certain limitations:

2.1   Support Vector Machine

Support Vector Machine is a supervised machine learning algorithm that can be used for classification problems involving two classes. SVM with the maximizing margin (i.e. the distance between the closest data point and the hyperplane) yields an improved outcome [10].

2.2   Neural Network

An Artificial Neural Network or Neural Network is structure and/or function as a set of interconnected identical units (neurons). With the help of interconnections are used to send signals from one neuron to the other neuron. Other than this, the weight of the interconnection is carried to increase the distribution between the neuron [11].

2.3   Naïve Bayes

Bayesian methods are those that exceptionally apply Bayes' theorem for problems such as classification and regression. The Bayesian classifier is designed in such a way that we use it only when its features are independent in each class, but this is not the case. Even if this is not a valid case, the Bayesian classifier works very well also [12].

2.4   Random Forest

Random Forest is a machine learning classifier. This classifier integrates with a series of tree predictors, each tree votes one unit for the most popular class, then integrating these results yields the final type of result. We use random forest classifiers when it comes to classification accuracy, overfitting, and tolerant utilities [13].

2.5   k Nearest Neighbor

k Nearest Neighbor is an instance-based learning model which is based on a decision problem with instances and the k-Nearest Neighbor classification algorithm is a non-parametric classification algorithm.

We propose a new method (figure 1) based on decision tree that offers better classification accuracy as compared to the above methods.

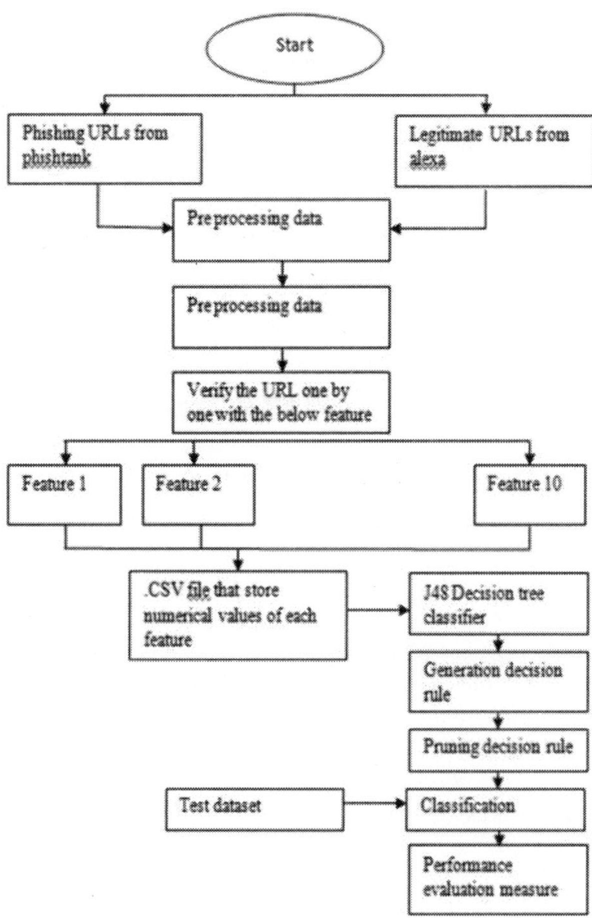

Figure 1 The proposed model

2.6   Decision Tree

Decision Tree is a supervised learning algorithm (pre-defined outcome) that is frequently used in classification problems. Whatever is output by the Decision Tree will be visible in binary tree format. The Decision Tree keeps such rules with which it can easily predict the target variable. Where the database has a lot of similarities in large-scale training replacements, the J48 algorithm works well and measures well. J48 is an extension of ID3. The additional features of the J48 algorithm usage greedy technique to the induced tree for classification. A Decision Tee is built by analyzing the training data and classify missing data [14].

2.6.1 Algorithm basics steps [15]

(a)   If in each case instances exist to the same features class, the tree produces a leaf so the leaf is returned with labeling with this same class.

(b)   Compute the potential information which is calculated for every attribute given for a test for the mode. After this compute the gain in information is that would get a result from analysis on the attribute.

(c)   Find the favorite attribute is based on the present procedure for attribute branching selection.

2.6.2 Counting gain

This process uses the "Entropy" which is a measure of the URLs phishing. The Entropy of is calculated

$$Entropy\left(\vec{y}\right) = -\sum_{j=1}^{n}\frac{|y_i|}{|\vec{y}|}\log\left(\frac{|y_i|}{|\vec{y}|}\right), Entropy\left(j|\vec{y}\right) = \frac{|y_i|}{|\vec{y}|}\log\left(\frac{|y_j|}{|\vec{y}|}\right)$$

$$Gain\left(\vec{y},j\right) = Entropy(\vec{y} - Entropy\left(j|\vec{y}\right))$$

Dividing by entire entropy due to split argument by value j for maximizing the gain.

2.6.3. Pruning

Pruning is used to reduce the classification errors that are caused by being specializing in training sets. This procedure has to done to make the Decision Tree classifier is more general.

3. Feature selection and model implementation

In this paper, we are implementing a machine learning-based approach for detecting phishing URLs. When compared to the other approaches, machine learning-based approaches can give better results. In machine learning-based approaches, first we have to choose the features and then we check whether that features are present in the given data or not for classification or clustering. Next, the very important thing is the dataset and without this, we can't work with machine learning. Training and testing are the other steps, where we train our classifier with the data and then it classifies the upcoming data automatically based on the training?. Better training can give a better outcome. By referring more than 20 research articles and the dataset (i.e. 418 phishing URLs from phishtank and 110 legitimate URLs from alexa) from phishtank and alexa, we found more than 70 features. From these features, we apply the Apriori algorithm to find the most frequent and very important features (i.e. 10 features). Later the 10 features are used for detecting the phishing, legitimate, and suspicious URLs by training the model these features. Decision Tree classifier is used to calculate the accuracy in classifying the phishing URLs from legitimate URLs. The implementation work can be further explained in detail in the following sections.

3.1 Features

For detecting the phishing URLs, the maximum number of features has been used earlier. We analyzed those features and found the minimum number of features for detecting the phishing URLs. 10 features are finalized from more than 70 features by using apriori algorithm. The proposed system is more flexible and can be added for additional features for better decision making when there is any new way of phishing attacks occur. All those features are URL length, number of dots in the path of the URL, number of hyphen in URL host, presence of SSL, number of slash present in host part of the URL, number of terms in the host part of URL, presence of IP based URL, presence of any special character in URL, presence of .exe in the URL, number of dots present in the host part of the URL. Most of the features are already implemented and we tried in our way to combine all these 10 features to detect the phishing URLs more accurately.

3.2 Classification Model

Once the features are selected, we train our model with those features to detect the phishing URLs more accurately. In the training process, we load the list of URLs to the model and for each URL, all the 10 features are extracted and the outcome (i.e. 1: phishing, -1: legitimate, 0: suspicious) and stored those results in a CSV file. For all the URLs, these 10 features are extracted and the outcome is stored in one CSV file. Later this

CSV file is used to calculate the accuracy of the model by using any classifier. In this work, we used Support Vector Machine, Neural Network, Naïve Bayes, Random Forest, k Nearest Neighbor, and Decision Tree.

3.3   Dataset

To implement the machine learning-based phishing detection approach, we choose the dataset (which is very important) from two different sources. Phishing URLs from phishtank.com and legitimate/binge URLs from alexa.com. We took 418 phishing URLs from phishtank.com and 110 legitimate URLs from alexa.com.

4.   Result Analysis

The machine learning classifier has generated better results for detecting phishing URLs and the output screenshot of our work has been included with the explanation. Among all machine learning classifiers, The Decision Tree classifier got 99.80 % accuracy in classifying the phishing URL from the legitimate one (Table 1). We gave 528 phishing and legitimate URLs for training and testing. The result may vary if we increase the size of the data for training and testing.

Table 1 Shows the accuracy rate based on different classifier

S.N.	Classifier	Accuracy in percent
1	Support Vector Machine	96.90
2	Neural Network	97.78
3	Naïve Bayes	96.25
4	Random Forest	98.80
5	k Nearest Neighbor	98.65
6	Decision Tree	99.80

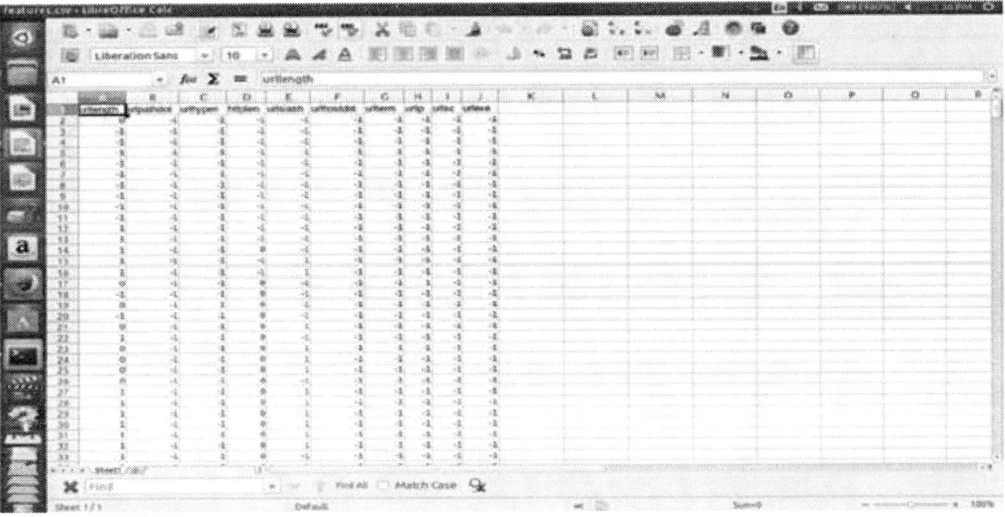

Figure 2 Screenshot of CSV file with 528 records based on 10 phishing feature

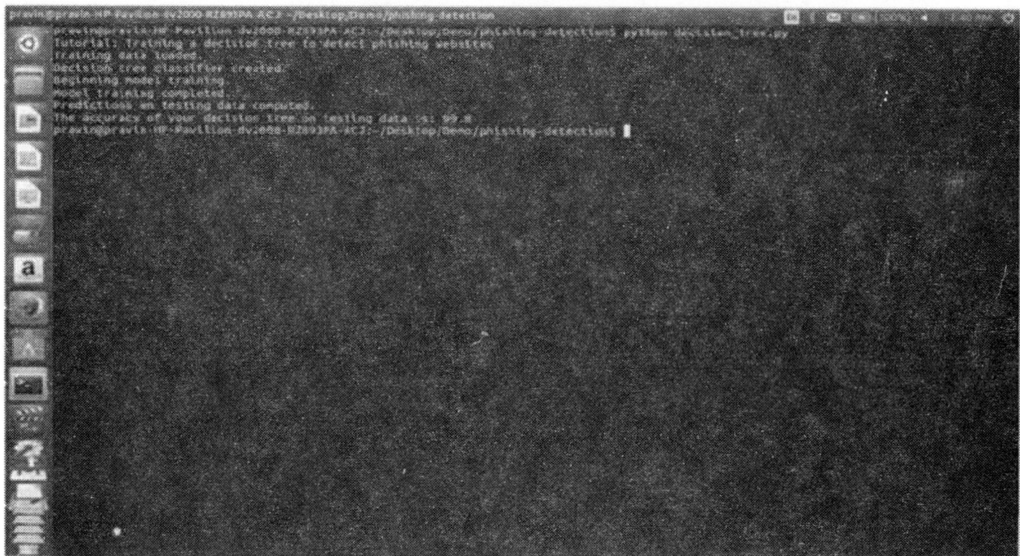

Figure 3 Screenshot of calculating accuracy with decision tree classifier

5. Conclusion

In this work, we used the Support Vector Machine, Neural Network, Naïve Bayes, Random Forest, k Nearest Neighbor, and proposed Decision Tree method. The table shows the comparative performance of different algorithms in the phishing detection problem. It is observed that the performance of the proposed Decision Tree method excels with the other techniques. It is also observed that the classification accuracy is significantly affected by the number of URLs / mails i.e. the size of available phishing data. It is also observed that the recognize 10 features govern the phishing detection problem most effectively. The Decision Tree utilizes these features in the best possible way to identify phishing.

In the future, supervised and unsupervised classifiers will be used to detect cell phone phishing, sound phishing, and phishing in many important areas.

6. References

1. Lininger, R., Vines, R. D. (2005). Phishing: Cutting the identity theft line. John Wiley & Sons.

2. H. Tout and W. Hafner, "Phishpin: An identity-based anti-phishing approach," Proc.- 12th IEEE Int. Conf. Comput. Sci. Eng. CSE 2009, vol. 3, pp. 347–352, 2009.

3. https://docs.apwg.org/reports/apwg_trends_report_q1_2019.pdf

4. Bhat, Sajid Yousuf, Muhammad Abulaish, and Abdulrahman A. Mirza. "Spammer classification using ensemble methods over structural social network features." Proceedings of the 2014 IEEE/WIC/ACM International Joint Conferences on Web Intelligence (WI) and Intelligent Agent Technologies (IAT)-Volume 02. IEEE Computer Society, 2014.

5. Zouina, Mouad, and Benaceur Outtaj. "A novel lightweight URL phishing detection system using SVM and similarity index." Human-centric Computing and Information Sciences 7.1 (2017): 17

6. Bahnsen, Alejandro Correa, et al. "Classifying phishing URLs using recurrent neural networks." 2017 APWG Symposium on Electronic Crime Research (eCrime). IEEE, 2017.

7. Suh, Jong Hwan. "Comparing writing style feature-based classification methods for estimating user reputations in social media." SpringerPlus 5.1 (2016): 261.

8.   Sonowal, Gunikhan, and K. S. Kuppusamy. "Masphid: a model to assist screen reader users for detecting phishing sites using aural and visual similarity measures." Proceedings of the International Conference on Informatics and Analytics. ACM, 2016.

9.   Tayal, Kshitij, and Vadlamani Ravi. "Particle swarm optimization trained class association rule mining: Application to phishing detection." Proceedings of the International Conference on Informatics and Analytics. ACM, 2016.

10.   Adewumi, Oluyinka Aderemi, and Ayobami Andronicus Akinyelu. "A hybrid firefly and support vector machine classifier for phishing email detection." Kybernetes 45.6 (2016): 977-994.

11.   Abu-Nimeh, Saeed, et al. "A comparison of machine learning techniques for phishing detection." Proceedings of the anti-phishing working groups 2nd annual eCrime researchers summit. ACM, 2007.

12.   Lakshmi, V. Santhana, and M. S. Vijaya. "Efficient prediction of phishing websites using supervised learning algorithms." Procedia Engineering 30 (2012): 798-805.

13.   RANDOM FORESTS, Leo Breiman. "Statistics Department." University of California, Berkeley, CA 94720 (2001).

14.   Lakshmi, V. Santhana, and M. S. Vijaya. "Efficient prediction of phishing websites using supervised learning algorithms." Procedia Engineering 30 (2012): 798-805.

15.   Korting, Thales Sehn. "C4. 5 algorithm and multivariate decision trees." Image Processing Division, National Institute for Space Research–INPE Sao Jose dos Campos–SP, Brazil (2006).

Polymer Blend Electrolytes Based on PVA-PVP-LiTf: Structural, Thermal and Ion Transport Properties Study

Pankaj Singh* and A.L.Saroj**

Department of Physics, Institute of Science, Banaras Hindu University, Varanasi-221005, India
*Email: *pankajjsingh04@gmail.com, **al.saroj@bhu.ac.in*

ABSTRACT

PVA-PVP-LiTf based polymer blend electrolytes (PBEs) films were prepared using solution cast technique. These films were characterized using thermo-gravimetric analysis (TGA), ATR-FTIR and AC impedance spectroscopic techniques. ATR-FTIR analysis reveals the interaction/complexation with the constituents of polymer blend and LiTf. TGA results show that the thermal stability of the PBEs changes with loading of LiTf, salt. The maximum conductivity at room temperature is found to be ~4.22×10⁻⁷ S/cm for the composition of 60PVP-40PVA-25wt%LiTf.

Keywords: Polymer Blend Electrolyte, Dielectric properties, TGA and Ionic conductivity.

1.   Introduction

Solid polymer electrolytes are of considerable interest for the last four decades, because of its importance and applications in many electrochemical devices such as Li-ion batteries, mobile phones, smart credit cards, electric vehicles, super capacitors, cellular telephones, electro chromic devices, etc. [1, 2]. The solid polymer electrolytes have many advantages compare to liquid electrolytes such as low costs, improved safety, ease of fabrication, and leakage free nature [3-6]. Ionic conductivity is the most important parameter in solid polymer electrolytes. For improvement in the ionic conductivity blending is the best method for Solid polymer electrolytes [7]. The polymer blend electrolytes (PBEs) are generally prepared by doping ionic salts, ionic liquids, alkali metal salts/or both with the polymer blends/co-polymers [8]. The work of ionic salts/ionic liquid in PBEs is to reduce the crystallinity of polymers and enhances the mechanical flexibility of polymer chains due to the plasticization effect of ILs/or salts [9]. In the Polymer electrolytes ion transport mechanism is directly associated with the segmental relaxation process of polymer as well as the segmental motion of polymer chains [10]. In the polymeric system the dielectric relaxation and frequency dependent conductivity both are highly sensitive for the orientation of dipoles and transportation of charge carriers [11]. The analysis of the dielectric properties such as dielectric constant, dielectric loss and electric modulus of polymer electrolytes are essential to get insights into the ion transport behaviour and the dopant materials interaction between the constituents of the polymer [8]. Polymer like polyvinyl alcohol (PVA) has some unique properties such as high chemical stability, water soluble, good charge storage capacity, good film making property, etc. Polymer, polyvinyl pyrrolidone (PVP) has also some properties such as easy good charge storage capacity, low scattering loss, high dielectric strength, and dopant-dependent properties. Due to the presence of pyrrole group (C=O) with the side chains of PVP, it is more attractive to PVA which has hydroxyl group (O-H) with its side chains [12].

In the present work, we have studies the effect of LiTf loading on PVA-PVP based polymer blend at room temperature.

2.   Experimental

2.1   Materials and Preparation of Polymeric films

Poly(vinyl) alcohol (PVA)-poly(vinyl) pyrrolidone (PVP)-Lithium triflate (LiTf) based polymeric blend films have been prepare by using solution casting technique. PVA average molecular weight~ 125,000 with purity >98%, PVP average molecular weight~ 44,000 with purity >99% are purchased from Merch, Germany. In this method we have taken 60PVA-40PVP i wt% ratio with x wt% LiTf (x=0, 10, 15, 25). All the materials were dissolved in distilled water in suitable wt% ratio and then kept this mixture in oven at 50^{0}C for 24 hours for swelling. Then the solution is stirred for 6 hours to obtain homogeneous slurry. The viscous slurry was poured into poly propylene Petri-dishes. These petri-dish containing slurry were kept in oven to dry at 45°C for 5 days, after that we got free standing films having uniform thickness of ~ 0.0526 cm.

3.   Results and Discussion

3.1   Electrical conductivity study

A Nyquist plot (Figure 1) was drawn between measured real part of impedance (Z') and imaginary part of impedance (Z") at different frequencies which gives a semicircular plot. From complex-impedance plot the bulk resistance (R_b) were estimated by the intersection of semicircle and long spike at real axis. The bulk conductivity (σ_{dc}) has been calculated using the relation; where R is the real part of impedance, is the thickness of sample and 'a' is the cross sectional area. In general, the electrical conductivity measurement is done by either pressed pellet membrane/film or single crystal sandwiched between two suitable electrodes. The usual geometry is: Electrode/sample/Electrode. The intercept on real axis gives the value of the bulk resistance and hence conductivity can be obtained using above relation. The electrical conductivity of polymer electrolytes is mainly due to the presence of ion species and their mobility.

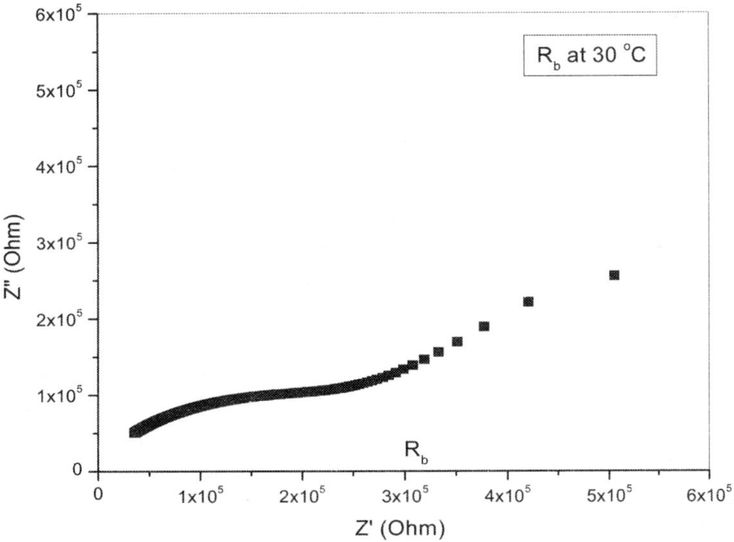

Fig. (1) Typical Nyquist plot of PVP-PVA-25wt % LiTf based polymeric blend.

3.2   FTIR analysis

Figure 2 (A-D) shows the FTIR spectra of PVA-PVP with x wt% LiTf (x=0, 10, 15, 25) based PBEs films. There is possibility to change in band frequencies of PVA (C-O stretching (842 cm^{-1}), O-H bending (1048 cm^{-1}), C-C stretching (1142 cm^{-1}), C=C stretching (1647 cm^{-1}), CH$_2$ assy. Stretching (2910 cm^{-1}) and O-H stretching (3455 cm^{-1})) [14], PVP (N-C=O bending (579 cm^{-1}), CH$_2$ bending (845 cm^{-1}), C-N stretching (1278 cm^{-1}), C=O stretching (1687 cm^{-1}), CH$_2$ assy. Stretching (2926 cm^{-1}), CH$_2$ ring sym. stretching (2958 cm^{-1})) [14] and CH$_2$ rock (777 cm^{-1}), C-O-O stretching (1064 cm^{-1}), CH$_2$ symmetric twist (1231 cm^{-1}) and C=O stretching (1639 cm^{-1}) of LiTf due to the complexation of salt with PVA-PVP polymer blend. The ATR-FTIR it has been found that thebdata of PVA-PVP polymer blend complexed with LiTf are N-C=O bending (572 cm^{-1}), CH$_2$ blending (845 cm^{-1}), C-H bending (1095 cm^{-1}), C-N stretching (1270 cm^{-1}), C=C stretching (1650 cm^{-1}), CH$_2$ assy. Stretch (2920 cm^{-1}), O-H stretch (3370 cm^{-1}) possible interactions between the polymers.

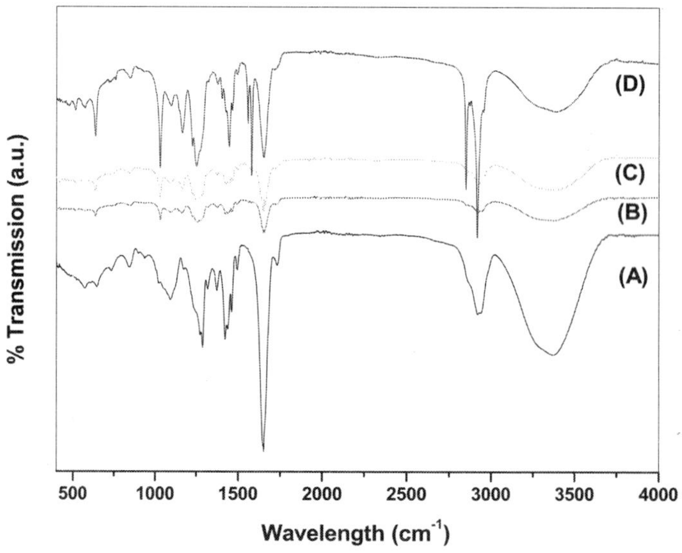

Fig. 2 (A-D) shows the FTIR spectra of PVA-PVP with x wt% LiTf (x=0, 10, 15, 25) based PBEs films.

3.3   Dielectric permittivity and electric modulus studies

The complex dielectric permittivity is defined as $\varepsilon^* = \varepsilon' - j\,\varepsilon''$, Where ε' is dielectric constant and ε'' is dielectric loss. Dielectric constant, ε' is associated with the storage of charge in electrolyte and ε'' is the measure of energy losses in movement of charge in the presence of electric field. The real and imaginary parts of dielectric permittivity i.e. ε' and ε'' are calculated as follows; $\frac{C\,l}{\varepsilon_o\,a}$ where C is the capacitance of sample, εo is the permittivity of free space, l is the thickness of the polymeric film and 'a' is the area of the blocking electrode. Frequency dependent ε' and ε'' at room temperatures are shown, respectively. From Figs. (3(A-B)) it has been observed that ε' and ε'' increase sharply in lower frequency range due to electrode polarization and decease towards higher frequency possibly due to fast periodic reversal of electric field . Therefore, polarization effect suppressed in high frequency region for PVP-PVA based polymer blend electrolyte film.

The electric modulus analysis reveals the effect of electrode polarization in polymeric systems and the conductivity relaxation can be analyzed from the complex electric modulus spectra. The electric modulus M* is defined as the reciprocal of complex relative permittivity. The electric modulus M* is defined as the reciprocal of complex relative permittivity, $M^* = \frac{1}{\varepsilon^*} = M' + j\,M'' = \frac{\varepsilon'}{(\varepsilon'^2+\varepsilon''^2)} + j\frac{\varepsilon''}{(\varepsilon'^2+\varepsilon''^2)}$ where M' is the real part and M'' is the imaginary part of the complex modulus M^*. The conductivity relaxation can be analyzed from the complex electric modulus spectra. From the electric modulus M' and M'' vs log f (Hz) spectra (Figs. 3(C) & (D)) it is clear that a long tail was observed at low frequencies due to the large capacitance associated with the electrodes. The behaviour suggests that the relaxation is thermally activated and charge carrier hopping is take place. In low frequency region, the value of M' and M'' approaches to zero indicating the electrode polarization in present polymer blend electrolyte system makes minimum contribution. At higher frequencies, M'' vs log f (Hz) spectra (Fig.3 (D)) shows peaks and the peak maximum shifted towards higher frequencies with increasing temperatures for polymer blend electrolyte system. This indicates that ionic conduction is predominated and thermally activated as observed in conductivity and loss tangent analysis.

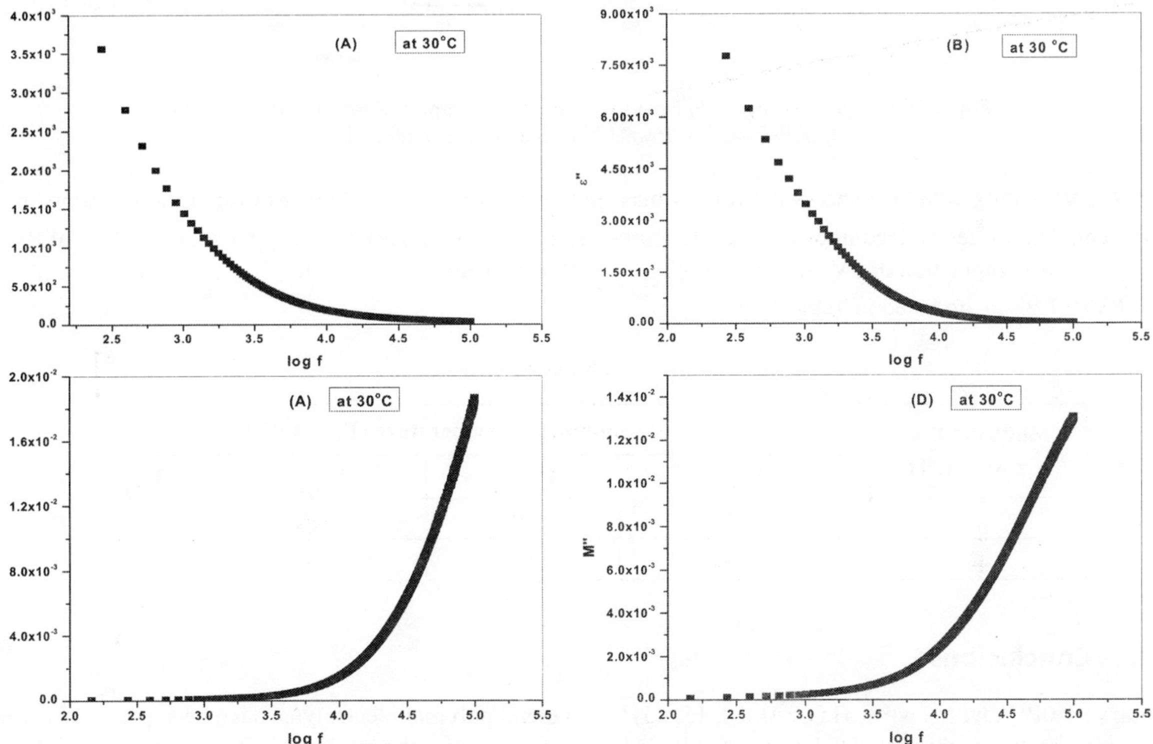

Figs. 3 (A-B) Log f vs. and ε', ε'' and (C-D) log f vs. M', M'' plots for PVP-PVA-25 wt%LiTf based polymer blend films, respectively.

3.4 TGA ANALYSIS

For thermal decomposition analysis of the prepared samples TGA was performed using *Mettler Toledo* TGA instrument (*TGA/DSC-1*) with scan rate 10K/min in the presence of nitrogen inert atmosphere (30 ml/min). 60PVP-40PVA with x wt% LiTf (x=0, 25) based blend polymer electrolytes have been prepared using solution casting technique. TGA supported by DTGA analysis gives the evidence of formation of 60 PVP-40PVA miscible blends with two step decomposition. TGA and 1st derivative of TGA curves for PVA-PVP-PEG with x wt% LiTf (x=0, 25) polymer blend electrolytes are shown in Fig. 4. The TGA (supported by 1st derivative of TGA) curves of

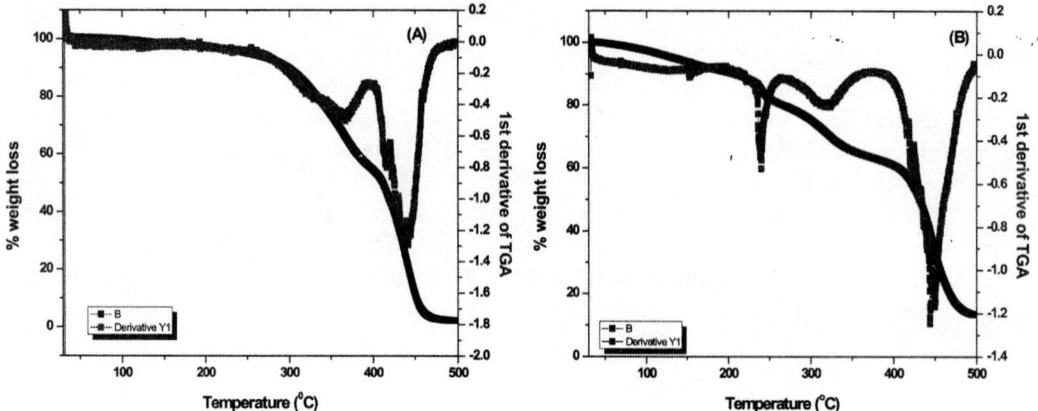

Fig. 4 TGA (supported by 1st derivative of TGA) thermo grams of (A) 60PVP-40PVA and (B) 60PVP-40PVA-25wt%LiTf based polymeric blend films.

PVA-PVP with x wt%LiTf shows the loss of mass between 30°C to 180°C due to evaporation of moisture/solvent. The values of decomposition temperatures i.e. onset decomposition ($T_{d, onset}$), decomposition of PVA ($T_{d1, peak}$), decomposition of PVA-PVP blend ($T_{d2, peak}$), decomposition of LiTf salt ($T_{d1, peak}$) and decomposition of PVP ($T_{d3, peak}$) are listed in Table 1.

Table 1

60PVP-40PVA x wt% LiTf	Decomposition temperature ($T_{d, peak}$) (°C)			
	$T_{d, onset}$	$T_{d1, peak}$	$T_{d2, peak}$	$T_{d3, peak}$
0	275	326	366	441
25	194	239	316	442

4. Conclusions

60PVP-40PVA with x wt%LiTf (x=0, 10, 15, 25) based blend polymer electrolytes have been prepared using solution casting technique. TGA supported by DTGA analysis gives the evidence of formation of PVP-PVA miscible blend with two step decomposition. ATR-FTIR results shows that the complexation/interaction with salt. The maximum conductivity at room temperature is found to be 4.22×10^{-7} S/cm for the composition of 60PVP-40PVA-25wt%LiTf.

5. References

1. Aihara Y, Kodama M, Nakahara K, Okise H, Marata K, Characteristics of a thin film lithium-ion battery using plasticized solid polymer electrolyte, J Power Sources 65, 143-147 (1997).

2. Armand M, The history of polymer electrolytes, Solid State Ionics 69, 309-319 (1994).

3. Angulakshmi N, Sabu Thomas KS, Nahm A, Manuel Stephan R, Nimma E Electrochemical and mechanical properties of nanochitin-incorporated PVDF-HFP-based polymer electrolytes for lithium batteries, Ionics 17, 407-414 (2011).

4.   Stephan M., A Review on gel polymer electrolytes for lithium batteries, Eur Polym J. 42, 21-42(2006).

5.   Mc Callum JR, Vincent C, A Polymer Electrolytes Reviews Elsevier, London (1987).

6.   Manuel Stephan A, Nahm KS, Review on composite polymer electrolytes for lithium batteries, Polymer 47, 5952-5964 (2006).

7.   S. Rajendra, M.R. Prabhu, M. Rani, Characterization of PVC/PEMA based polymer blend electrolytes, Int. J. Electrochem. Sci.,3 , 282–290 (2008).

8.   Singh P., Bharati D.C., Kumar H. and Saroj A. L., Ion transport mechanism and dielectric relaxation behavior of PVA-imidazolium ionic liquid-based polymer electrolytes, Phys. Scr., 94, 105801, (2019).

9.   Muchakayala R, Song S, Gao S, Wang X. and Fan Y., Structure and ion transport in an ethylene carbonate-modified biodegradable gel polymer electrolyte, Polymer Testing, 58, 116–125 (2017).

10.   Das S and Ghosh A., Ionic conductivity and dielectric permittivity of PEO-LiClO4 solid polymer electrolyte plasticized with propylene carbonate, AIP Advances, 5, 027125 (2015).

11.   MacCallum J R and Vincent C A (ed) Polymer Electrolyte Review-I (London: Elsevier) (1987).

12.   Singh P, Bharati D C, Gupta P N and Saroj A L, Vibrational, thermal and ion transport properties of PVA-PVP-PEGMeSO4Na based polymer blend electrolyte films, J. Non- Cryst. Solids, 494, 21–30 (2018).

Periodic Structure Containing Host Hyperbolic Material for Nano-Guiding, Sensing and Imaging Applications

Asish Kumar[1*], Pawan Singh, Sudesh K. Singh[2], Anil K. Yadav[1], and Khem B. Thapa[1*]

[1]Department of Physics, School of Physical and Decision Sciences, Babasaheb Bhimrao
Ambedkar Univeristy, Lucknow-226025, India
[3]Department of Physics, T.D.P.G. College, Jaunpur-222002, India.
* E-mail: khem.bhu@gmail.com

ABSTRACT

An anisotropy material having the permittivity tensor components with simultaneously different signs exhibits a unique optical phenomenon is called hyperbolic material (HM). Bulk plasmon polaritons and directional surface waves with the large wave vectors can localized in the HM as a host. This property is required in various applications in nano-guiding, sensing, and imaging. Another hand, the periodic structure of different materials is enhanced the optical property due to interference of the waves inside the structure. Hence, we have theoretically proposed to design the photonic device of symmetric structure of HM based on plasma photonic crystal which composed of traditional dielectric and plasma material. The optical properties like reflection, transmission and absorption spectra of the periodic structure with variation of variable parameters were investigated by using transfer matrix method (TMM).

Keywords: Nano-guiding, sensing, imaging, hyperbolic material, plasma material and TMM.

1. Introduction

Hyperbolic meta-materials, an anisotropic medium, which shows a hyperbolic shape of the dispersion relation in terahertz (THz), optical and near infrared frequency ranges of electromagnetic spectrum. Hyperbolic meta-materials have a variety potential applications including negative refraction, optical waveguide, and imaging hyper lens. The optical properties of hyperbolic meta-materials have been studied in the last several years due to abnormal behavior in the nanofabrication. A unique behavior of hyperbolic meta-materials at the far infrared frequency is composed of stacked graphene sheets separated by thin dielectric layers, which show that the graphene based hyperbolic meta-material can be worked as a super absorber for near fields. Hyperbolic meta-materials have clear potentials of enhancing the decay rate of emitters near its surface and also for designing efficient and innovative absorbers [1-6].

2. Theoretical Model and Methodology

We study a stacked of structure of hyperbolic meta-material photonic crystal by well known simple transfer matrix method (TMM) [7]. The wave angle of electromagnetic wave is Θ, A is hafnium dioxide and B is hyperbolic meta-material consisting of plasma and dielectric (air) material. For periodic structure formation, we use the effective medium theory to study the electromagnetic wave propagation in hyperbolic meta-material, which is an anisotropic medium with uniaxial dielectric tensor components and other all characteristics are follows [8].

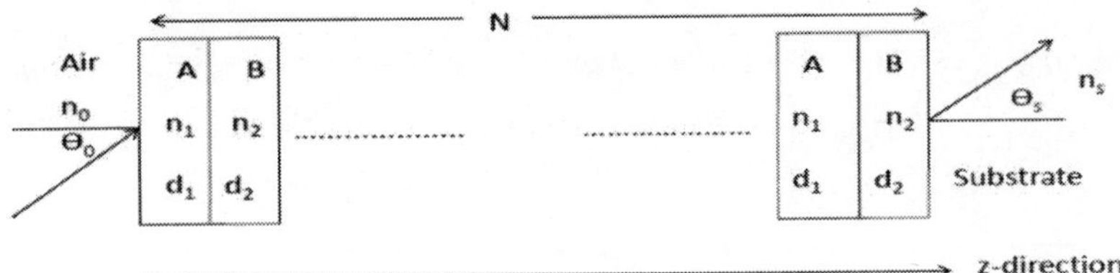

Fig. 1 One dimensional periodic structure of dielectric and hyperbolic material

The characteristic matrix for considered periodic structure-

$$M_i = \begin{bmatrix} \cos\gamma_i & -\dfrac{i}{p_i}\sin\gamma_i \\ -ip_i\sin\gamma_i & \cos\gamma_i \end{bmatrix}$$

Where $\gamma_i\left(\dfrac{}{}\right)n_i d_i \cos\theta_i$, c is the speed of light in vacuum, Θ_i is the ray angle inside layer i^{th} with a

refractive index as $\sqrt{\quad}$ $p_i = \sqrt{\dfrac{\varepsilon_i}{\mu_i}}\cos\theta_i$ and $\cos\theta_i = \sqrt{1-\dfrac{n_0^2\sin^2\theta_0}{n_i^2}}$ in which n_0 is the refractive index

of air where the incidence wave tends to enter the layer/material.

The reflection, transmission and absorption properties of the one-dimensional hyperbolic meta-material photonic crystal containing traditional dielectric and plasma are investigated.

The transfer matrix is given as-

$$M(d) = \begin{pmatrix} M_{1,1} & M_{1,2} \\ M_{2,1} & M_{2,2} \end{pmatrix}$$

$$M = (M_A M_B)^{10}$$

The reflection and transmission coefficient of the one-dimensional hyperbolic meta-material photonic crystal containing traditional dielectric and hyperbolic meta-material periodic structure calculated by-

$$t = \frac{2p_0}{\left(M_{11} + M_{12}/p_0 + M_{21}p_0 + M_{22}\right)}, t = \frac{\left(M_{11} + M_{12}/p_0 - M_{21}p_0 + M_{22}\right)}{\left(M_{11} + M_{12}/p_0 + M_{21}p_0 + M_{22}\right)}$$

The reflection, transmission and absorption spectra of the 1D photonic crystal containing dielectric and hyperbolic material is given by -

$$T = \left(\frac{p_s}{p_0}\right)|t|^2 \qquad R = |r|^2 \qquad A = 1 - R - T$$

3.   Results and Discussion

We have theoretically analyzed the reflection, transmission and absorption spectra of the 1D periodic structure containing Hafnium dioxide and hyperbolic material using simple matrix method [7]. Hyperbolic material is the composite material of dielectric and plasma material. We have taken the optical parameters of hafnium dioxide layer (A): $\varepsilon_A = 4.25$, $d_A = 1.4mm$, $\mu_A = 1$, $\Theta = 0^0$ and number of period (N=10). Now, we have taken the hyperbolic material layer (B), is the composite of the plasma and dielectric. The parameters of these materials are:

dielectric $\varepsilon_{die(air)} = 1$, $\mu_{die(air)} = 1$, $d_{die(air)} = 1.8mm$, $d_{HM} = 2.0mm f = \dfrac{d_{plasma}}{d_{HM}}$, $d_{plasma} = 0.2mm$, $\omega_p = 28.4GHz$, $\omega_p = 28.4$ GHz $\mu_{plasma} = 1$ respectively [8].

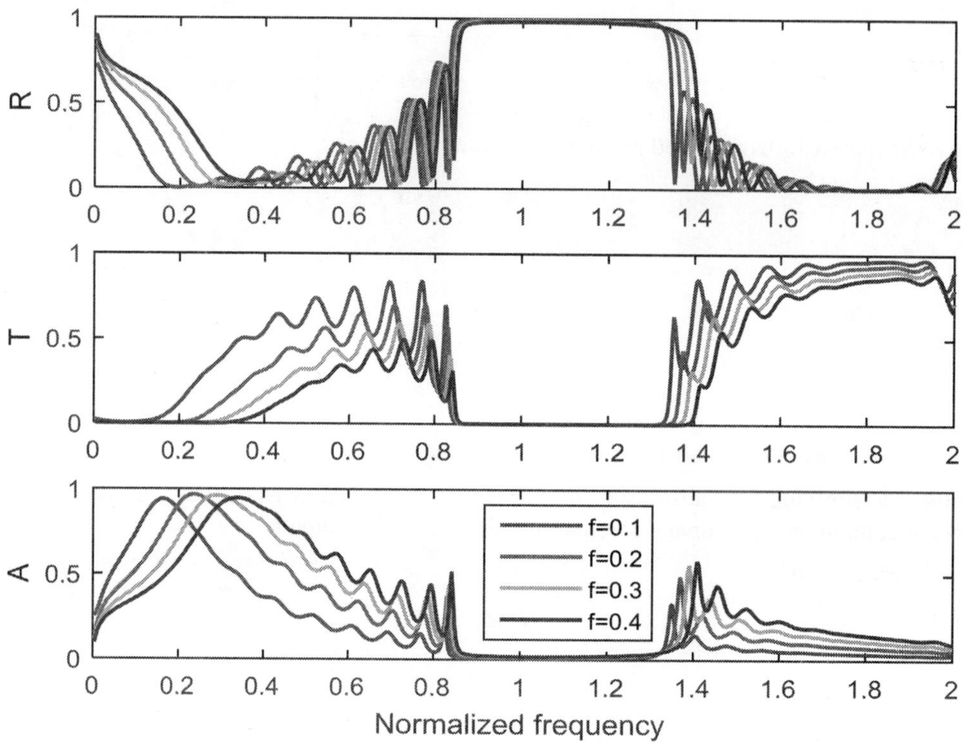

Figure 2 Shows the reflection and transmission spectra and absorption spectra against normalized frequency of one dimensional periodic structure with variation of filling fraction

The reflection, transmission and absorption spectra against normalized frequency has been analyzed of 1D periodic structure at a normal incident angle for transverse magnetic polarization with variation of filling fraction of hyperbolic material. Reflection spectra against normalized frequency with variation of filling fraction $f = 0.1, f = 0.2, f = 0.3,$ and $f = 0.4$ have been analyzed that at lower frequency range reflection will be less and higher frequency range forms a band gap at normalized frequency range (0.9-1.3). Transmission spectra against normalized frequency also varied corresponds to the variation of filling fraction $f = 0.1, f = 0.2, f = 0.3,$ and $f = 0.4$ at lower frequency (0.0-0.2) transmission nearly zero and at higher frequency transmission increases and forms a band gap in the previous range (0.9-1.3). Similarly, the absorption spectra against normalized frequency also analyzed with variation of filling fraction $f = 0.1, f = 0.2, f = 0.3,$ and $f = 0.4$ at lower frequency absorption becomes 90% which is very useful for optical applications and at higher normalized frequency forms an absorption band as shown in Fig.2. These calculated results proposed an innovative idea to design the tunable filter, optical window, optical logic gate, broadband reflector and absorption based devices.

4. Acknowledgement

Asish Kumar acknowledges to UGC, New Delhi for non-NET UGC fellowship and Dr Pankaj Singh, G.B. Pant University of Agriculture & Technology, Pantnagar (Uttarakhand) for his technical help to prepare the manuscript.

5. References

1. D. R. Smith and D. Schuring, Electromagnetic wave propagation in media with indefinite permittivity and permeability tensors, Phy. Rev. Lett. 90, 077405, (2003).

2. I. V. Iorsh, I. S Mukhin, I.V. Shadrivov, P.A. Belov, and Y.S. Kivshar, Hyperbolic metamaterial based on multilayer graphene structures, Phys. Rev. B 87, 075416 (2013)

3. M. A. K. Othman, C. Guclu, and F. Capolino, Graphene based tunable hyperbolic meta-materials and enhanced near-field absorption, Opt. Express 21, 7614 (2014).

4. L. Ferrari et.al. Hyperbolic meta-materials and their applications, Prog. Quant. Elect., 40, 01, (2015).

5. A. Kumar, K. B. Thapa and A. K. Yadav, Enhancement of absorption property of one-dimensional ternary periodic structure containing plasma based hyperbolic material for the application of microwave devices, J. Magn. Magn. Mater. 93, 165371 (2019).

6. A. Kumar, K. B. Thapa and G. N. Pandey, Tunable absorption property in hyperbolic meta-material, AIP Conference Proceeding, 2142, 050002 (2019).

7. P. Yeh, Optical Waves in Layered Media, John Wiley & Amp; Sons, New York, (1988).

8. Z. Jiao, R. Ning, Y. Xu, and J. Bao, Tunable angle absorption of hyperbolic meta-material based plasma photonic crystals, Phys. Plasma 23, 063301 (2016).

Effect of Structure Parameters on Optical Characteristics in One-dimensional Periodic Structure of GaAs and AlAs Materials

Sujata[1], Pawan Singh[1], Alok K. Gupta[2], Sudesh K. Singh[3], G. N. Pandey[4], and Khem B. Thapa[1,*]

[1]Department of Physics, School of Physical and Decision Sciences, Babasaheb Bhimrao
Ambedkar University, Lucknow-226025, India
[2]National Institute of Open Schooling, Regional Centre, Kochi-682036, India
[3]Department of Physics, T.D.P.G. College, Jaunpur- 222002, India
[4]Department of Physics, Amity University Uttar Pradesh, Noida-222002, India
*E-mail: khem.bhu@gmail.com

ABSTRACT

In this communication, we have studied the effect of structural parameters on transmission characteristics of one-dimensional periodic photonic(1DPC) of GaAs and AlAs materials. The optical properties of 1DPSof GaAs and AlAs multilayer system have been studied using transfer matrix method (TMM). The tunable characteristics of such GaAs and AlAs multilayer systemsstudied at different thickness ratios and various metal oxide thin film as defect layer in one-dimensional multilayer system. The proposed one-dimensional periodic structure can be used in solar cell device, integrated circuit and THz devices.

***Keywords:** GaAs, AlAs, transfer matrix method (TMM), one-dimensional periodic crystal (1DPC), solar Cell*

1.   Introduction

Photonic crystal is periodic dielectric structures, generally possessing photonic band gap regions (PBGs); a certain ranges of frequency in which light donot propagate inside the structure. This periodicity, which lengthscale is proportional to the wavelength of light in the band gaps, is the electromagnetic proportion of a crystalline atomic lattice, where the most recent acts on the electron wavefunction to produce the natural band gaps, semiconductors and so on, of solid state physics [1,2]. These structures are based on the interaction between optical field and material show periodicity on scale of wavelength of radiation, concede manipulating and direct the flow of light. One-dimensional periodiccrystal (1DPC) containsdifferent optical media with different dielectricpermittivity in one-dimension alternately. A lot of works has been done on 1DPC for different applications. 1DPC plays an important role in various device applications e.g. temperature sensorand material mixing sensor.

Semiconductor materials are very important in the study of technological devices and scientific applications such as rectifiers, optical filters, laser diodes and transistors. As they are technologically important, there is a huge studyon them and their combinations in the form of alloys. Gallium arsenide (GaAs) is III-V compound semiconductor is appropriate for optoelectronic devices. GaAs is considered asa prospective competitor silicon because of its wider band gap and higher electron mobility.GaAs is a direct band gap material and also used in switching, ultra high radio frequency applications detection of X-rays. Aluminum arsenide (AlAs) is an III-V compound semiconductor material which is used in the fabricated of photo electronic devices, such as high emitting diodes. This is same to lattice constant as aluminum and gallium arsenide and band gap is larger than gallium arsenide. AlAs and GaAs have almost the same lattice constant.

In this paper, we study the transmission, absorption and reflectance of one-dimensional periodic structure containing GaAs and AlAs semiconductor materialsare investigated.

2.   Theory and Methodology

To analyze the electromagnetic wave propagation inside 1DPC of GaAs and AlAs materials,as shown in Fig. 1, with thickness is d_1 and d_2 [3].By using the optics film theory, the light transmission characteristics in each layer of the medium can be expressed as 2x2 characteristic matrices.

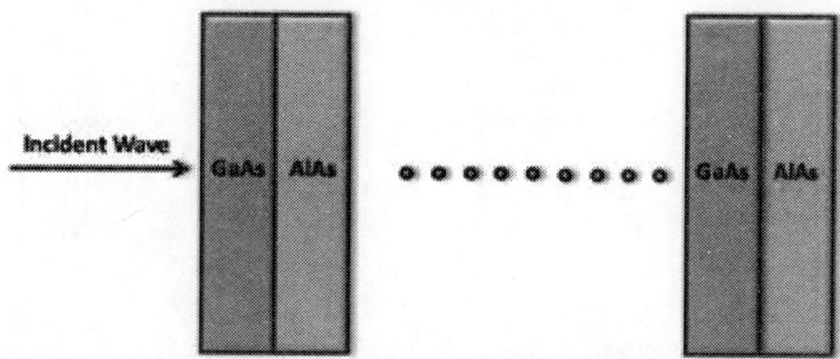

Fig. 1 One-dimensional periodic structure of GaAs and AlAs materials.

Where is the ray angle inside the layer and i=1, 2 for semiconductor layers and is the wavelength of incidence light in the air, is the refractive index of one medium layer in one-dimensional photonic crystal [3], the refractive index in the air = 1. Two medium layers from a basic cycle unit. The characteristic matrix can be written as [4];

$$M_i = \begin{pmatrix} cosk_{iz}d_i & -\dfrac{j}{p_i}sink_{iz}d_i \\ -jp_i sink_{iz}d_i & cosk_{iz}d_i \end{pmatrix}$$

where i=GaAs and AlAs,$p_i = \dfrac{k_{iz}}{\omega\mu_0}$ $for\ TE$ and $p_i = \dfrac{\omega\varepsilon_0\varepsilon_i}{k_{iz}}$ $for\ TM.$

Therefore, we can write the transfer matrix for N periods and is given as;

$$M = (M_G M_D)^N = \begin{pmatrix} m_{11} & m_{12} \\ m_{21} & m_{22} \end{pmatrix}$$

where r and t are the reflectance and transmittance coefficients which are given by;

$$\begin{cases} r = \dfrac{(m_{11} + m_{12}p_{N+1})p_0 - m_{21} - m_{22}p_{N+1}}{(m_{11} + m_{12}p_{N+1})p_0 + m_{21} + m_{22}p_{N+1}} \\ t = \dfrac{2p_0}{(m_{11} + m_{12}p_{N+1})p_0 + m_{21} + m_{22}p_{N+1}} \end{cases}$$

Where, for TE - polarization $p_o = n_o cos\theta_o$ and $p_{N+1} = n_{N+1} cos\theta_{N+1}$.Thus, total transmission (T) nd reflection (R) are represented to the transmission and re-flectance of the periodic structure respectively which can be expressed as;

$$R = |r|^2$$

$$T = \begin{cases} |t|^2 & For\ TE \\ \dfrac{p_0}{p_{N+1}}|t|^2 & For\ TM \end{cases}$$

Then, the total absorption can be calculated by;

$$A = 1 - T - R$$

3. **Results and Discussion**

In this portion, we study the optical properties of periodic structure composed of GaAs and AlAs at different thickness ratios because the thickness of the layers change the optical properties due to interference at the interface of the layers in 1DPS.

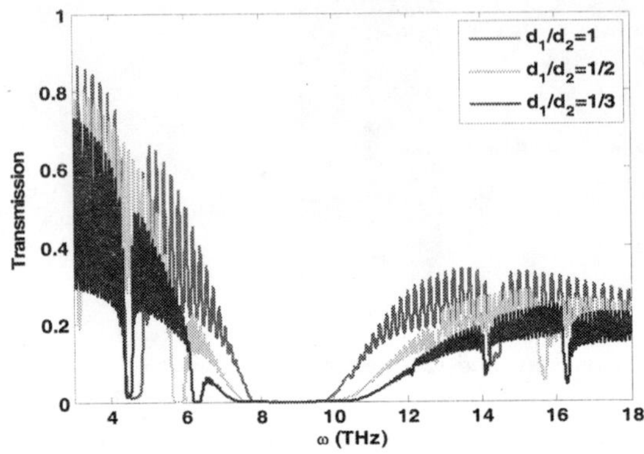

Fig. 2 Transmission of 1DPC of GaAs and AlAs at different thickness ratios

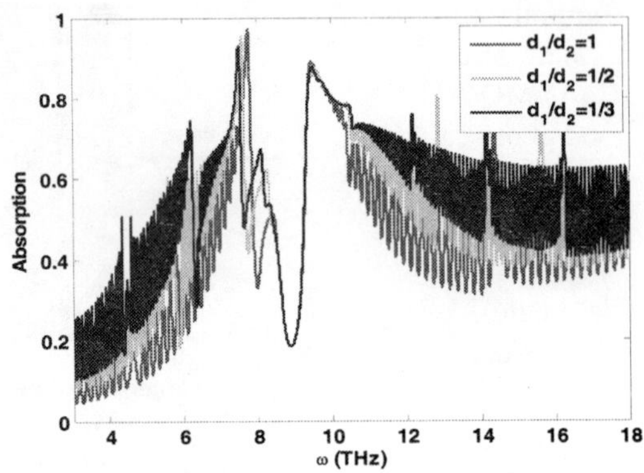

Fig. 3 Absorption of 1DPC of GaAs and AlAs at different thickness ratios

We have taken the ratio of thickness d_1/d_2 which are 1, ½ and 1/3 where d_1 and d_2 are the thicknesses of the GaAs and AlAs respectively. Using transfer matrix method methods (TMM), we have calculated transmission and absorption for these thicknesses. Figs. 2 and 3 show the transmittance and absorption of the considered structure with different thicknesses ratios. The study shows that periodic structure of the GaAs and AlAs has a band gap between 7.80-10THz with width of 2 THz. This band gap shows omni-directional behavior for the thickness ratio of the 1, ½ and 1/3.

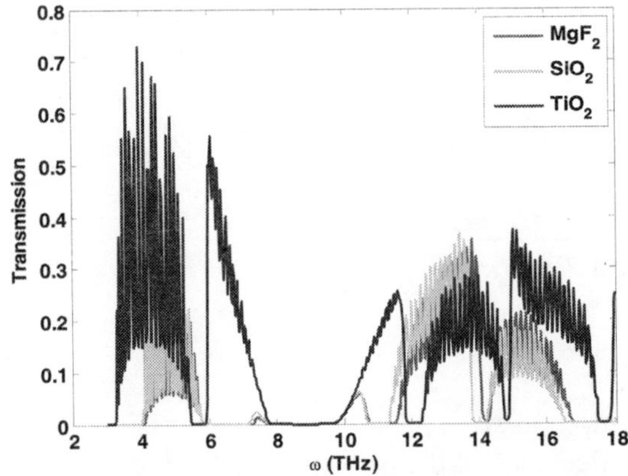

Fig. 4 Transmission of 1DPC of GaAs and AlAs at different defect layers

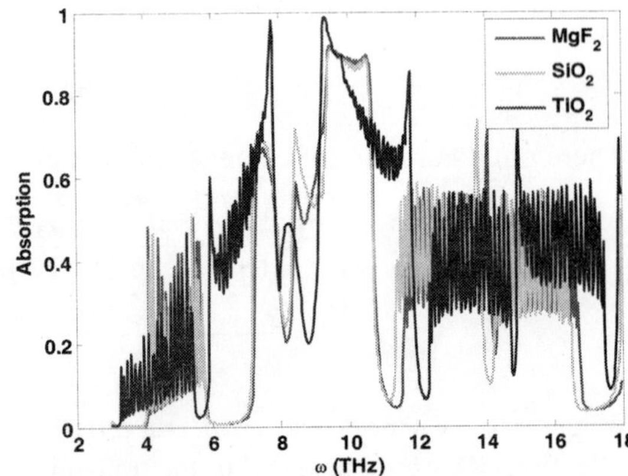

Fig. 5 Absorption of 1DPC of GaAs and AlAs at different defect layers

Now, we have consider the ternary periodic structure by inserting the new materials like MgF_2, SiO_2 and TiO_2 between GaAs and AlAs materials in 1DPS. The transmittance, reflectance and absorption of the ternary structure periodicaly in the $(GaAs/MO/AlAs)^N$, where MO is the MgF_2, SiO_2 and TiO_2 materials and N is the number of the periodic layer. The transmittance and absorption of the structure is shown in the Figs. 4 and 5 which shows a huge band gap in the same region. The ternary structure TiO_2 has largest band gap in the same frequency range.

4.   Conclusion

From our study, we conclude that thickness ratio of GaAs and AlAs layer (d_1/d_2) is 1, ½ and 1/3 for binary periodic structure gets maximum absorption for $d_1/d_2=1$ with common PBG band. The ternary structure $(GaAs/MO/AlAs)^N$ with MO= MgF_2, SiO_2 and TiO_2 gives maximum absorption for TiO_2 because TiO_2 is a good photo catalytic material.

5.   Acknowledgement

We would like to thank Dr. Pankaj Singh, G.B. pant University of Agriculture & Technology, Pantnagar (Uttarakhand) for his technical help to prepare the manuscript.

6.   References

1.   Joannopoulous, J. D., Johnson, S. G., Winn, J. N. and Meade, R. D.:Photonic Crystals Molding the Flow of Light. 2ndedn. Princeton University, Princeton and Oxford, 2008.

2.   Kumar R., Kushwaha, A. S.,Srivastava,S.K., One-dimensional nano layered SiC/TiO2 based photonic band gap materials as temperature sensor. Optik 126, 1324-1330 (2015).

3.   Wang, C. D. and Xiao, L. P., Effect of structure parameters on transmission characteristics in one-dimensional photonic crystals.Indian Journal of Pure & Applied Physics 49, 323-327 (2011).

4.   Suthar, B., Kumar, V., Kumar, A., Singh, Kh. S., Bhargava A., Thermal Expansion of Photonic Band Gap for One Dimensional Photonic Crystal. Progress In Electromagnetics Research Letters 32, 81-90 (2012).

Tunable Transmission Characteristics of One-Dimensional Periodic Structure of Dielectrics and Hyperbolic Metamaterials

Smriti Singh[1], Pawan Singh[1], Alok K. Gupta[2], Sudesh K. Singh[3], Anil K. Yadav[1], and Khem B. Thapa[1,*]

[1]Department of Physics, School of Physical and Decision Sciences,
Babasaheb Bhimrao Ambedkar University, Lucknow-226025, India
[2]National Institute of Open Schooling, Regional Centre, Kochi-682036, India
[3]Department of Physics, T.D.P.G. College, Jaunpur-222002, India
*E-mail: khem.bhu@gmail.com

ABSTRACT

In this paper, we study the formulation of the HM with negative index material (NIM) and plasma using effective medium theory. The optical properties of one-dimensional periodic structure of hyperbolic metamaterial have been studied using 4x4 transfer matrix method (TMM). The optical characteristics of such periodic structure are investigated at different filling fraction and different attenuation coefficient. The considered periodic structure can be used in THz devices applications.

Keywords: One-dimensional periodic structure (1DPS), hyperbolic metamaterial, negative index material (NIM), 4×4 TMM.

1. Introduction

Metamaterials are the artificially composite materials which shows excellent characteristics which are not found in nature. Left handed materials (LHM) are a subsection of metamaterials with an antiparallel relation between pointing vector and wave propagation vector leading to negative refraction [1]. LHM assemblies unusually show the negative refraction of electromagnetic wave on interaction with them. A subsection of LHM called as negative index materials (NIM) with negative values of the refractive index shows negative refraction. A subsection of NIM, double negative materials (DNM) with real parts of the permittivity and permeability are both having negative values which are sufficient but not necessary circumstances for NIMs [2]. Hyperbolic meta-materials are enormously anisotropic uniaxial materials, which show metallic behavior in one way and dielectric behavior in the orthogonal way [3-5].

In this paper, we have investigated the optical properties of hyperbolic metamaterial (HM) by 4x4 transfer matrix method (TMM) [6] due to their potential application in applied optics like nano-imaging and sub-surface imaging. We have studied transmittance (T), reflectance (R) and absorption (A) properties of periodic structure containing hyperbolic metamaterials for novel device application.

2. Theory and Methodology

To design one-dimensional multilayer structure, we have used effective medium theory to study the transmission of electromagnetic wave in hyperbolic meta-material (un iaxial anisotropic media) with dielectric tensor with diagonal elements as:

$$\varepsilon = \begin{pmatrix} \varepsilon_x & 0 & 0 \\ 0 & \varepsilon_y & 0 \\ 0 & 0 & \varepsilon_z \end{pmatrix}, \mu = \begin{pmatrix} 1 & 0 & 0 \\ 0 & 1 & 0 \\ 0 & 0 & 1 \end{pmatrix}$$

Where, $\varepsilon_x=\varepsilon_\parallel$, $\varepsilon_y=\varepsilon_z=\varepsilon_\perp$, $\varepsilon_\parallel$ and $\varepsilon_\perp$ are the perpendicular and parallel constituents of relative permittivity respectively, which can be written as follow:

$$\varepsilon_\perp = \frac{\varepsilon_p d_p + \varepsilon_m d_m}{\varepsilon_m d_p + \varepsilon_p d_m}, \ \varepsilon_\parallel = \frac{\varepsilon_p \varepsilon_m (d_p + d_m)}{\varepsilon_m d_p + \varepsilon_p d_m}$$

$$\mu_\perp = 1 \mu_\parallel = 1$$

With $d_{HM} = d_p + d_m$, f=d_p/d_m,$\varepsilon_\perp =(\varepsilon_p \varepsilon_m/ (\varepsilon_p f + \varepsilon_m (1\text{-}f))$, and$\varepsilon_\parallel = (\varepsilon_p f + \varepsilon_m (1\text{-f }))$, where ε_m and d_m, ε_p and d_p are the dielectric permittivity and thickness of GaP and plasma, respectively. For $\varepsilon_{xx}\varepsilon_{zz} < 0$, the dispersion relation have hyperbolic nature, and for $\varepsilon_{xx}\varepsilon_{zz} > 0$, it has elliptic nature [7]. For arbitrary values of oblique incidence of electromagnetic wave, the tangential constituents of electric and magnetic field of dielectric layer can be study using transfer matrix method (TMM). The propagation and dynamical matrices for the nth layers can be written as;

$$P_n = \begin{pmatrix} e^{-k_{z1}^n d_n} & 0 & 0 & 0 \\ 0 & e^{-k_{z2}^n d_n} & 0 & 0 \\ 0 & 0 & e^{-k_{z1}^n d_n} & 0 \\ 0 & 0 & 0 & e^{-k_{z1}^n d_n} \end{pmatrix}, D_n = \begin{pmatrix} \hat{e}_1^n.\hat{y} & \hat{e}_2^n.\hat{y} & \hat{e}_3^n.\hat{y} & \hat{e}_4^n.\hat{y} \\ \hat{h}_1^n.\hat{x} & \hat{h}_2^n.\hat{x} & \hat{h}_3^n.\hat{x} & \hat{h}_4^n.\hat{x} \\ \hat{h}_1^n.\hat{y} & \hat{h}_2^n.\hat{y} & \hat{h}_3^n.\hat{y} & \hat{h}_4^n.\hat{y} \\ \hat{e}_1^n.\hat{x} & \hat{e}_2^n.\hat{x} & \hat{e}_3^n.\hat{x} & \hat{e}_4^n.\hat{x} \end{pmatrix}$$

$$\text{Where, } Q = \begin{pmatrix} Q_{11} & Q_{12} & Q_{13} & Q_{14} \\ Q_{21} & Q_{22} & Q_{23} & Q_{24} \\ Q_{31} & Q_{32} & Q_{23} & Q_{34} \\ Q_{41} & Q_{42} & Q_{43} & Q_{44} \end{pmatrix} = M_{N+1,N} P_N M_{N,N-1} P_{N-1} \ldots\ldots M_{2,1} P_1 M_{1,0} P_0$$

The reflection and transmission coefficient can be calculated as:

$$r_{SS} = \frac{Q_{24}Q_{41} - Q_{21}Q_{44}}{Q_{22}Q_{44} - Q_{24}Q_{42}}, r_{SP} = \frac{Q_{21}Q_{42} - Q_{22}Q_{41}}{Q_{22}Q_{44} - Q_{24}Q_{42}}$$

$$t_{SS} = \frac{Q_{12}(Q_{24}Q_{41} - Q_{21}Q_{44}) + Q_{14}(Q_{21}Q_{42} - Q_{22}Q_{41})}{Q_{22}Q_{44} - Q_{24}Q_{42}}, t_{SP} = \frac{Q_{32}(Q_{24}Q_{41} - Q_{21}Q_{44}) + Q_{34}(Q_{21}Q_{42} - Q_{22}Q_{41})}{Q_{22}Q_{44} - Q_{24}Q_{42}}$$

Here,r_{SS}, r_{SP} are the reflection coefficients andt_{SS}, t_{SP} are transmission coefficients. The total absorption of periodic structure can be calculated as;

A=1-R-T

3.   Results and Discussion

In this part, we discuss the transmission characteristics of 1DPS of dielectric 1 (D1), dielectric 2 (D2) and NIM/Plasma (H) in which absorption coefficient (γ) is absent/present.

3.1 Without absorption i.e., γ = 0:

For this case, electrical permittivity components of the NIM are;

$$\varepsilon_M = 1 + \frac{70}{12.71^2 - f^2}, \varepsilon_p = 1 + \frac{22}{6.80^2 - f^2},$$

These parameters are applied to calculate the optical constant of the HM for both modes using the effective medium theory. The electric permittivity for perpendicular and parallel of the HM are studied graphically to exist the HM property with varying filling fraction [7].

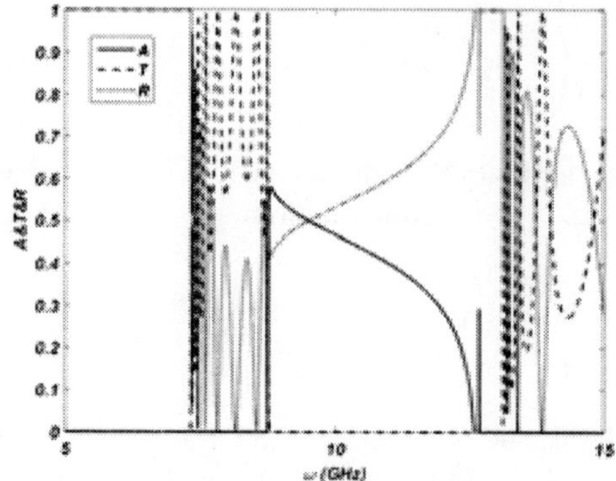

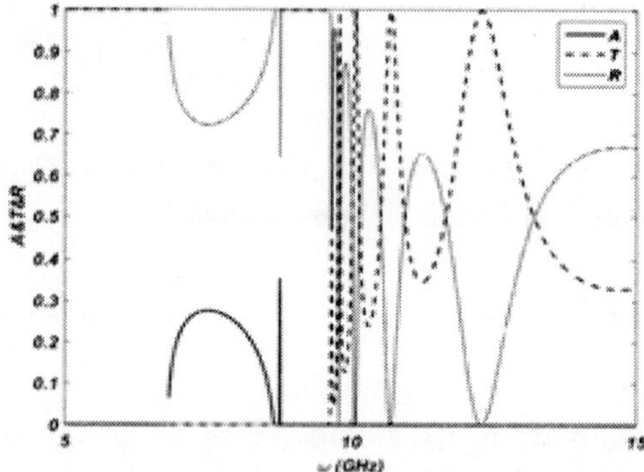

Fig. 1 Absorption (A), reflectance(R) and transmittance (T) of HM (DDH)^{10}vs. frequency for f = 0.1 with γ = 0

Fig. 2 Absorption (A), reflectance (R) and transmittance (T) of HM (DDH)^{10} vs. frequency for f=0.8 with γ = 0

The periodic structure of the HM and dielectric is represented by $(DDH)^{10}$ where D is dielectric material and H is hyperbolic material and composition parameters for these materials are: $\varepsilon_A = 43$, $d_A = 1.3$mm, $\varepsilon_B = 2.2$, $d_B = 3$ mm, $\mu_A = \mu_B = \mu_C = 1$, N=10, respectively. The absorption, transmittance and reflectance of $(DDH)^{10}$ are calculated by transfer matrix method (TMM). The absorption, transmittance and reflectance of $(DDH)^{10}$ are represented as Figs. 1 and 2 for f = 0.1 and f = 0.8, respectively. The optical property reveals that the HM periodic structure shows the absorption in a certain region without loss of the materials due to hyperbolic nature of the HM.

3.2   With absorption γ ≠ 0

To study of reflection (R), transmission (T) and absorption (A) of the HM for plamsa, we have chosen the composition parameters for these: $\varepsilon_A = 43$, $d_A = 1.3$mm, $\varepsilon_B = 2.2$, $d_B = 3$ mm, $\mu_A = \mu_B = \mu_C = 1$, N = 10, respectively. The plasma parameter for $\omega_p = 28.4$ GHz, $\gamma = 0.1\omega_p$.

The absorption (A), reflectance (R) and transmittance (T) of 1DPS containing HM for plasma are shown in the Figs 3 and 4. The optical properties periodic structure of $(DDH)^{10}$ are studied by calculating the reflectance, transmittance and absorption. The HM has already considered loss property. So the optical of the structure with HM has obtained the highly absorption inside the structure due to HM.

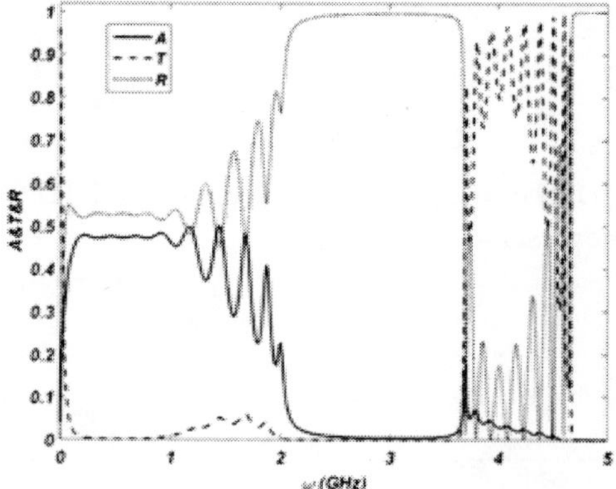

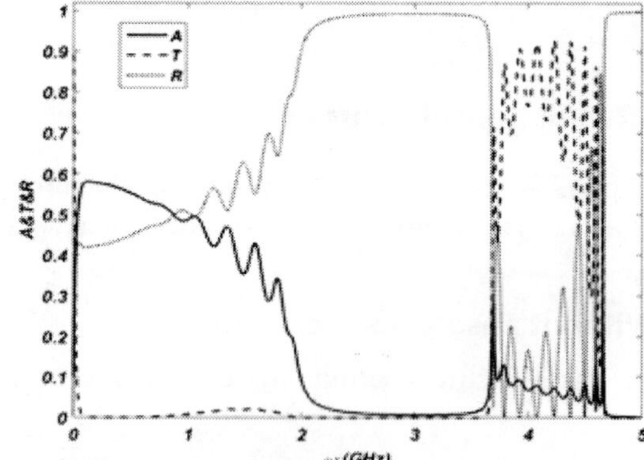

Fig. 3 Absorption (A), reflectance (R) and transmittance (T) of HM vs.frequency for f=0.8

Fig. 4 Absorption (A), reflectance (R) and transmittance (T) of HM vs.frequency for f=0.1

4.   Conclusion

Using effective medium theory, the HM is formulated by taking dielectric and NIM/Plasma material with considering the lossless and loss coefficient in the electric permittivity. The absorption, transmittance, reflectance of the HM structure studied for two conditions (i) without loss and (ii) with loss. The absorption of the considered structure shows the absorption property due to hyperbolic material.

5.   Acknowledgement

We would like to thank Dr Pankaj Singh, G.B. pant University of Agriculture & Technology, Pantnagar (Uttarakhand) for his technical help to prepare the manuscript

6.   References

1.   Shridhar, E. M., and Yogeshwar, P. K.: Metamaterial properties and applications, Int. J. Infor. Techn. and Knowledge Management, 0485-89 (2011).

2.   Eletheriades, G.V. and Balmain, K. G.: Negative refraction Metamaterials: Fundamental Principles and Applications. John Willey and Sons, USA, 2005.

3.   Ferrari, L., Wu, C., Lepage, D., Zhang, X., Liu, Z., Hyperbolic meta-materials and their applications. Prog. Quant. Elect. 40 01-40 (2015).

4.   Shekhar, P., Atkinson, J., and Jacob, Z., Hyperbolic metamaterials: fundamentals and applications. Nano Convergence 01, 2-17 (2014).

5.   Smolyaninov, I. I., Hyperbolic Metamaterials. Istedn. Morgan & Claypool Publishers, USA, (2018).

6.   Hau, J., and Zhou, L., Electromagnetic wave scatterings by anisotropic meta-materials: Generalised by 4x4 transfer matrix. Phys. Rev. B 77, 094201-12 (2008).

7.   Jiao, Z., Ning, R., Xu, Y., and Bao, J., Tunable angle absorption of hyperbolic metamaterials based on plasma photonic crystals. Phys. Plasma 23, 063301-6 (2016).

Specialized Simulation of Plan Drawings for Residential Sewage Purging Biogas Digesters

Siddharth and V.K. Pandey

Department of Environmental Science, VBS Purvanchal University, Jaunpur-222003, India

ABSTRACT

Through overviews, some delegate structures of residential sewage filtration biogas digesters have been gathered in India. In this paper, the specialized investigation of the attributes of five normal biogas plants is done so as to give a premise to the ideal structure of this innovation. The biogas tanks of India have basic specialized attributes, that is, the treatment methods of auxiliary anaerobic assimilation in addition to post-treatment (oxygen channel) are received, and however, there are contrasts in the unit plan. Contrasted and before structures, the ongoing plan utilizes progressively intersecting water gulfs and will, in general, rearrange the handling unit. In the cur-rent piece of the gadget structure, the parameters are discretionarily chosen, and the utilization of the filler is hazardous, which influences the impact of the gadget on residential sewage treatment.

Keywords: *Bio gas, decontamination, design process of recreation.*

1.   Introduction

Since the 1980s, as a supporting office for private and open toilets in little and medium-sized urban communities, the local sewage filtration biogas digesters have first created in dependent on the innovation of rustic biogas digesters and conventional septic tanks. This basic sewage treatment innovation for its speculation expansion, doesn't expend vitality, low working expenses, and land protection, and so forth steadily formed into a noteworthy specialized China Southern scattered sewage treatment, has been generally utilized before the finish of 2004, China's household sewage refinement biogas digesters have arrived at 137,013, with a complete pool limit of 5.74 million m3.

As of late, the anaerobic assimilation and scattering treatment innovation of residential sewage has grown quickly on the planet, and India and different nations call it DEWATS innovation.

2.   Representative Design Legend and its Main Parameters

2.1   General Standard Atlas of Domestic Sewage Purification Biogas Digesters (90SS-1)

The General Standard Atlas of Domestic Sewage Purification Biogas Digesters (90SS-1) together arranged by four units including the Sichuan Rural Energy Office in 1991 is China. The soonest set of structure drawings of local sewage decontamination biogas digesters, including strip, rectangular and cycle three arrangement of 10 details. Among them, 8 sorts of pools embrace the split sort water bay procedure, and 2 sorts of littler size pools are the joined stream type water gulf process. Figure 1 demonstrates a strip type A100 cleansing biogas tank with an all-out compelling volume of 100 m^3. It is a passage type partition tank and embraces a split stream process. The pretreatment zone incorporates a precipitation zone and an anaerobic processing zone. The anaerobic assimilation zone is separated into two units, anaerobic zone I and zone II, and delicate filler is given in the anaerobic zone II.

2.2   Processing unit partition and main parameters

The current domestic sewage purification biogas digesters are mainly composed of several processing units, namely: grit well, sedimentation zone, anaerobic zone I, anaerobic zone II, and post-treatment zone. The sedimentation tank mainly intercepts and precipitates refractory organic domestic waste, large solid particles, etc.; anaerobic zone I is mainly anaerobic digestion of organic matter; anaerobic zone II generally has soft filler as microbial carrier, cutting more The sludge further degrades the organic matter; the post-treatment zone is generally provided with a filler and a filter material to exert a facultative filtering effect, which is beneficial to reducing the SS concentration in the effluent and purifying the water quality. The author analyzed and summarized the selected five representative pools, and calculated the proportion of processing units. The results are shown in Table 1.

Table 1. Five Digester typical design atlas main parameters

No.	Hydraulic Retention time/h	Processing Step	Effective Volume /m³	Grit chamber	Volume occupied by the processing unit/%			
					Precipitation Area	Anaerobic Area 1	Anaerobic Area 2	Post processing Area
1	72	Diversion	100	No	10.2	33.5	31.7	24.6
2	72	confluence	50	Yes		40.0	26.6	33.4
3	48-72	confluence	17	Yes		35.0	35.0	30.0
4	96	confluence	90	Yes		66.7	27.1	6.20
5	96	confluence	60	No	12.5	18.8	56.2	12.5

2.3   Processing unit partition and main parameters

In the mid-1980s, the residential sewage sanitization biogas digesters were called biogas septic tanks, which advanced from customary septic tanks. The gadget comprises of two sections: a pre-treatment zone and a post-treatment zone. The pretreatment zone comprises of a coarseness chamber and a two-arrange anaerobic assimilation tank. The post-treatment zone comprises of a multi-organize anaerobic channel tank. This essential structure has been reached out right up 'til the present time. As indicated by various water delta modes, the pool kind of the sanitized biogas pool is typically partitioned into two sorts of procedures: conjunction type and preoccupation type. Juncture type implies that fecal sewage and other household sewage stream into the pool through a similar delta pipe. The split sort, that is, the fecal sewage and other household sewage is released independently and stream into the cleaned biogas tank through two separate channels.

The present residential sewage cleansing biogas digesters are predominantly made out of a few preparing units, to be specific: coarseness well, sedimentation zone, anaerobic zone I, anaerobic zone II, and post-treatment zone. The sedimentation tank fundamentally captures and encourages headstrong natural residential waste, huge strong particles, and so forth.; anaerobic zone I is predominantly anaerobic processing of natural issue; anaerobic zone II, by and large, has delicate filler as microbial bearer, cutting more The ooze further debases the natural issue; the post-treatment zone is for the most part given a filler and a channel material to apply a facultative separating impact, which is helpful to diminishing the SS fixation in the gushing and cleansing the water quality. The creator dissected and abridged chose five delegate pools, and determined the extent of handling units. The outcomes are appeared in Table 1.

Figure shows a circular arched series cell, which is a representative pool type. The anaerobic I zone is provided with a concentric return wall and a baffle wall. The sewage flows directly into the concentric small pool, and flows in an "S" shape under the action of the folding wall in the small pool, flowing from the other end of the small pool into the concentric.

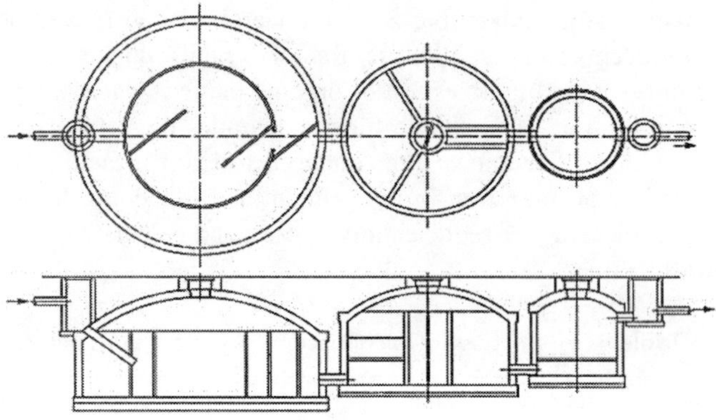

Figure 1 Sketch of sewage purification biogas digesters

Figure 1 is a passage type partition tank. The whole treatment framework is in an anaerobic state, and the anaerobic zone of the delicate filler is involved by a huge extent. The post-treatment zone is just a water outlet given a channel plate. The anaerobic I-arrange feed pipe is 45° descending, and the release pipe is set at 45° upward. The feed fluid can affect the base residue muck, and the ooze isn't anything but difficult to store and is very much blended. Simultaneously, a square gap is opened at the base of the release chamber to encourage the cleaning of the silt.

2.4   Effluent discharge compliance problem

In the advancement and application, it is constantly disputable whether the household sewage cleansing biogas digesters can meet the release prerequisites as indicated by the structure necessities. The finishes of different research and test reports are likewise unique. There are numerous components influencing the consistence of such residential sewage treatment gadgets, which are identified with variables, for example, structure, development, the executives and administration life.

3.   Conclusion

1.   The five local sewage cleaning biogas digesters chose to have the regular specialized qualities of such sewage treatment gadgets, that is, the treatment methods of auxiliary anaerobic absorption in addition to post-treatment (oxygen channel) are embraced, however, the treatment units are individual there are contrasts in structure. Contrasted and the early structure, the ongoing plan of the current undertaking has progressively blended water admission techniques and will, in general, improve the handling unit. Contrasted and the split sort water delta mode, the consolidated stream type speculation is progressively practical, however, it might influence the general sewage treatment impact.

2.   There are still a few issues with current gadgets and advancements. In the current piece of the gadget plan, the parameter choice is discretionarily enormous, and the level of institutionalization of the building configuration isn't high. It is earnest to complete plan advancement work and focused on exploratory research.

3.   It is one of the key specialized intends to put different fillers in the anaerobic zone II and the anaerobic channel tank to hold the dynamic microbial ooze. Existing fillers have numerous issues, which influence

the sewage treatment impact of the gadget. Subsequently, filler improvement ought to be the focal point of future advancement.

At present, the quantity of household sewage cleansing biogas digesters has arrived at an extensive scale.

After over 20 years of advancement, innovation is developing, and both the hypothesis and the training have amassed a lot of involvement and accomplishments. Through convenient summarizing background and fortifying specialized advancement and institutionalization work, the advancement and utilization of this innovation will be additionally advanced.

4.   References

1.   S. Prasad, D. Rathore, A. Singh,. Recent Advances in Biogas Production, 25 July 2017, ISSN: 2333-6633

2.   Ryckebosch E, Vervaeren H, Drouillon M. Techniques for transformation of biogas to biomethane. Biomass and Bioenergy , 2011, 35(5): 1633-1645.

3.   Ofoefule, Akuzuo U., Nwankwo, Joseph I., Ibeto, Cynthia N. Biogas Production from Paper Waste and its blend with Cow dung. Advances in Applied Science Research, 2010, ISSN: 0976-8610.

4.   Tamil Nadu Tsunami Resource Centre. Technical Orientation Training Workshop on DEWATS For implementing TWAD Engineers, 2007-5-9.

Anti-inflammatory and Antinociceptive Activity of Moringa Oleifera

Vinay Kumar Verma, Vijay Bahadur Maurya, Rajeev Kumar

Institute of Pharmacy, V. B. S. Purvanchal University, Jaunpur-222003, India

ABSTRACT

Moringa oleifera is commonly known as drumstick. It is found widely in the sub Himalayan range and commonly cultivated in all places of India. The powdered plant materials (1000g) was macerated with petroleum ether to remove fatty substances and the marc was further exhaustively extracted with 50% ethanol. The extracts obtained was further subjected to toxicological and pharmacological investigations. The antiinflammatory and antinociceptive activity of the 50% ethanolic extract of the Moringa oleifera leaf in animals is studied. The results obtained in the present study illustrate that correlations exist between the popular ancestral perception and genuine anti-inflammatory and antinociceptive activities of the whole plant of Moringa oleifera.

Key Words: *Moringa oleifera*, anti-inflammatory, antinociceptive

1. Introduction

There are about thirteen species of Moringa trees in the family Moringaceae. Moringa oleifera Lam. (synonym: Moringa pterygosperma Gaertn.) is the most widely known species but other species deserve further research as to their uses (M. L., 2000). Moringa oleifera is commonly known as drumstick. It is found widely in the sub Himalayan range and commonly cultivated in all places of India .It is a very popular backyard tree that grows to over 9 m height .It has soft, white corky trunk and branches bearing a gummy bark. Each tripinnately compound leaf bears several small leaflets. The flowers are white and the three winged seeds are scattered by the wind. The flowers, tender leaves and pods are eaten as vegetable. The leaves are rich in iron and therefore highly recommended for expectant mothers. Since all essential amino acids are present Moringa may be rightly called a complete food for total nutrition. The whole *Moringa oleifera* plant is used in the treatment of psychosis, eye diseases, fever and as an aphrodisiac, (Nadakami et al, 1973).

The aqueous extracts of roots and barks of it were found to be effective in preventing implantation, (Shukla et al, 1988) whereas the aqueous extracts of its fruits have shown significant anti-inflammatory activity. Methanolic extracts of its leaves have shown anti-ulcer activity while ethanolic extracts of seeds exhibited anti-tumour activity (Guevara et al, 1999). Different parts of this plant contain a profile of important minerals, and are a good source of protein, vitamins, β – carotene, amino and various phenolics acids (Farooq et al, 2007).

The *Moringa plant*, found in tropical and subtropical countries, provides a rich and rare combination of zeatin, quercetin, kaempferom and many other phytochemicals. It is very important for its medicinal value. Various parts of the plant such as the leaves, roots, seed, bark, fruit, flowers and immature pods act as cardiac and circulatory stimulants, possess antitumour (Makonnen et al, 1997), antipyretic, antiepileptic, anti-inflammatory and antiulcer (Pal et al, 1995).

In this study, the antiinflammatory and antinociceptive activity of the 50% ethanolic extract of the *Moringa oleifera* leaf in animals is described.

2. Methodology

2.1 Plant collection and identification

The plant leaves of *Moringa oleifera* Lam. (Family - Moringaceae) were collected from herbal garden of MGIP. Lucknow. The plant material was identified and authenticated taxonomically at Mahatma Gandhi Institute of Pharmacy, Lucknow. A voucher specimen of the collected sample was deposited in the departmental herbarium for future reference.

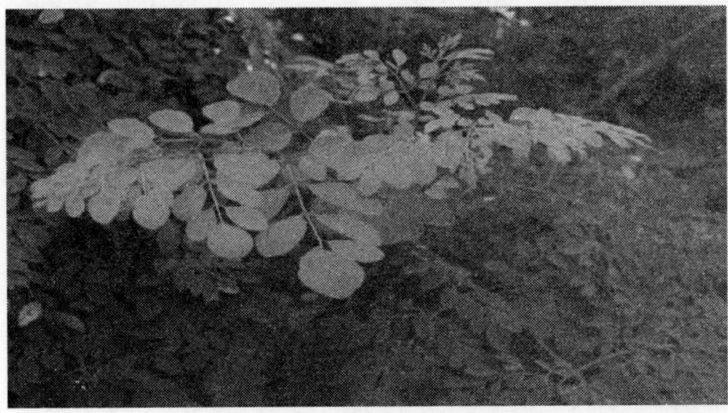

Figure 1 Moringa oleifera Leaves

2.2 Preparation of the Extracts

The freshly collected leaves (4 kg) of *Moringa oleifera* were first washed with distilled water dried in tray dryer under controlled conditions and powdered. The powdered plant materials (1000g) was macerated with petroleum ether to remove fatty substances and the marc was further exhaustively extracted with 50% ethanol for 3 days (3 X 5L). The extract was separated by filtration and concentrated on rotavapour (Buchi, USA) and then dried in lyophilizer (Labconco, USA) under reduced pressure. The yield of dried extract obtained was 95.0 g (9.5 % w/w MOE : 50% Ethanolic extracts of *moringa olifera* leaf). 50% ethanolic extracts obtained was further subjected to toxicological and pharmacological investigations. Preliminary qualitative phytochemical screening of extract for alkaloids, glycosides, flavonoids, saponins carbohydrates, protein, amino acids, lipids, steroids, phenolic acid and tannins were performed (Trease and Evans 1983). For the pharmacological tests the 50% ethanolic extract of leaves of *Moringa oleifera* (MOE) was suspended in double distilled water containing carboxymethyl cellulose (1%, w/v, CMC). For further studies 100, 200 and 400 mg/kg (p.o.) of maximum dose were employed.

2.3 Animals

Male Swiss albino mice weighing 20–25 g and Sprague–Dawley rats weighing 140–160 g were procured from the animal house of the Central Drug Research Institute, Lucknow. They were kept in departmental animal house in well cross ventilated room at 27±2°C, and relative humidity 44–56%, light and dark cycles of 10 and 14 h, respectively, for 1 week before and during the experiments. Animals were provided with standard rodent pellet diet (Amrut, India) and the food was with drawn 18–24 h before the experiment thought, water was allowed *ad libitum*. All the experiments were performed in the morning according to current guidelines for the care of the laboratory animals and the ethical guidelines for the investigation of experimental pain in conscious animals (Amresh et al., 2007a). The standard orogastric cannula was used for oral drug administration.

2.4 Antiinflammatory activity

2.4.3 Acetic acid–induced vascular permeability in mice

The Male Swiss albino were divided into five groups, each group had six mice. One hour after oral administration of the MOE 100,200 and 400 mg/kg, mice were injected with 0.25 ml (i.p.) of 0.6% solution acetic acid. Control mice received (1%, w/v, CMC) where as indomethacin (5mg/kg) served as the reference drug. Immediately after administration, 10 ml/kg of 10% Evan's blue was injected *i.v.* into all the mice.

Thirty minutes after Evan's blue injection, the mice were sacrificed, and the amount of dye that leaked into the peritoneal cavity was measured spectrophotometrically at 610 nm (Whittle, 1964).

2.5 Analgesic activity

2.5.1 Acetic acid–induced writhings in mice

Male Swiss albino were divided into five groups, each group had six mice. The MOE 100, 200 and 400mg/kg was administered orally 1 h before writhing induction with 10 ml/kg (0.6%) acetic acid in mice. Control groups received (1%, w/v, CMC) where as indomethacin (5mg/kg) was administered in the reference group. Writhings occurring between 5 and 15 min after acetic acid were counted (Koster et al., 1959).

3. Results

3.1 Phytochemical test

Preliminary qualitative phytochemical test of 50% ethanolic of leaves of *Moringa oleifera* extract give positive tests for alkaloids, glycosides, flavonoids, saponins carbohydrates, protein, amino acids, lipids, steroids, phenolic acid and tannins.

3.4 Acetic acid–induced vascular permeability in mice

Intraperitoneal administration of acetic acid into mice pretreated with control group resulted in the leakage of 63.7± 3.5 mg Evan's blue from the capillaries into the peritoneal cavity. However, pretreatment with the MOE 100, 200 and 400 mg/kg resulted in a significant and dose-related reduction in the amount of dye leakage, in comparison with the control animals. The percentage inhibition of dye leakage were inhibited by 27.49 (P <0.01), 40.03 (P <0.001), and 59.81 (P <0.001) with 100, 200 and 400 mg/kg of the MOE respectively. Indomethacin (5 mg/kg) produced the highest inhibition i.e. 68.13% (P <0.001) (Fig. 2).

3.5 Acetic acid–induced writhings in mice

50% ethanolic extract of *Moringa oleifera* (MOE) caused a statistically significant and dose-dependent reduction in the writhing response following injection with acetic acid. The percentage inhibition of writhings were 37.60 (P <0.05), 48.76 (P <0.01), 53.71 (P <0.01) at the dose of 100, 200 and 400 mg/kg of MOE while indomethacin (5 mg/kg) showed 60.74 (P <0.001) percent protection (Fig. 3).

4.   Discussion

The presence of edema is one of the prime signs of inflammation (Sur et al., 2002). Carrageenan induced paw edema is the most prominent acute experimental model in search for new anti-inflammatory drugs due to sensitive to cycloxygenase (COX) inhibitors and has been used to evaluate the effect of non-steroidal antiinflammatory agents (Rao et al., 2005; Morebise et al., 2002; Di-Rosa et al., 1971; Badilla et al., 2003; Asres et al., 2005; Loro et al., 1999).

The 50 % ethanolic extract of *Moringa oleifera* also produced significant inhibition of the acetic acid–induced increased vascular permeability in mice (Fig.3) as compared to control groups of animals. The acetic acid–induced writhings test is a highly sensitive and useful test for analgesic drug development, and it is a model of visceral pain (Vyklicky, 1979). The results strongly suggest that the mechanism of action of the extract may be linked partly to lipoxygenases and/or cycloxygenases. These writhings are related to the increase in the peritoneal fluid level of PGE_2 and $PGF_{2\alpha}$ (Deraedt et al., 1980). The maximum percentage inhibition of writhings was 53.71 (P <0.01) at the dose of 400 mg/kg of ALE while indomethacin (5 mg/kg) 60.74 (P <0.001) (Fig.4).

In phytochemical investigation of 50% ethanolic extract of leaf of *Moringa oleifera* contain various chemical constituents.

It confirms that 50% ethanolic extract contain alkaloids, glycosides, flavonoids, saponins, carbohydrates, protein, amino acids, lipids, steroids, phenolic acid and tannins. Some researchers have already reported that flavonoids have anti-inflammatory and antioxidant effects (Patak et al., 1991; Pelzer et al., 1998). Polyphenol and flavonoids are an important class of natural compounds that possess various biological activities which may be responsible for anti-inflammatory and analgesic activity of 50% ethanolic extract of leaf of *Moringa oleifera.*

Beta-Carboline alkaloids belonging to indole class of compounds was found to have antioxidant and free radical scavenging and ant allergic activity (Herraiz and Galisteo, 2003, 2004; Sun et al., 2004). No death or development of adverse reactions was observed on the animals within the study period. This is an indication that the 50% ethanolic extracts, from *Moringa oleifera* was not toxic at the doses employed in this study.

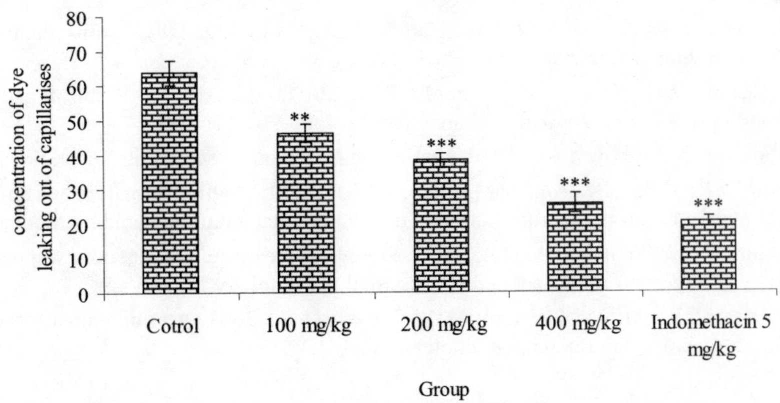

Figure 2 Effect of MOE on acetic acid induced vascular permeability in mice

100 mg/kg, 200 mg/kg and 400mg/kg represent the dose of 50% ethanolic extract of *Moringa oleifera* leaf (MOE).

Value expressed as ± S.E.M., n = 6 mice

* P < 0.05, ** P < 0.01, *** P < 0.001 compare to control group

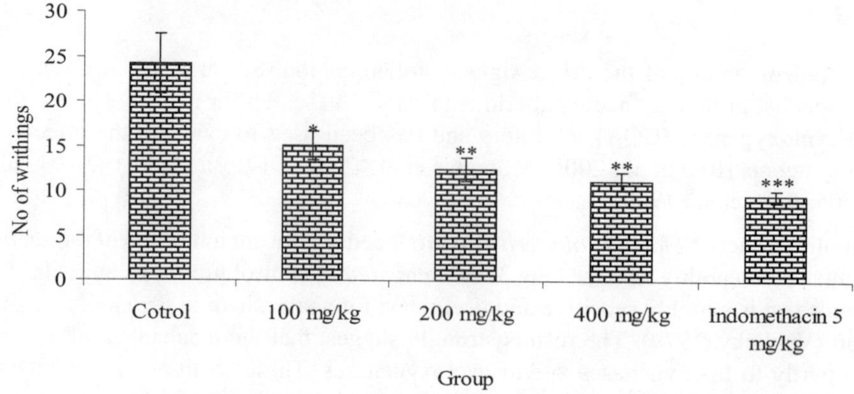

Figure 3 Effect of MOE on acetic acid induced writhings in mice

100 mg/kg, 200 mg/kg and 400mg/kg represent the dose of 50% ethanolic extract of Moringa oleifera leaf (MOE).

Value expressed as ± S.E.M., n = 6 rats.

* $P < 0.05$, ** $P < 0.01$, *** $P < 0.001$ compare to control group.

5.   Conclusion

The results obtained in the present study illustrate that correlations exist between the popular ancestral perception and genuine anti-inflammatory and antinociceptive activities of the whole plant of *Moringa oleifera*.

6.   References

1. Morebise, O., Fafunso, M.A., Makinde, J.M., Olajide, O.A., Awe, E.O., 2002. Anti-inflammatory and analgesic property of leaves of Gongronemalatifolium. Phytotherapy Research 16, 75–77.

2. Amresh, G., Reddy, G.D., Rao, Ch.V., Singh, P.N., 2007b. Evaluation of anti-inflammatory activity of Cissampelospareira root in rats. Journal of Ethnopharmacology 110, 526-531.

3. Koster, R., Anderson, M., De Beer, E.J., 1959. Acetic acid for analgesic screening. Federation proceedings 18, 412.

4. Rao, Ch.V., Kartik, R., Ojha, S.K., Amresh, G., Rao, G.M.M., 2005. Antiinflammatory and antinociceptive activity of stem juice powder of TinosporacordifoliaMiers. in experimental animals. Hamdard Medicus XLVIII, 102-106.

5. Di Rosa, M., Giroud, J.P., Willoughby, D.A., 1971. Studies of the acute inflammatory response induced in rats in different sites by carrageenan and turpentine. The Journal of Pathology 104, 15–29.

6. Badilla, B., Arias, A.Y., Arias, M., Mora, G.A., Poveda, L.J., 2003. Antiinflammatory and anti-nociceptive activities of Loasaspeciosain rats and mice. Fitoterapia 74, 45–51.

7. Asres, K., Gibbons, S., Hana, E., Bucar, F., 2005. Anti-inflammatory activity of extracts and a saponin isolated from Melilotus elegans. Pharmazie 60, 310–312.

8. Loro, J.F., del Rio, I., P`erez-Santa, L., 1999. Preliminary studies of analgesic and anti-inflammatory properties of Opunitadilleniiaqueous extract. Journal of Ethnopharmacology 67, 213–218.

9. Vyklicky, L., 1979. Techniques for the study of pain in animals. In: Bonica JJ, Liebeskind JC, Albe-Fessard DG, eds., Advances in Pain Research and Therapy. New York, Raven Press, pp. 727–745.

10. Deraedt, R., Jougney, S., Benzoni, J., Peterfalvi, M., 1980. Release of prostaglandins E and F in algogenic reaction and its inhibition. European Journal of Pharmacology 61, 17–24.

11. Pathak, D., Pathak, K., Singla, A.K., 1991. Flavonoids as medicinal agents—recent advances. Fitoterapia 62, 371–385.

12. Pelzer, L.E., Guardia, T., Ju´arez, A.O., Guerreiro, E., 1998. Acute and chronic antiinflammatory effects of plant flavonoids. Farmaco 53, 421–424.

13. Herraiz, T., Galisteo, J., 2003. Tetrahydro-beta-carboline alkaloids occur in fruits and fruit juices. Activity as antioxidants and radical scavengers. J. Agric. Food. Chem. 51, 7156.

14. Sun, B., Morikawa, T., Matsuda, H., Tewtrakul, S., Wu, L.J., Harima, S., Yoshikawa, M., 2004. Structures of new beta-carboline-type alkaloids with antiallergic effects from Stellariadichotoma. Journal of Natural Product 67,1464–1469.

Non Destructive Testing in Railway Industry by Ultrasonics

Vivek Kumar Khare[1], S K Shrivastava[1] and Kailash[2]

[1]Department of Physics, Bundelkhand University, Jhansi-284128, India
[2]Department of Physics, B.N.V. P.G. College, Rath, Hamirpur-210431, India

ABSTRACT

Ultrasonic testing is a Non destructive testing by using high frequency sound wave which frequency is above the range of audible sound. Ultrasound travels in different materials at different speed. Non destructive testing is widely used in railway industries for certification of manufactured products like wheels inspection and also use for effective repair or replacement of wheels with safety. Ultrasonic Non destructive testing inspection is presently very important for the inspection of different materials used in railway industries. In this paper Ultrasonic Nondestructive testing measurements will be presented and also discussion on quality control in welding of rail track

Keywords: Nondestructive testing, NDT in railway industries

1. Introduction

Indian Railways is considered as the lifeline of the nation. It fulfills vital transport necessity and large number of peoples travels daily on its network. The safety of the traffic is to be given paramount importance on a railway system. Lots of advancements have taken place in track infrastructure and better track maintenance practices have been evolved to improve the reliability of the system. The noteworthy among these are the conversion of free rails into long welded rails, use of pre-stressed concrete sleepers, mechanization of track maintenance, improvements in the rail manufacturing technology, improvements in the rolling stocks etc. The track structure today is sturdier and the track parameters are better maintained. This has certainly reduced the risk of accidents due to rail wheel interaction. However, discontinuity caused due to rail/ weld breakage is an area of concern for track maintenance engineers.

Any defect in the rail or any material which may lead to fracture or breakage is called a flaw or a defect. The development of flaws in rails is inevitable. The two main reasons for Occurrence of flaws are the inherent defects in the rails generated during manufacturing and fatigue of rails due to passage of traffic. The inherent weak spots or inherent defects in the rails such as non-metallic inclusions, hydrogen flakes, rolling marks, guide marks etc. at the manufacturing stage pose a threat in the form of rail breakages. The inherent defects can be taken care of by improving the rail metallurgy and the process of rail rolling during the manufacturing stage. On the other hand the defects due to fatigue in the rail during service will depend on the residual stresses in the rails, magnitude of the rail stresses and the number of load cycles.

2. Technique

It is essential that detection of flaws be carried out well in advance so that timely preventive action can be taken to avoid in-service breakage. This assumes importance as the consequences of in service failures may sometimes be disastrous.

Different types of Non-Destructive testing techniques presently available are

- Visual Inspection
- Dye Penetrant testing

- Magnetic particle Testing
- Radiography
- Eddy Current Testing
- Ultrasonic Testing

Apart from the visual inspection, ultrasonic testing has been considered to be the most effective means of ensuring the soundness of the rails and welds world over due to its versatility, accuracy, sensitivity, overall economy and flaw detection capabilities. Ultrasonic technique is having advantage of its high penetration power, estimation of severity of defect, feasibility of automation, scanning at high speed and requirement of access from one surface only. The use of the other techniques such as eddy current system for detection of surface defects, flaw detection using magnetic flux leakage, rail inspection using electro-magnetic acoustic transducers, rail inspection using alternating current field measurement, inspection using ultrasonic phased array are also in practice on limited scale on some railway systems. Some of these techniques are still in developmental stage.

Indian Railways, depend primarily on ultrasonic technique for reliable flaw detection. The ultrasonic testing of rails and welds is being used on Indian Railways for more than five decades. Testing procedures are continually being modified to suit the requirements of the newer kinds of flaws being noticed. For example, the detection of gauge face corner defects was started in 2005 by providing 70^0 gauge face side probe.

3.   Defects in Rails and Welds

These defects can be broadly classified as below:

1. Horizontal defects
2. Transverse defects
3. Gauge face corner defects
4. Longitudinal vertical defects
5. Bolt hole cracks.

In addition to these, there are certain defects which are specific to alumina thermic weld. These are:

1. Half moon defects
2. Porosity or blow holes
3. Lack of fusion
4. Slag inclusion

The defects in the rail are named as per their orientation i.e. the plane in which they lie - horizontal or vertical and their direction of propagation - longitudinal (i.e. along the length of the rail) or transverse (i.e. along the cross section of the rail).

3.1   Horizontal Defects (Hf)

These defects are horizontal and longitudinal i.e. they grow along the axis of the rail. They can develop in the head of the rail, at the head-web junction or at web-foot junction of the rail. High vertical stresses, high residual stresses and inclusions in the rails are responsible for initiation of these defects. These cracks can be easily detected using 0° probe during USFD testing. Fig. 1 shows a horizontal defect in the web of the rail through an AT welds.

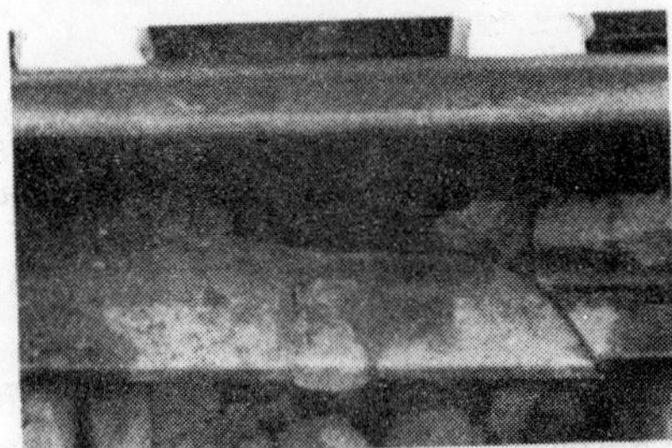

Figure 1 Horizontal Flaw in Web through Weld

3.2   Longitudinal Vertical Flaw (Lvf)

As the name suggests, these flaws are in vertical plane and run parallel to the longitudinal axis of the rail as shown in Fig. 2 and 3. These are caused by presence of non-metallic inclusions, poor maintenance of joints and high dynamic stresses. These defects cannot be easily detected in early stages by USFD due to their unfavourable orientation. These can be detected by 0^0 probe when grown up or by 45^0 tandem rig used on the side of the rail head.

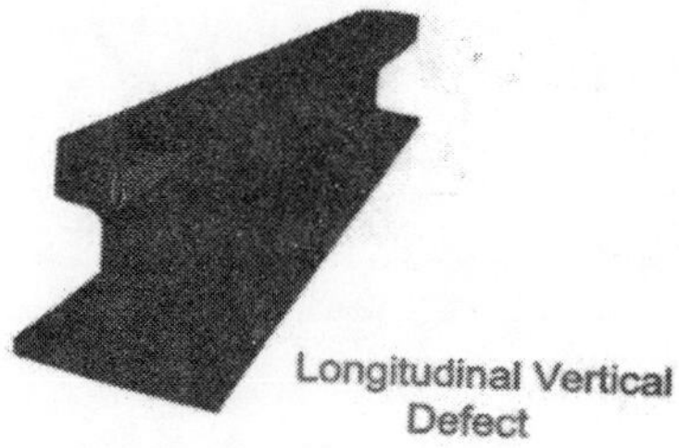

Figure 2 Schematic Diagram for Longitudinal Vertical Flaw

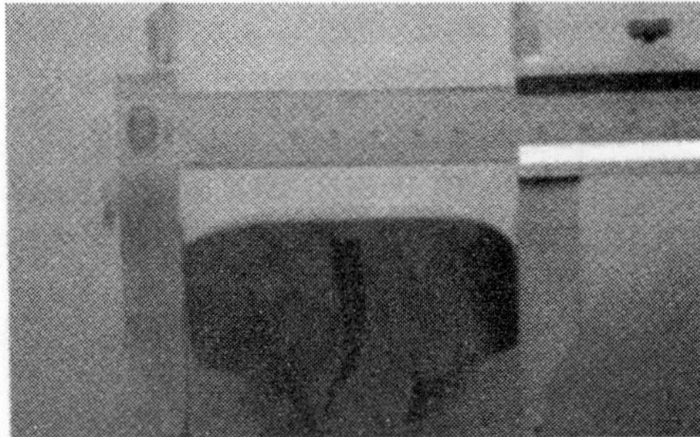

Figure 3 Longitudinal Vertical Flaw in Rail Head

3.3   Transverse Flaws in Rail Head (TF)

These flaws grow along the transverse plane i.e. along the cross section of the rail and their growth along the rail axis is quite small. These are mostly in the shape of a kidney when fully grown and hence, also known as kidney defects. They are generally inclined at an angle of $18\text{-}23^0$ to vertical plane and can be detected by 70^0 probes by USFD. Hydrogen accumulation and non-metallic inclusion coupled with high stresses are the main cause of this type of defect. A Transverse or kidney flaw is shown in Fig. 4.

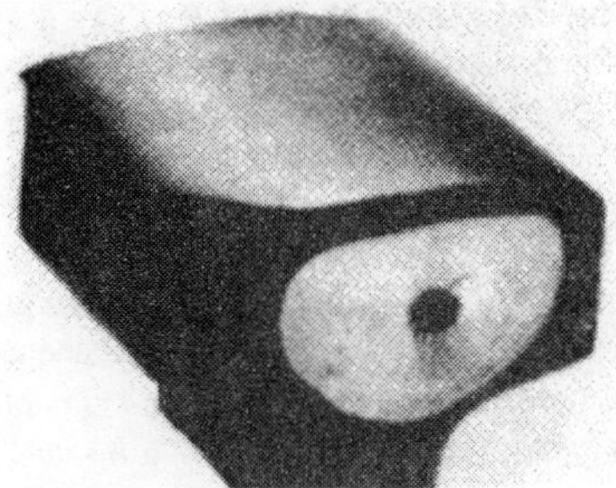

Figure 4 Transverse or Kidney Defect in Rail Head

4.   Conclusion

Indian Railways, depend primarily on ultrasonic technique for reliable flaw detection. The ultrasonic testing of rails and welds is being used on Indian Railways for more than five decades. Testing procedures are continually being modified to suit the requirements of the newer kinds of flaws being noticed. For example, the detection of gauge face corner defects was started in 2005 by providing 70° gauge face side probe.

USFD technique is successfully being used world over for the detection of internal flaws in the rails and welds. However, there are certain apprehensions about the capability of this technique on Indian railways. The reasons for this are more of administrative in nature rather than technical. The testing on Indian Railways is being carried out manually using hand testing equipment that brings in lot of subjectivity to the process. The results of testing thus depend upon the knowledge and sincerity of the USFD operator apart from the reliability of the equipment. The knowledge of track maintenance engineers is also one of the important issues that need to be addressed on our system. Without the complete and clear understanding of the technique in the minds of supervisors and officers, the doubts about its efficacy are natural. Understanding of the subject will expel most of the doubts regarding the capability and the limitations of the technique.

Anharmonic Behaviour of Lanthanum Selenide Crystal

Chandan Gupta[1] and Kailash[2]

[1]Department of Physics, Bundelkhand University, Jhansi-284128, India.
[2]Department of Physics, B.N.V. P.G. College, Rath, Hamirpur-210431, India.
Email: chandanphysics84@gmail.com, kailash.rath@yahoo.co.in

ABSTRACT

The elastic energy density for a deformed crystal can be expanded as a power series of strains using Taylor's series expansion. For the face centered cubic crystal; one can get this expansion starting from nearest neighbor distance and hardness parameter utilizing Coulomb and Born-Mayer potentials. The knowledge of the higher order elastic constants for a crystal is useful for obtaining the anharmonic properties of the crystals within the limit of the continuum approximation in a quantitative manner. The Lanthanum Selenide crystal possesses face centered cubic crystal structure. The theory is developed for obtaining second, third and fourth orders elastic constants (SOECs, TOECs and FOECs) of Lanthanum Selenide single crystals upto its melting point. With this theory SOECs, TOECs and FOECs of Lanthanum Selenide single crystals at an elevated temperature are evaluated. The data of SOECs, TOECs and FOECs are used to obtain the first order pressure derivatives (FOPDs) of SOECs and TOECs, second order pressure derivatives (SOPDs) of SOECs and partial contractions. The data of Lanthanum Selenide crystals obtained through different techniques give important and valuable information about internal structure and inherent properties of materials. The data thus obtained are compared with the experimental results whichever are available in literature.

Keywords: Anharmonic Behaviour, elastic constants, lanthanum compounds

1.   Introduction

A theory has been developed for obtaining higher order elastic constants of face centered cubic crystals. Experimental as well as theoretical work on different facts of anharmonic properties for several compounds has been reported in the recent years. Recent problems in material science often require values of elastic constants at elevated temperatures. In the last few years studies of anharmonic properties of monovalent compounds have attracted the attention of the physicists since they provide much valuable information regarding crystal structure. Elastic properties of divalent compounds are also equally important because they relate to the various fundamental solid state phenomena such as inter-atomic potentials, equation of state and phonon spectra. Inherent properties are strongly related thermodynamically with specific heat, thermal expansion and Debye temperature and Grüneisen numbers various measurements have been made on the anharmonic properties, such as second, third and fourth order elastic constants (SOECs, TOECs and FOECs), first order pressure derivatives (FOPDs) of SOECs and TOECs, second order pressure derivatives (SOPDs) of SOECs of several ionic crystals. Third and fourth order elastic constant are required to study many anharmonic properties of crystals and therefor their accurate evaluation is essential. Recently attempt has been made to calculate anharmonic properties of ionic crystals [1-6]. Only few of them are take account of the temperature dependents of these properties. The thermal contribution to elastic constants is very significant, the experimental data reveal that in going from O K to higher temperature, the values of second order elastic constants (SOECs) are changed considerable even for highly ionic solids like LaSe [7-10]. The complete experimental or theoretical efforts have been made so for in obtaining the temperature variation of anharmonic properties of divalent materials possessing different crystal structures in high temperature range

[11]. The elastic energy density for a deformed crystal can be expended as a power series of strains using Taylor's series expansion, the coefficients of the quadratic cubic and quartic terms are known as SOECs, TOECs and FOECs respectively. Several physical properties and crystal anharmonicities such as thermal expansion specific heat at higher temperature, temperature variation of acoustic velocity and attenuation and the FOPDs of SOECs and Grüneisen numbers are directly related to SOECs and TOECs. While discussing higher order anharmonicities such as the FOPDs of TOECs, the SOPDs of SOECs, partial contraction and deformation of crystals under present paper is mainly focused on the study of temperature variation of higher order elastic constants and their pressure derivatives up to an elevated temperature for LaSe using Born Mayer and coulomb potential starting from the nearest neighbor distance and hardness parameter. In the absence of any measured data on the elastic properties at higher temperature for this compound, comparison cannot be made. Lanthanum selenide has been found to be a very good system in which to investigate the dependence of superconductivity on various material parameters, since in this system one can vary these parameters in a relatively independent manner. This investigation reports on the behavior of the superconducting transition temperature as a function of electron concentration and on measurements of some relevant electronic and lattice properties of the system. Crystallographic, Hall-effect, Pauli-susceptibility, and specific-heat measurements have been made and were found to be in accord with a model of lanthanum selenide as a free-electron-like metal. Using this model, the electron-concentration dependence of the transition temperature was calculated and found to be in excellent agreement with experiment over the whole experimentally measured range of 1 to 10°K, corresponding to a variation of electron concentration between 0.8 and 5.4×1021 electrons/cc. [12-13].

2.   Formulation

The elastic energy density for a crystal of a cubic symmetry can be expanded up to quartic terms as shown below

$$U_0 = U_2 + U_3 + U_4$$

$$= [1/2!]\, C_{ijkl}\, \alpha_{ij}\alpha_{kl} + [1/3!]C_{ijklmn}\, \alpha_{ij}\alpha_{kl}\alpha_{mn} + [1/4!]C_{ijklmnpq}\, \alpha_{ij}\alpha_{kl}\alpha_{mn}\alpha_{pq} \tag{1}$$

Where C_{ijkl}, C_{ijklmn} and $C_{ijklmnpq}$ are the SOECs, TOECs and FOECs in tonsorial form; α_{ij} are the Lagrangian strain components; The SOECs, TOECs and FOECs are as given bellow:

$$C_{ijkl} = C_{IJ} = (\partial^2 U/\partial\alpha_{ij}\partial\alpha_{kl})_{\alpha=0}\,,$$

$$C_{ijklmn} = C_{IJK} = (\partial^3 U/\partial\alpha_{ij}\partial\alpha_{kl}\partial\alpha_{mn})_{\alpha=0}$$

and
$$C_{ijklmnpq} = C_{IJKL} = (\partial^4 U/\partial\alpha_{ij}\partial\alpha_{kl}\partial\alpha_{mn}\partial\alpha_{pq})_{\alpha=0}$$

C_{IJ}, C_{IJK} and C_{IJKL} are the SOECs, TOECs and FOECs in Brügger's definition and voigt notations.

$$C_{IJ} = C_{IJ}{}^0 + C_{IJK}{}^{vib}, \; C_{IJK} = C_{IJK}{}^0 + C_{IJK}{}^{vib}, \; C_{IJKL} = C_{IJKL}{}^0 + C_{IJKL}{}^{vib} \tag{2}$$

The first part is the strain derivative of internal energy U_0 and is known as "static" elastic constant and the second part is the strain derivative of the vibrational free energy U^{vib} and is called "vibrational" elastic constant. The superscript "0" has been introduced to emphasize that the static elastic constants correspond to 0K.

3.   Evaluation

The theory for the calculation of different anharmonic properties of the substances possessing FCC crystal structures is given in the preceding section. The TOECs for LaSe is evaluated from 300K to an elevated temperature (near melting point). Throughout this temperature range LaSe exhibits FCC crystal structure.

Selecting a few data obtained in this study, the values of TOECs at room temperature are given in Tables 2. The FOPDs of TOECs have been evaluated utilizing data of TOECs and SOECs and the results are shown in Table 3. The whole evaluation is based on the assumption that the FCC crystal structure of the material does not change when temperature varies up to their melting point. The values of the nearest-neighbor distance (r_0) and the hardness parameter (q) are given in Table 1.

Table 1 The Nearest Neighbor Distance (r_0) and Hardness parameter (q) in 10-8 cm and SOECs in 1011 dyne/cm2 of LaSe at room temperature

r_0	Q	C_{11}	C_{12}	C_{44}
2.9403	0.345	15.890	5.0775	5.2109

Table 2 The TOECs of LaSe in 1011 dyne/cm2 at room temperature

C_{111}	C_{112}	C_{123}	C_{144}	C_{166}	C_{456}
-218.35	-1.0336	9.0438	8.6883	8.7398	8.3750

Table 3 The FOECs of LaSe in 1012 dyne/cm2 at room temperature

C_{1111}	C_{1112}	C_{1122}	C_{1123}	C_{1144}	C_{1155}	C_{4444}	C_{4455}	C_{1255}	C_{1266}	C_{1456}
243.12	-1.6223	6.4023	-1.9879	-2.2283	9.6574	11.661	-1.9652	-2.2017	11.3894	-1.956

Table 4 The FOPDs of SOECs of LaSe at room temperature

dC_{11}/dP	dC_{12}/dP	dC_{44}/dP
-6.8133	-0.8527	-2.2047

Table 5 The FOPDs of TOECs of LaSe at room temperature

dC_{111}/dP	dC_{112}/dP	dC_{123}/dP	dC_{144}/dP	dC_{166}/dP	dC_{456}/dP
-63.9486	-1.9529	2.2481	0.5454	-2.0239	2.2892

Table 6 The SOPDs of SOECs of LaSe in 10-11 dyne/cm2

d^2C_{11}/dP^2	d^2C_{12}/dP^2	d^2C_{44}/dP^2
7.3053	-20.1648	-14.161

Table 7 The Partial Contraction of LaSe in 1012 dyne/cm2

Y_{11}	Y_{12}	Y_{44}
245.46	-0.3797	31.058

4.   Results and Discussion

The nearest neighbor distance, Hardness parameter and three Second order elastic constants in 10^{11} dyne/cm^2 for LaSe at room temperature are presented in Table 1. It is seen that the C_{11} is larger than other Second order elastic constants. There are six Third order elastic constants in 10^{11} dyne/cm^2 presented in Table 2. Among the calculated Third order elastic constants of this material, C_{123} is largest in their absolute values and an order of magnitude larger than the SOECs. Magnitude of other C_{ijk}'s are markedly smaller than those of C_{123}. For LaSe, the values of C_{123}, C_{144}, C_{166} and C_{456} are positive in nature, while C_{111} and C_{112} is negative in nature. There are eleven Fourth order elastic constants presented in Table 3. Among the calculated fourth order elastic constants for LaSe, C_{1111} is the largest in their values. Magnitudes of other C_{ijkl}'s are smaller than those of C_{1111}. The values of C_{1111}, C_{1122}, C_{4444}, C_{1155} and C_{1266} are positive in nature, while C_{1112}, C_{1123}, C_{1144}, C_{1456}, C_{4455} and C_{1255} are negative in nature. There are three First order pressure derivatives of second order elastic constants are shown in Table 4. There are six First order pressure derivatives of third order elastic constants are presented in Table 5. Among the calculated first order pressure derivatives of third order elastic constants for LaSe dC_{111}/dP is larger than other values in magnitude. The values of dC_{123}/dP, dC_{144}/dP and dC_{456}/dP are positive in nature, while dC_{111}/dP, dC_{112}/dP and dC_{166}/dP are negative in nature. The second order pressure derivatives of second order elastic constants are shown in Table 6.

5.   References

1.   J. Kumar, Kailash, S.K.Shrivastava, Anharmonic properties of CdO, CoO, FeO, Applied Ultrasonics, Shree Publishers & Distributors, 38 (2011).

2.   J. Kumar, Kailash, V. Kumar, Anharmonic properties of CdO, FeO and TeO in high Temparature, Applied Ultrasonics, Shree Publishers & Distributors, 132 (2011).

3.   S. Khanjani and A. Morsali, Journal of Molecular Liquids, 153, 129 (2010).

4.   Y. Liu, X. Liu, L. Zhao and Y. Lyu, Journal of Catalysis, 347, 170 (2017).

5.   J. Yang, J. Hu, Y. Zheng, J. Gao and C. Wu, Journal of Alloys and Compounds, 697, 25 (2017).

6.   A. K. Verma, S. Kaushik, D. Singh, R. R. Yadav, Journal of Physics and Chemisty of Solids, 133, 21 (2019).

7.   K. P. Jayachamdran and C. S. Menon, Physica C, 454, 27 (2007).

8.   J. Yang, J. Hu, Y. Zheng, J. Gao and C. Wu, Journal of Alloys and Compounds, 697, 25 (2017).

9.   M. do Carmo Rangel, P. Santos Querino, S. Maria Santana Borges and S. Gustavo Marchetti, Catalysis Today, 296, 262 (2017).

10.   J. Kumar, V. Kumar, Kailash, S. K. Shrivastava, J. Pure Appl. Ultrason., 34, 30 (2013).

11.   J. D. Pandey, V. Sanguri, R. K. Mishra and A. K. Singh, J. Pure Appl. Ultrason., 26, 18 (2004).

12.   R. P. M. Krishna and A. Chatterjee, Physica B, 358, 191 (2005).

13.   J. Kumar, Kailash, V. Kumar and S. K. Shrivastava, Global : International Journal of Research & Development, 1, 12 (2011).

Elastic, Mechanical and Ultrasonic Properties of Terbium Chalcogenides

Aayushi Tomar[1], Shivani Kaushik[2, *], Vyoma Bhalla[1] and Devraj Singh[1]

[1]*Department of Physics, Amity Institute of Applied Sciences, Amity University Uttar Pradesh, Noida-201313, India*
[2]*State Council of Educational Research & Training, Gurugram-122002, India*
**E-mail: kaushikshivani16@gmail.com*

ABSTRACT

The present paper describes the elastic, mechanical, and ultrasonic properties of terbium chalcogenides TbX (X: S, Se) along <100>, <110> and <111> at room temperature. The second order elastic constants have been evaluated using Ghate's approach. The second order elastic constants are used to compute the mechanical constants such as Young's modulus, shear modulus, bulk modulus, tetragonal modulus, Zener anisotropy ratio, Pugh's ratio. On the basis of mechanical properties of TbX, we predicted that these materials are brittle in nature and stable at room temperature. The second order elastic constants are further used to find out the ultrasonic velocity of TbX. Obtained results of present investigation have been discussed with other NaCl-type materials.

Keywords: Terbium chalcogenides, elastic constants, mechanical parameters, ultrasonic velocity.

1.   Introduction

The unusual behaviour of rare-earth compounds due to their partially filled f-orbitals has attracted the researchers to study the thermodynamic and lattice dynamical properties[1-5]. Various ultrasonic methods can be applied to study the physical and mechanical properties of rare earth materials[6-7]. The polycrystalline Tb_xS and Tb_xTe having NaCl – type structure were studied through neutron diffraction by Fischer et al [8]. Nakanishi et al[9] investigated the elastic and magnetic properties of TbSb using high field magnetization and ultrasonic measurements. The magnetic and quadrupolar interactions were explained using the (H-T) phase diagram. Terbium chalcogenides and pnictides (TbS, TbSe, TbTe and TbBi) were studied to investigate the temperature dependence of trigonal lattice distortions by Hulliger[10]. It was observed that the rocksalt cell is rhombohedrally elongated below Neel point. The terbium chalcogenides were studied using full-potential linear augmented plane wave (FP-LAPW) method based on density functional theory[11]. The ground state properties such as lattice parameter, bulk modulus and its pressure derivatives were obtained. The results obtained were in good agreement with the available data. The mechanical and thermodynamical properties were also studied in the temperature range 0-1200K.

The present paper deals with the theoretical computation of higher order elastic constants, ultrasonic velocities for longitudinal and shear modes of propagation, mechanical, thermal and ultrasonic properties of terbium chalcogenides TbX (X: S, Se) along <100>, <110> and <111> directionsin the temperature range 0-300K.

2.   Theoretical Approach

The various theoretical approaches used are described in the following steps:

2.1   Calculation of second order and third order elastic constants

The second- and third- order elastic constants (SOECs and TOECs) of terbium chalcogenides have been calculated using Coulomb and Born Mayer potentials as given in literature[12-13]. The lattice parameter for TbS and TbSe are 5.43 Å and 5.654Å [11]. The hardness parameter is considered to be 0.303 Å [14]. The density, Poisson's ratio (v), Zener's anisotropy(A) and tetragonal moduli (C_S) are also evaluated using equations given in literature[7].

2.2   Orientation dependence of ultrasonic velocity

There are three types of ultrasonic velocities- one longitudinal (V_L) and two shear (V_{S1} and V_{S2}) for each direction in the cubic crystal. The expressions are given in literature [15].

3.   Results and Discussion

3.1   The SOECs and TOECs

The SOECs and TOECs have been evaluated using two basic parameters i.e., lattice parameter and hardness parameter. The values of SOECs and TOECs are calculated for the temperature range 0-300K and listed in Table1.

Table 1 Computed values of SOECs and TOECs (in the order $10^{10}N/m^2$)

Materials	Constants	C_{11}	C_{12}	C_{44}	C_{111}	C_{112}	C_{123}	C_{144}	C_{166}	C_{456}
	100K	5.66	1.66	1.75	-89.55	-6.84	2.41	2.9	-7.19	2.88
TbS	**200K**	5.83	1.58	1.76	-90.21	-6.54	1.94	2.92	-7.21	2.88
	300K	6.01	1.5	1.77	-91.08	-6.23	1.47	2.94	-7.24	2.88
	100K	5.23	1.38	1.47	-84.74	-5.67	1.97	2.47	-6.01	2.45
TbSe	**200K**	5.41	1.3	1.48	-85.56	-5.36	1.5	2.49	-6.03	2.45
	300K	5.59	1.22	1.48	-86.48	-5.05	1.02	2.51	-6.06	2.45

From Table 1, it is observed that the values of C_{11}, C_{44}, C_{111}, C_{166} and C_{144} increases with temperature while C_{12}, C_{112} and C_{123} decreases with temperature. The values of C_{456} remains constant. These variations are shown in Fig 1.

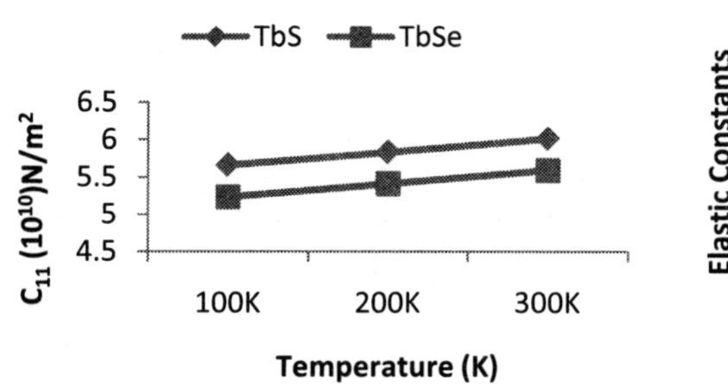

Figure 1. Variation of C_{11} with temperature

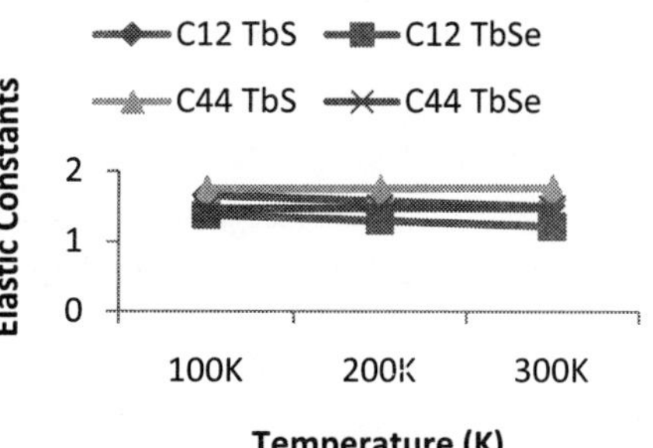

Figure 2. Variation of C_{12} and C_{44} with temperature

These values are in agreement with monochalcogenides of lanthanum [16], neptunium [17].

3.2 Mechanical Constants

The values of Bulk Modulus (B), Tetragonal Modulus (C_S), Zener's Anisotropy Ratio(A), Young's Modulus (Y), Isotropic shear modulus(G)and Poisson's ratio at room temperature are shown in Table 2.

Table 2 Mechanical Constants- B, C_S, A, Y, v at room temperature

Material	B	C_S	A	Y	N	G
TbS	3	2.25	0.78	4.8	0.23	1.95
TbSe	2.67	2.18	0.67	4.27	0.23	1.73

The Born criterion $C_S = (C_{11} - C_{12})/2 > 0$, $B = (C_{11} + 2C_{12})/3 > 0$ and $C_{44} > 0$ for stability is satisfied for all these materials. Hence these materials are mechanically stable. The ratio of isotropic shear modulus to bulk modulus i.e., G/B (toughness/fracture) is greater than 0.57, so the materials have brittle nature. The nature of bonding forces can be analysed from Poisson's ratio. For central forces, the value of Poisson's ratio should lie in region $0.25 < v < 0.5$. For the material considered in our study the value does not fall in thisrange which means that the forces are non-central. The value of Young's modulus is greater for TbS and hence TbS is stiffer than TbSe.

3.3 Ultrasonic Velocities

The calculated values for ultrasonic velocities are given in Table 2 along the three crystallographic directions- <100>, <110> and <111>.

Table 3 Ultrasonic velocities (in 10^3 m.s^{-1}) alongcrystallographic directions in the temperature range 100-300K

Material	Temp	<100>			<110>			<111>		
		V_L	V_{S1a}	V_{S2b}	V_L	V_{S1b}	V_{S2d}	VL	V_{S1c}	V_{S2c}
TbS	100	2.67	1.49	1.49	2.61	1.49	2.24	2.59	1.55	1.55
	200	2.71	1.49	1.49	2.63	1.49	2.31	2.6	1.59	1.59
	300	2.75	1.49	1.49	2.64	1.49	2.38	2.6	1.62	1.62
TbSe	100	2.44	1.29	1.29	2.33	1.3	2.09	2.3	1.42	1.42
	200	2.48	1.3	1.3	2.35	1.3	2.16	2.3	1.45	1.45
	300	2.52	1.3	1.3	2.36	1.3	2.23	2.3	1.49	1.49

[a]shear waves polarized along <010> direction [b]shear waves polarized along <001> direction
[c]shear waves polarized along <10> direction   [d]shear waves polarized along<10>direction

It is seen that the value of ultrasonic velocity is more for TbS than TbSe. The longitudinal wave velocity is maximum along <100> and minimum along <111> direction. The longitudinal wave velocity is maximum for TbS along <100> direction and minimum for NpSb along <111> direction.

4. Conclusion

- The ultrasonic behaviour of terbium monochalcogenides is studied in the temperature range 0-300K using Coulomb and Born Mayer potentials.

- SOECs and TOECs are highest for TbS so its mechanical properties are better than TbSe.
- The compounds follow the Born-Criterion so these are mechanically stable.
- Ultrasonic velocity is found higher for TbS so it can be considered better among the chosen materials for ultrasonic wave propagation.
- G/B' values are greater than 0.57, so these materials are brittle in nature.

The obtained results of present study will be utilised further to study the Ultrasonic Gruneisen parameter, thermal conductivity, relaxation time, acoustic coupling constant and ultrasonic attenuation of these materials. These achieved results can also be used for industrial and engineering applications.

5. References

1. Verma C M.Mixed valence compounds, Rev Mod Phy.48(2), 219 (1976).

2. Jefferson J H, Stevens K W H.Intermediate valence – a view of the theoretical situation, J Phys C. 11(19), 3919(1976).

3. Srivastava V, Bandopadhyay A K, Jha P K, Sanyal S P.: High pressure phase transition and elastic properties of cerium chalcogenides and pnictides, J Phy Chem Solids.64(6), 907(2003)

4. Bouhemadou A, Khenata R, Sahnoun M, Baltache H, KharoubiM.First-principles study of structural, electronic and high-pressure properties of cerium chalcogenides, Physica B..363(1-4), 255(2005)

5. Vaitheeswaran G, Kanchana V, Heathman S, Idoro M, Bihan T Le, Svane A, Delin A., Elastic constants and high pressure structural transitions in lanthanum monochalcogenides from experiment and theory, Phy Rev B.75(18), 184108(2007)

6. Singh D, Pandey D K, Yadawa P K, Ultrasonic wave propagation in rare-earth monochalcogenides. Cent Eur J Phys.7(1), 198-205(2009).

7. Singh D, Kaushik S, Pandey S K, Mishra G, Bhalla V.Mechanical and thermo-physical properties of neptunium monopnictides.. VNU J. of Sci-Math. 32(2), 43-53(2016)

8. Fischer P, Schobinger P, Kaldis E, Ernst A., Magnetic ordering of rare earth monochalcogenides II. neutron diffraction investigation of terbium sulphide, telluride and holmium telluride. J Phy C, Solid State Physics.10(18), 3601-3612(1977)

9. Nakanishi Y, Sakon T, Motokawa M, Ozawa M, Suzuki T., Elastic properties and phase diagram of rare-earth monopnictide TbSb. Phy Rev B.68(14), 144427-144432(2003).

10. Hulliger F, Stucki F., Lattice distortions in terbium chalcogenides and pnictides, Z Phys B.31, 391-393 (1978).

11. Tripathi S N, Srivastava V, Sanyal S P., First principle mechanical and thermodynamic properties of some TbX (S, Se) compounds, Journal of Superconductivity and Novel Magnetism. (2019)

12. Born M., Mayer J.E., ZurGittertheorie der Ionenkristalle. Z. Phys. 75, 1(1931).

13. Mori S, Hiki Y, Calculation of the third- and fourth-order elastic constants of alkali halide crystals. J. Phys. Soc. Jpn.45 1449 (1975).

14. Philip J, Breazeale M.A. Third- order elastic constants and Grüneisen parameter of silicon and germanium between 3 and 300K. J.Appl.Phy.54, 752(1983).

15. V. Bhalla, D. Singh, S.K. Jain. Mechanical and thermophysical properties of cerium monopnictides. Int. J. Thermophys. 37, 33(2016).

16. Yadav R R, Singh D. Ultrasonic attenuation in lanthanum monochalcogenides J. Phys. Soc. Jpn.70, 1825 (2001).

17. Singh D, Pandey D K, Singh D K, Yadav R R. Propagation of ultrasonic waves in neptunium monochalcogenides, Appl. Acoust. 72, 737 (2011).

Cyber Security Techniques on Mobile Devices

Krishna Kumar Yadav[1*], Surya Kant Asthana[2]

[1]Department of Computer Science & Engineering, UNSIET, V.B.S. Purvanachal University, Jaunpur-222003, India
[2]Department of Electrical Engineering, UNSIET, V.B.S. Purvanachal University, Jaunpur-222003, India
*E-mail: kkyadav.vbspu@yahoo.com

ABSTRACT

Smartphone turns into the most common and popular cellular device in recent years. Mobile devices are the predominant platform for the users to switch and change various data for communication. These devices are variably used for applications like banking, personal digital assistance, remote working, m-commerce, net access, enjoyment and medical usage. However humans are still hesitant to use mobile devices because of its protection issue. Mobile devices are turning into a technique to furnish an environment friendly and convenient way to access, discover and share information; however, the availability of this facts has brought on an amplify in cyber attacks. Traditional protection software discovered in computing device computing platforms, such as firewalls, antivirus, and encryption, is broadly used by the popular public in cell devices. Moreover, cell gadgets are even greater prone than non-public computing device computer systems due to the fact extra humans are using cell devices to do non-public tasks. The ease with which protection flaws in today's mobile devices can be exploited underscores the need for cell security research. The creation of the Internet of Things (IoT)—where interacting heterogeneous units encompass cell customers and manage points in buildings and automobiles—increases the need for robust safety mechanisms that can withstand a range of attacks. The technological advancements in mobile connectivity offerings such as GPRS, GSM, 3G, 4G, Blue-tooth, WiMAX, and Wi-Fi made cell phones a essential issue of our everyday lives. Also, cellular telephones have grown to be clever which let the customers operate movement's duties on the go. However, this speedy make bigger in technological know-how and gorgeous utilization of the smart phones make them vulnerable to malware and other protection breaching attacks. This various range of mobile connectivity services, device software program platforms, and standards make it integral to appear at the holistic image of the cutting-edge developments in smart phone safety research.

Keyword: Pass code, iPhone, IoT, iOS.

1. Introduction

Mobile units are the quickest developing client technology, with worldwide unit sales expected to increase from 16 million in 1995, to 4536 million in 2019 [1]. In June 2011, for the first time ever, humans on average spent extra time the usage of cell applications (81 minutes) than browsing the cellular internet (74 minutes) [2]. While as soon as restrained to easy voice communication, the mobile machine now enables additionally sending textual content messages, get entry to email, browse the web, and even function economic transactions. Even extra significant, applications are turning the mobile gadget into a general-reason computing platform. Apple i-phone SDK was added in 2008, within a short span of three years Apple boasts over 425,000 applications for i-OS devices. Similarly explosive growth of Android Market additionally now carries over 200,000 purposes after only a brief period of time [3]. As mobile units grow in popularity, it will be the incentives for attackers. In addition to economic information, mobile devices store splendid amounts of non-public and commercial data that may attract both centered and mass-scale attacks. Security is a fundamental venture for IT departments as cell devices, specially smart telephones and tablets, emerge as key productiveness equipment in the workplace. [5] Currently, cellular units are the preferred gadget for internet browsing, emailing, using social media and making purchases. Due to their size, cellular gadgets are without difficulty carried in people's pockets, purses or briefcases. [8] Unfortunately, the reputation of cell devices is a breeding floor for cyber attackers. As smartphone presents the full-size services, thus are saddled with some challenges like protection and privacy as well. Since most of the operations smartphones operate are on the Internet, so it is imperative to ensure protection and security of records and information. [6] For smartphone authentication, a sample like password, code password, PIN password, and face unencumbered can be used [11]. But these authentication methods are not secured at excessive ratio due to the fact with brute forcing and guessing such measures should be penetrated.

2.   Smartphone Security

This area illustrates the characteristic and protection trouble of three sorts of popular smartphone in the market: Android, iPhone and BlackBerry.

3.   Google Android

Features

Android is a well-known running system for cell device. Its name is from the first developing company, Android Inc [Android]. In October 2003, Android Inc. was once founded, whose center of attention is on growing software program for mobile devices. After two years, Android Inc. used to be acquired through Google, and grew to be wholly subsidiary of Google. [6] This was once the first signal that Google would amplify their services to cellular telephone market. Figure 1 indicates the images of Android Smartphone devices. [8] Android was once revealed on November 5, 2007. On the same day, the news that Open Handset Alliance is centered was announced. [3]

The most captivating part of Google Android is that Google releases most of supply code. Google permits the organizations within Open Handset Alliance freely install this running system. This movement leads to widespread growth of the cellular market of Android, from 2.8% market share in 2009 to 48% market share in 2011 in smartphone's market. Google Android has become the excellent promoting cellular device platform. [8]

Table : Android version history (Source [Android Histroy] [8])

Code name	Version numbers	Initial release date	API level
No codename	1	September 23, 2008	1
Petit Four (only internally used)	1.1	February 9, 2009	2
Cupcake	1.5	April 27, 2009	3
Donut	1.6	September 15, 2009	4
Eclair	$2.0 - 2.1$	October 26, 2009	$5 - 7$
Froyo	$2.2 - 2.2.3$	May 20, 2010	8
Gingerbread	$2.3 - 2.3.7$	December 6, 2010	$9 - 10$
Honeycomb	$3.0 - 3.2.6$	February 22, 2011	$11 - 13$
Ice Cream Sandwich	$4.0 - 4.0.4$	October 18, 2011	$14 - 15$
Jelly Bean	$4.1 - 4.3.1$	July 9, 2012	$16 - 18$
KitKat	$4.4 - 4.4.4$	October 31, 2013	$19 - 20$
Lollipop	$5.0 - 5.1.1$	November 12, 2014	$21 - 22$

Marshmallow	6.0 − 6.0.1	October 5, 2015	23
Nougat	7.0 − 7.1.2	August 22, 2016	24 − 25
Oreo	8.0 − 8.1	August 21, 2017	26 − 27
Pie	9	August 6, 2018	28
Queen Cake	10	September 3, 2019	29

Security Issues

Android additionally affords application safety thru "sandbox" which isolates applications from every other. Without permission, one application can no longer get right of entry to different application's data or non-public facts in the cellular device [Android].

Since Android is an open platform working system, it provides extra freedom to the users to set up their wish applications. However, it causes the machine less complicated to be attacked at the same time. There are some kinds of protection issues as below. [3]

The second type of security difficulty is that malicious functions can steal users' private data. Because some of purposes may additionally want user's permission to get right of entry to SD card, ship messages, or access contacts, some malicious purposes faux to be innocent to get admission to and steal data. [4] This may motive a serious harm to users, in particular when the machine shops plenty of personal information. Although these sorts of malwares suggests up occasionally, Google removes them quickly.

The 0.33 kind of protection issue is Root Trojans. [8] Android default setup is to disable of access root, but many customers like to root their cellular device. This increases the possible of being attack. Some malwares can steal users' private statistics or even remotely control the users' device. Whenever Google finds out these bad applications, it will eliminate them quickly. [7] But still, this sort of Trojan does now not stop, so it is higher for customers to ensure root security through themselves.

Sometimes a flaw of software program can motive vast matter. The common method to solve the trouble is that the builders recognize the flaws and supply replace version of software. For example, Skype as soon as used to be sincerely careless to keep username, contacts and some other personal information. [5] Also in late 2010, a research located that there was once a flaw in Android that allowed attacker to down load documents on Secure Digital (SD) card thru JavaScript or HTML. [6] The latest one was once that researchers determined out that nearly all Android gadgets had a safety gap in their authentication token. It was once possible to man-in-the-middle attack to the Android devices. Now Google has already fixed this flaw.

4. Apple iPhone

Features

The iPhone is one of the most popular smartphones in the world marketed via Apple Inc. The first technology iPhone was once launched on June 29, 2007 [iPhone]. Now it definitely launched five generations, the fifth generation, iPhone 4S, was released on October 14, 2011. Figure 1 suggests the photographs of iPhone 4S. As a smartphone, iPhone helps video call, textual content message, media player, email, internet looking through 3G and Wi-Fi connectivity. The users interface is touchscreen, which is designed for one finger or a couple of fingers.

The operating machine of iPhone is iOS [iOS Version]. This operating machine is additionally used in other Apple's cell devices, such as iPad or iPod. Table three suggests the history of iOS version. Apple customers can update their working system thru iTunes. iOS model 5.0 supports wi-fi records synchronization through iCloud service. These capacity customers do no longer want USB connection with iTunes to replace data. Table four shows some one-of-a-kind aspects provided by way of iPhone.

Any third-party issuer who wants to enhance applications for iPhone needs SDK [SDK]. After paying ninety-nine dollar per yr for membership fee, a third-party developer can add their utility to Apple store. Apple store can grant voluntary free download and set a fee to their utility including 30% revenue which will go to Apple. [11] Developers have to use C, C++, or Objective-C to boost all iPhone applications.

There are also some restrictions of iOS SDK. First, it doesn't permit builders run Java on the iPhone, so builders can now not write Java functions and load onto Apple store. Second, it can no longer installation .NET framework. Thus developers can no longer use their .NET software program environment. Third, neither Adobe Flash nor Adobe Flash Lite is supported with the aid of iOS.

Security Issues

According to the booklet from Apple website, Apple considers the protection of iPhone for personal or commercial enterprise use from 4 aspects: machine security, community security, facts protection and software safety [iPhone Security]. [4]

For system security, it broadly speaking focuses on preventing unauthorized use of device. It requires each user to have a unique pass code to generate encryption key. This is used to guard the personal information stored on the iPhone. [3] Also, organization can set some unique settings or restrictions when iPhone used in the commercial enterprise environment. The pass code policy provides some specific requirements, such as pass code reuse history, minimal length and complicated of pass code, most failure tries and so on. These polices can be enforced through installation in the configuration profiles, which are XML files.

For community security, Apple considers both approved use and safe information transmission via Wi-Fi or cellar facts connection. iPhone makes use of general X.509 digital certificates to authentication which stop unauthenticated get right of entry to on private resource of the company. [9] iPhone integrates two-factor token, RSA Secure ID and CRYPTO Card, to protect company's resource.[10] In addition, iPhone supports many Virtual Private Network (VPN) technologies, such as IPsec, L2TP, Cisco and PPTP. It also supports Secure Sockets Layer (SSL) VPN, which provides a greater level of protection to transmit data. [4]

For statistics security, there are two types of information wished to be encrypted. One is transmitted records and the other is stored information on the device. iPhone makes use of AES-256 to grant the hardware encryption. Users can not disable this encryption. It also encrypts the data and lower back it up to the iTunes. Through producing a sturdy key, iPhone can encrypt the transmission data. Pass code additionally plays a necessary position in information protection; accordingly placing a strong pass code is critical. If customers by accident lose the device, issuing a far off wipe command can deactivate the device and erase all the information. In order to grant brute pressure pass code attempts, local wipe command can additionally erase data after many failed attempts. [7] The default attempts putting through Apple are ten times. Of course, customers can set unique wide variety by using themselves.

For utility security, a "sandboxed" strategy prevents one software get admission to data of different applications. If software desires to read different application's data, it wants to use utility programming interface (APIs) whose offerings are supported via iOS.

Although Apple claims to provide high security of iPhone, new safety holes nonetheless open up [Security Issue]. Recently German information confirmed that flaws in software strolling on the gadgets can be a serious problem. [9] After clicking a contaminated PDF file, the attacker can steal all the exclusive facts saved on the device.

5. BlackBerry

Features

BlackBerry is the title of one form of Smartphone machine developed by means of Research In Motion (RIM), which is an Canadian enterprise [BlackBerry]. The first BlackBerry Smartphone was unveiled in 2003. In this first version, it supports web browsing, mobile telephone, textual content messaging, net faxing, push email, and different web services. Figure three shows some pictures of BlackBerry devices. [5] The most famous feature is that BlackBerry gives excessive level of safety through complicated encryption approach to push e-mail and on the spot message.

The running device of BlackBerry is BlackBerry OS [BBOS] written by using C++. BlackBerry OS supports multitasking and specialized enter device, such as trackball, track wheel, track pad and touch screen. This working gadget supports WAP1.2, Mobile Information Device Profile (MIDP) 1.0 and a subset of MIDP2.0. This helps Wi-Fi synchronization trade tasks, email, and different commercial enterprise schedule through BlackBerry Enterprise Server (BES). BES is a software package supporting companies' e-mail system. It can be use in Google Apps, Lotus Domino, Novell GroupWise and Microsoft Exchange. The BlackBerry running device can be routinely up to date via their Wi-Fi carriers. [8]

Like other Smartphone devices, third-party utility can be run on BlackBerry devices. All third-party developers must be digitally signed to make certain the security of the application. One big news is that now android applications can run on unmodified most recent BlackBerry Smartphone on BlackBerry OS7. This news is introduced by using RIM on October 20, 2011.

Security Issues

BlackBerry Enterprise Solution provides industry-leading security on both saved data and Wi-Fi transmitted data. It additionally presents some superior protection facets for government users.

For stored data, BES makes mandatory password authentication. After ten times of failed attempts, all the memory on the system will be erased. All the messages, contact information, duties and schedules will be encrypted via AES and Password Keeper. Administrator can remotely alternate the password. All local facts can be locked or deleted by administrator after receiving file of phone lost. Only authenticated command can be execute on the machine and solely decrypted communication can be permitted. BES never stores users' personal data. Only server and the users' cell device can decrypt data. This prevents unauthorized parties' assault [Security Feature].[11]

For wireless data, Blackberry Enterprise Solution makes use of each AES and 3DES to encrypt the transmitted data. Each Smartphone consumer has a secret key saved each on invulnerable employer account and on their device. This secret key can be regenerated via the user. BES and the Smartphone device use the secret key to encrypt or decrypt the transmitted data. [9] Through the whole transmission process, information is encrypted. If customers prefer to get admission to company intranets, RSA Secure ID offers two-factor authentication, each username and token care be request. Both proxy mode and quit to stop mode of HTTPS conversation are supported by means of BlackBerry.

BlackBerry also gives advanced protection elements for authorities customers [Advance Security]. BlackBerry affords gadgets which encrypt Federal Information Processing Standard 140-2 validation and Secure/Multipurpose Internet Mail Extensions (S/MIME) and public key infrastructure. [10] This meets the requirement of Department of Defense. S/MIME gives a excessive stage of Smartphone safety and use non-public and public key to encrypt messages. PGP additionally objectives to improve an excessive level of security. BlackBerry Smart Card Reader permits customers add extra security characteristic to current security architecture. Through all above methods, BlackBerry affords a safety protection for users.

6.   Conclusion

The purpose of this paper is to give a huge photo of current popular smart phones and help users pick out one of a kind brands primarily based on their unique needs on security. [7] In the first section, this paper introduces the definition of mobile device. In the 2nd section, it compares specific points and safety problems of three famous smart phones: Google Android, Apple iPhone and BlackBerry. For Google Android, the most benefit is that it presents open platform which makes the merchandise grab the biggest market share quickly.[11] The programming language is Java as well as C/C++. The improvement of SDK is free. These free platform and free SDK also cause some safety problems. The mobile device and functions are inclined to be attacked. This requires customers to be extra responsible and careful to defend their private records when downloading applications. For iPhone, its interface is very attractive; as a result it can entertain users better. [5] The platform is closed and the programming language is only goal C. Third birthday celebration providers need to pay member price to upload their functions to Apple store. The protection degree of iPhone is pretty exact due to the fact of the control by means of Apple keep and the closed platform. For BlackBerry, it is an enterprise device alternatively of a exciting device. It provides a excessive degree of security on both saved facts and wireless transmitted data. [10] To enterprise users, it provides many functions and methods to make certain the security of enterprise information. In addition, it offers superior security points for government. Therefore, BlackBerry would be a exact preference if customers have high requirement on confidentiality and security.

7.   References

1.   S. Farhan, M. Ali, M. Kamran, Q. Javaid, and S. Zhang, "A Survey on Security for Smartphone Device," Int. J. Adv. Comput. Sci. Appl., vol. 7, no. 4, pp. 206–219, 2016.

2.   A. Koohang and M. Georgia, "Security policy and data protection awareness of mobile devices in relation to employees ' trusting beliefs," vol. 6, no. 2, pp. 7–22, 2018.

3.   M. Dawson, J. Wright, and M. Omar, "Mobile devices: The case for cyber security hardened systems," Mob. Comput. Wirel. Networks Concepts, Methodol. Tools, Appl., vol. 2–4, no. September 2015, pp. 1103–1123, 2015.

4.   S. M and P. G, "Mobile Device Security: A Survey on Mobile Device Threats, Vulnerabilities and their Defensive Mechanism," Int. J. Comput. Appl., vol. 56, no. 14, pp. 24–29, 2012.

5.   V. Vylegzhanina, D. C. Schmidt, and J. White, "Gaps and future directions in mobile security research, MobileDeLi 2015 - Proc. 3rd Int. Work. Mob. Dev. Lifecycle, pp. 49–50, 2015.

6.   R. Jain, "Table of Contents Table of Contents اماب ساما ت - ىذرنشذ," pp. 2–4.

7.   "Mobile Protection using cyber security," no. June 2011.

8.   Android version history, "Android version history," Wikipedia, Free Encycl., no. Api 11, pp. 1–45, 2019.

9.   Wikipedia, "iOS Version History," no. June 2007, pp. 1–106, 2019.

10. L. Gupta, R. Jain, and G. Vaszkun, "Survey of Important Issues in UAV Communication Networks," IEEE Commun. Surv. Tutorials, 2016.

11. D. Goel and A. K. Jain, "Mobile phishing attacks and defense mechanisms: State of art and open research challenges," Computers and Security. 2018.

Influence of Copper and Zinc Nanoparticles on the Production of Lignolytic Enzme by White Rot Fungi

V. K. Pandey*, A. Kushwaha and A. K. Bhardwaj

Department of Environmental Science, V.B.S. Purvanchal University, Jaunpur-222003, India,
*E-mail: drvivekpandey4@gmail.com

ABSTRACT

Nanoparticle is a small object that behaves as a whole unit in term of its transport and properties. Nanotechonology involves the tailoring of materials at atomic level to attain unique properties, which can be suitably manipulated for the desired applications. Recently, biosynthetic methods employing microorganisms such as bacteria and fungus and plant extract have emerged as a simple and viable alternative to more complex chemical synthetic procedures. In the present work, role of Nanoparticles in term of radial growth rate of Pleurotus species on petri plate media which have Cu, and Zn is observe. Pleurotus ostreatus and P. eryngii shows no inhibitory effect on Cu nanopartilcles containing media, however, in the case of Zn nanopartilcles containing media shows less inhibitory effect for the P. Ostreatus but in the case P. Eryngii, Zn containing media shows inhibitory effect. In the case of broth culture both nanoparticles increases the activity of laccase enzyme in comparison with control. The maximum laccase activity was found in Cu nanoparticles followed by Zinc supplemented media. In whole work it was found that the Cu and Zn nanopaticles enhanced the enzymatic activity and radial growth of both species. Low concentration of Cu and Zn nanoparticles increase the growth and enzyme production of the fungus positively because, that nanoparticles working as metal co-factors for enzymes (metaloenzyme) activity enhancement. Besides enzymes, other metalloproteins are involved in non-enzyme electron transfer reactions (cytochromes), may act as storage or transport proteins.

Keywords: Pleurotus, nanoparticles, enzymes

1. Introduction

A nanoparticle is a small object that behaves as a whole unit in term of its transport and properties. Nanoparticles have very unique physico-chemical properties. Fine particles of nanoparicles cover a range between 100 and 2500 nanometers (nm), while ultrafine particles are sized between 1 and 100 nm. Application of nanoparticle in science and technology for the purpose of manufacturing. widely use of nanoparticles in different sectors like industry, fabrics, personal care products and for environmental remediation. The increase in the production and use of engineered nanoparticles makes exposure to the natural environment. Microorganisms play an important role in proper functioning of most ecosystems, one aspects of evaluation of the toxicity of nanoparticles on the physiology of the microorganisms. *Pleurotus* species of oyster mushroom play an important role in conversion of organic material in to humus, carbon and nitrogen. complex organic compounds converted into humus is carried out by the secretion of extracellular lignin degrading enzymes, as well as cellulose degrading enzymes. Metal nanoparticles have anti-microbial property. Iron and copper nanoparticles could be presumed to react with peroxidase present in the environment to generate free radicals which is highly toxic to microorganisms. However the radicals influence the production of enzymes significantly to *Pleurous* species. Heavy metal nanoparticle releases to the environment increasing continuously as a result of industrial activities and technological developments, which effect environment and public health because of their toxicity, accumulation in the food chain and persistence cause of carcinogenic and mutagenic in nature [1]. According to the WHO (World Health Organization), the metals like cadmium, chromium, cobalt, copper, lead, nickel, mercury and zinc,the presence of above metals >5 g cm^3 in water effect human life, aquatic life, and microbial and cause severe disease like brain damage, reproductive failure, nervous system failures, tumor formation, etc [2,3,4] The current study evaluates the effect of copper and iron nanoparticles on the growth and enzymes activity of fungus *Pleurotus* species. Fungal biomass secretes higher amounts of proteins during culture and growth on organic matter

2.   Objectives

Keeping in the goal of the present investigation is to role of heavy metal nanoparticles using white rot fungi (Pleurotus species). The objectives of present work are as follows-

- To select the suitable nanoparticles for better growth of *Pleurotus* species.
- Evaluate the effect of iron and copper nanoparticles on the growth and extracellular enzymes activity of fungus *Pleurotus* species.

3.   Materials and Methods

Cultures and their maintenance

The pure cultures *Pleurotus ostreatus* and *P. eryngii* were used in present experiments were procured from centre of Biotechnology Allahabad University, Allahabad. Throughout the study, the stock cultures was maintained on Potato Dextrose Agar slants at 27± 20C and sub cultured at regular interval of three weeks.

Metal nanoparticle

Two different types, Zinc (ZnNPs), copper (CuNPs) which were provided by Physics Department, University of Allahabad. Metal nanoparticles were diluted at different concentrations of (i.e., 5, 10, 15, 20, 25, 30, 35 mg L-1) using distilled water [5]. All solutions were stored at 4°C until further use.

Chemicals and Glasswares

All chemicals used were analytical grade and purchased from Hi Media Company. The Borosil glass wares and pure water (Millipore's pure water) were used in the present investigation. The glass wares were washed with exalin, which is neutral biodegradable which is eco- friendly.

Sterilization

Glass wares were sterilized in an oven at 180 ± 50C for 90 minutes. The media were sterilized for disinfection by steam sterilization process at 15 lb/inch2 at 1210C for 25 minutes. The dyes are sterilized by membrane filtration method.

Recording growth rate

The mycelial growth rate of *P. ostreatus* and *P. eryngii*, on solid media having 5, 10, 25 and 35ppm Cu and Zn nanoparticls, were recorded in term of ratio of the mycelial growth rate in the presence of metal nano particle (R_M) to the growth rate on a control plate without adding metal nanoparticl (R_C). R_M / R_C value of <1.0 indicates that the nano particle of heavy metal compound inhibit the growth of the *Pleurotus* species [6,7,8,9]. The growth extent was dependent on the concentration of the metals added to the medium. A decrease in growth (measured in terms of R_M/R_C) was observed upon increasing nano particle of heavy metal concentration at any given time interval compared to the control without Nano particle of heavy metal amendment. Throughout the experiment three replicates of each treatment were used and their average was taken as quantitative measure for studying the vegetative growth under different conditions.

Liquid media composition

Synthetic media	
Glucose	0.05%
CaCl2	0.05%
Wheat bran	1%
Cu NPs or Zn NPs	1-50 ppm
pH	6.0-6.5

Enzymatic study
Laccase (EC 1.10.3.2)

Laccase was assayed by following the method of [10] using a reaction mixture consisting of 1ml of enzyme filtrate and 3ml of guicol substrate prepared in 0.1M sodium phosphate buffer (pH 6.0). Change in absorbance was observed at 495 nm with the help of UV-visible spectrophotometer model Elico SL -218, per minute. One unit (U) was defined as the amount of enzyme that oxidised 1µM guicol in 1min and the activities were reported as Ul-1.

4.   Results and Discussion

Recording growth rate

Table 1 Pleurotus species growth rate (RC=RM/RC) on heavy metals nano particles containing media; RM/RC value of <1.0 indicates that the metal compound inhibit the growth

Species	Nanopaticles of Heavy Metal	Growth Rate					
		5ppm	10ppm	15ppm	20ppm	25ppm	30ppm
P. ostreatus	Copper	0.9	0.86	0.84	0.8	0.78	0.77
	Zinc	1.0	1.0	1.0	1.0	1.0	0.96
P. eryngii	Copper	0.82	0.74	0.72	0.72	0.70	0.68
	Zinc	1.0	1.0	0.96	0.93	0.88	0.88

The effect of nanoparticles i.e. Cu and Zn in term of growth rate ratio (RM/RC) of *P. ostreatus* and *P. eryngii* is presented in Table 1. *P. ostreatus* shows no inhibitory effect in zinc containing media at 5 to 25ppm while at 30ppm less inhibitory effect was observed ie.0.96. Whereas, in the case of *P. eryngii* that shows inhibitory effect above 10ppm, ranged 0.96, 0.93, 0.88 and 0.88 at 15ppm, 20ppm, 25ppm and 30ppm Zn containing media, respectively. In copper containing media the less inhibitory effect was observed by *P. ostreatus* ranged 0.9, 0.86, 0.84, 0.8, 0.78 and 0.77 as compared with *P. eryngii* ranged 0.82, 0.74, 0.72, 0.72, 0.70 and 0.68 at 5ppm, 10ppm, 15ppm, 20ppm, 25ppm, 30ppm respectively.

Enzymatic study

Table 2: Laccase enzymes activity (µM/ml/min) of *P. ostreatus* and P. eryngii in heavy metals nano particles containing synthetic media.

Species	Nanopaticles	Days interval			
		5	**10**	**15**	**20**
P. ostreatus	Control	143.25	245.7	354.26	403.98
	Copper	155.09	201.49	400.83	427.22
	Zinc	192.04	170.36	375.92	413.53
P. eryngii	Control	141.687	278.358	412.15	415.54
	Copper	129.07	167.823	195.139	275.68
	Zinc	119.993	147.056	386.50	371.40

Laccase (EC 1.10.3.2)

Table 2 depict that the laccase activity of *P. ostreatus* in the liquid culture filtrate of synthetic media containing heavy metals nano particles at the concentration of 20 ppm. All metals nano particles enhance the laccase activity in comparison with control. The maximum laecase activity was found in copper nanopariticles conaining media i.e. 427.22 µM/ml/min followed by Zinc (413.53 µM/ml/min). In the case of *P. eryngii* the liquid culture filtrate of synthetic media containing heavy metals nano particles at the concentration of 20 ppm. The maximum laccase activity was observed in media supplemented with Zinc i.e. 386.50µM/ml/min followed by copper (275.68 µM/ml/min). In whole work it is found that *P.ostreatus and P.eryngii* shows higher laccase enzyme activity in the presence of copper and zinc nanoparticles. Laccase belongs to the blue multi copper oxidase and participates in cross-linking of monomers.

5.   Conclusion

The effect of nanoparticles of Cu, and Zn in term of growth rate ratio of *pleurotus species*, *P. ostreatus* show no inhibitory effect in Zinc nanopartilcles containing media whereas, *P. eryngii* show inhibitory effect in Zinc nanopartilcles containing media. In copper containing media the less inhibitory effect was observed by *P. ostreatus* as compared with *P. eryngii*. In zn containing media the less inhibitory effect was found by *P. eryngii* followed by *P. ostreatus*. The lack of growth was observed by *P. ostreatus* above 15ppm whereas *P. eryngii* shows above 20ppm in containing media.

Cooper nanoparticles increase the laccase activity in comparison with control. The maximum laccase activity was found in Cu nanoparticles followed by Zinc. In whole work it is found that Cu nanopaticles inhance the enzymatic activity and zn nanopaticles enhance growth rate. Low concentration of Cu and Zn nanoparticles increase the positive effect on the growth and enzyme production of the fungus because cu particles working as metal co-factors for enzymes (metaloenzyme) activity enhancement. Besides enzymes, other metalloproteins are involved in non-enzyme electron transfer reactions (cytochromes), may act as storage or transport proteins. Laccases are generally produced in low concentrations by laccase-producing fungi [11] but higher concentrations were obtained with the addition of various supplements such as xenobiotic compound to media [12] Recently laccase have been efficiently applied to nanobiotechnology due to their ability to catalyze electron transfer reactions without additional cofactor.

6.   References

1.   Pandey, V. K., Singh, M.P., Srivastava, A. K., Vishwakarma S. K., and Takshak, S.: Biodegradation of sugarcane bagasse by white rot fungus Pleurotus citrinopileatus. Cell. Mol biol.58(1), 8-14 (2012).

2.   Pandey, VK, Chakrabarti, DK, Pandey, A.: Fusarium moniliforme - enzyme induced ripening of banana fruits. Journal of food science and technology-mysore 43 (1), 46-48 (2006).

3.   MP Singh, VK Pandey, AK Pandey, SK Singh.: Effect of temperature and ph on mycelial growth of oyster mushroom (Pleurotus species) Journal of Mountain Research 1, 15-20 (2006).

4.   Anderson, N. A., Wang, S. S. and Schwandt, J. W.: Regional Differences. Marine Pollution Bulletin in press. Mycologia, 65: 28-35 (1973).

5.   Aust, S. D., Swaner, P. R. and Stalh, J.D.: Detoxification and metabolism of chemicals by white rot fungi. In: Pesticide Decontamination and Detoxification, Washington DC Oxford University Press, 3-14 (2003).

6.   Pandey, VK and Singh, MP.: Biodegradation of wheat straw by pleurotus ostreatus. Cell Mol biol. 60 (5), 29– 34 (2014).

7.   Mahavi P.: Use of tea waste as bioabsorbent for removal of heavy metals from waste water. Chemosphere 54: 1522-29 (2005).

8.   Hamman, S.Bioremediation capabilities ofwhite rotfungi. BI570–review article. Journal of Molecular Biology, 23, 234-238 (2004).

9.   Kim, S,H., Kim EM , Lee, Chang-Moon, Kim, D. W. ,1,2,3 Lim S.T., Sohn M.H , and Jeong, H.J., Journal of Nanomaterials Volume , Article ID 504026, 9, (2012)

10.   Dhaliwal, R. P. S., Garcha, H. S. and Khanna, P. K..: Regulation of lignocellulotic enzyme system in Pleurotus ostreatus. Indian J. Microbial., 31 (2): 181-184 (1991).

11.   Vasconcelos, F. D., Barbosa,A. M., Dekker, R. F. H., Scarminio, I. S. and Rezende, M. I.: Optimization of laccase production by Botryosphaeria sp. in the presence of veratryl alcohol by the response-surface method," Process Biochemistry, 35, 1131–1138 (2000).

12.   Lee I. Y., Jung,K. H., Lee, C. H. and Park, Y. H.: Enhanced production of laccase in Trametes vesicolor by the addition of ethanol," Biotechnology Letters, 21, 65–968 (1999).

A Study of Association of ABO Blood Group types with Cancer Risk

Vishal Singh, UpendraYadav, Vandana Rai and Pradeep Kumar*

Department of Biotechnology Veer Bahadur Singh Purvanchal University,Jaunpur 222003, India
*Email: pradipk14@yahoo.co.in

ABSTRACT

More than 30 blood group systems have been recognized by International Society of Blood Transfusion (ISBT). ABO blood group is one of the most studied blood group system. ABO blood group system consist of three alleles A, B and O, out which A and B are co- dominant and O is recessive. Many researchers and investigators have found association between ABO blood group and cancer risk. It was found from the recent data that blood group A and AB is associated with increased pancreatic and gastric cancer risk. In the present study data of ABO blood group of 243 patients, both males and females, with confirmed cases of cancer was obtained from Sir Sunderlal hospital, Institute of Medical Science (IMS), Banaras Hindu University (BHU) and Apex hospital, DLW Road, Varanasi. 250 Samples of both males and females were taken as control. Out of 243 cancer patients 117 were males and 126 were females. In 243 cases enrolled in present study, highest number of cases were of breast cancer among women and lowest were rectal cancer. It was found that A blood group was associated with breast cancer, oral cancer, liver cancer and ovarian cancer as compared to other blood group and blood group O was associated with lung cancer, gastric cancer, colon cancer, skin cancer and endometrial cancer.

1. Introduction

ABO blood group system contains three antigens (i.e. A, B and H) and is clinically most important blood group system among 33 blood group systems (1). Blood groups classification refers to the antigens present or absent on the red blood cells (RBCs) surface. The gene for ABO is located on chromosome 9 at 9p34.1-q34.2. ABO gene has 7 exons. ABO locus has three main allelic forms A, B and O. The frequency of A and B blood groups differs among the population of the world (2, 3, 4). Several studies have been carried out to find the frequency and association of ABO blood groups with different types of diseases in different population of the world (5-34)

Table.1 Association of ABO Blood Group with Different Type of Cancer

S.N.	Cancer	Sample Size	Blood Group Association	Country and State	References/ study
1	Breast Cancer	1713	A	Korea	Park et. al., 2017
2	Breast Cancer	206	A	Rajasthan	Saxena et. al., 2015
3	Breast Cancer	166	A	Greece	Meo et. al., 2017
4	Breast Cancer	197	A	Iran	Shiryazadi et. al., 2015
5	Pancreatic Cancer	166	A	Germany	Pelzer et. al., 2013
6	Pancreatic Cancer	633	A	Turkey	Engin et. al., 2012
7	Pancreatic Cancer	627	A	Germany	Rahbari et. al., 2012
8	Pancreatic Cancer	274	A	U.S	Greer et. al., 2010
9	Liver Cancer	88	A	Bangladesh	*Hosen et. al, 2018*
10	Gastric Cancer	1412	A	China	Xu et. al., 2016
11	Gastric Cancer	1045	A	China	Wang et. al., 2012

12	Gastric Cancer	3245	A	Korea	Song et. al., 2013
13	Colorectal Cancer	1620	A	Turkey	Urun et. al., 2012
14	Esophageal Cancer	480	A	India	Kumar et al., 2014
15	Lung Cancer	307	A	Turkey	Oguz et. al., 2013
16	Lung Cancer	2044	A	Turkey	Urun et. al., 2013
17	Lung Cancer	458	A	Jordan	Alqudah et al., 2018

2. Data Collection

Data was collected from Sir Sunderlal Hospital, IMS, BHU, Varanasi and Apex Hospital, Varanasi. Out of 243 confirmed diagnosed cancer patients, 117 were males and 126 were females. Out of which 57 sample were patients suffering from breast cancer, 17 were patients suffering from kidney cancer, 29 were patients suffering from lung cancer, 27 were patients suffering from oral cancer, 9 were patients suffering from liver cancer, 21 were patients suffering from blood cancer, 6 were patients suffering from brain tumor, 3 were patients suffering from prostate cancer, 10 were patients suffering from endometrial cancer, 17 were patients suffering from ovarian cancer, 18 were patients suffering from gastric and stomach cancer, 17 were patients suffering from colorectal and colon cancer, 2 were patients suffering from Rectal and anal canal node and 10 were patients suffering from skin cancer. Data of 250 Samples were taken as control. Out of which 160 were male and 90 were female.

3. Results

Blood group A was highest among the total 243 cancer patients. The distribution of ABO blood groups among the patients suffering with breast cancer were blood group type A(49.12 %), blood group type B(15.78 %), blood group type AB (8.77 %) and blood group type O (26.31%). Blood group A was found more in patients suffering from breast cancer as compared to the other blood groups (P value 0.0005).

Table. 2 Distribution of ABO Blood Group in Cancer Patients (n=243).

Blood Group	Number	Percentage
A	86	35.39
B	55	22.63
AB	25	10.28
O	77	31.68
Total	243	100

Table 3. Distribution of ABO blood group in normal population

Blood Group	Number	Percentage
A	45	18
B	94	37.6
AB	25	10
O	86	34.4
Total	250	100

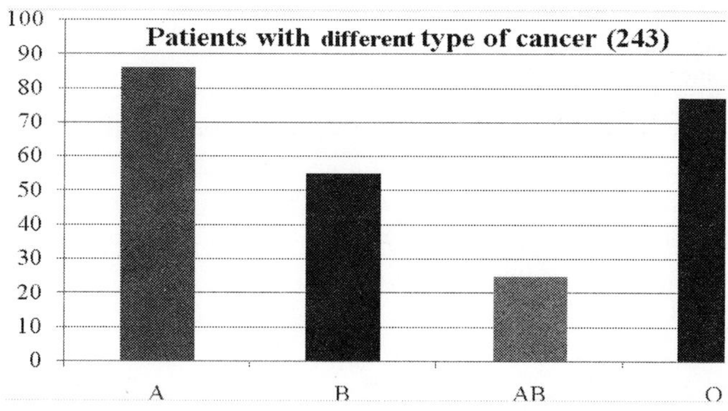

Figure 1. Distribution of ABO Blood Group in Cancer Patients(n=243).

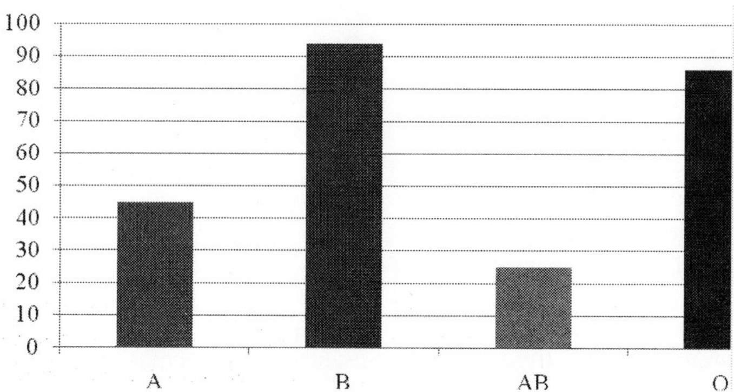

Figure 2. Distribution of ABO blood group in normal population (Control n=250).

Table 4. Distribution of ABO blood group in breast cancer patients.

Blood Group	Number	Percentage	P-Value
A	28	49.12	0.0005
B	9	15.78	0.015
AB	5	8.77	0.89
O	15	26.31	0.382
Total	57	100	

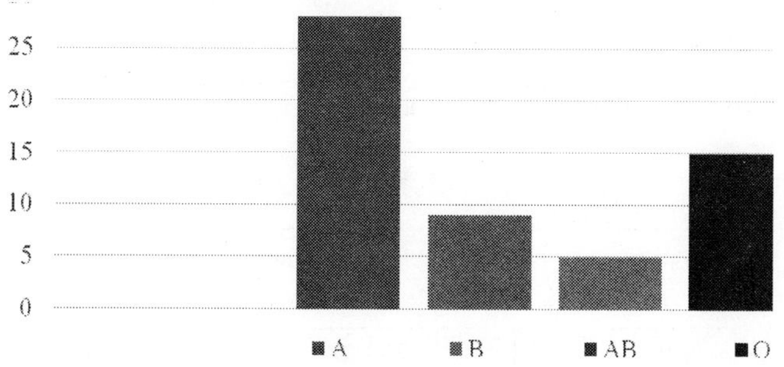

Figure 3. Distribution of ABO blood group in breast cancer patients

4.   Discussion

This study aimed to investigate the association between ABO blood groups and risk of cancer. In the present study, data from 243 number of cases and 250 controls, we found significant associations of blood group A with increased risk of Cancer in Eastern (U.P.). Studies across the word has shown association of blood group A with, Breast Cancer (18-21), pancreatic cancer(22-25), liver Cancer(26) gastric and lung Cancer (27,28,29,32,33,34) risk. Data from a these studies have shown that blood group A is associated with breast cancer, liver and pancreatic cancer, and lung cancer risk.

5.   Conclusion

In conclusion, is found that different ABO blood groups are associated with different type of diseases. Our study also showed that blood type A was more associated to cancer patients and blood type AB having least association and risk of cancer patients.

6.   References

1.   Mitra, R., Mishra, N., Rath, G., P.: Blood group systems. Indian J Anaesth 58(5), 524-528(2014)

2.   Anstee, D.J.:The relationships between blood groups and disease. Blood 115(23), 4635-4643(2010).

3.   Hirszfeld, L., Hirszfeld, H.: Serological differences between the blood of different races. Lancet 197, 675-679(1919).

4.   Mourant, A., E, Kopec, A., C.,Domaniewska-Sobczak, K.: Blood groups and diseases.,Oxford University Press, Oxford (1978).

5.   Kumar, P., Yadav, M., Rai, V.: ABO and Rh(D) blood groups among yadav of district Jaunpur. Pb. Univ. Res. J. Sci. 58, 79-81(2008).

6.   Kumar, P., Singh, V., K., Rai, V.: Study of ABO and Rh(D) blood groups in kshatriya (Rajput) of Jaunpur district, Uttar Pradesh. Anthropologist. 11, 303-304(2009).

7.   Kumar, P., Maurya, S., Rai,V.: Distribution of ABO and Rh(D) clood groups among Koari (Backward Caste) Population of Jaunpur District. Anthropologist. 11, 309-310 (2009).

8.   Kumar, P., Saima, Rai, V.: Study of ABO and Rh(D) blood groups in Sunni muslims of Jaunpur district. Anthropologist. 12: 225-226 (2010).

9.   Rai, V., Kumar, P.: The Incidence of ABO Blood Group in Muslim Population of Uttar Pradesh, India. J. Appl. Biosci. 36, 191-195(2010).

10.   Rai, V., and Kumar, P.: Genetic Analysis of ABO and Rh Blood Groups in Backward Caste Population of Uttar Pradesh, India. Not Sci Biol. 3, 07-14 (2011).

11.   Rai, V., Jahan, S., Kumar, P.: Demographic study of ABO and Rh (D) Blood Groups among Muslim Population of Jaunpur District (U P). Asian Jr. Microbiol. Biotech. Env. Sc. 12, 429-432 (2010).

12.   Rai, V., Maurya, S., K., Kumar, P.: ABO and Rh(D) Blood Groups Distribution Among Khatik (Scheduled Caste) Population of Jaunpur District (U P). Pb. Univ. Res. J. Sci. 59, 107-109 (2009).

13.   Rai, V., Patel, RP., Kumar, P., Study of ABO and Rh(D) blood groups in Scheduled Caste of Jaunpur district. Anthropologist. 11, 151-152(2009).

14.   Rai, V., Verma, A., K., Kumar, P.: A study of ABO and Rh(D) blood groups among Kurmi (Backward caste) of Jaunpur district. Anthropologist. 11, 305-306(2009).

15.   Kumar, P., Kumar, P., Rai, V.: Distribution of ABO Blood Groups in malaria patients belonging to OBC population of eastern Uttar Pradesh. J.Exp.Zoo.India 18(1), 31-33(2015).

16.   Kumar, P., Maurya, A.K., Rai, V.: ABO and Rh(D) blood groups among maurya(backward caste) population of Jaunpur District(UP), India. Asian Jr. Microbiol. Biotech. Env. Sc. 11(4), 723-726(2009)

17.   Kumar, P., Rai, V.: Red blood cell antigen distribution in Scheduled Caste population of Uttar Pradesh India. Asian Jr. Microbiol. Biotech. Env. Sc. 14(2), 217-222(2012).

18.   Park, S., Kim, KS., Kim, JS., et al.: Prognostic value of ABO blood types in young patients with breast cancer; A nationwide study in Korean Breast Cancer Society. Med Oncol. 346, 118(2017).

19.   Saxena, S., Chawla, VK., Gupta, KK., Gaur, KL.: Association of ABO blood group and breast cancer in Jodhpur. Indian J Physiol Pharmacol. 591, 63-68(2015).

20.   Meo, S, A., Suraya, F., Jamil, B.: Association of ABO and Rh blood groups with breast cancer; Saudi J Biol Sci. 247, 1609-1613 (2017).

21.   Shiryazadi, S., M, Kargar, S., Dehghan, M., A, Nematzadeh, H., Jahromi, M., A.: Frequency distribution of ABO/ Rh blood group systems in breast cancer, Yazd. 2007–2013. Zahedan J. Res. Med. Sci. 17-8 (2015).

22.   Pelzer, U., Klein, F., Bahra, M., et al.: Blood group determinates incidence for pancreatic cancer in Germany. Front Physiol. 24, 118 (2013).

23.   Engin, H., Bilir, C., Ustun, H., Gokmen A.: ABO blood group and risk of pancreatic cancer in a Turkish population in Western Blacksea region. Asian Pac J Cancer Prev. 13,131–3 (2012).

24.   Rahbari, N,N., Bork, U., Hinz, U., Leo, A., Kirchberg, J., Koch, M., et al.: AB0 blood group and prognosis in patients with pancreatic cancer. BMC Cancer 12, 319 (2012).

25.   Greer, JB., Yazer, MH., Raval, JS., et al.:Significant association between abo blood group and pancreatic cancer. World J Gastroenterol. 16, 5588-91(2010).

26.   Hosen, S,M ,Yusuff., S, Barua., A, Chowdhury.: ABO Blood Type and threat of git cancer and liver cancer in Bangladeshi populations; jmbas. 10, 15520-105(2018).

27.   Xu, YQ., Jiang, TW., Cui, YH., Zhao, YL., Qiu, LQ.: Prognostic value of ABO blood group in patients with gastric cancer. J Surg Res. 201, 188–95 (2016).

28.   Wang, Z., Liu, L., Ji, J., et al.: ABO blood group system and gastric cancer: a case-control study and meta-analysis Int J Mol Sci. 13, 13308-21(2012).

29.   Song, HR., Shin, MH., Kim, HN., et al.: Gender-specific differences in the association between ABO genotype and gastric cancer risk in a Korean population. Gastric Cancer. 16, 254–60. (2013).

30.   Urun, Y., Ozdemir, NY., Utkan, G., et al.: ABO and Rh blood groups and risk of colorectal adenocarcinoma . Asian Pac J Cancer Prev. 13, 6097-6100(2012).

31.   Kumar, N., Kapoor, A., Kalwar, A., Narayan, S., Singhal, MK., Kumar, A., et al.: Allele frequency of ABO blood group antigen and the risk of esophageal cancer. Biomed Res Int. 28, 6810(2014).

32.   Oguz, A., Unal, D., Tasdemir, A., et al.: Lack of any Association between Blood Groups and Lung Cancer Independent of Histology. Asian Pac J Cancer Prev. 14, 453-6(2013).

33.   Urun, Y., Utkan, G., Cangir, AK., Oksuzoglu, OB., Ozdemir, N., Oztuna, DG., et al.: Association of ABO blood group and risk of lung cancer in a multicenter study in Turkey. Asian Pac J Cancer Prev. 145, 2801–3(2013).

34.   Alqudah, M., Allouh, M., Hamouri, S., Zaitoun, A., Ghamdi, N, A., et al.: Is. Rh Positivity a Possible Risk Factor for Lung Cancer. Jordan J. Biol. Sc 11, 281-284(2018).

Author Index